COMPLETE TRANSPOSITION OF THE GREAT ARTERIES

Complete Transposition of the Great Arteries

Reda M. Shaher, M.B.Ch.B., M.R.C.P.E., Ph.D. (London)

Division of Pediatric Cardiology
Albany Medical Center Hospital
and
Albany Medical College
Albany, New York

ACADEMIC PRESS New York and London   1973

A Subsidiary of Harcourt Brace Jovanovich, Publishers

ACADEMIC PRESS, INC.
111 Fifth Avenue, New York, New York 10003

United Kingdom Edition published by
ACADEMIC PRESS, INC. (LONDON) LTD.
24/28 Oval Road, London NW1

LIBRARY OF CONGRESS CATALOG CARD NUMBER: 72-7687

PRINTED IN THE UNITED STATES OF AMERICA

Dedicated to

Drs. John D. Keith and William T. Mustard

CONTENTS

FOREWORD

Although transposition of the great arteries has been recognized for over 150 years, no one paid much attention to its ravages until the era of cardiac catherization and modern cardiac surgery made it one of the major challenges in pediatric cardiology. The reports of the nineteenth century received little attention, and even the excellent writings of Dr. Maude Abbott were not fully appreciated until after her death.

A Blalock–Hanlon operation provided a partial step forward and led to the survival of many infants who otherwise would have succumbed in the first few months of life. The Baffes operation produced another method of mixing the circulation. It was not until the Mustard operation, however, that a breakthrough was provided and a curative procedure provided.

Dr. Reda Shaher's interest in this condition began about fifteen years ago, first in Egypt, then in London and in Toronto, and now in Albany, New York. During this time he persistently collected important data on all aspects of transposition of the great arteries. The anatomic details, the physiological response, the history, the various subdivisions of classification, surgery, and ultimate followup have all come under his attentive and persistent eye. His immense drive and energy have been turned to collating the data which comprises this book. So much has been written in recent years that it was time someone collected a summation of these thoughts, and Dr. Shaher has done this in a very thorough and conscientious manner, presenting the various points of view involved, indicating, in many cases, where his preference lies.

The author has set out the anatomic and embryological considerations in a well-organized, readable, and instructive manner. He has dealt with the non-controversial and controversial areas in a dispassionate way, leaving the reader with an understanding of the difficulties in reaching firm conclusions.

Every authority in the field has his own definition of what constitutes transposition of the great arteries, and while they argue about this, the average observer needs a statement of definition as he attempts to clarify his approach to this complicated subject. Dr. Shaher has helped us in this regard.

Transposition of the great arteries is still a developing field, with more knowledge needed in anatomy, embryology, hemodynamics, incidence, identification, and understanding of the reasons for the occurrence of pulmonary vascular disease, and early in life in many cases. Surgical correction has proved successful, but it has produced even more problems than it has solved. Unusual arrhythmias, unexplained sudden death, effects of stitches and baffles on the atria, long-term effects on the tricuspid valve, problems of complete surgical correction in early life, particularly in the first year, continue to plague the path of the cardiologist and surgeon.

No previous publication on transposition of the great arteries has assembled such a wealth of material, and Dr. Shaher is to be congratulated on this major effort which should prove helpful to anyone interested in congenital heart disease, and in particular, transposition of the great arteries. Someone once said: "If you are going to write about anything, do it about something with which you are thoroughly familiar." One has only to read a few pages to realize that Dr. Reda Shaher has done just this, and very successfully.

John D. Keith, M.D.
The Hospital for Sick Children
Toronto, Canada

PREFACE

In 1960, when I was working as a House Officer at the Cardiac Unit, Western Hospital, Southampton, England, I saw an unusual case of a 5-year-old child with transposition of the great arteries. His electrocardiogram showed left axis deviation and left ventricular hypertrophy. Since it was accepted at that time that this electrocardiographic pattern was diagnostic of tricuspid atresia, this unusual finding in a patient with transposition intrigued me. In 1961, to observe more patients with cyanotic heart disease and, in particular, transposition, I took a position in the Cardiac Department, Guy's Hospital, London, England. A large number of patients with cyanotic heart disease were being followed at this hospital by Dr. Maurice Campbell. After working there for nearly three years I moved to Toronto, Canada (1964) to work with Dr. John Keith. At that time Dr. William Mustard had just published his surgical procedure for total correction of transposition. The huge number of patients seen at the Hospital for Sick Children, Toronto and the success of the Mustard operation gave me the insentive I needed to continue my work on transposition. At the Hospital for Sick Children I got to know Dr. William Mustard well. Together we spent days and nights in the autopsy room, in the Pathology Department, with the microscope, studying medical records, and in the operating room investigating transposition. In December 1966 I moved to Albany, New York where I accumulated more material and started assembling the data for this book.

Twenty chapters comprise this volume. Four are devoted to anatomy and embryology. The experimental production of transposition is discussed in one chapter and the pathology of transposition in two. The clinical aspects of the disease are presented in the remaining chapters. Since transposition of the great arteries is a disease of infancy and its clinical picture changes with age, data were studied in relationship to various age groups with particular emphasis on the neonate. In most chapters I have summarized my own experience and then referred to the literature. In the eighth on the experimental production of transposition I refer to the literature only. In a growing field such as transposition of the great arteries, several points are still controversial. I have endeavored to present the various views but have also indicated where my preference lies.

It is my earnest hope that this book will be of help to cardiologists and cardiac surgeons and others interested in transposition of the great arteries.

Reda M. Shaher

ACKNOWLEDGMENT

It is hardly possible to acknowledge everyone who helped me in writing this book. I am particularly indebted to Dr. John D. Keith, Head of the Cardiology Department, Hospital For Sick Children, Toronto, Canada for his generous support of this work. Not only did I study a significant number of patients in this book in his department, but his impressive organization made it possible for me to obtain all details about these patients. I would like to recognize a particular debt to my friend Dr. William Mustard, Head of the Department of Thoracic Surgery, Hospital For Sick Children, Toronto, Canada. The success of his operation was a major stimulus for the completion of this work. He was a constant source of interest, support, information, and encouragement. I am also indebted to Dr. Frederick Moes, Senior Staff Radiologist, Hospital For Sick Children, Toronto, who helped me with the initial interpretation of a large number of roentgenograms and angiocardiograms. It is a pleasure to acknowledge his assistance.

My personal thanks to Dr. Ralph Alley, Clinical Professor of Thoracic Surgery, Albany Medical College, and Dr. Paul Patterson, Professor of Pediatrics, Albany Medical College, for having given me, directly or indirectly, the opportunity to complete this work. I am also grateful to Drs. D. C. Deuchar, Head of Cardiology Department, Guy's Hospital, London; R. V. Gibson, Head of Cardiology Department, Brompton Hospital, London; and Rodney Fowler and George Trusler, Hospital For Sick Children, Toronto, for having furnished me with important information. I am also grateful to Drs. George Khoury, Professor and Chairman of Pediatric Cardiology, West Virginia University School of Medicine; Ian H. Porter, Professor and Chairman of Pediatrics, Albany Medical College; Herbert Strauss, Associate Professor of Pediatrics, Albany Medical College; and E. Hook, Associate Professor of Pediatrics, Albany Medical College, for having read portions of the manuscript.

I am also grateful to Drs. Harold Wiggers, Dean of Albany Medical College; Thomas Hawkins, Director of Albany Medical Center; and

William Kinnard, Associate Director of Albany Medical Center, for having given the Division of Pediatric Cardiology, Albany Medical Center, constant physical and moral support. To them I wish to record my deep gratitude. Their reasoned approach has stimulated the Division of Pediatric Cardiology over the years. It is a great pleasure to acknowledge the value of this assistance.

I have had first-rate technical help in the Pediatric Cardiac Catheterization Laboratory at Albany Medical Center from Mrs. Geraldine Wiley, Miss Elizabeth Davenport, and Mrs. Patricia Giglio, whose dedication has ensured top performance of radiologic, hemodynamic, and recording equipment. The smooth operation and pleasant atmosphere in the Pediatric Cardiac Catheterization Laboratory are closely related to their ability and technical competence.

I am grateful to the Staff of Medical Illustration at Albany Medical Center, Hospital for Sick Children, Toronto, and Guy's Hospital, London, who took such care with the preparation of the figures.

To my devoted secretary, Sally Kunkel, I owe a special tribute. Her patience, skill, and organization deserve more thanks than I can ever provide.

My most important collaborators were my wife, Hayat, and my children, Dina, Ahmed, and Sharif, whose patience was commendable and whose confidence in the outcome of my work was always far greater than mine.

Chapter 1

INTRODUCTION

In 1797 Baillie described the first recorded case of transposition of the great arteries in a 2-month-old child.

> The aorta in this heart arose out of the right ventricle, and the pulmonary artery out of the left. There was no communication between the one vessel and the other, except through the small remains of the ductus arteriosus which was just large enough to admit a crow quill. The foramen ovale was a little more closed than in a child newly born. The heart was of the common size for a child of two months old, and except for the circumstances which have been stated, had nothing remarkable in its structure. In this child a florid blood must have been always circulating between the lungs and the left side of the heart, except for the admixture of the dark blood which passed through the small communication of the foramen ovale; and a dark blood must have been always circulating between the right side of the heart and the general mass of the body, except for the very small quantity of florid blood which passed into the aorta by the remains of the ductus arteriosus. Life must, therefore, have been supported for a very considerable length of time with hardly any florid blood distributed over the body.

Subsequently, sporadic cases of transposition were reported by Langstaff (1811), Wistar (1814), von Tiedemann (1824), Duges (1827), Coliny (1834), Stedman (1841), King (1844), Ward (1850), Johnson (1850), Meyer (1857), Buchanan (1857), Martin (1859), Peacock (1866), Semple (1870), Kelly (1871), Pye-Smith (1872), von Rokitansky (1875), Janeway (1877), Lees (1879), Dorning (1890), Theremin (1895), and others. In 1863, Cockle analyzed 42 reported cases, including 2 cases occurring in a lamb and a calf.

In the earlier part of the nineteenth century, writers became interested in the morphology of the ventricles in transposition. Thus, Farre (1814), Gamage (1815), Walshe (1842), and Stoltz (1851) described cases of transposition of the great arteries with "transposition of the ventricles."

In 1875 in his epoch-making investigation into the pathogenesis of cardiac spetal defects *"Die Defecte der Scheidewande des Herzens,"* von Rokitansky described corrected transposition of the great arteries and differentiated it from uncorrected or complete transposition. Lochte (1894) pointed out that the position of the great arteries in corrected transposition in situs solitus is identical with that in complete transposition in situs inversus, and the position of the great arteries in corrected transposition in situs inversus is the same as that in complete transposition in situs solitus. Extensive description of the pathology and embryogenesis of transposition appeared in the German literature in the early part of the twentieth century. Thus, Giepel (1903) and Monckeberg (1924) divided transposition into pure and corrected forms, each occurring in situs solitus and in situs inversus. Depending on the position of the ventricles, each type was further subdivided into two types. This resulted in four types in situs solitus and four types in situs inversus. Spitzer (1923) evolved a phylogenetic theory of normal cardiac development of the heart as well as of abnormal development in transposition of the great arteries.

For some time, transposition of the great arteries remained only of pathological interest, but Fanconi (1932) and Taussig (1938) revived the clinicians' interest by describing its clinical and radiological pictures. Until recently, complete transposition was believed to be uncommon (Jacobson, 1921; Still, 1924; Kato, 1930; Feldman and Chalmers, 1933; Abbott, 1936; Cardell, 1956). In 1951, however, Gardner and Keith pointed out, that complete transposition is the second leading cause of death from congenital malformations of the heart in the birth to 15-year-old group. Ober and Moore (1955) found that among congenital heart disease complete transposition is the most frequent cause of death in the first month of life. In 1958, Keith, Rowe, and Vlad pointed out that 90% of patients with complete transposition of the great arteries die during the first year of life.

In 1950, Blalock and Hanlon suggested that the surgical therapy for transposition might be to create an atrial septal defect. Since then this procedure has been the operation of choice for palliating most patients with transposition of the great arteries. In 1966, Rashkind and Miller introduced the technique of balloon atrial septostomy for nonsurgical creation of an atrial septal defect. This procedure is now being performed as a part of the initial cardiac catheterization on almost all infants with transposition. Total correction of transposition was attempted by various workers since the early 1950's but it was not until 1964, when Mustard described his operation of interatrial transposition of the venous return, that a breakthrough in the hemodynamic correction of this condition was achieved. The success of this operation in this country and abroad, stimulated extensive research in the embryological, pathological, and clinical aspects of transposition. Only a few years ago the condition was regarded as being inoperable, and uncorrectable. Today surgeons successfully correct the hemodynamic problem of children with transposition at a younger and younger age. It is gratifying to see so many children with complete transposition lose their cyanosis and develop like normal children. There is much to be learned, however, about the long-term follow-up of patients with surgically "corrected" transposition. There is much to be known about the cause, prevention, and management of pulmonary vascular disease, and left ventricular outflow tract obstruction in this condition. As yet more information is needed to learn if the right ventricle and tricuspid valve will support systemic pressure for a long time. Considerable time and experience will be needed before we know the answer to some or all of these problems. It is hoped that this work, which is based on the pathological, clinical, and surgical experience with 409 patients, will be of some help to those who diagnose and those who treat transposition of the great arteries.

References

Abbott, M. E. (1936). "Atlas of Congenital Heart Disease." American Heart Association, New York.

Baillie, M. (1797). "The Morbid Anatomy of Some of the Most Important Parts of the Human Body," 2nd Ed. Johnson and Nicol, London.

Blalock, A., and Hanlon, C. R. (1950). The surgical treatment of complete transposition of the aorta and the pulmonary artery. *Surg. Gynecol. Obstet.* **90**, 1.

Buchanan, G. (1857). Malformation of the heart. Cyanosis. *Trans. Pathol. Soc. London* **8**, 149.

Cardell, B. S. (1956). Corrected transposition of the great vessels. *Brit. Heart J.* **18**, 186.

Cockle, J. (1863). A Case of transposition of the great vessels of the heart. *Med. Chir. Trans.* **46**, 193.

Coliny, M. (1834). Vice de Conformation du Coeur. *Arch. Gen. Med.* **5**, 284.

Dorning, J. (1890). A case of transposition of the aorta and pulmonary artery with patent foramen ovale; death at 10 years of age. *Trans. Amer. Pediat. Soc.* **2**, 46.

Duges. (1827) . *J. Gen. Med.* **101**, 88 [Cited by K. Kato, (1930) *Amer. J. Dis. Child* **39**, 363]

Fanconi, G. (1932). Die Transposition der Grossen Gefasse (Das charakteristische Rontgenbild). *Arch. Kinderheilk.* **95**, 202.

Farre, J. R. (1814). "Pathological Researches." Essay #1, Malformations of the Human Heart. Longman, London, p. 29.

Feldman, W. M., and Chalmers, A. (1933). A case of complete transposition of the great vessels of the heart with a patent foramen ovale. *Brit. J. Child. Dis.* **30**, 27.

Gamage, W. (1815). Case of malformation of the heart. *N. Engl. J. Med. Surg.* **4**, 244.

Gardner, J. H. and Keith, J. D. (1951). Prevalence of heart disease in Toronto children. 1948–1949 Cardiac Registry. *Pediatrics* **7**, 713.

Giepel, P. (1903). Weitere Beitrage zum situs transversus und zur hehre von den transposition der grossen Gefasse des Herzens. *Arch. Kinderheilk.* **35**, 112, 222.

Jacobson, V. C. (1921). Deviation of the aortic septum: complete transposition of great vessels with report of two cases in infants. *Amer. J. Dis. Child.* **21**, 176.

Janeway, E. G. (1877). Malposition of aorta and pulmonary artery thrombus in heart and cerebral embolism; death from intestinal hemorrhage. *Med. Rec.* **12**, 811.

Johnson, C. P. (1850). Cyanosis produced by transposition of the orifices of the aorta and pulmonary artery. *Amer. J. Med. Sci.* **20** [N.S.], 370.

Kato, K. (1930). Congenital transposition of cardiac vessels: a clinical and pathologic study. *Amer. J. Dis. Child.* **39**, 363.

Keith, J. D., Rowe, R. D., and Vlad, P. (1958). "Heart Disease in Infancy and Childhood." MacMillan, New York.

Kelly, C. (1871). Malformation of the heart; transposition of the great vessels; cyanosis. *Trans. Pathol. Soc. London* **22**, 92.

King, T. W. (1844). Case of transposition of the aorta, and pulmonary artery, with remarks on the causes of communication between the two sides of the heart. *London Edinburgh Monthly J. Med. Sci.* **4**, 32.

Langstaff, G. (1811). Case of a singular malformation of the heart. *London Med. Rev.* **4**, 88.

Lees, D. B. (1879). Case of malformation of the heart with transposition of the aorta and pulmonary artery. *Trans. Pathol. Soc. London* **31**, 58.

Lochte, E. H. T. (1894). Bertrag zur Keuntniss des situs transversus partialis und der angeborenen Dextrocardie. *Beitr. Pathol. Anat. Allg. Pathol.* **16**, 189.

Martin. (1859). *Muller's Arch. J.* **5**, 222, [Cited by J. Cockle (1863). *Med. Chir. Trans.* **46**, 193.]

Meyer, H. (1857). *Virchows Arch. Pathol. Anat. Physiol.* **12**, 364, 497. (Cited by J. S. Harris and S. Farber, *Arch. Pathol.* **28**, 427, 1939.)

Monckeberg, J. G. (1924). Die Missbildungen des Herzes. *In* "Handbuch der Speziellen Pathologischen Anatomie und Histologie" (F. Henke and O. Lubarsch, eds.), Vol. 2, pp 1–183. Springer, Berlin.

Mustard, W. T. (1964). Successful two-stage correction of transposition of the great arteries. *Surgery* **55**, 469.

Ober, W. B., and Moore, T. E., Jr. (1955). Congenital cardiac malformations in the neonatal period; an autopsy study. *N. Engl. J. Med.* **253**, 271.

Peacock, T. B. (1866). "On Malformation of the Human Heart," 2nd Ed., pp. 143–149. Churchill, London.

Pye-Smith, P. H. (1872). Transposition of the aorta and pulmonary artery. *Trans. Pathol. Soc. London* **23**, 80.

Rashkind, W. J., and Miller, W. W. (1966). Creation of an atrial septal defect without thoracotomy. *J. Amer. Med. Ass.* **196**, 991.

Semple, H. (1870). Malformation of the heart; patent foramen ovale: imperfection ventriculosum; aorta given off from the right ventricle; ductus arteriosus giving off the right and left pulmonary arteries; cyanosis. *Trans. Pathol. Soc. London* **21**, 80–82.

Spitzer, A. (1923). Über den Bauplan des normalen und missbildeten Herzens. *Virchows Arch. Pathol. Anat. Physiol.* **243**, 81. (Translated by M. Lev and A. Vass, Thomas, Springfield, Illinois, 1951).

Stedman, S. S. (1841–1842). Cyanosis; transposition of the great vessels of the heart. *Lancet i*, 645.

Still, G. F. (1924). "Common Disorders and Diseases of Children," 4th Ed. Oxford Univ. Press, New York.

Stoltz, J. A. (1851). Vice de conformation du coeur, consistant dans la transposition des ventricules du coeur; mort très peu de temps après la naissance. *Arch. Gen. Med.* **27, 213.**

Taussig, H. B. (1938). Complete transposition of the great vessels. Clinical and pathologic features. *Amer. Heart J.* 16, 728.

Theremin, E. (1895). "Etudes sur les Affections Congénitales du Coeur." Asselin and Houzeau, Paris.

von Rokitansky, C. F. (1875). "Die Defecte der Scheidewände des Herzens." Braumüller, Vienna.

von Tiedemann, B. (1824). "Zeitschrift für Physiologie," Vol. 1, p. 111. Heidelberg.

Walshe, W. H. (1842). Case of cyanosis, depending upon transposition of the aorta and pulmonary artery. *Med. Chir. Trans.* 25, 1.

Ward, O. (1850). Transposition of the aorta and pulmonary artery. *Trans. Pathol. Soc. London.* 3, 63.

Wistar, C. (1814). "System of Anatomy," Vol. 2, p. 78. Dobson, Philadelphia, Pennsylvania.

Chapter 2

ANATOMICAL AND EMBRYOLOGICAL CONSIDERATIONS

Comparative Anatomy of the Heart

According to Robertson (1913), Spitzer (1923), Walmsley (1929), and Neal and Rand (1947), the most primitive heart is tubular in shape, e.g., in many of the Annelida. In all Vertebrata, the simple tubular heart is divided transversely to its long axis into four chambers: sinus venosus, atrium, ventricle, and bulbus cordis. During its further evolution, and associated with changes in the respiratory apparatus, the heart undergoes a division parallel to its long axis into bilateral halves so that within it the pulmonary and systemic circulations are separated from one another. This division affects the atrium, ventricle, and bulbus cordis, but not the sinus venosus, and can be followed gradually in its successive stages through the vertebrate series until it reaches its completion in the birds and the mammals.

FISHES

The heart in fishes is a simple tubular structure divided into the four primary parts: sinus venosus, atrium, ventricle, and bulbus cordis. The contraction of the heart begins in the sinus venosus. The atrium is a comparatively thin-walled chamber, expanded laterally in the form of appendices. The ventricle is characterized by its thick muscular wall; it is the essential propulsory chamber of the heart. The blood from the ventricle is thrown into the bulbus cordis when the ventricle contracts. The future division into the pulmonary and systemic hearts as seen in higher animals is foreshadowed in the fish heart. The most primitive type of bulbus cordis is found in the elasmobranch fishes. It consists of a comparatively straight muscular tube whose cavity is subdivided by four longitudinal ridges. These ridges extend throughout the length of the bulbus and are jammed together as the cardiac contraction passes along the muscular walls of the bulbus, thus preventing any regurgitation toward the ventricle. The ganoid fish, Lepidosteus, presents a somewhat similar condition, with one difference. Instead of four longitudinal ridges, the bulbus cordis possesses eight longitudinal rows of pocket valves, four of which are prominent and four less conspicuous rows alternate with them. These two fishes have simple heart tubes, with single atrial and ventricular cavities; the respiratory system is entirely branchial (Fig. 2.1).

A marked modification occurs, however, in the dipnoan fish, ceratodus. It is correlated with the appearance of a pulmonary system of respiration and circulation, and at the same time with the development of incomplete atrial, ventricular, and bulbar septa. In this fish, the bulbus cordis has become kinked on itself, and its middle part has assumed a somewhat transverse position, so that the bulbus may now be divided into distal, transverse or middle, and proximal portions. A solid spiral valve has appeared, apparently derived from the fusion of certain of the pocket valves, and extends from about the middle of the distal to the proximal part of the proximal segment of the bulbus. The valvular structures have disappeared on the expanded walls of the transverse part of the bulbus, and elsewhere have become smaller and more irregular except at the distal extremity of the distal part of the bulbus, where they remained large and apparently functional. Thus, simultaneously with the atrial and ventricular chambers, the bulbus cordis is being adapted to meet the requirements of the differentiated systemic and pulmonary circulations. In *Lepidosiren* there is a similar arrangement of the bulbus with a few further modifications toward the more efficient separation of the two blood streams. The spiral ridge or valve extends from the distal to the proximal end of the bulbus. In the distal segment there is a longitudinal ridge opposite the spiral valve, that renders the division of this part into anterior and posterior compartments.

Amphibia

The cavity of the atrium is partially divided into right and left chambers by an incomplete septum. The sinus venosus opens into the right atrium and the pulmonary vein into the left atrium. There is a single atrioventricular opening. The mixing of the two streams in the ventricle is hindered by the trabecular formation of its musculature. The bulbus cordis arises from the right side of the ventricular cavity and the two streams of blood are kept considerably separate within it by an incomplete spiral septum formed by valves in its interior.

REPTILES

The division of the heart is further advanced. The atrium is divided by a complete septum into right and left chambers which are entirely separate from one another, each having its own opening into the ventricle. The sinus venosus opens into the right atrium while the single pulmonary vein opens into the left atrium. The ventricle is partly divided by a septum in lower reptiles and more or less completely divided in the crocodiles and alligators. A peculiarity of the reptilian circulation is manifested in the triple splitting of the truncus arteriousus. Three arteries leave the heart. One of these is the pulmonary artery carrying venous blood from the right ventricle to the lungs, while the remaining two vessels are the systemic arteries, one of which comes from the right and the other from the left ventricle. The left ventricular aorta is connected to the right 4th aortic arch, while the right ventricular aorta is connected to the left 4th aortic arch. Semilunar valves are present at the bases of the great vessels. In some reptiles a foramen connects the two aortae (foramen of Panizza). A further modification, therefore, has occurred in the bulbus cordis of the reptilia. Here the bulbus is considerably shortened and straightened and the spiral valve is replaced by a spiral septum. The disappearance of the musculature of the middle and distal segments of the bulbus is complete and semilunar valves have developed at the bases of the great vessels. Thus the contractile muscular function of the distal two-thirds of the bulbus has now been replaced by a mechanical arrangement of valves.

MAMMALS

The sinus venosus cannot be distinguished from the exterior as a separate chamber of the mammalian heart. The venae cavae open into the right atrium and the single pulmonary vein (monotremes) or the four pulmonary veins (human) open into the left atrium. The atrium and ventricle are completely divided into right and left chambers. The mammalian bulbus cordis merely presents further modification along the same lines as the reptilian heart. There is shortening and straightening of the bulbus and there is diminution of the spiral twisting of the bulbar septum. The bulbar musculature is reduced to a minimum and the bases of the great vessels are guarded by semilunar valves.

EVOLUTION OF THE HEART

The chief changes which the heart has undergone in phylogenesis may be briefly summarized as follows. Primarily the heart had neither valves nor chambers but consisted of a two-layered tube with a muscular wall and endothelial lining. The first subdivision of the heart was into a receiving chamber or atrium and an anterior propulsive division or ventricle. Later a posterior sinus division and an anterior bulbus were added. Heart septation began with the development of pulmonary respiration and both are intimately related phylogenetically. Pulmonary respiration is essentially the primary and cardiac septation the secondary mechanism. Septation of the heart began in the dipnoan fish and was complete in mammals. The purpose of heart septation is not only to separate both circulations from each other, but also because they must be diverted in such a manner that the blood passes from the right heart to the lungs and from these to the left heart before finally reaching the body. For this reason the dividing septum underwent rotation so the oxygenated blood from the left ventricle was directed to the systemic circulation and deoxygenated blood from the right ventricle was directed to the pulmonary circuit. During the process of septation one septum divided the atria and ventricles into right and left halves. In reptiles two septa divided the truncus arteriosus into two aortae and one pulmonary artery, whereas in mammals one septum divided the truncus into one aorta and one pulmonary artery. During evolution there was diminution in the muscular power of the bulbus cordis. The functions of this chamber were taken over by other parts of the heart tube. Its valve function, to prevent regurgitation of blood into the ventricles, was taken over by the semilunar valves. Most of its musculature disappeared, as contractile power was concentrated in the ventricles. The portion of the bulbus which remained as the infundibulum of the right ventricle retained its functions as a shock absorber of the pulmonary circulation (Keith, 1909).

The Situs Solitus and the Situs Inversus Hearts

In the situs solitus heart the superior and inferior vena cava and the coronary sinus enter the right atrium which presents a limbus and a fossa ovalis on its septal surface. It communicates with the right ventricle through the right atrioventricular valve. The right ventricle is divided into two parts: the inflow or body which lies below the tricuspid valve, and the outflow or conus which lies below the pulmonary valve. The two parts of the right ventricle are separated by the crista supraventricularis which is a prominent muscular bundle which arches across the outflow tract of the right ventricle. Its right (parietal band) anterior limb originates in the anterior wall of the right ventricle at the level of the tricuspid ring, arches upward and to the left, to pass across the upper wall of the outflow tract between the papillary muscle of the conus below and posteriorly and the pulmonary valve above and anteriorly. Its left limb (septal band) arches from under the pulmonary valve downward along the ventricular septum. The interior of the right ventricle has large thick trabeculae. The right atrioventricular valve (the tricuspid valve) is divided into three leaflets, anterior, posterior, and septal. Three sets of papillary muscles are attached to it—anterior muscle, posterior muscle, and the papillary muscle of the conus. Another important element in the right ventricle is the anterior papillary muscle which is united to the right septal surface of a band of myocardium, the moderator band. The ventral aspect of the ventricular septum lies more to the left than it does at its dorsal aspect, consequently, the right ventricle lies anteriorly and to the right and the left ventricle posteriorly and to the left. The membraneous septum is divided by the line of attachment of the septal leaflet of the tricuspid valve into a lower interventricular portion and an upper atrioventricular portion separating the left ventricle from the right atrium. The pulmonary artery originates from the right ventricle anteriorly and to the left of the aorta. The pulmonary veins are connected to the left atrium which has on its septal surface the irregular configuration of the septum primum as it is adherent to the septum secundum. The left atrium communicates with the left ventricle through the left atrioventricular valve. The left ventricle is finely trabeculated in contrast to the heavy trabeculations of the right ventricle. The left atrioventricular valve (the mitral valve) is divided into two leaflets, anterior and posterior. The large anterior leaflet, forming a portion of both the inflow and outflow tracts of the left ventricle, is firmly connected to the aortic root by being continuous with it and with portions of the left anterior and posterior cusps of the aortic valve. Two papillary muscles are attached to the mitral valve, an anterior muscle and a posterior muscle. The aorta originates from the left ventricle posteriorly and to the right of the pulmonary artery. Thus the outflow tracts of the two ventricles cross each other. If the heart is removed from the body and held so that the ventricular septum forms its median plane, the pulmonary trunk lies almost directly ventral to the aorta, and the semilunar valves of the pulmonary artery are named right posterior, left posterior, and anterior; while those of the aorta are named right anterior, left anterior, and posterior or noncoronary. The right coronary artery arises from the right anterior sinus of Valsalva and proceeds to the right. It appears on the surface of the heart between the pulmonary artery and the right atrial appendage. It runs in the right atrioventricular sulcus and gives off a right marginal branch and continues as the posterior descending coronary artery which descends in the posterior interventricular groove. The left coronary artery arises from the left anterior sinus of Valsalva and passes behind the pulmonary artery. It gives off an anterior descending coronary artery which descends in the anterior interventricular groove, and the left circumflex artery which runs to thes left in the atrioventricular sulcus to reach the diaphragmatic surface of the heart.

The situs inversus heart is in all respects a mirror-image of the situs so- litus heart. Thus, the superior and inferior vena cava drain into the mor- phological right atrium which lies on the left. It communicates with the left-sided, but morphologically right ventricle, through a tricuspid left atrioventricular valve. The crista supraventricularis separates the left-sid- ed tricuspid valve and the pulmonary valve. The pulmonary artery origi- nates from the left-sided ventricle and is situated anteriorly and to the right of the aorta. The right-sided morphologically left atrium receives the pulmonary veins and is connected with the right-sided morphological- ly left ventricle through a bicuspid atrioventricular valve. The anterior leaflet of the right atrioventricular valve is continuous with the aortic valve. The aorta takes origin from the right-sided ventricle and is situated posteriorly and to the left of the pulmonary artery. The aortic arch is right-sided. The coronary arteries are mirror-image of the normal situs solitus heart.

Conducting System of the Heart

The impulse initiating cardiac contraction originates in the sino-atrial (S-A) node which lies at the junction of the superior vena cava and the right atrium. From the S-A node the impulse spreads through the atria to the atrioventricular (A-V) node. According to Merideth and Titus (1968) the A-V node lies on the tricuspid valve ring, posterior to the membranous septum and anterior to the ostium of the coronary sinus. Atrial conduction pathways between the S-A and A-V nodes have been described in the normal heart by Wenckebach (1907), Thorel (1909, 1910), James (1963), and Merideth and Titus (1968). These authors described three internodal pathways—anterior, middle, and posterior. According to James (1963), these connecting pathways between the S-A node and the A-V node contain Purkinje fibers, but also many myocar- dial fibers. The anterior internodal tract passes from the sinus node to sweep anterior to the superior vena cava into Backmann's bundle, where it divides to distribute to the left atrium and to curve back into the inter- atrial septum and descend to the A-V node. The Backmann's bundle is an interatrial tract which extends from the junction of the superior vena cava with the right atrium toward both right and left atrial appendages. The middle internodal tract leaves the dorsal and posterior margins of the sinus node and courses behind the superior vena cava through the sinus intercavarum to the crest of the interatrial septum, and there descends to the A-V node, merging with fibers of the anterior tract as it approaches the node. The posterior internodal tract follows the crista terminalis from the sinus node to the Eustachian ridge and thence through the ridge to the posterior margin of the A-V node. From the A-V node, impulses are conducted down the A-V bundle to the ventricles. This bundle of specialized conducting tissue divides into right and left branches which pass down on either side of the interventricular septum and ramify widely beneath the endocardium in a syncytial network, which extends outward toward the pericardium. The S-A node has a special blood vessel which arises from the right coronary artery in 55% of cases and from the circumflex artery in 45% of cases. The A-V nodal artery, which supplies the A-V node, arises from the right coronary artery in 90% of cases and from the circumflex artery in 10% of cases. The A-V bundle and its proximal two branches receive their blood supply from the A-V nodal artery. Beyond the lower portion of the membranous septum, the two branches of the A-V bundle receive their blood supply from the septal branches of the anterior descending coronary artery.

Normal Development of the Situs Solitus and Situs Inversus Hearts

According to Davis (1927), Kramer (1942), Streeter (1948), de la Cruz and da Rocha (1956), de la Cruz *et al.* (1959), and Hamilton *et al.* (1962), the dilated termination of each vitelline vein joins the caudal extremity of the endocardial heart tube. Each dilatation is joined by the corresponding umbilical vein to form the right or left primitive sinus venosus which later receives the termination of the common cardinal vein of the same side. The cranial end of the heart tube continues on each side with the first aortic arches which join the corresponding dorsal aortae. After the disappearance of the mesocardium, the primitive heart is fixed to the pericardial wall only at the venous entrance or caudal end and arterial outlet or cranial end. The primitive heart now undergoes differential expansion so that several dilatations separated by grooves result (Fig. 2.1). These dilatations from the caudal end are the right and left sinus venorum, the right and left primitive atria (which soon fuse to form a single atrium), the ventricle, the bulbus cordis, and the aortic bulb. These areas are separated by the right and left atrioventricular sulci, the right and left bulboventricular sulci, and the right and left interbulbar sulci, respectively. As the venous and arterial ends are fixed by the pericardium, an elongation of the cardiac tube, which is more rapid than the enlarge-

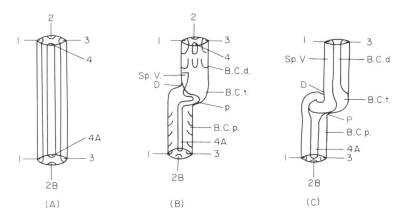

Fig. 2.1. Diagram of the bulbus cordis of the heart of an elasmobranch fish (A); ceratodus (B); and *Lepidosiren paradoxa* (C), the two latter being dipnoan fishes. 1, Right bulbar ridge; 2 distal, and 2B proximal part of dorsal bulbar ridge; 3, left bulbar ridge; 4 distal and 4A, proximal part of ventral ridge; B.C.d., distal segment of bulbus cordis; B.C.p., proximal segment of bulbus cordis, B.C.t. transverse segment of bulbus cordis; D, distal constriction of bulbus cordis; P, proximal constriction of bulbus cordis; Sp.V., spiral valve. From Robertson (1913), with permission of *J. Pathol. Bacteriol.* **18,** 191.

ment of the pericardial cavity, causes the heart to bend into a compound S-shaped curve which nearly fills the pericardial cavity. As the loop involves mainly the dilatations of the ventricles and the bulbus cordis it is called the bulboventricular loop. The atrial region can be recognized as the transversely dilated portion of the cardiac tube into which the great veins converge. This part of the heart remains dorsally located, being anchored to the body wall by a persistent portion of the dorsal mesocardium and the entering veins. On the other hand, the bulboventricular part of the cardiac tube loses its dorsal mesocardium and is thus free to bend laterally. Cephalically, the depth of the interbulbar sulci decreases and finally disappears. The transition from the bulbus to the truncus is regarded as taking place at the level where the aortic and the pulmonary valves are formed. The bulboventricular loop has two limbs: the dextroventral, formed by the bulbus cordis (right ventricle), and the sinistrodorsal, represented by the primitive (left) ventricle. The convexity of the bulboventricular loop is directed toward the right and its concavity toward the left. The progressive changes of the sulci are as follows: the left bulboventricular sulcus becomes deeper, while the right bulboventricular sulcus disappears. On the other hand, the right atrioventricular sulcus becomes deeper than the one on the left. The fate of these sulci determines

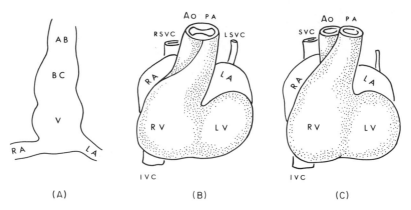

Fig. 2.2. Schematic representation of the various stages of the normal development of the situs solitus heart. (A) The straight heart tube. (B) Formation of the bulboventricular loop. (C) Completion of division of the conotruncus with the aorta arising from the left ventricle and pulmonary artery from the right ventricle. AB, Aortic bulb; Ao, aorta; BC, bulbus cordis; IVC, inferior vena cava; LA, left atrium; LSVC, left superior vena cava; LV, left ventricle; PA, pulmonary artery; RA, right atrium; RSVC, right superior vena cava; RV, right ventricle; SVC, superior vena cava; V, ventricle. From Shaher *et al.* (1967), by permission of *Amer. Heart J.*

the orientation of the convexity of the bulboventricular loop toward the right and its concavity toward the left. During the development of the bulboventricular loop the apex of the heart is oriented toward the right because the loop convexity is also directed toward the right. At a latter stage of development the apex of the heart has a left-sided position (Fig. 2.2).

The caudal part of the cardiac tube now undergoes further differentiation. Fusion of the primitive atrial dilatations gives rise to a single transversely dilated atrium which, as it is gradually freed from the septum transversum, comes to lie in the pericardial cavity dorsal and to the left of the bulboventricular loop. A continuation of the separation process results in almost complete freeing of the right and left sinus venosus from the septum transversum so that they, in turn, come to be situated in the pericardial cavity dorsal to the atrium. Here they undergo partial fusion to form a confluent sinus venosus which opens by a sinuatrial orifice into the atrial cavity. The most caudal portions of the venous sinuses remain unfused as the right and left horns of the definitive sinus venosus. Because of a rearrangement of the veins in the septum transversum, the left horn is reduced in size and becomes the coronary sinus. The ductus venosus sends most of the blood entering the heart to the right sinus horn which consequently enlarges, and the sinuatrial orifice moves to the right side of the dorsal surface of the atrium. The atrium, ventricle, and bulbus cordis now expand rapidly and at the same time undergo some rearrangement in position. The atrium expands transversely and extends laterally and ventrally and appears on either side of the cephalic part of the bulbus cordis. With continuing growth of the cardiac tube, the left bulboventricular sulcus becomes reduced in depth and the bulbus gradually shifts toward the left and appears in a midline position on the ventral surface of the developing heart. During these changes the atrioventricular grooves become accentuated to form a narrow waist, the lumen of which is called the atrioventricular canal. The medial shift of the bulbus is of great importance in bringing the septa in the truncus arteriosus and the bulbus cordis into line with the muscular interventricular septum. During development of the atrial septum, the sinus venosus is absorbed into the right atrium and the pulmonary vein into the left atrium.

At a time when the atrial and muscular ventricular septa are being formed, there is a concentration of the endocardial cushion tissue into two longitudinal ridges extending into a clockwise spiral path from cephalic end of the truncus throughout the bulbus cordis to the ventricles. Although these ridges are by no means equally developed at all levels, some endocardial cushion tissue is present throughout the length of the truncus and bulbus. There are three levels in which the ridge system of the truncus and bulbus are best developed: (1) in the ventral aortic roots at the level where the 4th and 6th arches are being separated; (2) in the truncus arteriosus at the level where the aortic and pulmonary valves are being formed; and (3) in the bulbus cordis. At the cephalic end of the truncus and at the caudal end of the bulbus these ridges have the same direction as the muscular interventricular septum and are situated in a dextrodorsal and sinistroventral positions. Accordingly, the cephalic end of the truncoconal septum has an oblique orientation from right to left and from back toward the front. It divides the cephalic end of the truncus into two regions—sinistrodorsal, which is in continuity with the 6th aortic arch (main pulmonary artery), and dextroventral, which is in continuity with the 4th aortic arch (the aortic arch). At its caudal end, the truncoconal septum has the same orientation, i.e., from right to left and from back toward the front, because it is formed by the dextrodorsal and sinistroventral conus ridges. The direction of the caudal end of the spiral septum is similar to that of the muscular portion of the interventricular septum. In this way the 6th aortic arch, which is in a sinistrodorsal position, is in continuity with the right ventricle in a dextroventral position, and the 4th aortic arch, which is in a dextroventral position, is in continuity with the left ventricle in a sinistrodorsal position.

In 1962, de Vries and Saunders made an exhaustive study of the literature and also carefully examined their own series of embryos between the age groups IX and XV. They agreed with His (1885) and Waterston (1918) that the right and left ventricles arise in series rather than in parallel. They pointed out that the bulbus cordis of Davis (1927) gives rise to the infundibulum distally and to the trabeculated right ventricle proximally. They agreed with Kramer (1942) that the infundibulum gives rise to the outflow tracts of both ventricles. They pointed out, however, that the assumption of Keith (1906), Kramer (1942), and de la Cruz and da Rocha (1956) that the conoventricular flange interferes with the egress of blood from the left ventricle, is erroneous both in observation and in interpretation. This fold is, in fact, the forerunner of the ventrocephalic portion of the interventricular septum. The medial shift of the infundibulum (conus), therefore, is not related to absorption of the conoventricular flange, but is due to expansion of the right atrium, right ventricle, medial displacement of the elongating infundibulum, and linear growth of the truncus arteriosus. The lateralization of the atrioventricular canal to the left during the early stages of development appears to result from a greater linear growth of the right atrium than that of the left atrium. Later, bulging of the left wall of the myocardial heart tube on either side of the atrioventricular junction, results in a medial position of the atrioventricular canal in relation to the lateral borders of the heart.

The idea that the two endocardial spiral ridges are the chief agents in the formation of the aorta and the pulmonary artery has been rejected by Shaner (1962). His study of pig embryos of 15 to 50 mm length, which are roughly equivalent to human embryos of the first trimester, lead him to believe that these ridges take little part in the formation of the aorta and the pulmonary artery and that they are concerned mostly with the semilunar valves and with the aortic and pulmonary orifices beneath them. Thus in a 7-mm pig embryo two longitudinal spiral ridges are present in the bulbus and are labeled 1 and 3. Ridge 1 begins proximally in front of the interventricular foramen, while ridge 3 begins opposite it in the endocardial tissue around the atrioventricular canal. Each ridge spirals distally so that ridge 1 begins on the left side of the proximal bulbus and ends on the right side of the distal bulbus and aortic sac. As the bulbus leaves the pericardial sac, two small cushions labeled 2 and 4 appear and mark the site of the future semilunar valves. The aortic sac is divided into aorta and pulmonary artery by the aorticopulmonary septum, an extracardiac fold of connective tissue, which passes down between the 4th and 6th arterial arches. It descends in the frontal plane and joins the tips of ridges 1 and 3 and follows them as far as the semilunar valves. When it reaches the valve level it divides the tissue of ridge 1 and 3 and lays down the rudiments of the six semilunar cusps. The aorta and the pulmonary artery are lengthened and twisted by two events in the bulbus. First, the distal end of the bulbus and its valve rudiments rotate clockwise about half a circle, and, second, the entire bulbus shrinks and is absorbed into the right ventricle thus pulling the semilunar valves down upon the base of the ventricle. Shaner points out that the two spiral ridges have little to do with the great vessels distal to the valves, since rotation of the bulbus untwists these ridges and reduces them into two short thick cushions which fuse and form the aortic and the pulmonary inlets. Together with the adjacent endocardial tissue, they also form the membranous interventricular septum.

Van Mierop, *et al.* (1963) pointed out that, at first, the truncus swellings (dextrosuperior and sinistroinferior) grow much faster than the conus swellings. The dextrosuperior swelling grows distally and to the left while the sinistroinferior swelling grows distally and to the right. They soon fuse to form the truncus septum which divides the proximal truncus into aortic and pulmonary channels. The undivided distal truncus and adjacent portion of the ventral aorta dilate concomitantly (truncoaortic sac). The sixth arches are shifted to the left; the ventral aorta, to the right. The posterior wall of the truncoaortic sac invaginates to form a vertically disposed septum, the aorticopulmonary septum, which meets and fuses with the truncus septum. Thus, the truncus is divided into pulmonary artery and aorta. The conus swellings (dextrodorsal and sinistroventral) now grow rapidly in size and bulk until they also have fused with each other and distally with the truncus swellings, thus completing the division of the truncoconus. Meanwhile, enlargement of the atrioventricular canal transversely and to the right, and a relative shift and flattening out of the conoventricular flange have brought the posteromedial (aortic) portion of the conus in line with the left ventricle to form the aortic vestibule. The authors emphasized that the proximal ascending aorta, the aortic vestibule, the proximal pulmonary artery, and the entire right ventricle are all derived from the bulbus cordis. In the young embryo, therefore, both the aorta and the pulmonary artery originate from the right ventricle, the aorta being transferred secondarily to the left ventricle. The characteristic twist of the two great arteries around each other in the normal adult heart is the result of four developmental processes: (1) torsion due to formation of the cardiac loop, (2) the mode of division of the truncoaortic area, (3) the transfer of the aortic root to the left ventricle, and (4) growth and dilatation of the two arteries.

Relationship between Two Blood Streams and Heart Septation

Baer (1828) recognized the significance of blood streams in relation to the position of the aorta and the pulmonary artery, and pointed out that both appear to have formed from two different blood streams. [The idea of this causation of the heart septa has been discussed by Spitzer (1919, 1921, 1923)]. Beneke (1920) suggested that the blood stream is directly responsible for the shape of the heart, the kink of the atrium against the ventricle, and the formation of the ventricular septum. He emphasized the relation between blood streams and the genesis of stenosis or atresia of the valves, and the width of the great vessels. His views, however, have been rejected by Stohr (1925), Bredt (1935), and Goerttler (1956) on the grounds that asymmetry of the shape of the heart begins before blood transportation. Bremer (1928) suggested that the subdivision of the heart into right and left halves of the adult was due to the presence of two more or less parallel streams of blood flowing through the early simple heart tube. The two blood streams might remain as separate entities, and between them would be linear areas of lessened internal pressure. He suggested that the two opposed endocardial cushions and the paired internal bulbar ridges represented these areas where lessened internal pressure had encouraged the thickening of the inner wall by the multiplication of its component cells. In 1931, Bremer demonstrated, in the chick embryo of about 48 hours or older, that the two streams enter the heart from the right and left vitelline veins and run through the chick embryonic heart in definite spiral courses. Between them the endocardial cushions and the interventricular and bulbar septa develop. The interatrial septum apparently develops across one of the streams. In the chick, while the young heart tube is in the loop form, the bulging right wall of the common atrium overlaps the ascending limb of the ventricle, and with each peristaltic heart beat this right side of the atrium is lifted dorsally, until, with continued growth, the atrium as a whole is tilted transversely, its right side more dorsal than the left. Consequently, the veins entering from the left tend to be directed ventrally, while those from the right are directed dorsally. Thus the stream from the right veins passes to the right side of the atrioventricular canal, while that from the left veins flows spirally around it, at first ventral, then to the right of it, dorsal to it, and finally on its left side in the canal. Because of the spiral twist of the distal portion of the heart, the stream from the left veins would be carried to the ventral side of the bulb and the more cranially situated aortic arches. The stream from the right veins would pass to the dorsal part of the bulb and the future pulmonary arches. Thus the asymmetry of the atrium, due to simple mechanical causes, leads to the production of two individual streams of blood within the young heart. The propulsive force for the two streams is provided by the waves of peristaltic contraction, beginning in the veins and transmitted first to the right atrial wall, as the next cranial segment of the tube, and then to the left atrial wall, and so the atrioventricular canal and the ventricles. Bremer, however, pointed out that it is not yet proved that the presence of the streams is the cause of the development of the septa, and that heart development is purely the result of mechanical or hydrodynamic forces. There may be inherited tendencies to form septa around which the streams arrange themselves, or which will form without the presence of any stream. Moreover, he mentioned that the experiments of Stohr (1925), Ekman (1925), and Copenhaver (1926) showed that hearts growing without circulation, or with a single entering vein only, develop the usual division of atria ventricles and bulb, but none of these hearts, however, were old enough to demonstrate whether subdivisions of the heart could have occurred under these circumstances. On the other hand, Fales (1946), working on Amblystoma, pointed out that there was no evidence to indicate that the external shape of the heart depended on the presence of blood flow, since hearts in which very little blood flow was taking place had a normal shape. He concluded that the flow of blood was necessary for the hollowing-out effect. Hearts without blood frequently had thicker walls, particularly in the ventricles, and the conus might be partially solid or only have a very narrow cavity. Patten *et al.* (1948) agreed with Bremer that spiral blood streams may have an internal molding effect since an excised chick heart kept alive by tissue culture methods does not differentiate morphologically under the influence of its "inherent developmental potencies." On the other hand, Streeter (1948) stated "One naturally associates the formation of two separate channels with the growth and activity of the two ventricular pouches, . . . as one can see in horizon xvi, as they become large and their positions prove favorable for producing directional thrusts or currents toward the pulmonary and aortic outlets, respectively. Consideration of the wide variety of anomalies that occur in these large arteries warns one, however, that ventricular thrusts, if a factor at all, may be only one of many in the development of this, our most important organ." Doerr (1952) stressed that the normal migration of the conotruncus (the vectorial conus torsion) has three components: (1) migration of the conus from right to left, (2) torsion of the truncus along its longitudinal axis, and (3) angular bending of the conus from right and ventral to left and dorsal. Goerttler (1956) thought that because of this bent form of the conotruncus, the spiraling of the blood streams is maintained in this region.

Using glass models of undivided embryonic human hearts between 4 and 7 mm (3½ to 4½ weeks) and colored water as a perfusing solution, Goerttler (1956) observed two different routes taken by the fluid. The direction of the flow from the left sinus horn was across the front of the atrium, then it turned spirally below the atrial roof to the auricular canal. It flowed through the ventral part of the left ventricle and turned dorsally to pass obliquely across the posterior wall of the bulbus and along its right edge, turned to the front, and finally left the heart. The flow from the right sinus horn and later from the enlarged right superior vena cava flowed first along the posterior atrial wall and along the "base" of the atrioventricular canal to the posterior wall of the left ventricle. It turned along the base of the ventricular loop to the frontal wall of the right ventricle, crossed the first stream, passed in the left frontal bulbus section, and left it medially and posteriorly. Between these two streams "lateral pressure-free zones" were formed with minimal acceleration of flow. The position of these zones was identical with the position of the endocardial ridges which form the truncal septum. Goerttler pointed out that the first stream represented in all detail the direction of the flow of the arterial blood, while the second represented in all respects the flow of the venous blood.

de Vries and Saunders (1962) found that in human embryos between age group XII and age group XVI, two longitudinal spiral ridges develop in the infundibulotruncal outflow tract following the period of peristaltic contraction and coinciding with the development of the two ventricular pumps. These ridges which spiral distally in a clockwise direction, arise from a conformation of the plastic gelatinous layer around a spiral stream. The spiral ridges become deeper and are largely approximated before the descent of the spur between the 4th and 6th aortic arches. Spiral septation of the outflow tract, therefore, precedes its histological segmental differentiation but follows considerable morphological differentiation of the two trabeculated ventricles. The authors believed that the spiral streams result from the junction of two columns or streams of blood in the proximal infundibulum. These two streams are brought about by the ejection of blood from contraction of the right and left trabeculated ventricles, both of which are proximal to the infundibulum at this stage of development and, therefore, lie more parallel than in series. They studied junctioning streams and found that a left stream, slightly behind, junctioning with a right stream slightly to the front, will form a clockwise spiral. They pointed out that the morphological position of the ventricles in age group XIII would, in the normal course of development, allow the junctioning of the streams in such a manner so as to produce a clockwise spiral. The development of spiral septation can be viewed, not only as a result of the action of a spiralling stream moulding the plastic subendocardial tissue, but primarily as a function of the morphological development of the two ventricles so located as to produce flow vectors which will join in a specific manner. The ventricular relationship required for the genesis of a fluid form, spiraling clockwise in a distal direction, is that of a left ventricular stream which joins dorsally with a right ventricular stream. Foxon (1959), commenting on the two views of cardiac development, pointed out that in the extreme mechanical view genetic control does not seem to be envisaged after the blood stream has started to move, as, from that time onward, all development follows quite mechanically. The alternative view is one that envisages a prolongation of the gene action. Based on this view, the blood flowing through the heart is a part of the environment of the developing heart and not a proved chief determinant. He concluded that heart development, as the development of all organs, must be a mixture of hereditary factors and the factors imposed in the immediate environment, of which the blood stream is one.

Positional Variation of the Apex of the Heart

From its inception, the atria are fixed to the posterior body wall by the entering veins and by the persistent portion of the mesocardium. On the other hand, the apex of the heart is not a fixed structure and can move from right to left or remain in the midline. The situs solitus heart develops with its venous atrium on the right and arterial atrium on the left. If the apex remains on the right there is dextroversion of the ventricles or dextrocardia with solitus atria. If it remains in the midline there is mesocardia with solitus atria, and if it takes a left-sided position we speak of the normal situs solitus heart (Fig. 2.4). Developmentally, therefore, dextrocardia with solitus atria, mesocardia with solitus atria, and the normal situs solitus heart are one and the same. The essential feature of this group is a venous atrium on the right and an arterial atrium on the left.

The situs inversus heart develops with its venous atrium on the left and arterial atrium on the right. The early bulboventricular loop of this heart points toward the left but later takes a right-sided position. If the apex of this heart remains on the left there is levoversion of the ventricles or levocardia with inversus atria, if it remains in the midline there is mesocardia with inversus atria, and if it takes a right-sided position we speak of the normal situs inversus heart (Fig. 2.4). Developmentally, therefore, levo-

DEXTROCARDIA		MESOCARDIA		LEVOCARDIA	
Dextroversion	Situs inversus heart	Situs inversus atria	Situs solitus atria	Situs solitus heart	Levoversion

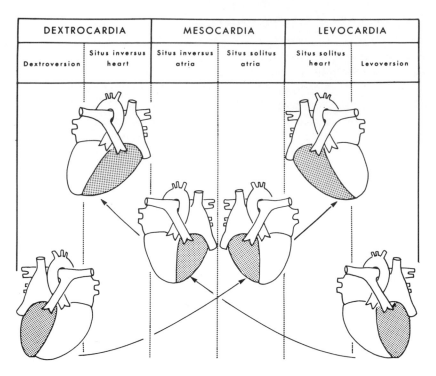

Fig. 2.4. Positional variation of the apex of the normal situs solitus and situs inversus hearts. Arrows indicate the direction of shifting of the cardiac apex during normal development. Note the occurrence of the two types of levocardia, mesocardia, and dextrocardia. A third type exists if the situs of the atria is not known. From Shaher *et al.* (1967), by permission of *Amer. Heart J.*

cardia with inversus atria, mesocardia with inversus atria, and the normal situs inversus heart are one and the same. The essential feature of this group is a venous atrium on the left and an arterial atrium on the right.

From the forementioned, three types of dextrocardia, mesocardia, and levocardia exist— (1) with situs solitus atria, (2) with situs inversus atria, and (3) with indeterminable atrial situs (Shaher *et al.* 1967).

Positional Variation of the Ventricles: Ventricular Inversion

The normal situs solitus heart develops with the convexity of the bulboventricular loop to the right and its concavity to the left. Occasionally, however, the bulboventricular loop of a situs solitus heart develops a convexity to the left and a concavity toward the right (de la Cruz *et al.*,

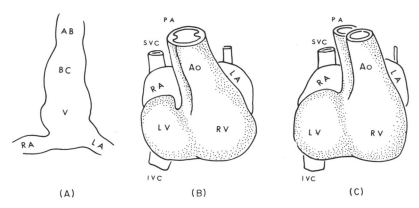

Fig. 2.5. Schematic representation of the various stages of the development of in-version of the ventricles in situs solitus heart. (A) The straight heart tube (note right atrium on the right, and left atrium on the left). (B) Bending of the bulboven-tricular loop to the left. (C) Completion of the process of inversion of the ventricles and the development of corrected transposition of the great arteries; the right atrium communicates with the morphological left ventricle, and the left atrium communi-cates with the morphological right ventricle; the aorta originates from the morpholog-ical right ventricle, and the pulmonary artery from the morphological left ventricle. (Abbreviations as in Fig. 2.2.) From Shaher *et al.* (1967), by permission of *Amer. Heart J.*

1959). This type of loop will have two limbs: a sinistroventral which gives rise to the morphological right ventricle and the bulbus cordis, and a dextrodorsal which gives rise to the morphological left ventricle (Fig. 2.5). Since the atria are normally situated for this type of heart, the right atrium will communicate with the morphological left ventricle in a dex-trodorsal position, and the left atrium will communicate with the mor-phological right ventricle in a sinistroventral position. The interventricu-lar septum will be oriented from back toward the front and from left to right. When the bulboventricular loop of a situs solitus heart develops a convexity to the left, transposition of the great arteries nearly always re-sults. Since the convexity of the bulboventricular loop is toward the left, the apex of this heart initially points toward the left, but later takes a right-sided position. In other words, situs solitus hearts with this type of loop, after complete development, should have dextrocardia with solitus atria. If the apex of this heart fails to point to the right and instead points to the left or to the midline, situs solitus heart or mesocardia with solitus atria, respectively, result (Fig. 2.6).

The embryological basis of inversion of the ventricles in situs inversus hearts is the same as that of inversion of the ventricles in situs solitus

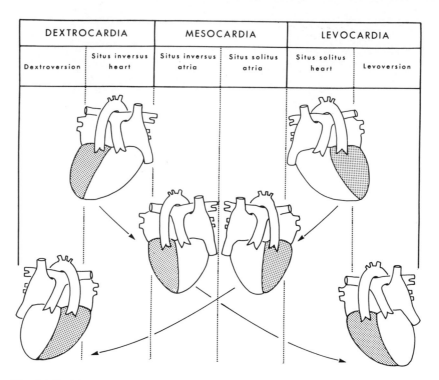

DEXTROCARDIA		MESOCARDIA		LEVOCARDIA	
Dextroversion	Situs inversus heart	Situs inversus atria	Situs solitus atria	Situs solitus heart	Levoversion

Fig. 2.6. Positional variation of the apex of the situs solitus and situs inversus hearts with inversion of the ventricles. Arrows indicate the direction of shifting of the cardiac apex during the various stages of development. Note that either dextroversion or levoversion results if development is completed. From Shaher *et al.* (1967), by permission of *Amer. Heart J.*

hearts. Thus a heart which is going to be a situs inversus heart, develops with the venous atrium on the left and the arterial atrium on the right. The bulboventricular loop, however, develops a convexity to the right and a concavity to the left (Fig. 2.7). Thus, the left-sided venous atrium communicates with the morphological left ventricle situated in a sinistro-dorsal position, while the right-sided arterial atrium communicates with the morphological right ventricle situated in a dextroventral position. The interventricular septum is oriented from back toward the front and from right to left. When the bulboventricular loop of a situs inversus heart develops a convexity to the right, transposition of the great arteries nearly always results. Since the convexity of the bulboventricular loop is toward the right, the apex of this heart initially points toward the right but later takes a left-sided position. In other words, situs inversus hearts with this type of loop should develop with levocardia and with inversus atria. If the apex, however, fails to point to the left and remains on the right or points in the midline, situs inversus heart or mesocardia with inversus atria, respectively, result (Fig. 2.6).

Significance of the Atrial Situs in the Diagnosis of Positional Anomalies of the Heart

During cardiac development the position of the ventricles and that of the great vessels are subject to deviation from the normal pattern. Thus, the bulboventricular loop of either the situs solitus or the situs inversus heart may develop a convexity to the right or to the left. In other words, the right ventricle of either heart may be situated on the right or on the left. Similarly the great vessels may be transposed or both vessels may originate from one ventricle. The apex of the heart may point to the right, to the midline, or to the left. On the other hand, from the very beginning the atria are fixed structures. They are anchored to the posterior abdominal wall by the entering great veins and by the persistent portions of the mesocardium. The atria are the only cardiac compartments whose development is not affected by the shape of the bulboventricular loop. The relationship of the atria to each other, therefore, characterizes each of the two types of heart (Shaher *et al.*, 1967). Thus, if the venous atrium is situated on the right, regardless of the position of the cardiac apex, this

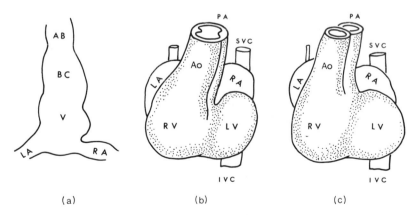

(a)　　　　　　　　(b)　　　　　　　　(c)

Fig. 2.7. Schematic representation of the various stages of development of inversion of the ventricles in situs inversus heart. (a) Straight heart tube (note right atrium on the left and the left atrium on the right). (b) Bending of the bulboventricular loop to the right. (c) Completion of the process of inversion of the ventricles and the development of corrected transposition of the great arteries. (Abbreviations as in **Fig. 2.2.**) from Shaher *et al.* (1967), by permission of *Amer. Heart J.*

heart is a situs solitus heart. On the other hand, if the venous atrium is situated on the left, regardless of the position of the cardiac apex, this heart is a situs inversus heart.

The position of the viscera in relation to the atria deserves a special mention. Although in the majority of cases the situs of the atria corresponds to that of the abdominal viscera and the situs of the abdominal viscera may be taken as indicative of that of the atria, there are the unusual cases, however, where discordance between the position of these structures occurs. Here again, if the situs of the atria is known, it matters very little if the abdominal viscera are concordant or discordant. Moreover, the undeterminable visceral situs in some cases of asplenia should not be a deterrent against making a complete cardiac diagnosis if the position of the atria is known. On the other hand, in the condition of isomerism of the atria (Van Mierop and Wiglesworth, 1962: Van Mierop *et al.*, 1964), where both atria are morphologically right atria, the presence of inversion of the ventricles or the type of transposition of the great arteries cannot be determined.

References

Baer, K. E. V. (1828). Cited by Goerttler, K. (1956). *Virch. Arch.* **328**, 391.

Beneke, R. (1920). Über Herzbieldung und Herzurifsbildung als Funktionen primärer Blutstrom formem. *Beitr. Pathol. Anat. Allg. Pathol.* **67**, 1.

Bredt, H. (1935). Cited by Goerttler, K. (1956). *Virch. Arch.* **328**, 391.

Bremer, J. L. (1928). An interpretation of the development of the heart. *Amer. J. Anat.* **42**, 307.

Bremer, J. L. (1931–1932). The presence and influence of two spiral streams in the heart of the chick embryo. *Amer. J. Anat.* **49**, 409.

Copenhaver, W. M. (1926). *J. Exp. Zool.* **43**, 321. (Cited by J. L. Bremer, 1931–1932.)

Davis, C. L. (1927). Development of the human heart from its first appearance to the stage found in embryos of 20 paired somites. *Contrib. Embryol.* **19**, 245.

de la Cruz, M. V., and da Rocha, J. P. (1956). An ontogenetic theory for the explanation of congenital malformation involving the truncus and conus. *Amer. Heart J.* **51**, 782.

de la Cruz, M. V., Anselmi, G., Cisneros, F., Reinhold, M., Portillo, B., and Espino-Vela, J. (1959). An embryologic explanation for the corrected transposition of the great vessels. Additional description of the main anatomic features of this malformation and its varieties. *Amer. Heart J.* **57**, 104.

de Vries, P. A., and Saunders, J. B. D. M. (1962). Development of the ventricles and spiral outflow tract in the human heart. A contribution to the development of the human heart from age group IX to age group XV. *Contrib. Embryol.* **37**, 89.

Doerr, W. (1952). Pathologische Anatomie typischer Grundformen angeborener Herzfehler. *Monatsschr. Kinderheilk.* **100**, 107.

Elman, G. (1925). *Arch. Entro. Organismen* **106**, 320. (Cited by J. L. Bremer, 1931–1932.)

Fales, D. E. (1946). A Study of double hearts produced experimentally in embryos of Amblystoma Punctatum. *J. Exp. Zool.* **101**, 281.

Foxon, G. E. H. (1959). Some possible causes of congenital heart malformation. *Brit. Heart J.* **21**, 51.

Goerttler, K. (1956). Hämodynamische Untersuchun über die Entstehung der Missbidungen des arteriellen Herzendes. *Virch. Arch.* **328**, 391.

Hamilton, W. J., Boyd, J. D., and Mossman, H. W. (1962). "Human Embryology," 3rd Ed. Heffer, Cambridge.

His, W. (1885). "Anatomie Menschlicher Embryonen." Leipzig. (Cited by de Vries and Saunders, 1962.)

James, T. N. (1963). Connecting pathways between the sinus node and A-V node and between the right and the left atrium in the human heart. *Amer. Heart J.* **66**, 498.

Keith, A. (1906). Malformation of the bulbus cordis. *In* "Studies in Pathology," (William Bullock, ed.), Vol. 21, p. 57. Aberdeen University Studies, Aberdeen, Scotland.

Keith, A. (1909). The Huntarian lectures on malformations of the heart. *Lancet ii*, 359, 433, 519.

Kramer, T. C. (1942). The partitioning of the truncus and conus and the formation of the membraneous portion of the interventricular septum in the human heart. *Amer. J. Anat.* **71**, 343–370.

Merideth, J., and Titus, J. L. (1968). The anatomic atrial connections between sinus and A-V node. *Circulation* **37**, 566.

Neal, H. V., and Rand, H. W. (1947). "Comparative Anatomy." Blakeston, Philadelphia, Pennsylvania.

Patten, B. M., Kramer, T. C., and Barry, A. (1948). Valvular action in the embryonic chick heart by localized opposition of endocardial masses. *Anat. Rec.* **102**, 299.

Robertson, J. I. (1913). The comparative anatomy of the bulbus cordis with special reference to abnormal positions of the great vessels in the human heart. *J. Pathol. Bacteriol.* **18**, 191.

Shaher, R. M., Duckworth, J. W., Khoury, G. H., and Moes, C. A. F. (1967). The significance of the atrial situs in the diagnosis of positional anomalies of the heart. I. Anatomical and embryological considerations. *Amer. Heart J.* **73**, 32.

Shaner, R. F. (1962). Anomalies of the heart bulbus. *J. Pediat.* **61**, 223.

Spitzer, A. (1919). I. Über die Urasachen und den Mechanismus der Zweiteilung des Wirbeltienherzens. *Arch. Entwicklungsmech. Organismen* **45**, 686.

Spitzer, A. (1921). II. Über die Urasachen und den Mechanismus der Zweiteilung des Wirbeltienherzens. *Arch. Entwicklungsmech. Organismen* **47**, 510.

Spitzer, A. (1923). Über den Bauplan des normalen und missbildeten Herzens. *Virch. Arch. Pathol. Anat. Physiol.* **243**, 81. (Translated by M. Lev, and A. Vass, Thomas, Springfield, Illinois, 1951.)

Stohr, P., Jr. (1925). *Arch. Entwichlungsmech. Organismen* **106**, 409. (Cited by J. L. Bremer, 1931–1932.)

Streeter, G. L. (1948). Developmental horizons in human embryos. Description of age groups XV, XVI, XVII, and XVIII, being the third issue of a survey of the Carnegie Collection. *Contrib. Embryol.* **32**, 133.

Thorel, C. (1909). *Munchen Med. Wochschr.* **56**, 2159. (Cited by Merideth and Titus, 1968).

Thorel, C. (1910). *Munchen Med. Wochschr.* **57**, 183. (Cited by Merideth and Titus, 1968).

Van Mierop, L. H., and Wiglesworth, F. W. (1962). Isomerism of the cardiac atria in the asplenia syndrome. *Lab. Invest.* 11, 1303.

Van Mierop, L. H. S., Alley, R. D., Kausel, H. W., and Stranahan, A. (1963). Pathogenesis of transposition complexes. I. Embryology of the ventricles and great arteries. *Amer. J. Cardiol.* 12, 216.

Van Mierop, L. H. S., Patterson, P. R., and Reynolds, R. W. (1964). Two cases of congenital asplenia with isomerism of the cardiac atria and the sinoatrial nodes. *Amer. J. Cardiol.* 13, 407.

Walmsley, T. (1929). *In* "Quain's Elements of Anatomy." (E. A. Schäfer, J. Symington, and T. H. Bryce, eds.), 11th Ed., Vol. 4, Part 3, The Heart. Longman, London.

Waterston, D. (1918). The development of the heart in man. *Trans. Roy. Soc. Edinburgh* (Part 2), p. 257.

Wenckebach, K. F. (1907). *Arch. Physiol.*, p. 1. (Cited by Merideth and Titus, 1968).

Chapter 3

CLASSIFICATION OF TRANSPOSITION

In 1875, von Rokitansky assumed that the normal truncal septum begins as a swelling in the left and posterior part of the truncus. It grows toward the right and anterior part of the truncus usually with an anterior convexity. The aorta lies on the concave side of the septum and the pulmonary artery on the convex side. At first the aorta and the pulmonary artery arise from the right ventricle. Later, with the growth of the ventricular septum, the aorta is transferred into the left ventricle. He believed that the ventricle on the side from which the ventricular septum takes origin will be the morphological left ventricle with a bicuspid atrioventricular valve. The other ventricle will be the morphological right ventricle with a tricuspid atrioventricular valve and a crista supraventricularis. He recognized two types of transposition of the great arteries (Fig. 3.1) ; corrected (Series A) and uncorrected or complete (Series B). In corrected transposition of the great arteries the aorta arises from the correct or the corresponding ventricle, i.e., the aorta from the left-sided ventricle and the pulmonary artery from the right-sided ventricle. He considered a ventricle as "right" so long as it occupied a position to the right of the other ventricle, and similarly, with regard to the left ventricle. In uncorrected or complete transposition (Series B) the aorta arises from the right-sided ventricle and the pulmonary artery from the left-sided ventricle. Since the ventricular septum may originate from the right or left, this gives rise to eight possible variations in his scheme. In Series A5 to 8 and Series B5 to 8 the ventricle septum originates from the right so that the ventricles are inverted. Whereas, A1 is normal, the rest of the series up to and including 8 show variable types of transposition of the great arteries whose erroneous relations to the ventricles are corrected by a spiral adjustment of the ventricular septum, the aorta always opening from the correct or the corresponding ventricle. Regardless of the morphology of the ventricle (for von Rokitansky) the correct or corresponding ventricle was the left for

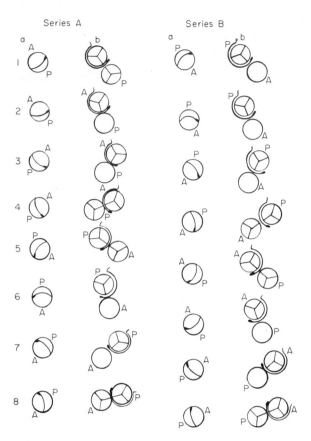

Fig. 3.1. Schematic representation of von Rokitansky's transposition of the great arteries. Scheme A shows his series of "corrected" transpositions; scheme B his series of "anomalous" uncorrected transpositions of the great arteries. A, Aorta; P, pulmonary artery. Column (a) shows the variations of the truncus septum, the rounded knob indicating the point of origin of the septum; column (b) shows the position of the vessels consequent upon their separation and the relations of the interventricular septum; the rounded knob indicates the insertion of the ventricular septum round the posterior vessel, corresponding with point of origin of the truncus septum. The spindle-shaped thickening represents the membranous septum. From Robertson (1913), by permission of *J. Pathol. Bacteriol.* **18,** 191.

the aorta and the right for the pulmonary artery. Similarly in Series B, von Rokitansky considered diagram 1 (Fig. 3.1), where the aorta is situated in front of the pulmonary artery as the starting point for a series of transpositions that cannot be corrected throughout the series so that the pulmonary artery arises from the left-sided ventricle and the aorta from the right-sided ventricle.

Robertson (1913) pointed out that in von Rokitansky's Series A, as far as diagram 4 (Fig. 3.1), the whole heart is practically normal except that the bulbus cordis appeared to have reverted to the dipnoan degree of torsion of the great vessels. Accordingly, no marked errors of development of the interventricular septum need be expected or any unusual egress of the great vessels from the ventricles. She found that the lower half of von Rokitansky's Series B corresponds exactly to a mirror picture of the upper half of Series A, and suggested that von Rokitansky's statement that the whole of his Series B consisted of uncorrected anomalous

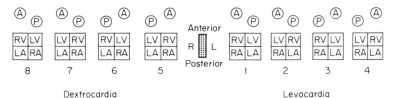

Fig. 3.2. Schematic representation of the various types of uncorrected and corrected transpositions. A, Aorta; LA, left atrium; LV, left ventricle; P, pulmonary artery; RA, right atrium; RV, right ventricle.

Geipel (1903) and Mockberg (1924)

A. Pure Transportation
1. Situs solitus
2. Situs solitus and transposition of the ventricles
5. Situs transversus
6. Situs transversus and transposition of the ventricles

B. Corrected Transposition
3. Situs solitus
4. Situs solitus and transposition of the ventricles
7. Situs transversus
8. Situs transversus and transposition of the ventricles

Pernkopf (1926)

A. Crossed Transposition
1. Without correction
2. With pure anatomic correction
8. With functional correction
7. With complete functional and anatomic correction

B. Crossed Inverse Transposition
5. Without correction
6. With pure anatomic correction
4. With functional correction
3. With complete functional and anatomic correction

Spitzer (1927)

1. Pure crossed transposition in situs solitus
2. Crossed transposition with inversion of the ventricles
3. Crossed transposition with bulbus inversion
4. Crossed transposition with ventricular and bulbar inversion
5. Inverse crossed transposition
6. Crossed transposition with sinoatrial and bulbar inversion
7. Crossed transposition with sinoatrial and ventricular inversion
8. Crossed transposition with sinoatrial inversion

positions of the great arteries must be modified since the lower half of this series can only be explained as "corrected" transposition in cases of situs inversus. Moreover, she argued that von Rokitansky's lower half of Series A is a mirror picture of the upper half of his Series B. If the latter, as von Rokitansky stated, is "uncorrected," therefore, the lower half of Series A being its mirror picture, must be regarded as cases of "uncorrected" transposition in situs inversus. She pointed out, however, that in cases of situs inversus in Series A, the condition of dextrocardia is partial; only the ventricular loop is involved, the auricles may be unaffected, and the aortic arch appears always to curve over the left bronchus.

Geipel (1903) reviewed the views of von Rokitansky (1875) and Lochte (1898) on the embryological basis of corrected transposition and classified transposition of the great arteries into two types: pure and corrected. Depending on the position of the ventricles and the presence of situs solitus or situs transversus (inversus) of the viscera, each is further subdivided into four types (Fig. 3.2) :

Type 1
  a. Pure Transposition
        Aorta right in front from right ventricle
        Pulmonary artery left behind from left ventricle
        Right ventricle tricuspid atrioventricular valve
        Left ventricle bicuspid atrioventricular valve
  b. Pure Transposition in Situs Transversus (Inversus)
        Aorta left in front from left ventricle
        Pulmonary artery right behind from right ventricle
        Right ventricle bicuspid atrioventricular valve
        Left ventricle tricuspid atrioventricular valve
Type 2
  a. Pure Transposition with Transposition of the Ventricles
        Aorta right in front from right ventricle
        Pulmonary artery left behind from left ventricle
        Right ventricle bicuspid atrioventricular valve
        Left ventricle tricuspid atrioventricular valve
  b. Pure Transposition with Transposition of the Ventricles in Situs
      Transversus (Inversus)
        Aorta left in front from left ventricle
        Pulmonary artery right behind from right ventricle
        Right ventricle tricuspid atrioventricular valve
        Left ventricle bicuspid atrioventricular valve

Type 3

a. Corrected Transposition of the Great Vessels with Transposition of
the Ventricles

    Aorta left in front from left ventricle

    Pulmonary artery right behind from right ventricle

    Right ventricle bicuspid atrioventricular valve

    Left ventricle tricuspid atrioventricular valve

b. Corrected Transposition of the Great Vessels with Transposition of
the Ventricles in Situs Transversus (Inversus)

    Aorta right in front from right ventricle

    Pulmonary artery left behind from left ventricle

    Right ventricle tricuspid atrioventricular valve

    Left ventricle bicuspid atrioventricular valve

Type 4

a. Corrected Transposition of the Great Vessels without Transposition
of the Ventricles

    Aorta left in front from left ventricle

    Pulmonary artery right behind from right ventricle

    Right ventricle tricuspid atrioventricular valve

    Left ventricle bicuspid atrioventricular valve

b. Corrected Transposition without Transposition of the Ventricles in
Situs Transversus (Inversus)

    Aorta right in front from right ventricle

    Pulmonary artery left behind from left ventricle

    Right ventricle bicuspid atrioventricular valve

    Left ventricle tricuspid atrioventricular valve

The views of Monckeberg (1924) on the classification of transposition
of the great vessels are similar to those of Geipel. Two types of transposition occur with situs solitus hearts, namely, pure and corrected transposition. Each type is further subdivided into two types depending on whether the ventricles are normally situated or "transposed." Mirror-image of
these two types and also of their subdivisions occurs with situs inversus
(Fig. 3.2) .

A. Pure Transposition

1. In Situs Solitus

    Aorta right in front from right tricuspid ventricle

    Pulmonary artery left behind from left mitral ventricle

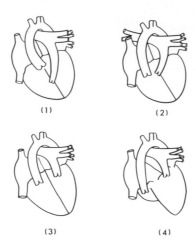

(1)   (2)

(3)   (4)

Fig. 3.3. Spitzer's four grades of transposition. (1) Overriding aorta; (2) simple transposition of the aorta into the right ventricle; (3) crossed transposition of both arterial trunks; (4) mixed transposition of the arterial trunks.

 2. In Situs Transversus (Inversus)
        Aorta left in front from left tricuspid ventricle
        Pulmonary artery right behind from right mitral ventricle
 3. In Situs Solitus and Transposition of the Ventricles
        Aorta right in front from right mitral ventricle
        Pulmonary artery left behind from left tricuspid ventricle
 4. In Situs Transversus (Inversus) and Transposition of the Ventricles
        Aorta left in front from left mitral ventricle
        Pulmonary artery right behind from right tricuspid ventricle
B. Corrected Transposition
   1. In Situs Solitus
        Aorta left in front from left mitral ventricle
        Pulmonary artery right behind from right tricuspid ventricle
   2. In Situs Transversus (Inversus)
        Aorta right in front from right mitral ventricle
        Pulmonary artery left behind from left tricuspid ventricle
   3. In Situs Solitus and Transposition of the Ventricles
        Aorta left in front from left tricuspid ventricle
        Pulmonary artery right behind from right mitral ventricle
   4. In Situs Transversus (Inversus) and Transposition of the Ventricles
        Aorta right in front from right tricuspid ventricle
        Pulmonary artery left behind from left mitral ventricle

On the other hand, Spitzer (1923) recognized four types of pure or common transposition of the great vessels (Fig. 3.3).

Type 1. Riding Aorta

The pulmonary artery originates from the right ventricle while the aorta overrides the ventricular septum. The infundibulum of the right ventricle is partially separated posteriorly from the right side of the aortic ostium by the protruding crista supraventricularis. The pulmonary artery may be narrowed and its valve occasionally possesses two semilunar cusps. A small ventricular septal defect, below the aorta, is present.

Type 2. Simple Transposition of the Aorta into the Right Ventricle

Both aorta and pulmonary artery emerge from the right ventricle with the aortic ostium lying to the right of the pulmonary artery ostium. The ventricular septal defect is larger than in the last type and there is more hypertrophy of the crista supraventricularis.

Type 3. Crossed Transposition of Both Arterial Trunks

The aorta, situated anteriorly and to the right, emerges from the right ventricle, and the pulmonary artery, situated posteriorly and to the left, emerges from the left ventricle. The pulmonary artery is usually narrow and possesses two cusps. The ventricular septal defect is still larger than in the previous two types. Both atrioventricular valves open into their corresponding ventricles. There are two variants of this type: (A) with a single ventricle, and (B) with a closed ventricular septum. In type (B) the pulmonary artery may widen again; its valve possesses three cusps.

Type 4. Mixed Transposition of the Arterial Trunks

This type is similar to the last type, but, in addition, the tricuspid valve, as well as the mitral valve, opens into the left ventricle. The right ventricle contains only the aortic ostium which is more situated anteriorly and to the right, so that the right ventricle protrudes above the level of the anterior surface of the ventricular region in the form of a "hump." The ventricular septal defect is smaller than in the last type, the aortic ostium may be narrowed, and the pulmonary artery ostium may be widened and possesses three cusps.

Spitzer pointed out that inverted transposition occurs when these four types are combined with "situs inversus of the heart bow." Thus, in Type 1 the aorta overrides the septum, whereas the pulmonary artery arises from the left ventricle. In Type 2 the two great vessels originate from the left ventricle. In Type 3 the aorta arises anteriorly and to the left from the left ventricle, whereas the pulmonary artery arises posteriorly and to the right from the right ventricle. Type 4 is similar to Type 3, but, in addition, the left-sided atrioventricular valve opens into the right ventricle and the aortic hump is formed by the small left ventricle.

In 1926, Pernkopf criticized von Rokitansky's classification on the grounds that he failed to realize that some of his types could be explained best on the basis of situs inversus. He pointed out that Geipel and Monckeberg used the term "corrected" transposition in a different sense from that of von Rokitansky, since according to these two authors, the corresponding ventricle to the aorta is the "mitral" ventricle, and to the pulmonary artery is the "tricuspid" ventricle. He accepted Spitzer's nomenclature, but not his theory. To simplify Geipel's "clumsy" nomenclature, Pernkopf recognized three types of corrected transposition: functional, anatomical, and complete functional and anatomical. With functional correction the aorta arises from the "tricuspid" ventricle and is situated on the same side as the pulmonary (arterial) atrium. With anatomical correction, the aorta arises from the "mitral" ventricle but is situated on the same side as the caval (venous) atrium. While with complete functional and anatomical correction, the anteriorly situated aorta arises from the "mitral" ventricle and is situated on the same side as the pulmonary (arterial) atrium. He classified transposition into usual and inverse forms depending on whether these are related to a normal (situs solitus) or to an inverse (situs inversus) truncus septation, respectively (Fig. 3.2).

Usual Transpositions

1. Riding Aorta (usual form)
       Pulmonary artery from right ventricle
2. Mixed Usual Transposition with a Pulmonary Ventricle
       Pulmonary artery left anterior from left ventricle
       Aorta right posterior from right ventricle
       Atrioventricular valves open into right ventricle
3. Riding Pulmonary Artery
       Aorta right posterior from right ventricle
4. Simple Usual Transposition
       Aorta right, pulmonary artery left
       Both arteries from right ventricle, left ventricle receives an atrioventricular valve.
       Arterial ostia lie obliquely behind each other
5. Crossed Usual Transposition
       Pulmonary artery ostium left posterior
       Aortic ostium right anterior

    a. Without Correction
        Aorta from right tricuspid ventricle
        Pulmonary artery from left bicuspid ventricle
        Caval atrium on the right
        Pulmonary atrium on the left.
    b. With Functional Correction
        Pulmonary artery from left bicuspid ventricle
        Aorta from right tricuspid ventricle
        Pulmonary atrium on the right
        Caval atrium on the left
    c. With Complete Functional and Anatomical Correction
        Aorta from right bicuspid ventricle
        Pulmonary artery from left tricuspid ventricle
        Caval atrium on the left
        Pulmonary atrium on the right
    d. With Pure Anatomical Correction
        Aorta from right bicuspid ventricle
        Pulmonary artery from left tricuspid ventricle
        Caval atrium on the right
        Pulmonary atrium on the left
6. Crossed Usual Transposition
    a. With Riding Aorta
        Aorta right anterior from both ventricles
        Pulmonary artery left posterior from left ventricle
    b. With Riding Pulmonary Artery
        Aorta right anterior from right ventricle
        Pulmonary artery left posterior from both ventricles
7. Mixed Usual Transposition with an Aortic Ventricle
        Aorta right anterior from right aortic ventricle
        Pulmonary artery left posterior from left ventricle
        Atrioventricular valves open into left ventricle

Inverse Transpositions

1. Riding Aorta (Inverse Form)
        Pulmonary artery from left ventricle
2. Mixed Inverse Transposition with Pulmonary Ventricle
        Pulmonary artery right anterior from right ventricle
        Aorta left posterior from left ventricle
        Atrioventricular valves open into left ventricle
3. Riding Pulmonary Artery (Inverse Form)
        Aorta left posterior from left ventricle

4. Simple Inverse Transposition
      Aorta left, pulmonary artery right
      Both arteries from left ventricle; right ventricle receives an atrio-
      ventricular valve
      Arterial ostia lie obliquely behind each other
5. Crossed Inverse Transposition
      Pulmonary artery ostium right posterior
      Aortic ostium left anterior
   a. Without Correction
         Aorta from left tricuspid ventricle
         Pulmonary artery from right bicuspid ventricle
         Caval atrium on the left
         Pulmonary atrium on the right
   b. With Functional Correction
         Aorta from left tricuspid ventricle
         Pulmonary artery from right bicuspid ventricle
         Caval atrium on the right
         Pulmonary atrium on the left
   c. With Complete Functional and Anatomical Correction
         Aorta from left bicuspid ventricle
         Pulmonary artery from right tricuspid ventricle
         Caval atrium on the right
         Pulmonary atrium on the left
   d. With Pure Anatomical Correction
         Aorta from left bicuspid ventricle
         Pulmonary artery from right tricuspid ventricle
         Caval atrium on the left
         Pulmonary atrium on the right
6. Crossed Inverse Transposition
   a. With Riding Aorta
         Aorta left anterior from both ventricles
         Pulmonary artery right posterior from right ventricle
   b. With Riding Pulmonary Artery
         Aorta left anterior from left ventricle
         Pulmonary artery right posterior from both ventricles
7. Mixed Inverse Transposition with an Aortic Ventricle
      Aorta left anterior from left aortic ventricle
      Pulmonary artery right posterior from right ventricle
      Atrioventricular valves open into right ventricle

In 1927, Spitzer disagreed with the nomenclature and explanations of
the types of transposition suggested by Geipel, Monckeberg, and Pern-

kopf. He thought that Monckeberg's use of the term "ventricular transposition" showed that Monckeberg did not know the difference between inversion and transposition. He criticized the terms "corrected transposition" and "corresponding ventricle" since these could have more than one meaning. In addition, he pointed out that in Monckeberg's classification there are corrected forms of transposition in which the position of the great vessels is exactly similar to some of the pure forms. He objected to Geipel–Monckeberg's definition of ventricular transposition in situs inversus and thought that there was no reason to assume a uniform situs of the whole heart determined by the position of the atria. These cases could be viewed as examples of inversion of the atria with situs solitus of the ventricles. He strongly criticized Pernkopf's nomenclature and classification on the following grounds.

1. Pernkopf accepted Spitzer's four grades of usual and inverse forms of transposition as well as von Rokitansky's term "corrected transposition," but, in addition, tried to enlarge on both, thus causing new confusion.

2. Pernkopf misinterpreted the definition of Spitzer's pure and inverse forms and related them to mixed forms of transposition.

3. Although Pernkopf emphasized the independence of inversion of the single heart sections (truncus, ventricles, and atria), he contradicted himself and repeated Geipel–Monckeberg's principal error of accepting the situs of a section of the heart (the bulbus in case of Pernkopf) as being characteristic of the whole situs of the organ. As a result, Monckeberg's inverse forms become Pernkopf's usual or noninverse forms, and vice versa; Monckeberg's situs solitus forms become Pernkopf's inverse forms.

4. Equally wrong and confusing is Pernkopf's use of term "corrected transposition." His term "functional correction" is a new name for an old definition, because in Monckeberg's view the success of correction depends on the transposed aorta being perfused with arterial blood and the pulmonary artery with venous blood. This process results from the placement of the aorta on the same side as the pulmonary atrium, and the pulmonary artery on the same side as the caval atrium. Again, the term "anatomic correction" is a new name for an old definition and is identical with Monckeberg's "corresponding ventricle" which means origin of the aorta from the mitral ventricle and the pulmonary artery from the tricuspid ventricle. As a result of Pernkopf's definition, the term corrected transposition now has three different meanings. Moreover, even the apparent pure functionally corrected cases are as much anatomically corrected as the apparent pure anatomical forms. Anatomical correction in

functionally corrected cases takes the form of hypertrophy of bands or formation of abnormal septa. Similarly, anatomical correction may have a functional side to it, if, for instance, the ventricular septal defect affects the supply of arterial blood to the aorta. Spitzer stressed that his old suggestion of dropping the term "corrected transposition" gains new strength and justification through Pernkopf's use of this term.

Spitzer (1927) assumed that the four compartments of the heart: sinus, atrium, ventricle, and bulbus, are capable of isolated inversion either singly or in combination, and thought that it would be more logical to simply add to his term "transposition Type 3" the inverted sections of the heart. Accordingly, there are two extreme forms of Type 3 (crossed) transposition. The first is the usual or the pure form while the second one is an inverse form. In between these two extremes there are mixed types which would best be named as follows (Fig. 3.2) :

1. Crossed transposition with primary inversion of the ventricles alone
2. Crossed transposition with bulbus inversion alone
3. Crossed transposition with sinoatrial inversion alone
4. Crossed transposition with primary bulboventricular inversion
5. Crossed transposition with sinoatrial and primary ventricular inversion without bulbus inversion
6. Crossed transposition with sinoatrial and bulbus inversion without ventricular inversion

Spitzer pointed out that of these mixed types, 1 and 2 are closer to the pure transposition, while 5 and 6 are closer to the inverse transposition, since in 1 and 2 only one of the four heart compartments is inverted. Types 3 and 4 lie in the middle between pure and inverse transposition. He stressed that the allocation of half of the mixed forms to the pure type of transposition and the other half to the inverse type of transposition is not permissible since all six types show partial inversions, but, at the most, could be counted as inverse forms of transposition. Spitzer, therefore, recognized two forms of his Type 3 crossed transposition: (1) a pure form in which the morphologically right chambers of the heart are situated on the right and the morphologically left chambers on the left, with the aorta arising anteriorly and to the right from the right ventricle and the pulmonary artery arising posteriorly and to the left from the left ventricle and (2) an inverse form in which there is inversion of all the compartments of the heart; sinus, atria, ventricles, and bulbus. The morphologically left chambers are situated on the right. The aorta originates anteriorly and to the left from the left-sided ventricle (which is a morphologically right ventricle) while the pulmonary artery originates posteriorly and to the right from the right-sided ventricle (which is a morphologically left ventricle). In between there are mixed forms each having one, two, or three inverted compartments of the heart. Spitzer concluded that the advantage of his classification is that at a glance one can see the factors and symbols, and that it has eliminated multiple meaning confusing terms like "inverse forms," "corrected transposition," "situs solitus," and "situs inversus."

Writers more recently tended to classify transposition either on the basis of Spitzer's four grades, or on the basis of the associated defects. In an analysis of 1000 cases of congenital heart disease, Abbott (1936) classified transposition as follows.

1. Dextroposition of Aorta
    a. Aorta from left ventricle, ventricular septum entire
    b. Aorta from both ventricles
    c. Aorta from right ventricle
    d. Aorta from right ventricle, double conus
2. Complete Transposition
    a. Closed ventricular septum
    b. Defect ventricular septum
3. Partial Transposition
4. Corrected Transposition

Emerson and Green (1942) added overriding aorta with pulmonary atresia to the four types of transposition of Spitzer. Lev and Saphir (1945) added other anomalies to Spitzer's Type 4 and classified transposition as follows:

Type 1 (Spitzer). Riding Aorta (von Rokitansky)
    a. With an aneurysm of the membranous septum
    b. With a defect of the ventricular septum
Type 2 (Spitzer). Partial Transposition (von Rokitansky)
    The aorta and the pulmonary artery arise from the right ventricle
Type 3 (Spitzer). Complete Transposition (von Rokitansky)
    The aorta arises from the right ventricle and the pulmonary artery from the left ventricle
Type 4 (Spitzer). Miscellaneous Group
    Truncus communis, truncus solitaris aorticus with transposition
    Truncus solitaris pulmonalis with transposition, and transposition with atresia of the tricuspid valve

On the other hand, in 1962, Lev *et al.* divided transposition into two main types: simple (with normal ventricular architecture) and other types. According to the anatomy of the associated defects the simple type was further subdivided into six types:

1. Without ventricular septal defect
   With large atrial septal defect
   With patent ductus arteriosus
   Without patent ductus arteriosus
   With patent ductus arteriosus without large atrial septal defect
2. With ventricular septal defect
3. With pulmonary stenosis or atresia
4. With common ventricle
   With pulmonary stenosis
5. With single ventricle and small outlet chamber
6. With abnormal atrioventricular orifices
   With tricuspid stenosis or atresia
   With mitral stenosis or atresia
   With common atrioventricular orifice

Recently, Van Mierop and Wiglesworth (1963) studied pathologically eighty-five specimens of transposition of the great arteries and stressed that only two types of "true" transposition exist; one without inversion of the ventricles (complete transposition) and the other with inversion of the ventricles (corrected transposition). They pointed out that these two types occur in situs solitus, and their mirror-images in situs inversus also occur. The authors analyzed the series of twenty-four cases collected from the literature by earlier workers and by Cardell (1956) and concluded that the other types of true transposition do not exist because they are embryological impossibilities.

Van Praagh *et al.* (1964a,b) defined transposition of the great arteries as the condition in which there is mitral–aortic valve discontinuity and designated the type of transposition of the great arteries in which the transposed aortic valve is situated to the right of the transposed pulmonary valve as *d*-transposition, and the type of transposition in which the transposed aortic valve is situated to the left of the transposed pulmonary valve as *l*-transposition. As to the reversal of the lateral relationships of the ventricles, they preferred the term "transposition of the ventricles," since the term "inversion" is probably based on embryological uncertainties. The authors pointed out that there are *d*-bulboventricular loops, *l*-bulboventricular loops, and *x*-bulboventricular loops. A *d*-loop means that following the straight tube stage, the primitive heart protrudes initially to the right, an *l*-loop means that it protrudes initially to the left, while an *x*-loop is present if the initial protrusion is uncertain. In a *d*-loop the right ventricle is situated on the right and the left ventricle on the left, while in an *l*-loop the right ventricle is situated on the left and the left ventricle on the right. When transposition occurs it is *d*-transposition in a *d*-bulboventricular loop, and *l*-transposition in *l*-loop. A cardiac loop is concordant or is discordant relative to the type of visceroatrial situs. A concordant loop conforms or corresponds to the type of the visceroatrial situs, whereas a discordant loop does not. Concordant loops are a *d*-loop with situs solitus, and an *l*-loop with situs inversus. Conversely discordant cardiac loops are an *l*-loop with situs solitus, and a *d*-loop with situs inversus. Uncorrected transposition is a concordant cardiac loop; *d*-loop with *d*-transposition of the great arteries. Corrected transposition is the discordant *l*-loop; situs solitus with an *l*-loop and *l*-transposition.

References

Abbott, M. E. (1936). "Atlas of Congenital Cardiac Disease." American Heart Association, New York.

Cardell, B. S. (1956). Corrected transposition of the great vessels. *Brit. Heart J.* **18**, 186.

Emerson, P. W., and Green, H. (1942). Transposition of the great cardiac vessels. *J. Pediat.* **21**, 1.

Geipel, P. (1903). Weitere Beitrage zum situs transversus and zur hehre von den transposition der grossen Gefasse des Herzens. *Arch. Kinderheilk.* **35**, 112, 222.

Lev, M., and Saphir, O. (1945) . A theory of transposition of the arterial trunks based on the phylogenetic and ontogenetic development of the heart. *Arch. Pathol.* **39**, 172.

Lev, M., Paul, M. H., and Miller, R. A. (1962) . A classification of congenital heart disease based on the pathologic complex. *Amer. J. Cardiol.* **10**, 733.

Lochte, E. H. T. (1898). Ein Fall von situs viscerum irregularis nelst einem Beitreg zur Lehre von der Transposition der arteriellen grossen Gefassetamme des Herzens. *Beitr. Pathol. Anat. Allg. Pathol.* **24**, 187.

Monckeberg, J. G. (1924). Die Missbildungen des Herzens. In "Handbuch der Speziellen Pathologischen Anatomie und Histologie" (F. Henke and O. Lubarsch, eds.), Vol. 2, pp 1–183. Springer, Berlin.

Pernkopf, E. (1926). Der partielle situs inversus der Eingeweide beim Menschen. *Z. Anat. Entwicklungsgesch.* **79**, 577.

Robertson, J. I. (1913). The comparative anatomy of the bulbus cordis with special reference to abnormal positions of the great vessels in the human heart. *J. Pathol. Bacteriol.* **18**, 191.

Spitzer, A. (1923). Über den Bauplan des normalen und missbildeten Herzens. *Virch. Arch. Path. Anat. Physiol.* **243**, 81. (Translated by M. Lev and A. Vass, Thomas, Springfield, Illinois, 1951.)

Spitzer, A. (1927). Zur Kritik der phylogenetischen Theorie der normalen und missbildeten Herzarchitektur. *Z. Anat. Entwicklungsgesch.* 84, 30.

Van Mierop, L. H. S. and Wiglesworth, F. W. (1963). Pathogenesis of transposition complexes. III. True transposition of the great vessels. *Amer. J. Cardiol.* 12, 233.

Van Praagh, R., Ongley, P. A., and Swan, J. C. (1964a). Anatomic types of single or common ventricle in man. *Amer. J. Cardiol.* 13, 367.

Van Praagh, R., Van Praagh, S., Vlad, P., and Keith, J. D. (1964b). Anatomic types of congenital dextrocardia. Diagnostic and embryologic implications. *Amer. J. Cardiol.* 13, 510.

von Rokitansky, C. F. (1875). "Die Defecte der Scheidewände des Herzens." Braumüller, Vienna.

Chapter 4

DEFINITION OF COMPLETE TRANSPOSITION OF THE GREAT ARTERIES

The term "transposition of the great arteries" has been used in two different senses in the literature. Earlier writers used it when the great arteries were altered in their relation to their respective ventricle. In this sense, the earliest observation of transposition where the aorta arose from both ventricles is probably that of Stenonis (1671). In his case there was a small pulmonary artery and a large ventricular septal defect. Von Rokitansky (1875) considered that all forms of transposition were the result of abnormal rotation of the aortic septum, which being unable to meet the ventricular septum, resulted in one or both vessels apparently arising from the wrong ventricle. Reversal of the anteroposterior relationship of the aorta and the pulmonary artery in transposition was commented upon by various workers as early as the nineteenth century. Kürschner (1837) observed that in transposition there was a reduction in, or lack of, the normal spiral twist of the pulmonary artery about the aorta. The anterior position of the aorta in transposition was also noted by Keith (1909) who pointed out that in transposition the aortic portion of the bulbus expands and the pulmonary portion atrophies and such a process results in an anteriorly situated aorta and in the right ventricle. Geipel (1903), Monckeberg (1924), and Pernkopf (1926) described rare types of transposition in which an anterior aorta arose from a morphological left ventricle, and a posterior pulmonary artery from a morphological right ventricle. In 1927, Abbott defined transposition as "an alteration in the position of the two great vessels relative to the ventricles of the heart, or to each other at their origin, so that they spring either from reversed ventricles—the aorta from the right, and the pulmonary artery from the left chambers (complete transposition) —or from the ventricles to which they normally belong, but in reverse relationship (corrected transposition)."

the truncus the pulmonary artery originates from the right ventricle and is situated anteriorly and to the left, and the aorta originates from the left ventricle and is situated posteriorly and to the right. As early as the Nineteenth Century, almost all authors agreed that in transposition the great arteries descend without twisting or spiraling around each other. Transposition of the great arteries should be regarded as the condition in which the two great arteries fail to twist around each other with the result that their relationship remains unchanged from the cephalic to the caudal end of the truncus. In transposition of the great arteries, therefore, the aorta lies anterior to the pulmonary artery. This anatomical relationship between the aorta and the pulmonary artery may exist with the two vessels arising from the same ventricle or from opposite ventricles. The term "complete" signifies the latter relationship between the aorta and the pulmonary artery.

There are two types of transposition of the great arteries. In noninverted transposition (Rosenbaum, 1964) in situs solitus, the aorta is anterior and to the right of the pulmonary artery. In situs inversus, the aorta lies anterior and to the left of the pulmonary artery. In inverted transposition (Spitzer, 1923) in situs solitus the aorta is anterior and to the left of the pulmonary artery. In situs inversus the aorta is anterior and to the right of the pulmonary artery. Noninverted complete transposition in situs solitus means that the aorta originates from the right-sided ventricle and the pulmonary artery from the left-sided ventricle. The reverse is true in situs inversus. Most authors refer to this type as "complete transposition of the great arteries." Inverted complete transposition in situs solitus means that the aorta arises from the left-sided ventricle and the pulmonary artery from the right-sided ventricle. The reverse is true in situs inversus. Most authors refer to this type as "congenitally corrected transposition of the great arteries."

In almost all patients with these two types of complete transposition the aorta arises from the morphological right ventricle, and the pulmonary artery from the morphological left ventricle. Very rarely, however, the transposed aorta arises from the morphological left ventricle, and the transposed pulmonary artery from the morphological right ventricle. Accordingly, each of the two types of complete transposition could be divided into two types as follows.

1. Noninverted Complete Transposition (Fig. 4.1)

    a. With solitus ventricles; complete transposition of the great arteries.

    b. With inversion of the ventricles; anatomically corrected transpo-

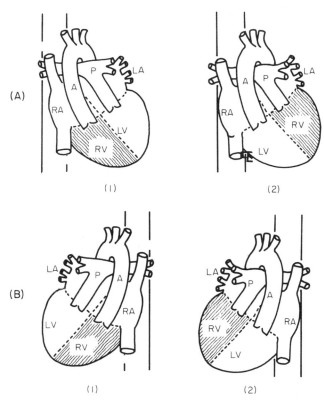

Fig. 4.1. (A) Noninverted complete transposition in situs solitus. 1, With solitus ventricles; 2, with inversion of the ventricles. (B) Noninverted complete transposition in situs inversus. 1, Without inversion of the ventricles; 2, with inversion of the ventricles. A, aorta; LA, left atrium; LV, left ventricle; P, pulmonary artery; RA, right atrium; RV, right ventricle.

sition (Geipel, 1903; Monckcberg, 1924; Lev and Rowlatt, 1961; Shaher, 1964; Van Praagh and Van Praagh, 1967; Anderson *et al.,* 1972).

   2. Inverted Complete Transposition (Fig. 4.2)

   a. With solitus ventricles (Cardell, 1956; Shaher, 1964; Raghib *et al.,* 1966).

   b. With inversion of the ventricles; congenitally corrected transposition (Anderson *et al.,* 1957; Lev and Rowlatt, 1961).

In this system the normal situs solitus and situs inversus hearts have been used as frames of reference. As a result, mirror-image lesions with levocardia and dextrocardia have the same anatomical name. In contrast

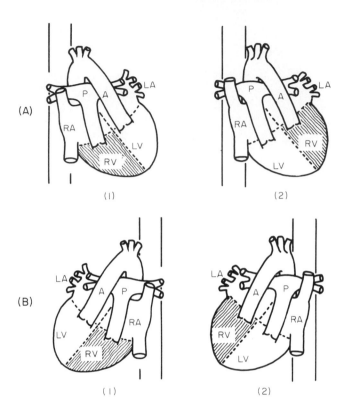

Fig. 4.2. (A) Inverted complete transposition in situs solitus 1, Without inversion of the ventricles; 2, with inversion of the ventricles. (B) Inverted complete transposition in situs inversus. 1, Without inversion of the ventricles; 2, with inversion of the ventricles. Abbreviations are the same as in 4.1.

to Geipel–Monckeberg's nomenclature, only anatomical names have been used in the present classification. Pernkopf's terms functional, anatomical, and complete functional and anatomical corrected transpositions have been avoided. Spitzer (1927) attached conditions to his terms "pure crossed transposition" and "crossed inverse transposition" by including the position of the cardiac chambers in these terms. Consequently, there were mixed forms as well as two extreme forms. From a terminology point of view, the terms "crossed transposition of the great arteries" and "crossed inverse transposition of the great arteries" signify changes in the position of the great arteries only and not of the cardiac chambers. Spitzer abolished the terms "in situs solitus" and "in situs inversus." He considered that the venous chambers were normally situated, so long as they were situated on the right, and inverted if they were situated on the left.

It has been pointed out that from the very beginning the atria are fixed structures. They are anchored to the posterior abdominal wall by the entering great veins and by the persistent portions of the mesocardium. The atria are the only cardiac compartments whose development is not affected by the shape of the bulboventricular loop. The relationship of the atria to each other, therefore, characterizes each of the two types of heart. With these points in mind, the term inversion of the atria becomes embryologically unsound for neither in the situs solitus nor in the situs inversus hearts are the atria capable of inversion. Whether the venous atrium develops on the right as in the situs solitus heart or on the left as in the situs inversus heart, it does so in the normal position for either of these two hearts. As far as Spitzer's remaining three grades of transposition, most recent authors used descriptive names for these anomalies, i.e., tetralogy of Fallot for grade 1, double outlet right ventricle for grade 2, and common ventricle for grade 4. Van Mierop and Wiglesworth's (1963) concept of transposition is mainly in accord with the present classification.

The statement that transposition can be present or absent but never partial (Van Praagh 1967), the terms d- and l-transposition (Van Praagh et al., 1964), and the concept of transposition with posterior aorta deserve special consideration. Von Rokitansky's term "partial transposition" when used by various authors signified transposition of only one vessel, in most cases the aorta to the right ventricle. In this sense, it differentiated this anomaly from complete or crossed transposition in which both aorta and pulmonary artery are transposed. Having defined transposition of the great arteries as aortic–mitral valve discontinuity, Van Praagh (1967) went on to say that transposition can be present or absent but never partial. As far as I can tell, no author, except Van Praagh, ever used the term partial transposition to signify partial aortic–mitral valve discontinuity. Moreover, his use of the term complete d- or l-transposition (Van Praagh et al. 1971) implies that both of these transpositions could be incomplete or partial. The terms d- or l-transposition, when used in the sense of noninverted and inverted transposition, respectively, are probably simpler. Van Praagh (1967) defined transposition as mitral–aortic valve discontinuity or subaortic infundibulum. In d-transposition, the transported aortic valve is to the right of the transposed pulmonary valve, while in l-transposition the aortic valve is to the left of the transposed pulmonary valve. However, Van Praagh failed to define what a transposed pulmonary valve is, with the result that his definition of the terms d- and l- is meaningless. Moreover, the use of these terms as defined by Van Praagh could be confusing, for as pointed out by Shaher et al. (1967), in 32% of the angiocardiograms of patients with noninverted complete transposition and pulmonary stenosis, the aorta occupies a position to the left of the pulmonary artery. His statement that transposition in the d-loop is d-transposition and in l-loop is l-transposition (Van Praagh et al., 1964) will not explain double outlet right ventricle (Kirklin 1972) or left ventricle (Van Praagh et al. 1972 with solitus ventricles but with l-transposition. Neither will it explain anatomically corrected transposition (Van Praagh and Van Praagh, 1967) or corrected transposition with isolated bulbar inversion (Raghib et al., 1966). His statement that transposition is not a reversal of the anteroposterior relationship of the aorta and the pulmonary artery because in one-third of these cases the two great arteries may originate side by side (Van Praagh, 1971) does not have much support from angiocardiographic studies. Although he emphatically rejected the definition of transposition as reversal of the anteroposterior relationship of the aorta and the pulmonary artery, his theory on the embryogenesis of transposition (Van Praagh, 1967; Van Praagh et al., 1971) is based entirely on the concept that in transposition the aorta moves anterior to the pulmonary artery. His recent definition of transposition as the condition in which the two great arteries are placed across the ventricular septum compared to normal does not emphasize the conotruncal origin of the problem; and after all, one of the theories suggests that in transposition truncal septation proceeds normally but the pulmonary part of the truncus is held in continuity with the mitral ring (Grant 1962). In addition, this definition excludes anatomically corrected transposition and corrected transposition with isolated bulbar inversion. The case for defining transposition as the condition in which the two great arteries are placed across the ventricular septum compared to normal has been rather weakened by Van Praagh's description of a case of transposition of the great arteries with "overriding aorta" (Van Praagh et al., 1972). His concept of transposition with posterior aorta and an anterior pulmonary artery and his proposition of the terms d- and l-malposition (Van Praagh et al., 1971) compound the existing confusion in terminology. According to his concept, any relationship of the great arteries, including the normal, in single ventricle, qualifies for the term malposition. Rashkind (1971) pointed out that "such terms as subaortic conus, l- and d-loops, valve discontinuity and the concepts behind them have done little to clarify the hemodynamic disorder."

References

Abbott, M. E. (1927). Congenital cardiac disease. In "Modern Medicine," (W. Osler and T. McCrae, eds.) 3rd Ed.. Vol. 4. Lea and Febiger, Philadelphia, Pennsylvania.

Anderson, R. C., Lillehei, C. W., and Lester, R. G. (1957). Corrected transposition of the great vessels of the heart. *Pediatrics* **20**, 626.

Anderson, R. H., Arnold, R., and Jones, R. S. (1972). *d*-Bulboventricular loop with *l*-transposition in situs inversus. *Circulation* **46**, 173.

Cardell, B. S. (1956). Corrected transposition of the great vessels. *Brit. Heart J.* **18**, 186.

Edwards, J. E. (1960). Congenital malformations of the heart and great vessels. *In* "Pathology of the Heart" (S. E. Gould, ed.), pp. 354, 2nd Ed. Charles C. Thomas, Springfield, Illinois.

Geipel, P. (1903). Weitere Beiträge zum situs transversus and zur hehre von den transposition der grossen Gefässe des Herzens. *Arch. Kinderheilk.* **35**, 112, 222.

Grant, R. P. (1962). The morphogenesis of transposition of the great vessels. *Circulation* **26**, 819.

Harris, J. S., and Farber, S. (1939). Transposition of the great cardiac vessels with special reference to the phylogenetic theory of Spitzer. *Arch. Pathol.* **28**, 427.

Ivemark, B. I. (1955). Implications of agenesis of the spleen on the pathogenesis of cono-truncus anomalies in childhood; analysis of heart malformations in splenic agenesis syndrome, with 14 new cases. *Acta Paediat.* **44** (Suppl. 104), 1.

Janeway, E. G. (1877). Malposition of aorta and pulmonary artery—thrombus in heart and cerebral embolism—death from intestinal hemorrhage, *Med. Rec.* **12**, 811.

Keith, A. (1909). The Huntarian lectures on malformations of the heart. *Lancet* ii, 359, 453, 519.

Kirklin, J. W. (1972). Lewis A. Conner memorial lecture. Evaluating the results of cardiac surgery. *Circulation* **46**, Suppl. 2, 1.

Kürschner, T. (1837). Commentatio de corde cuius ventricule inter se communicant. (Cited by J. W. Brown, "Congenital Heart Disease." Staples Press, London, 1950.)

Lev, M. (1953). The pathologic anatomy of cardiac complexes associated with transposition of the arterial trunks. *Lab. Invest.* **2**, 296.

Lev, M., and Saphir, O. (1937). Transposition of the large vessels. *J. Tech. Methods* **17**, 126.

Lev, M., and Rowlatt, U. F. (1961). The pathologic anatomy of mixed levocardia. A review of thirteen cases of atrial or ventricular inversion with or without corrected transposition. *Amer. J. Cardiol.* **8**, 216.

Monckeberg, J. G. (1924). Die Missbildungen des Herzes. *In* "Handbuch der Speziellen pathologischen Anatomie und Histologie" (F. Henke, and O. Lubarsch, eds.), Vol. 2, pp. 1–183. Springer, Berlin.

Pernkopf, E. (1926). Der partielle situs inversus der Eingeweide beim Menschen. *Z. Anat. Entwicklungsgesch.* **79**, 577.

Raghib, G., Anderson, R. C., and Edwards, J. E. (1966). Isolated bulbar inversion in corrected transposition. *Amer. J. Cardiol.* **17**, 407.

Rashkind, W. J. (1971). Transposition of the great arteries. *Pediat. Clin. N. Amer.* **18**, 1075–1090.

Robertson, J. I. (1913). The comparative anatomy of the bulbus cordis with special reference to abnormal positions of the great vessels in the human heart. *J. Pathol. Bacteriol.* **18**, 191.

Rosenbaum, H. D. (1964). A simplified basic classification of spatial alignments of the heart, its chambers and the great vessels. *Circulation* **30**, 194.

Shaher, R. M. (1964). Complete and inverted transposition of the great vessels. *Brit. Heart J.* **26**, 51.

Shaher, R. M., Moes, F., and Khoury, G. (1967). Radiologic and angiocardiographic findings in complete transposition of the great vessels with left ventricular outflow tract obstruction. *Radiology* **88**, 1092.

Spitzer, A. (1923). Über den Bauplan des normalen und missbildeten Herzens. *Virch. Arch. Path. Anat. Physiol.* **243**, 81. (Translated by M. Lev and A. Vass, Thomas, Springfield, Illinois, 1951.)

Spitzer, A. (1927). Zur Kritik der phylogenetischen Theorie der normalen und missbildeten Herzarchitektur. *Z. Anat. Entwicklungsgesch.* **84**, 30.

Stenonis, N. (1671). *Acta Hafmensa* **71** (Obs. 3). (Cited by J. W. Brown, "Congenital Heart Disease." Staples Press, London, 1950.)

Van Mierop, L. H. S. (1971). Transposition of the great arteries. 1. Clarification or further confusion. *Amer. J. Cardiol.* **28**, 735.

Van Mierop, L. H. S. and Wiglesworth, F. W. (1963). Pathogenesis of transposition complexes. III. True transposition of the great vessels. *Amer. J. Cardiol.* **12**, 233.

Van Praagh, R. (1967). Complete transposition of the great arteries. *In* "Heart Disease in Infancy and Childhood". (J. D. Keith, R. D. Rowe, and P. Vlad, eds.), 2nd Ed. MacMillan, New York.

Van Praagh, R. (1971). Transposition of the great arteries. II. Transposition clarified. *Amer. J. Cardiol.* **28**, 739.

Van Praagh, R., and Van Praagh, S. (1967). Anatomically corrected transposition of the great arteries. *Brit. Heart J.* **29**, 112.

Van Praagh, R., Calder, A. L., Delisle, G., and Izukawa, T. (1972). Transposition of the great arteries with overriding aorta and pulmonary stenosis: new entity and its surgical management. *Circulation* **46**, Suppl. 2, 96.

Van Praagh, R., Pérez-Trevino, C., López-Cuellar, M., Baker, F., Zuberbuhler, J. R., Quero, M., Perez, V. M., Moreno, F., and Van Praagh, S. (1971). Transposition of the great arteries with posterior aorta, anterior pulmonary artery, subpulmonary conus and fibrous continuity between aortic and atrioventricular valves. *Amer. J. Cardiol.* **28**, 621.

Van Praagh, R., Van Praagh, S., Vlad, P., and Keith, J. D. (1964). Anatomic types of congenital dextrocardia. Diagnostic and embryologic implications. *Amer. J. Cardiol.* **13**, 510.

von Rokitansky, C. F. (1875). "Die Defecte der Scheidewände des Herzens." Braumüller, Vienna.

Chapter 5

MATERIAL

The pathological, clinical, and surgical chapters are based on the experience of the author with 409 cases with noninverted complete transposition of the great arteries. These cases were studied in three institutions: The Hospital for Sick Children, Toronto, Canada, 336 cases; Guy's Hospital, London, England, 44 cases; and Albany Medical Center, Albany, New York, United States, 29 cases. Noninverted complete transposition in situs solitus, as defined in the previous chapter, was present in 407 cases, and in situs inversus in 2 cases. Excluded from this study are patients with mitral atresia, tricuspid atresia, or pulmonary atresia. As the term "complete" implies, patients with a common or a single ventricle were not included. Since the so-called "anatomically corrected transposition" was not seen in this study, the condition of all patients will be simply referred to as "complete transposition of the great arteries."

Of the 409 patients in this series the diagnosis has been established by autopsy examination in 183, by angiocardiography in 132, and by combined autopsy and angiocardiography in 94. Patients in whom the diagnosis has been suggested by only hemodynamic data have not been included.

Depending on the presence or absence of a ventricular septal defect or left ventricular outflow tract obstruction, patients were divided into four groups as follows.

Condition	No.
1. With an intact ventricular septum	209
2. With an intact ventricular septum and left ventricular outflow tract obstruction	16
3. With a ventricular septal defect	138
4. With a ventricular septal defect and left ventricular outflow tract obstruction	46
Total	409

TABLE 5.1
Age Distribution of 409 Patients [a]

Group	Months												Years												
	0-1	1-2	2-3	3-4	4-5	5-6	6-7	7-8	8-9	9-10	10-11	11-12	1-2	2-3	3-4	4-5	5-6	6-7	7-8	8-9	9-10	10-15	15-20	20-25	25-30
Group 1 (209)	115	24	9	10	3	3	6	3	0	0	0	1	13	4	4	3	2	0	0	0	3	4	1	1	0
Group 2 (16)	3	1	1	0	0	0	0	0	2	0	0	0	1	2	3	0	1	1	0	0	0	1	0	0	0
Group 3 (138)	24	21	12	6	5	5	2	2	1	3	2	0	15	5	5	7	2	5	2	1	2	6	2	2	1
Group 4 (46)	5	0	0	0	0	1	0	1	1	0	2	1	8	5	3	1	2	4	3	2	1	3	0	1	2
Total (409)	147	46	22	16	8	9	8	6	4	3	4	2	37	16	15	11	7	10	5	3	6	14	3	4	3

[a] Within the total of 409 patients 101 patients are alive, 308 are deceased.

A ventricular septal defect was accepted as being present if this defect was demonstrated by autopsy or angiocardiographical examinations, or if the pulmonary artery was intubated from the right ventricle during cardiac catheterization. Left ventricular outflow tract obstruction was diagnosed if there was autopsy or angiocardiographical evidence of stenosis of the pulmonary valve or the subvalvular area, or if a gradient of 40 mm Hg or more between the pulmonary artery and left ventricle was demonstrated at cardiac catheterization.

At the conclusion of the study 308 patients were deceased, while 101 patients were living. The age distribution of the 409 patients in this series is shown in Table 5.1. Of the total number of 409 patients, 208 underwent heart surgery while the remaining 201 were not operated upon. Further analysis of these figures will be given in Chapter 18.

Of the 409 patients in this series there were 280 males and 129 females; a male incidence of 67% or a male:female ratio of about 2.2.

The available pathological, clinical, and surgical data and the criteria employed for analysis of these informations are discussed in the appropriate chapters. Heart specimens, lung sections, electrocardiograms, vectorcardiograms, chest roentgenograms, and angiocardiograms, which form the basis of most of the pathological and clinical chapters, have been personally examined by the author. Material not examined by the author has been excluded.

Since complete transposition of the great arteries is essentially a disease of infancy, and its clinical presentation, and prognosis seem to be related to the type of the associated defects, all available data were studied in terms of the group of the patient and the age at which the information was obtained.

Chapter 6

INCIDENCE OF TRANSPOSITION

According to Keith *et al.* (1958) the prevalence of transposition of the great arteries in the age group of birth to 14 years of age is 1:11,000. Among 58,105 live-born children in Gothenberg, Sweden, during the years 1941 to 1950, Carlgren (1959) found 369 cases of congenital heart disease. Of these 369 cases, there were 20 with transposition with an overall incidence of 1:3000 births. Liebman *et al.* (1969) estimated the minimal incidence of transposition as one per 4500 births. The reported incidence of complete transposition of the great arteries in autopsied cases of congenital heart disease is shown in Table 6.1. This incidence varied between 1.3 (White, 1955) and 20.2% (Keith *et al.*, 1958). The incidence of transposition in clinical cyanotic heart disease, and in clinical congenital heart disease is shown in Tables 6.2 and 6.3, respectively. The incidence of transposition among autopsied neonates with congenital heart disease was 27% reported by Ober and Moore (1955), 10% by Rowe and Cleary (1960), 11% by Mehrizi *et al.* (1964), and 15% by Lambert, *et al.* (1966). Of the 100 consecutive patients with congenital heart disease seen in the neonatal period by Rowe and Mehrizi (1968), 14 had complete transposition of the great arteries. According to Coleman (1965) 16% of infants with symptoms secondary to congenital heart disease have transposition of the great arteries.

Transposition of the great arteries is predominantly a male disease. Of the 409 patients in this series, 280 were males and 129 were females. Becker and Brill (1948) pointed out that among patients with complete transposition males outnumber females by 4 to 1. A high incidence of experimentally produced transposition in male rats was reported by Monie *et al.* (1966). The reported sex incidence of complete transposition is shown in Table 6.4. The percentage of males with transposition varied between 57 (Wells, 1963; Boesen, 1963), and 88% (Sherman, 1963; Shaher, 1963).

TABLE 6.1

INCIDENCE OF TRANSPOSITION IN AUTOPSIED CASES OF CONGENITAL HEART DISEASE

Total congenital heart disease	Trans-position	Per-centage	Author
106	26	24.40	Theremin (1895)
383	76	20.00	Vierordt (1898)
270	25	9.50	Keith (1909)
44	1	2.20	Still (1924)
75	7	9.50	Leech (1935)
1000	49	4.90	Abbott (1936)
44	1	2.25	Nicholson (1936)
21	1	4.70	Terplan and Sanes (1936)
80	4	5.00	Philpott (1936)
111 (PFO 49) [a]	2	1.80	Szypulski (1937)
36	5	13.90	Rannels and Propst (1937)
49 (PFO 9) [a]	1	2.00	Roberts (1937)
105	9	8.60	Gibson and Clifton (1938)
87	5	5.70	Ingham (1938)
131 (PFO 77) [a]	4	3.00	Jacobius and Moore (1938)
141	—	5.70	Clawson (1944)
141	—	7.10	Sommers and Johnson (1951)
100	18	18.00	Soulié (1952)
95	8	8.40	Donzelot and D'Allaines (1954)
223	—	1.30	White (1955)
520	108	20.80	Keith *et al.* (1958)
357	24	6.70	Fontana and Edwards (1962)

[a] PFO = Patent foramen ovale.

TABLE 6.2

INCIDENCE OF TRANSPOSITION IN CLINICAL CYANOTIC CONGENITAL HEART DISEASE

Congenital heart disease with cyanosis	Trans-position	Percentage	Author
400	25	6.26	Campbell and Suzman (1951)
72	16	22.20	Astley and Parsons (1952)
691	28	4.10	Donzelot and D'Allaines (1954)
1500	138	9.20	Keith *et al.* (1958)

TABLE 6.3

INCIDENCE OF TRANSPOSITION IN CLINICAL CONGENITAL HEART DISEASE

Congenital heart disease	Trans-position	Percentage	Author
1395	64	4.58	Gasul and Fell (1956)
1000	—	1.00	Wood (1956)
577	36	6.20	Nadas (1957)

TABLE 6.4

SEX INCIDENCE OF COMPLETE TRANSPOSITION OF THE GREAT ARTERIES

Total	Males	Females	Percentage males	Author
47	35	12	74	Kato (1930)
34	27	7	79	Abbott (1936)
111	78	33	71	Abrams et al. (1951)
13	9	4	69	Cooley and Sloan (1952)
44	31	13	71	Keith et al. (1953)
15	10	5	67	Edwards (1953)
29	17	12	61	Lillehei and Varco (1953)
47	34	13	72	MacMahon et al. (1953)
56	33	23	59	Polani and Campbell (1955)
138	97	41	70	Keith et al. (1958)
15	10	5	67	Kjellberg et al. (1959)
20	13	7	65	Carlgren (1959)
50	39	11	78	Noonan et al. (1960)
83	69	14	83	Warkaney (1960)
70	52	18	74	Landing et al. (1961)
45	33	12	73	Ochsner et al. (1961)
24	15	9	63	Fontana and Edwards (1962)
35	31	4	88	Shaher (1963)
60	36	24	60	Apitz and Beuren (1963)
145	83	62	57	Boesen (1963)
35	31	4	88	Sherman (1963)
30	17	13	57	Wells (1963)
40	31	9	77	Morgan et al. (1965)
358	238	120	67	Keith et al. (1967)
742	476	266	64	Liebman et al. (1969)
409	280	129	67	Present series

References

Abbott, M. E. (1936). "Atlas of Congenital Cardiac Disease." American Heart Association, New York.

Abrams, H. L., Kaplan, H. S., and Purdy, A. (1951). Diagnosis of complete transposition of the great vessels. *Radiology* **57**, 500.

Apitz, V. J., and Beuren, A. J. (1963). Congenital heart defects during the first year of life. Survey of 630 infants with heart disease. *Arch. Kreislaufforsch.* **42**, 264.

Astley, R., and Parsons, S. (1952). Complete transposition of the great vessels. *Brit. Heart J.* **14**, 13.

Becker, M. C., and Brill, R. M. (1948). Complete transposition of the great vessels. *Arch. Pediat.* **65**, 249.

Boesen, I. B. (1963). Complete transposition of the great vessels: importance of septal defects and patent ductus; analysis of 132 patients dying before age 4. *Circulation* **28**, 885.

Campbell, M., and Suzman, S. (1951). Transposition of the aorta and pulmonary artery. *Circulation* **4**, 329.

Carlgren, L. (1959). The incidence of congenital heart disease in children born in Gothenburg 1941–1950. *Brit. Heart J.* **21**, 40.

Clawson, B. J. (1944). Types of congenital heart disease in 15,597 autopsies. *Lancet* **64**, 134.

Coleman, E. N. (1965). Serious congenital heart disease in infancy. *Brit. Heart J.* **27**, 42.

Cooley, R. N., and Sloan, R. D. (1952). Angiocardiography in congenital heart disease of cyanotic type. III. Observations on complete transposition of the great vessels. *Radiology* **58**, 481.

Donzelot, E., and D'Allaines, F. (1954). "Traité des Cardiopathies Congénitales." Masson et Cie, Paris.

Edwards, J. E. (1953). Congenital malformations of the heart and great vessels. *In* "Pathology of the Heart" (S. E. Gould, ed.). 1st Ed. p. 344. Thomas, Springfield, Illinois.

Fontana, R. D., and Edwards, J. E. (1962). "Congenital Cardiac Disease: A Review of 357 Cases Studied Pathologically." Saunders, Philadelphia, Pennsylvania.

Gasul, B. M., and Fell, E. H. (1956). Salient points in the clinical diagnosis of congenital heart disease. Based on a nine-year study of 1,395 patients. *J. Amer. Med. Ass.* **161**, 39.

Gibson, S., and Clifton, W. M. (1938). Congenital heart disease. A clinical and post mortem study of one hundred and five cases. *Amer. J. Dis. Child.* **55**, 761.

Ingham, D. W. (1938). Congenital heart disease: incidence at the Mayo Clinic. *J. Tech. Methods* **18**, 131.

Jacobius, H. L., and Moore, R. A. (1938). Incidence of congenital cardiac anomalies in the autopsies of the New York Hospital. *J. Tech. Methods* **18**, 133.

Kato, K. (1930). Congenital transposition of cardiac vessels: a clinical and pathologic study. *Amer. J. Dis. Child.* **39**, 363.

Keith, A. (1909). The Huntarian lectures on malformations of the heart. *Lancet* **2**, 359, 453, 519.

Keith, J. D., Rowe, R. D., and Vlad, P. (1958). "Heart Disease in Infancy and Childhood," 1st Ed. MacMillan, New York.

Keith, J. D., Rowe, R. D., and Vlad, P. (1967). "Heart Disease in Infancy and Childhood." 2nd Ed. MacMillan, New York.

Kjellberg, S. R., Mannheimer, E., and Rudhe, U. (1959). "Diagnosis of Congenital Heart Disease," 2nd Ed. Year Book Publ. Chicago, Illinois. 1959.

Lambert, E. C., Canent, R. V., and Hohn, A. R. (1966). Congenital cardiac anomalies in the newborn. A review of conditions causing death or severe distress in the first month of life. *Pediatrics* **37**, 343.

Landing, B. H., Nakai, H., Margaretten, W., Kobayashi, N., and Beavely, P. H. (1961). Some genetic and biochemical implications of congenital heart disease. *Quart. Rev. Pediat.* **16**, 160.

Leech, C. B. (1935). Congenital heart disease. Clinical analysis of seventy-five cases from the Johns Hopkins Hospital. *J. Pediat.* **7**, 802.

Liebman, J., Cullun, L., and Belloc, N. B. (1969). Natural history of transposition of the great arteries. Anatomy and birth and death characteristics. *Circulation* **40**, 237–262.

Lillehei, C. W., and Varco, R. L. (1953). Certain physiologic, pathologic and surgical features of complete transposition of the great vessels. *Surgery* **34**, 376.

MacMahon, B., McKeown, T., and Record, R. G. (1953). Incidence and life expectation of children with congenital heart disease. *Brit. Heart J.* **15**, 121.

Mehrizi, A., Hirsch, M. S., and Taussig, H. B. (1964). Congenital heart disease in the neonatal period. Autopsy study of 170 cases. *J. Pediat.* **65**, 721.

Monie, I. W., Takacs, E., and Warkany, J. (1966). Transposition of the great vessels and other cardiovascular abnormalities in rat fetuses induced by trypan blue. *Anat. Rec.* **156**, 175.

Morgan, A. D., Krovetz, L. J., Schiebler, G. L., Shanklin, D. R., Wheat, M. W., Jr., and Bartley, T. D. (1965). Diagnosis and palliative surgery in complete transposition of the great vessels. *Ann. Thorac. Surg.* **1**, 711.

Nadas, A. S. (1957). "Pediatric Cardiology," 1st Ed. Saunders, Philadelphia, Pennsylvania.

Nicholson, M. M. (1936). Relative incidence of cardiac anomalies found in autopsies performed in Washington hospitals. *J. Tech. Method* **15**, 100.

Noonan, A., Nadas, A. S., Rudolph, A. M., and Harris, G. B. C. (1960). Transposition of the great arteries. A correlation of clinical, physiologic, and autopsy data. *N. Engl. J. Med.* **263**, 592.

Ober, W. B., and Moore, T. E., Jr. (1955). Congenital cardiac malformations in the neonatal period; An autopsy study. *N. Engl. J. Med.* **253**, 271.

Ochsner, J. L., Cooley, D. A., Harris, L. C., and McNamara, D. G. (1961). Treatment of complete transposition of the great vessels with the Blalock-Hanlon operation. *Circulation* **24**, 51.

Philpott, N. W. (1936). Relative incidence of congenital cardiac anomalies in Montreal hospitals. *J. Tech. Methods* **15**, 96.

Polani, P. E., and Campbell, M. (1955). Aetiological study of congenital heart disease. *Ann. Human Genet.* **19**, 209.

Rannels, H. W., and Propst, J. H. (1937). Incidence of congenital cardiac anomalies found at autopsies performed in Hospital of University of Pennsylvania. *J. Tech. Methods* **17**, 113.

Roberts, J. T. (1937). The incidence of congenital heart disease in the New Orleans Charity Hospital. *J. Tech. Methods* **17**, 108.

Rowe, R. D., and Cleary, T. E. (1960). Congenital malformation in the newborn period. Frequency in a Children's Hospital. *Can. Med. Ass. J.* **83**, 299.

Rowe, R. D., and Mehrizi, A. (1968). "The Neonate with Congenital Heart Disease." p. 80. Saunders, Philadelphia, Pennsylvania.

Shaher, R. M. (1963). Prognosis of transposition of the great vessels with and without atrial septal defect. *Brit. Heart J.* **25**, 211.

Sherman, F. E. (1963). "An Atlas of Congenital Heart Disease." Lea and Febiger, Philadelphia, Pennsylvania.

Sommers, S. C., and Johnson, J. M. (1951). Congenital tricuspid atresia. *Amer. Heart J.* **41**, 130.

Soulié, P. (1952). "Les Cardiopathies Congenitales." L'Expansion Scientifique Francaise, Paris.

Still, G. F. (1924). "Common Disorders and Diseases of Childhood," 4th Ed. Oxford University Press, New York.

Szypulski, J. T. (1937). Study of congenital heart disease of Philadelphia General Hospital. *J. Tech. Methods* **17**, 108.

Terplan, K., and Sanes, S. (1936). The incidence of congenital heart lesions in infancy. A comparative statistical study based on post mortem examination. *J. Tech. Methods* **15**, 86.

Theremin, E. (1895). "Etudes sur les Affections Congénitales du Coeur." Asselin and Houzeau, Paris.

Vierordt, H. (1898). Die angeborenen Herzkrankheiten. *Nothnagel's Spez. Pathol. Therap.* **15**, 244.

Warkany, J. (1960). Etiologic factors in congenital heart disease. *In* "Congenital Heart Disease" (A. D. Bass and G. K. Moe, eds.). Publication No. 63 of the American Association for the Advancement of Science, Washington.

Wells, B. (1963). The sounds and murmurs in transposition of the great vessels. *Brit. Heart J.* **25**, 748.

White, P. D. (1955). The history of congenital cardiovascular defects. *In* "Congenital Heart Disease," pp. 61–70. Report of the fourteenth M and R Pediatric Research Conference, M and R Laboratories, Columbus, Ohio.

Wood, P. (1956). "Diseases of the Heart and Circulation," 2nd Ed. Eyre and Spottiswoode, London.

Chapter 7

ETIOLOGICAL FACTORS IN TRANSPOSITION

Birth Rank, Maternal Age, Consanguinity of Parents, Previous Miscarriages, Seasonal Incidence, and Race

The birth rank of 295 patients in this series is shown in Table 7.1. Of these 295 patients 28% were first born, 32% second born, and 18% third born. The average age of the fathers was 30.6 years, and the average age of the mothers was 27.8 years. Table 7.2 shows the average age of the parents in the four groups. Patients with left ventricular outflow tract obstruction (Groups II and IV), had older parents than patients without left ventricular outflow tract obstruction (Groups I and III). There was no particular seasonal incidence of transposition. Consanguinity of parents was noted on one occasion, and previous miscarriages on thirty-seven (Table 7.3). All patients in this series were Caucasians.

Similar findings suggesting that the majority of infants with transposition are either first or second born were reported by MacMahon (1952). Of his 33 patients with transposition, 10 were first born, 13 second born, 7 third born, while 3 were fourth born or over. While Polani and Campbell (1955) found no statistically significant differences between the expected and observed members of affected children with congenital heart disease in general in the various birth ranks, Lamy et al. (1957) pointed out that the mean birth rank is significantly higher in the congenital heart disease group (including transposition) than in the control group. MacMahon (1952) pointed out that there was no apparent association between maternal age and the incidence of transposition. Polani and Campbell (1955) and Lamy et al. (1957) agreed that maternal age does not appear to correlate with the incidence of congenital heart disease in offsprings if cases of mongolism are omitted. On the other hand, of the 50 patients with transposition reported by Noonan et al. (1960) only 4 were first born and in two of these the mothers were 39 and 41 years old,

TABLE 7.1

BIRTH RANK OF 295 PATIENTS

	Group											
	1	2	3	4	5	6	7	8	9	10	11	12
Intact septum (157 patients)	33	50	36	12	10	6	3	3	2	1	1	0
Intact septum and pulmonary stenosis (13 patients)	7	4	0	1	0	1	0	0	0	0	0	0
Ventricular septal defect (96 patients)	32	33	12	7	5	3	2	1	0	1	0	0
Ventricular septal defect and pulmonary stenosis (29 patients)	12	8	5	1	1	0	1	1	0	0	0	0
Total (295 patients)	84	95	53	21	16	10	6	5	2	2	1	0

respectively, at the time of delivery. In the whole group there were six mothers over the age of 35 years at the time of delivery, and previous miscarriages were recorded in nine cases. Excess miscarriages or still-births in families of children with congenital heart disease was not found by Polani and Campbell (1955). Liebman *et al.* (1969) pointed out that transposition of the great arteries is not related to maternal age, but the frequency of this disease increases when the mother had three or more previous children. In one series only (Lamy *et al.*, 1957), the amount of

TABLE 7.2

AVERAGE AGE OF PARENTS

	Intact septum	Intact septum and pulmonary stenosis	Ventricular septal defect	Ventricular septal defect and pulmonary stenosis	Total
Average age of fathers (in years)	30.7 (50)	36.5 (2)	29.4 (34)	33.6 (9)	30.6
Average age of mothers (in years)	28.0 (83)	32.8 (7)	26.4 (39)	28.3 (12)	27.8

parental consanguinity was significantly higher in the congenital heart disease group than in controls. Although a seasonal incidence for patent ductus arteriosus and coarctation of the aorta has been observed by Rutstein *et al.* (1952), Record and McKeown (1953), and Rowe and Mehrizi (1968), most authors agree that there is, in general, no particular seasonal incidence for congenital heart disease (MacMahon, 1952; Polani and Campbell, 1955; Lamy *et al.*, 1957). In the study performed

TABLE 7.3

PRENATAL FACTORS [a]

1. Sibs with congential heart disease (5)	a. Tetralogy of Fallot b. Cyanotic spell, died at 6 months c. Probable corrected transposition of the great vessels, died d. Died at home, congenital heart disease e. Twin sister died of congenital heart disease at 4 months
2. Sibs with other diseases (5)	Four stillborn One muscular dystrophy
3. Relative with congenital heart disease (4)	a. Cousin with cyanotic congenital heart disease, died b. Mother with ventricular septal defect c. Cousin with ventricular septal defect d. Cousin with congenital heart disease
4. Relative with other diseases (3)	a. Uncle retarded b. Uncle hydrocephalic c. Cousin with spina bifida
5. Diabetes (3)	Two grandmothers One mother
6. Rubella (4)	Two contacts One definite One probable
7. Prematurity (8)	36–37 weeks
8. Twins (3)	One with congenital heart disease
9. Bleeding, first trimester (9)	
10. Viral infection, first trimester (7)	
11. Drugs, first trimester (4)	
12. X-ray exposure, first trimester (2)	
13. Previous abortions (37)	

[a] Number in parenthesis indicates number of cases.

by Mitchell *et al.* (1971) the only cardiac lesion found to have a significantly skewed racial distribution for whites was transposition of the great arteries.

Birth Weight, Prematurity, Multiple Births, and Stillbirths

The average birth weight of patients studied in this series was 6.7 pounds. A control study was not available. Infants with left ventricular outflow tract obstruction (Groups II and IV) had a lower birth weight than infants without left ventricular outflow tract obstruction (Groups I and III). The average birth weight was 7.2 pounds in Group I, 6.7 pounds in Group II, 7.2 pounds in Group III, and 6.9 pounds in Group IV. The distribution of birth weight by sex is shown in Table 7.4. Eight patients were born prematurely (36–37 weeks gestation) and 4 were stillborn. There were three pairs of twins in this series; only one member of each was affected with transposition. The other member of one pair died of probable congenital heart disease at the age of 4 months (Table 7.3).

TABLE 7.4

BIRTH WEIGHT

Weight (pounds)	Group I		Group II		Group III		Group IV		Total
	Male	Female	Male	Female	Male	Female	Male	Female	
3 to 3.9	0	0	0	0	1	0	0	0	1
4 to 4.9	1	0	0	2	2	1	0	1	7
5 to 5.9	4	4	1	1	4	5	1	0	20
6 to 6.9	29	15	3	0	16	6	5	2	76
7 to 7.9	38	10	5	1	18	11	9	4	96
8 to 8.9	28	10	2	0	12	9	2	2	65
9 to 9.9	5	3	0	1	6	2	2	0	19
10 or more	3	0	0	0	1	0	0	1	5

It is generally accepted that infants with transposition of the great arteries have high birth weight (Noonan *et al.*, 1960). Mehrizi and Drash (1961) found the average weight of 117 newborns with transposition of the great arteries was 7.6 pounds compared with 6.87 pounds for newborns in the general Baltimore white population. Naeye (1965) found that babies with congenital heart disease weighed 91.1% of their predicted normal, whereas in transposition of the great arteries the weights were 103%. In 26 newborn infants with transposition, Naeye (1966) described body and organ enlargement due to an increased cytoplasmic mass in individual parenchymal cells. In addition to this cellular abnormality there was pancreatic islet hyperplasia and fetal zone adrenal enlargement. The author explained these findings on the basis of hyperglycemia in the fetal pancreatic perfusate brought about by an abnormal prenatal circulatory pattern. On the other hand, Liebman *et al.* (1969) pointed out that their study did not support the hypothesis that children with transposition are heavier at birth. The average birth weight among their 564 cases of transposition collected from the State of California was 7.12 pounds compared to a birth weight of 7.26 pounds of infants in the general population in California. Mitchell *et al.* (1971) found that the average birth weight, with standard error, of the patients with transposition, none of whom had major extracardiac malformations was 3235 ± 124 gm; that of the matched cardiac control subjects, 6 of whom had major extracardiac malformations, was 2779 ± 234 gm; that of the offspring of the maternal control subjects, none of whom had cardiac or extracardiac malformations was 3263 ± 99 gm. The average gestational age of her patients with transposition was 40 ± 0.68 weeks, that of cardiac control subjects 36 ± 1.35 weeks, and of maternal control subjects 40 ± 0.3 weeks. That transposition does not create a serious hemodynamic problem to the fetus, has been emphasized by Lillehei and Varco (1953) and Liebman *et al.* (1969). However, of the 16 necropsied cases of transposition in the neonatal period reported by Mehrizi *et al.* (1964) there were 3 stillborn.

Genetic Factors, Chromosomal Aberrations, and Single Gene Disorders

Neither repeated occurrence of transposition through several generations nor repeated occurrence in siblings has been observed in the present series. However, a sib with congenital heart disease was noted on five occasions, and with muscular dystrophy on one (Table 7.3). Relatives with congenital diseases were noted on seven occasions (Table 7.3).

While it is generally accepted that several types of congenital heart disease may occur through several generations, e.g., ductus arteriosus (Ekstrom, 1952; Burman, 1961), ventricular septal defect (Lund, 1948; Tucker and Kinney, 1954; Rubenstein and Weaver, 1965), atrial septal defect (Campbell, 1965), coarctation of the aorta (Walker, 1934), pulmonary stenosis (Lewis *et al.*, 1958), and dextrocardia (Cockayne, 1938; Campbell, 1959), transposition of the great arteries has no familial predisposition. The occurrence of transposition or other congenital heart disease among sibs of patients with transposition is rare. Sorenson (1951) reported transposition of the great arteries in a patient and truncus arteriosus in a sib with a postmortem confirmation on both. He also reported transposition and patent ductus arteriosus in another patient and tetralogy of Fallot in a sib both confirmed by postmortem examination. McKeown *et al.* (1953), described two families, in each of which a member had transposition. In the first family one sib also had transposition and in the second family a sib had a patent ductus. Polani and Campbell (1955) reported a family in which tetralogy of Fallot occurred in one sibling and transposition of the great arteries in another. Among the 50 patients with transposition of the great arteries reported by Noonan *et al.* (1960), a sibling of one of the affected patients had a history of cyanotic congenital heart disease. In 3 additional patients a history of congenital heart disease was reported in their uncles, 2 of whom were cyanotic. Chelius *et al.* (1962) reported transposition of the great arteries in a girl while the maternal aunt had tricuspid stenosis, pulmonary stenosis, ventricular septal defect, and drainage of the coronary sinus into the left atrium. Lynch *et al.* (1964) reported an autopsy confirmation of complete transposition of the great arteries in two siblings. The authors pointed out that with a reported incidence of one in 11,000 live births for complete transposition of the great arteries, the likelihood of this occurring twice, by chance, in a sibship is less than 1 in 100 million times. In the face of this rare likelihood, coupled with the absence of any known extragenetic factors during utero in the family, the authors postulated an autosomal recessive gene.

Nora and Meyer (1966) studied the familial nature of congenital heart disease. There were 7 probands with transposition. There were 7 members affected with congenital heart disease other than a proband. In these 7 individuals the cardiac lesion was concordant in 1, partially concordant in 2, and the concordance was unknown in 5. Of the 26 pairs of twins affected by congenital heart disease studied by Uchida and Rowe (1957), transposition of the great arteries was present in one member of a dizygotic pair of twins. Since the 26 pairs were discordant for congenital heart disease, the authors concluded that this finding does not support the theory of genetic transmission of congenital heart disease. However, on the basis of family studies, Nora (1971) pointed out that the expected recurrence risk in first-degree relatives of patients with transposition is 2.2%.

The reported incidence of congenital heart disease in Down's syndrome varies widely. Thus, Comby (1906) reported an incidence of 7.1%, Rowe and Uchida (1961) 40.4%, Berg *et al.* (1960) 56.2%, and Engler (1949) 70%. While it is generally agreed that atrioventricular canal defects and ventricular septal defects are the most common lesions in mongolism (Abbott, 1936; Strauss, 1953; Rowe, 1962; Shaher *et al.*, 1972), the occurrence of transposition of the great arteries is very rare in this condition. No example of transposition of the great arteries is found in the large series of congenital heart disease in mongolism reported by Evans (1950), Berg *et al.* (1960), or Rowe and Uchida (1961). A case of transposition of the great arteries in association with mongolism, however, was reported by Doxiades and Portius (1938) and Mannheimer (1949). Müller (1955) reported the necropsy findings in 18 mongoloid children nearly all under 6 months of age. Transposition of the great arteries was encountered once. On the other hand, Hambach (1953) found a relatively high incidence of transposition of the great arteries among his patients with mongolism and congenital cardiac defects. Of his group of 17 necropsied cases, 6 had transposition of the great arteries.

Cardiovascular malformations are known to occur in the XO Turner syndrome (Kosenow, 1960; Lemi and Smith, 1963), and in the autopsmal trisomies 13–15 (Smith, 1963) and 17–18 (Smith, 1962; Townes *et al.*, 1963), but much less frequently in XXY Klinefelter syndrome. Among the 10 cases of 18 trisomy reported by Cummings and Uchida (1963), 1 case (Case 8) had transposition of the great arteries with a ventricular septal defect. McKusick (1964) discussed and listed all single gene mutants which give rise to cardiovascular involvement. Transposition of the great arteries has not been reported with Marfan's syndrome (McKusick, 1955; Wagenvoort *et al.*, 1962) or Kartagener's syndrome (Katz *et al.*, 1953). These two conditions being the most common single gene mutants with high incidence of cardiovascular malformations. Ellis and van Creveld (1940) described the syndrome comprised of ectodermal dysplasia, chondrodysplasia, polydactyly, and congenital heart defect. Fusion of the hamate and capitate are typical (McKusick, 1964; McKusick *et al.*, 1964). The most frequent cardiac lesion is single atrium (Giknis, 1963). Smith and Hand (1958) reported two cases of this syndrome. In their Case 2 there was common atrium and ventricle and transposition of the great arteries.

Anomalies of the skeletal system occurring in conjunction with atrial septal defect was first reported by Oppenheimer and colleagues (1949). In 1960, Holt and Oram elaborated on the association of atrial septal defect with skeletal abnormalities of the upper extremities and reported on four members of the same family with such a combination of lesions (now known as the Holt–Oram syndrome). The syndrome is the result of autosomal dominant inheritance with variable expressivity acting at about the fifth week of gestation when the heart and upper limbs are differentiating. The scope of cardiovascular abnormalities in Holt–Oram syndrome was widened by Holmes (1965), who described a family with a ventricular septal defect, and Lewis and associates (1965), whose family of eighteen members in three generations was affected by atrial and ventricular septal defects, anomalous coronary artery, and retroesophageal right subclavian artery. Their Case 11 was a male who died at the age of 3 months. Cyanosis was noted shortly before death. There was syndactyly of the right thumb and forefinger and a curved left thumb. Both hands deviated to the radial side of the forearm. Clinical examination revealed cyanosis and a systolic murmur. The liver was enlarged. The chest X ray showed extreme cardiac enlargement and an increase in the pulmonary vascularity. The electrocardiogram showed first degree A-V block and interventricular conduction defect. The clinical diagnosis was probable complete transposition of the great arteries. This diagnosis, however, was not confirmed by angiocardiography or autopsy.

The association of lower facial paralysis with congenital heart disease was first reported by Cayler (1969). Of his 14 cases that displayed this combination pulmonary stenosis was present in 1, tetralogy of Fallot in 3, ventricular septal defect in 7, atrioventricularis communis in 1, coarctation in 1, and single ventricle in 1. Chromosome investigations in 3 revealed a large number of breakages. Chantler and McEnery (1971) reported 3 other patients with the cardiofacial syndrome. Their case KK had transposition of the great arteries, ventricular septal defect, and pulmonary stenosis. Chromosome studies, however, were not performed on this patient.

Viral Infections or Other Illnesses during Pregnancy

Viral infections and other illnesses occurring during the first trimester of pregnancy are shown in Table 7.3. It is worth noting that two mothers had German measels contact but did not develop clinical signs of infection during this period of pregnancy. One mother developed German measles and gave birth to an infant with transposition, microphthalmia, and a malformed left ear. There were 7 other instances of viral infections occurring in the early part of pregnancy mostly described as influenza or flu. A positive history of diabetes in the maternal side of the family occurred on three occasions. Bleeding during the first trimester of pregnancy occurred on nine occasions and exposure to X rays on two (Table 7.3).

In 1941, Gregg reported 78 cases of congenital cataract occurring after rubella in the mother during the first 2 months of pregnancy. Congenital heart disease was noted in 44 of these 78 cases. Swan *et al.* (1943) pointed out that if the rubella occurred during the first or second month of pregnancy 100% were affected, but during the third month only 50 and after this only 12.5% were affected. Among the 31 cases they collected there were 13 with congenital cataract, 7 deaf–mutes, and 17 with cardiac defects. On the other hand, Greenberg *et al.* (1957) summarized the results of prospective studies and concluded that the available data indicate that after maternal rubella in the first trimester about 12% of the children born are affected by congenital malformation. According to Greg (1941) and Swan *et al.* (1943) a patent ductus arteriosus was the leading malformation in the maternal rubella syndrome. Rutstein *et al.* (1952) reviewed the reported cases in which specific heart lesions were mentioned. In 77 cases patent ductus arteriosus was diagnosed 42 times and septal defects 36 times. Rare diagnosis of tetralogy of Fallot and coarctation of the aorta was also made. Of the 16 cases of congential heart disease attributable to maternal rubella in early pregnancy reported by Gibson and Lewis (1952), 14 had patent ductus arteriosus, 1 tetralogy of Fallot, and 1 an atrial septal defect. All 4 patients with a history of rubella reported by Campbell (1949) showed signs of Fallot's tetralogy. Recently it has been shown that peripheral pulmonary artery stenosis may occur in this syndrome (Gyllensward *et al.,* 1957; Williams *et al.,* 1957; Arvidsson *et al.,* 1961; Rowe, 1963; Venables, 1965). Of the 27 patients reported by Stuckey (1956) a patent ductus arteriosus occurred in 13, ventricular septal defect in 4, atrial septal defect in 3, tetralogy of Fallot in 2, and each of aortic stenosis, coarctation of the aorta, pulmonary stenosis, and Eisenmenger's syndrome in 1. He recorded one instance of transposition of the great arteries. In a study of 136 cases of rubella syndrome, Campbell (1961) mentions one case with transposition of the great arteries.

Three other viral infections have been associated with anomalies in embryo and fetuses: mumps, influenza, and Coxsackie B. Dogramaci and Green (1947) recorded two examples of ventricular septal defect in children whose mothers had influenza in the second and third months of pregnancy. Clayton-Jones (1959) described 2 cases of postinfluenza congenital malformations. The first patient developed diffuse pigmentation of the retina while the second was born with a "heart lesion" and a "curious face." Coffey and Jessop (1959) suggested that influenza in the first trimester was most likely teratogenic. They reported a 2½ times greater incidence of congenital malformations in offsprings of 220 mothers who had the illness compared to the same number of pregnancies in a control group. Other studies have suggested that Coxsachie B virus and mumps may be an etiological factor in the production of congenital cardiovascular malformations. (Fruhling *et al.*, 1962; Mehrizi *et al.*, 1965; Aagenaes, 1965; Mitchell *et al.*, 1966; Brown and Evans, 1967). Dogramaci and Green (1947) described 8 cases in which the mother had a nonexanthematous infection during pregnancy. The mother of their Case 7, with transposition of the great arteries had infected teeth during this period. Of the 50 patients with complete transposition of the great arteries reported by Noonan *et al.* (1960) a history of exposure to viral agents during the first trimester was obtained in 4. Another mother had a low grade fever for 3 or 4 days during the first trimester, and another had a "flu" at the fifth week.

The increased risk of fetal maldevelopment in association with maternal diabetes mellitus has been reported by White (1944), Dekaban and Baird (1959), Gellis and Hsia (1959), Driscoll *et al.* (1960), Pedersen *et al.* (1964, 1965) and Rusnak and Driscoll (1965). Pedersen *et al.* (1964) found congenital malformations in 6.4% of the diabetic group and 2.1% of the control group. Gross limb deformities appear to be characteristic malformations of infants born to diabetic mothers. Of the 104 dying infants of diabetic mothers reported by Gellis and Hsia (1959) a ventricular septal defect was present in 3 and each of transposition of the great arteries, atrial septal defect, coarctation of the aorta, and corbilocular in 1. Rusnak and Driscoll (1965) reported 3 children with congenital malformations born to diabetic mothers. Apart from spinal deformities, which were present in the 3 patients, Case 1 had transposition of the great arteries with an intact ventricular septum and pulmonary atresia. It is of interest that in 16 of 50 patients with complete transposition of the great arteries reported by Noonan *et al.* (1960) a history of diabetes was recorded in at least one grandparent.

The possibility that maternal–fetal incompatibility could be a cause of congenital anomalies was studied by Terasaki *et al.* (1970). These authors demonstrated that a large proportion of the sera from 574 parous women contained cytotoxic antibodies against *HL-A* tissue antigens. After their second pregnancies, one-quarter of the women had cytotoxins, and after the sixth one-half of the women had these antibodies. Retrospective studies of the outcome of pregnancies showed that women with antibodies had a significantly higher incidence of infants with congenital anomalies than did those without antibodies. Transposition of the great arteries occurred in an infant born to a mother with antibodies against *HL-A* tissue antigens. The authors postulated that antibodies produced by the mother against these antigens of the fetus may have a deleterious effect upon the fetus in subsequent pregnancies.

Hypoxia

Experimental and clinical evidence suggest that congenital heart disease in the offspring may result if the mother is exposed to hypoxia at certain stages of gestation. Ingalls *et al.* (1950, 1952) investigated the effects of anoxia on fetal development of mice. Pressure, used an an indirect measure of anoxia on pregnant rats, was held at two levels equivalent to 25,000 and 27,000 feet of altitude. Anencephaly and multiple skeletal deformities in fetuses followed exposure to a rarefied atmosphere on about the ninth day and cleft palate on around the fifteenth day. Defects of the interventricular septum were observed in 4 (1.9%) of 210 fetuses from mice subjected to anoxia during the fifth to seventh day. In general, induced defects were more numerous and severe at higher altitudes. Reports exist showing that patent ductus arteriosus is more common in populations living at high altitudes than in those living at sea level. Alzamora-Castro *et al.* (1953) reported from Lima, Peru, that in their clinical material of 42 cases of patent ductus arteriosus 26 were born at an altitude of 3000 meters or more. Of their 51 cases with an "interatrial communication" 13 were born at an altitude of 3500 or more. In an analysis of 110 patients with a patent ductus arteriosus from Peru, Alzamora-Castro *et al.* (1960) found that 19 (17.8%) were born in areas where the altitude was between 3000 and 3500 meters, 11 (10%) between 3500 and 4000 meters, and 22 (20%) in areas where the altitude was over 4000 meters. The authors pointed out that 20% of patients with patent ductus arteriosus come to the hospital from an altitude in which only 2.04% of the total population of Peru live (above 4000 meters). Sime *et al.* (1963) investigated 32 healthy children living at high altitudes and reported mild pulmonary hypertension and increased pulmonary vascular resistance in all. They pointed out that at high altitudes there is a delay in the evolution of the pressures with aging and that pulmonary hypertension and chronic hypoxia are factors related to patency of the ductus arteriosus. Penaloza *et al.* (1964) confirmed these findings and demonstrated that pulmonary hypertension is principally related to structural changes of the pulmonary vasculature, while arteriolar vasoconstriction and polycythemia are secondary factors. While these experimental and clinical observations suggest that there is some relationship between hypoxia and congenital heart disease, such relationship has not been demonstrated to exist in transposition of the great arteries.

Drugs

In the present series four mothers received a medication during the first trimester of pregnancy; medication for cystitis in one, nausea pills in two, and pain pills in one.

There are two drugs that have a cardiac teratogenic effect on fetuses if given in the early part of pregnancy; thalidomide (Lenz and Pliess, 1963), and dextroamphetamine (Nora *et al.*, 1971). Lenz and Pliess (1963) reported their findings in 562 clinical cases and 15 autopsies of thalidomide congenital malformations. Skeletal deformities appear to be the most common abnormalities. A relationship occurs between the time the drug was taken by the mother and the type of congenital malformations. Cardiac anomalies occurred in 27 of 121 clinical cases reported by Lenz and Pliess (1963) and in 4 of 47 cases studied by d'Avignon *et al.*, (1965). The most common lesion was a ventricular septal defect followed by persistent ductus arteriosus (Lenz and Pliess, 1963). Transposition of the great arteries has not been described among thalidomide congenital malformations. A possible relationship between dextroamphetamine and transposition of the great arteries was reported by Nora (1971). He described 3 mothers of infants with transposition of the great arteries who had taken this medicine early in their pregnancy.

Conclusions

The following conclusions appear warranted.

1. The precise causes of transposition are unknown.

2. It is probable that both environmental and genetic factors contribute to the lesion but the relative role of each is undetermined.

References

Aagenaes, O. (1965). Embryonic environment as a cause of congenital malformations. *Acta Paediat. Scand. Suppl.* **159**, 30.

Abbott, M. E. (1936). "Atlas of Congenital Heart Disease." American Heart Association, New York.

Alzamora-Castro, V., Rotta, A., Battilana, G., Abugattas, R., Rubio, C., Bouroncle, J., Zapata, C., Santa-Maria, E., Binder, T., Subiria, R., Paredes, D., Parido, B., and Graham, G. (1953). On the possible influence of great altitudes on the determination of cardiovascular anomalies. *Pediatrics* **12**, 259.

Alzamora-Castro, V., Battilana, G., Abugattas, R., and Sialer, S. (1960). Patent ductus arteriosus and high altitude. *Amer. J. Cardiol.* **5**, 761.

Arvidsson, H., Carlsson, E., Hartmann, A., Jr., Argyrios, T., and Grawford, C. (1961). Supravalvular stenoses of the pulmonary arteries. *Acta Radiol.* **56**, 466.

Berg, J. M., Crome, L., and France, N. E. (1960). Congenital cardiac malformations in mongolism. *Brit. Heart J.* **22**, 331.

Brown, G. C., and Evans, T. N. (1967). Serologic evidence of coxsackievirus etiology of congenital heart disease. *J. Amer. Med. Ass.* **199**, 183.

Burman, D. (1961). Familial patent ductus arteriosus. *Brit. Heart J.* **23**, 603.

Campbell, M. (1949). Genetic and environmental factors in congenital heart disease. *Quart. J. Med.* **18**, 379.

Campbell, M. (1959). The genetics of congenital heart disease and situs inversus in sibs. *Brit. Heart J.* **21**, 65.

Campbell, M. (1961). Place of maternal rubella in the aetiology of congenital heart disease. *Brit. Med. J.* **1**, 691.

Campbell, M. (1965). Causes of malformations of the heart. *Brit. Med. J.* **2**, 895.

Cayler, G. G. (1969). Cardiofacial syndrome. Congenital heart disease and facial weakness, a hitherto unrecognized association. *Arch. Dis. Child.* **44**, 69.

Chantler, C., and McEnery, G. (1971). Cardiofacial syndrome. *Proc. Roy. Soc. Med.* **64**, 20.

Chelius, C. J., Rowe, G. G., and Crumpton, C. W. (1962). Familial aspects of congenital heart disease. *Amer. J. Cardiol.* **9**, 508.

Clayton-Jones, E. (1959). Maternal influenza and congenital deformities. *Lancet* **ii**, 1086.

Cockayne, E. A. (1938). The genetics of transposition of the viscera. *Quart. J. Med.* **7**, 479.

Coffey, V. P., and Jessop, W. J. E. (1959). Maternal influenza and congenital deformities. A prospective study. *Lancet* **ii**, 935.

Comby, J. (1906). *Arch. Med. Enfants* **9**, 193 (Cited by J. M. Berg, L. Crome, and N. E. France, *Brit. Heart J.* **22**, 331, 1960.)

Cumming, G. R., and Uchida, I. (1963). Cardiopatia en pacientes con anomalies cromosomales. Memorias Del IV Congreso Mundral De Cardiologia, Tomo 1-A, Mexico, p. 5.

d'Avignon, M., Hellgren, K., and Juhlin, I. M. (1965). Thalidomide damaged children, experiences from Eugeniahemmet. *Acta Pediat. Scand. Suppl.* **159**, 79.

Dekaban, A., and Baird, R. (1959). The outcome of pregnancy in diabetic women. *J. Pediat.* **55**, 563–576.

Dogramaci, I., and Green, H. (1947). Factors in the etiology of congenital heart anomalies. *J. Pediat.* **30**, 295.

Doxiades, L., and Portius, W. (1938). *Z. Menschl. Vererbungs. Konstitutionslehre* **21**, 384. (Cited by Berg *et al.*, 1960.)

Driscoll, S. G., Benirschke, K., and Curtis, G. W. (1960). Neonatal deaths among infants of diabetic mothers. *Amer. J. Dis. Child.* **100**, 818.

Ekstrom, G. (1952). The surgical treatment of patent ductus arteriosus; a clinical study of 290 cases. *Acta Chir. Scand. Suppl.* **169**.

Ellis, R. W. B., and van Creveld, S. (1940). A syndrome characterized by ectodermal dysplasia, polydactylia, chondrodysplasia and congenital morbus cordis. *Arch. Dis. Childhood* **15**, 65.

Engler, M. (1949). "Mongolism (Peristalic Amentia)," pp. 49–50. Wright, Bristol. (Cited by Berg *et al.*, 1960).

Evans, P. R. (1950). *Brit. Heart J.* **12**, 258. (Cited by Berg, *et al.*, 1960.)

Fruhling, L., Korn, R., Laviellaureix, J., Surjus, A., and Foussereau, S. (1962). La myo-endocardite chronique fibro-élastique du nouveau-né et du nourrison (fibro-élastose). *Ann. Anat. Pathol.* **7**, 227.

Gellis, S. S., and Hsia, Y. (1959). The infant of the diabetic mother. *Amer. J. Dis. Child.* **97**, 1–41.

Gibson, S., and Lewis, K. C. (1952). Congenital heart disease following maternal rubella during pregnancy. *Amer. J. Dis. Child.* **83**, 317.

Giknis, F. L. (1963). Single atrium and the Ellis-van Creveld syndrome. *J. Pediat.* **62**, 558.

Greenberg, M., Pellitteri, O., and Barton, J. (1957). Frequency of defects in infants whose mothers had rubella during pregnancy. *J. Amer. Med. Ass.* **165**, 675.

Gregg, N. M. (1941). Congenital cataract following German measles in mother. *Trans. Ophthalmol. Soc. Austr.* **3**, 35.

Gyllensward, A., Lodin, H., Lundberg, A., and Moller, T. (1957). Congenital multiple peripheral stenosis of the pulmonary artery. *Pediatrics* **19**, 399.

Hambach, R. (1953). *Ann. Paediat.* **181**, 27. (Cited by Berg *et al.*, 1960).

Holmes, L. B. (1965). Congenital heart disease and upper extremity deformities. *New Engl. J. Med.* **272**, 437.

Holt, M., and Oram, S. (1960). Familial heart disease with skeletal malformations. *Brit. Heart J.* **22**, 236.

Ingalls, T. H., Curley, F. J., and Prindle, R. A. (1950). Anoxia as a cause of fetal death and congenital defects in the mouse. *Amer. J. Dis. Child.* **80**, 34.

Ingalls, T. H., Curley, F. J., and Prindle, R. A. (1952). Experimental production of congenital anomalies: Timing and degree of anoxia as factors causing fetal deaths and congenital anomalies in the mouse. *N. Engl. J. Med.* **247**, 758.

Katz, M., Benzier, E. E., Nangeroni, L., and Sussman, B. (1953). Kartagener's syndrome. *N. Engl. J. Med.* **248**, 730.

Kosenow, W. (1960). Das Ullrich Turner Syndrome in heutiger Sicht. *Muenchen. Med. Wochenschr.* **102**, 24, 83.

Lamy, M., de Grouchy, D., and Schweisguth, O. (1957). Genetic and non-genetic factors in etiology of congenital heart disease. Study of 1,188 cases. *Amer. J. Human Genet.* **9**, 17.

Lemi, L., and Smith, D. W. (1963). The XO syndrome: a study of the differential phenotype in 25 patients. *J. Pediat.* **63**, 577.

Lewis, K. B., Bruce, R. A., Baum, D., and Motulsky, A. (1965). The upper limb–cardiovascular syndrome. An autosomal dominant genetic effect on embryogenesis. *J. Amer. Med. Assoc.* **193**, 1080.

Lenz, W., and Pliess, G. (1963). The pathology of thalidomide embryopathy and associated defects of the heart. Memorias Del IV Congreso Mundial De Cardiologia. Tomo 1-A, Mexico, p. 150.

Lewis, S. M., Sonnenblick, B. P., Gilbert, L., and Biber D. (1958). Familial pulmonary stenosis and deaf-mutism. Clinical and genetic considerations. *Amer. Heart J.* **55**, 458.

Liebman, J., Cullum, L., and Belloc, N. B. (1969). Natural history of transposition of the great arteries. Anatomy and birth and death characteristics. *Circulation* **40**, 237–262.

Lillehei, C. W., and Varco, R. L. (1953). Certain physiologic, pathologic and surgical features of complete transposition of the great vessels. *Surgery* **34**, 376.

Lund, C. J. (1948). Maternal congenital heart disease as obstetric problem. *Amer. J. Obstet. Gynecol.* **55**, 244.

Lynch, H. T., Grisson, R. L., Moorneng, P., and Krush, A. (1964). Complete transposition of great vessels. Manifestation in two siblings confirmed at autopsy. *J. Amer. Med. Ass.* **190**, 95.

Mannheimer, E. (1940). Morbus Coeruleus. An analysis of 114 cases of congenital heart disease with cyanosis. *Bibl. Cardiol.* 4 Suppl., Fasc. 4.

McKeown, T., MacMahon, B., and Parsons, C. G. (1953). The familial incidence of congenital malformation of the heart. *Brit. Heart J.* **15**, 273.

McKusick, V. A. (1955). The cardiovascular aspects of Marfan's syndrome. *Circulation* **11**, 321.

McKusick, V. A. (1964). A genetical view of cardiovascular disease. *Circulation* **30**, 326.

McKusick, V. A., Egeland, J. A., Eldridge, R., and Krusen, D. E. (1964). Dwarfism in the Amish. I. The Ellis-van Creveld syndrome. *Bull. Johns Hopkins Hosp.* **115**, 306.

MacMahon, B. (1952). Association of congenital malformation of the heart with birth rank and maternal age. *Brit. J. Soc. Med.* **6**, 178.

Mehrizi, A., and Drash, A. (1961). Birth weight of infants with cyanotic and acyanotic congenital malformations of the heart. *J. Pediat.* **59**, 715.

Mehrizi, A., Hirsch, M. S., and Taussig, H. B. (1964). Congenital heart disease in the neonatal period. *J. Pediat.* **65**, 721.

Mehrizi, A., Hutchins, G. M., Medearis, D. N., Jr., and Rowe, R. (1965). Enterovirus infection and endocardial fibroelastosis. *Circulation* **32**, 150.

Mitchell, S. C., Froehlich, L. A., Banas, J. S., Jr., and Gilkeson, M. R. (1966). An epidemiologic assessment of primary endocardial fibroelastosis. *Amer. J. Cardiol.* **18**, 859.

Mitchell, S. C., Sellmann, A. H., Westphal, M. C., and Park, J. (1971). Etiologic correlates in a study of congenital heart disease in 56,109 births. *Amer. J. Cardiol.* **28**, 653–657.

Müller, K. (1955). *Z. ärztl Fortbild.* **49**, 408. (Cited by Berg *et al.*, 1960).

Naeye, R. L. (1965). Unsuspected organ abnormalities associated with congenital heart disease. *Amer. J. Pathol.* **47**, 95.

Naeye, R. L. (1966). Transposition of the great arteries and prenatal growth. *Arch. Pathol.* **82**, 412.

Noonan, A., Nadas, A. S., Rudolph, A. M., and Harris, G. B. C. (1960). Transposition of the great arteries. A correlation of clinical, physiologic and autopsy data. *N. Engl. J. Med.* **263**, 592.

Nora, J. J. (1971). Etiologic Factors in congenital heart disease. *Pediat. Clin. N. Amer.* **18**, 1059–1074.

Nora, J. J., and Meyer, T. C. (1966). Familial nature of congenital heart diseases. *Pediatrics* **37**, 329–334.

Nora, J. J., Vargo, T. A., Nora, A. H., Love, K. E., and McNamara, D. G. (1971). Dexamphetamine, a possible environmental trigger in cardiovascular malformations. *Lancet* **i**, 1290.

Oppenheimer, B. S., Block, N. S., and Grishman, A. (1949). The association of interatrial septal defects and anomalies of the osseous system. *Trans. Assoc. Am. Physicians* **62**, 284.

Pedersen, L. M., Tygstrup, I., and Pedersen, J. (1964). Congenital malformations in newborn infants of diabetic women. *Lancet* **i**, 1124.

Pedersen, L. M., Tygstrup, I., and Pedersen, J. (1965). Congenital malformations in newborn infants of diabetic women. Correlation with maternal diabetic vascular complications. *Acta Paediat. Scand. Suppl.* **159**, 40.

Penaloza, D., Alias-Stella, J., Sime, F., Recavanen, S., and Marticorena, E. (1964). Heart and pulmonary circulation in children of high altitudes. *Pediatrics* **34**, 568.

Polani, P. E., and Campbell, M. (1955). Aetiological study of congenital heart disease. *Ann. Human Genet.* **19**, 209.

Record, R. G., and McKeown, T. (1953). Observations relating to aetiology of patent ductus arteriosus. *Brit. Heart J.* **15**, 376.

Rowe, R. D. (1962). Cardiac malformation in mongolism. *Amer. Heart J.* **64**, 567.

Rowe, R. D. (1963). Maternal rubella and pulmonary artery stenosis. Report of eleven cases. *Pediatrics* **32**, 180.

Rowe, R. D., and Mehrizi, A. (1968). "The Neonate with Congenital Heart Disease." Saunders, Philadelphia, Pennsylvania.

Rowe, R. D., and Uchida, I. A. (1961). Cardiac malformations in mongolism. A prospective study of 184 mongoloid children. *Amer. J. Med.* **31**, 726.

Rubenstein, H. J., and Weaver, K. H. (1965). Monozygotic twins concordant for ventricular septal defect. Case report and review of the literature of congenital heart disease in monozygotic twins. *Amer. J. Cardiol.* **15**, 386.

Rusnak, S. L., and Driscoll, S. G. (1965). Congenital spinal anomalies in infants of diabetic mothers. *Pediatrics* **35**, 989.

Rutstein, D. D., Nicherson, R. J., and Herald, F. P. (1952). Seasonal incidence of patent ductus and maternal rubella. *Amer. J. Dis. Child.* **84**, 199.

Shaher, R. M., Farina, M. A., Porter, I., and Bishop, M. (1972). Clinical aspects of congenital heart disease in mongolism. *Amer. J. Cardiol.* **29**, 497.

Sime, F., Banchero, N., Penaloza, D., Gamboa, R., Cruz, J., and Marticorena, E. (1963). Pulmonary hypertension in children born and living at high altitudes. *Amer. J. Cardiol.* **11**, 143.

Smith, D. W. (1962). The No. 18 trisomy syndrome. *J. Pediat.* **60**, 513.

Smith, D. W. (1963). The D1 trisomy syndrome. *J. Pediat.* **62**, 326.

Smith, H. L., and Hand, A. M. (1958). Chondroectodermal dysplasia (Ellis-van Creveld syndrome). *Pediatrics* **21**, 298.

Sorenson, H. R. (1951). Familial occurrence of congenital heart disease. *Nord. Med.* **46**, 1402.

Strauss, L. (1953) . *Trans. Amer. Coll. Cardiol.* **3**, 214. (Cited by Berg *et al.* 1960).

Stuckey, D. R. (1956). Congenital heart defects following maternal rubella during pregnancy. *Brit. Heart J.* **18**, 519.

Swan, C., Tostevin, A. L., Moore, B., Mayo, H., and Black, G. H. B. (1943). Congenital defects in infants following infectious diseases during pregnancy with special reference to relationship between German measles and cataract, deaf mutism, heart disease, and microcephaly and to period of pregnancy in which occurrence of rubella is followed by congenital abnormalities. *Med. J. Aust.* **2**, 201.

Terasaki, P. I., Mickey, M. R., Yamazaki, J. N., and Vredevoe, D. (1970). Maternal-fetal incompatibility. I. Incidence of HL-A antibodies and possible association with congenital anomalies. *Transplantation* **9**, 538.

Townes, P. L., Krentner, K. A., Krentner, A., and Manning, J. (1963). Observations on the pathology of the trisomy 17-18 syndrome. *J. Pediat.* **62**, 703.

Tucker, A. W., Jr., and Kinney, T. D. (1954). Interventricular septal defect (Roger's disease) occurring in mother and her 6 months fetus. *Amer. Heart J.* **30**, 54.

Uchida, L. A., and Rowe, R. D. (1957). Discordant heart anomalies in twins. *Amer. J. Human Genet.* **9**, 133.

Venables, A. W. (1965). The syndrome of pulmonary stenosis complicating maternal rubella. *Brit. Heart J.* **27**, 49.

Wagenvoort, C. A., Neufeld, H. N., and Edwards, J. E. (1962). Cardiovascular system in Marfan's syndrome and in idiopathic dilatation of ascending aorta. *Amer. J. Cardiol.* **9**, 496.

Walker, W. G. (1934). Coarctation of the aorta in father and son. *N. Engl. J. Med.* **211**, 1192.

White, P. D. (1944). "Heart Disease." 3rd Ed., p. 1025 MacMillan, New York.

Williams, C. B., Lange, R. L., and Hecht, H. H. (1957). Post valvular stenosis of the pulmonary artery. *Circulation* **16**, 195.

Chapter 8

EXPERIMENTAL PRODUCTION OF TRANSPOSITION

Complete transposition of the great arteries has been reported in cows (Cockle, 1863; Kast, 1970). Congenital anomalies have been produced in the fetuses of rats and other animals by subjecting the mother or the fetuses at a critical period to folic acid deficiency (Baird et al., 1954; Nelson et al., 1952; Monie et al., 1955), folic acid antagonists (Hogan et al., 1950), vitamin A deficiency (Wilson and Warkany, 1949; Wilson et al., 1953c), vitamin E deficiency (Cheng and Thomas, 1954), and riboflavin deficiency (Nelson et al., 1956). The results of these experiments showed that ventricular septal defects and aortic arch abnormalities occurred with considerable regularity in these instances. Abnormal origin of the right subclavian artery from the distal part of the aortic arch was more common after folic acid deficiency.

The teratogenic effects of the influenza A virus in the early chick embryos has been demonstrated by Hamburger and Habel (1947) and Williamson et al. (1956). A specific syndrome comprising microcephaly, and impairment of the growth of the amnion results from injecting the unattenuated virus in chick embryos 48 hours after incubation (Hamburger and Habel, 1947). de la Cruz et al. (1963) used the influenza A virus at supra- and suboptimal temperatures to produce cardiovascular lesions in developing chick embryos. Whereas both supra- and suboptimal temperatures resulted in significant mortality of the embryos, suboptimal temperature gave rise to congenital heart lesions, particularly, ventricular septal defect. Activated influenza A virus caused high mortality as well as central nervous system lesions when injected at the beginning of incubation. On the other hand, injection of allantoid liquid together with the inactivated virus gave rise to a high incidence of congenital heart disease. Valvular abnormalities and ventricular septal defects were common.

Rychter and Lemez (1957, 1958) and Rychter (1962), working on chick embryos, were able to produce transposition and aortic arch abnormalities by suppressing the heart loop or aortic arches by a microclip. Suppression of both pulmonary arches or of all left aortic arches produced a distinct type of ventricular septal defect. Suppression of the left atrium resulted in left ventricular hypoplasia and marked narrowing of the aortic arch. By placing a large clamp in the bulboventricular groove of the heart loop on the third day of incubation, the movement of the bulbus to the left was prevented and the aortic and pulmonary trunks remained in their original spatial relation to the right ventricle. If the clip is put in place on the fourth day of incubation partial transposition of the aorta is produced. This type differs from the former by a more pronounced shift of the bulbus to the left. These experiments suggested to the authors that transposition is due to restriction of the morphogenetic movement of the bulbus to the left.

In 1951, Wilson and Karr pointed out that direct irradiation of rat embryos on the tenth day of gestation, through an abdominal incision in the mother, gives rise to congenital abnormalities in these embryos. Dosage with 100 R slightly increased the incidence of intrauterine death and in the survivors reduced the rate of growth and caused retarded or anomalous development of the eyes in 75% of embryos. The brain and urinary organs were also occasionally the site of malformations. Reversed asymmetry of the aortic arches and tail in a few instances suggested a tendency toward situs inversus. When embryos were irradiated on the ninth day, Wilson *et al.* (1953b) produced aortic arch and other congenital anomalies, in 9 fetuses and in 1 term animal. Transposition of the aorta and the pulmonary artery occurred five times and was the most common single defect. It was associated with other aortic arch abnormalities in all but one instance. Double aortic arch was seen in 3 (2 with transposition), right aortic arch in 4 (2 with transposition), and truncus arteriosus in 3. Malformations of the heart occurred in 17 instances. Eight of these had defective development of one or more of the cardiac septa or atrioventricular valves. In 8 embryos the interatrial septum failed to develop perforation. Abnormal termination of the major veins occurred in 2. Fifteen animals were affected by some degree of reversed asymmetry of the viscera. Of the individual organs the heart was most often affected. It was the only organ involved in five instances. Many of these defects were found as often in term animals as in the embryo removed at earlier age, but anomalies involving the central nervous system and the cardiovascular system were less frequent in term animals and appeared to be associated with, if not responsible for, the high rate of prenatal mortality.

Treatment of pregnant rats with trypan blue was used by various authors to produce cardiovascular abnormalities in embryos (Gillman *et al.,* 1948, 1951; Waddington and Carter, 1952, 1953; Hamburgh, 1954; Wilson, 1954, 1955; Fox and Goss, 1956, 1957, 1958; Richman *et al.* 1957; Monie *et al.* 1966). Fox and Goss (1956) reported that trypan blue injections in pregnant rats of a Long-Evans substrain on the 8½ days of gestation resulted in a syndrome of severe cardiovascular malformations which occurred in 23 (43.5%) of their 53 fetuses affected by cardiovascular abnormalities. The syndrome included the following: (1) displacement of major portions of atrial appendages to either the right or left of the arterial trunks; (2) elongation and craniocaudal orientation of heart; (3) counterclockwise rotation of ventricles; (4) interventricular septal defect; and (5) dextroposition of the aorta usually accompanied by subpulmonary stenosis or some degree of pulmonary transposition. Aortic arch abnormalities, malformations of the atrioventricular valves, and unilateral eye defects were also present in the majority of the fetuses exhibiting the syndrome. Complete transposition of the great arteries was present in 7 fetuses. In 1958, Fox and Goss reported in detail the results of trypan blue injections of 1ml of 1% solution in pregnant rats on the 7½ and 8½ days of pregnancy. Of the 186 fetuses recovered from dams injected with dye, 53 had variable grades of transposition of the aorta and pulmonary artery. Complete transposition of the great arteries was observed in 11 fetuses. The incidence of this anomaly was higher in the 8½ days series (7 fetuses) than in the 7½ days series (4 fetuses). Certain features, which are unusual in congenital complete transposition, occurred in transposition following trypan blue injection in the mother. All 11 fetuses had a ventricular septal defect. The root of the pulmonary artery was situated dorsal and to the right (rather than to the left in the congenital group) of the aorta. Hypoplasia of the pulmonary and aortic trunks were observed each in 4 cases. In the 7 fetuses in which the coronary artery pattern was studied, there was an interchange of the distribution patterns so that the anterior descending coronary artery was taken over by the right artery. Appreciable "auricular displacement" with both atrial appendages situated on the right or on the left of the great vessels was observed in all but 1 case. Subpulmonary stenosis was not observed and 10 fetuses had some form of abnormality of the atrioventricular valves. In 6 a single atrioventricular valve which communicated with one or both ventricles was present. Aortic arch abnormalities occurred in 8 fetuses. This took the form of double systemic arches in 2, complete interruption proximal to the left subclavian artery in 1 and distal to it in 2, and right ductus arteriosus in 3. The authors pointed out that the experimental production of congenital transposition complexes in rats depends on three factors. First, it is determined by the nature of the teratogenic agent. Transposition of the arterial trunks is the most common fetal vascular malformation which results from maternal trypan blue injections on the seventh or eighth day of pregnancy. Maternal pteroylglutamic acid or vitamin A deficiencies operative during this period results in truncus or aortic arch malformations but not in arterial transposition. Second, it is influenced by the developmental state of the embryo during the period of teratogenic activity. The incidence of transposition complexes was considerably higher when trypan blue was administered on the eighth day rather than on the seventh day. Direct fetal X-ray radiation shows a similar limitation. Exposure causes transposition on the ninth day of gestation but not on the eighth (Wilson *et al.,* 1953a) or tenth (Wilson and Karr, 1951). Third, substrains of rats appear to differ in their susceptibility to this malformation. Monie *et al.* (1966) produced complete and partial transposition of the great arteries, dextrocardia, tricuspid stenosis, or atresia in rat fetuses from mothers injected with trypan blue solution subcutaneously on the eighth and ninth day of gestation. Hearts with transposition of the great arteries were usually characterized by shortness of the aorta and pulmonary trunk, cranial location of the aortic valve, displacement of the coronary arteries, and a channel or track extending from the infundibulum of the right ventricle to the commencement of the transposed pulmonary trunk. Inadequate expansion of the atrioventricular ring about the twelfth or thirteenth day of gestation possibly leads to deformity of the atrioventricular cushions and absence or stenosis of the tricuspid or mitral valves. Sinuosity of the truncus arteriosus seen in many thirteenth day and older embryos of the trypan blue series was considered by the authors to be a significant factor in the development of transposition of the great arteries. Truncal sinuosity and shortening are probably responsible for the sinistral location of the truncus observed in some embryos in which the lumen of that structure lay over the cranial edge of the ventricular septum. As a consequence of this, either from derotation or from altered bloodflow, spiraling of the truncobulbar cushions is minimal or absent which leads to the dorsally placed pulmonary trunk communicating directly with the left ventricle while the ventrally located aorta retains its connection with the right ventricle. The authors, as well as Wilson (1960), pointed out that although many teratogens are known to affect cardiovascular development, only x-irradiation and trypan blue have been shown to produce transposition of the great arteries in quantity and consistently.

References

Baird, C. D. C., Nelson, M. M., Monie, I. W., and Evans, H. M. (1954). Congenital cardiovascular anomalies induced by pteroylglutamic acid deficiency during gestation in the rat. *Circ. Res.* **2**, 544.

Cheng, D. W., and Thomas, B. H. (1953). Relationship of time of therapy to teratogeny in maternal avitaminosis E. *Proc. Iowa Acad. Sci.* **60**, 290.

Cockle, J. (1863). A case of transposition of the great vessels of the heart. *Med. Chir. Trans.* **46**, 193.

de la Cruz, M. V., Sainz, C. C., Armas, S. M., Chavez, A. P., and Bandera, R. Z. (1963). Cardiopatias congenitas producidas experimentalment por variaciones de temperatura y por virus de influenza en el embrion de pollo. Memorias del IV Congreso Mundial De Cardiologia. Tomo 1-A, Mexico, p. 12.

Fox, M., and Goss, C. M. (1956). Experimental production of a syndrome of congenital cardiovascular defects in rats. *Anat. Rec.* **124**, 189.

Fox, M., and Goss, C. M. (1957). Experimentally produced malformation of the heart and great vessels in rat fetuses. Atrial and caval abnormalities. *Anat. Rec.* **129**, 309.

Fox, M. H., and Goss, C. M. (1958). Experimentally produced malformations of the heart and great vessels in rat fetuses. Transposition complexes and aortic arch abnormalities. *Amer. J. Anat.* **102**, 65.

Gillman, J., Gilbert, C., Gillman, T., and Spence, I. (1948). A preliminary report on hydrocephales, spina bifida and other congenital anomalies in the rat produced by trypan blue: significance of these results in the interpretation of congenital anomalies following maternal rubella. *S. Afr. J. Med. Sci.* **13**, 47.

Gillman, J., Gilbert, C., Spence, I., and Gillman, T. (1951). A further report on congenital anomalies in the rat produced by trypan blue. *S. Afr. J. Med. Sci.* **16**, 125.

Hamburger, V., and Habel, K. (1947). Teratogenic and lethal effects of influenza—A and mumps viruses on early chick embryos. *Proc. Soc. Exp. Biol. Med.* **66**, 608.

Hamburgh, M. (1954). The embryology of trypan blue induced abnormalities in mice. *Anat. Rec.* **119**, 409.

Hogan, A. G., O'Dell, B. L., and Whitley, J. R. (1950). Maternal nutrition and hydrocephalus in newborn rats. *Proc. Soc. Exp. Biol. Med.* **74**, 293.

Kast, A. (1970). Angeborene transposition en von aorta und a. pulmonalis beim rind. *Zentrabl. Veterinaermed.* **17A**, 780.

Monie, I. W., Nelson, M. M., Baird, C. D. C., and Evans, H. M. (1955). Pathogenesis of cardiovascular abnormalities in fetal rats following transitory maternal pteroylglutamic acid deficiency. *Circulation* **12**, 750.

Monie, I. W., Takacs, E., and Warkany, J. (1966). Transposition of the great vessels and other cardiovascular abnormalities in rat fetuses induced by trypan blue. *Anat. Rec.* **156**, 175.

Nelson, M. M., Asling, C. W., and Evans, H. M. (1952). Production of multiple congenital abnormalities in young by maternal pteroylglutamic acid deficiency during gestation. *J. Nutr.* **48**, 61.

Nelson, M. M., Baird, D. C., Wright, H. V., and Evans, H. M. (1956). Multiple congenital abnormalities in the rat, resulting from riboflavin deficiency induced by the antimetabolite galactoflavin. *J. Nutr.* **58**, 125.

Richman, S. M., Thomas, W. A., and Konikov, N. (1957). Survival of rats with induced cardiovascular anomalies. *Arch. Pathol.* **63**, 43.

Rychter, Z. (1962). Experimental morphology of the aortic arch and the heart loop in chick embryos. *Advan. Morphog.* **2**, 333.

Rychter, Z., and Lemez, L. (1957). Experimentelle untersuchung über die Entstehung sowie über die Lage und Grösse von Kammerseptumdefekten am Herzen von Hühnembryonen. *Verhandl. Anat. Ges.* **54**, 97.

Rychter, Z., and Lemez, L. (1958). Experimenteller Beitrag zur Entstehung der Transposition von Aorta in die rechte Herzkammer der Hühnembryonen. *Verhandl. Anat. Ges.* **55**, 310.

Waddington, C. H., and Carter, T. C. (1952). Malformations in mouse embryos induced by trypan blue. *Nature (London)* **169**, 27.

Waddington, C. H., and Carter, T. C. (1953). A note on abnormalities induced in mouse embryos by trypan blue. *J. Embryol. Exp. Morphol.* **1**, 167.

Williamson, A. P., Simonsen, L., and Blattner, R. J. (1956). Specific organ defects in early chick embryos following inoculation with influenza A virus. *Proc. Soc. Exp. Biol. Med.* **92**, 334.

Wilson, J. G. (1954). Congenital malformation produced by injecting Azo Blue in pregnant rats. *Proc. Soc. Exp. Biol. Med.* **85**, 319.

Wilson, J. G. (1955). Teratogenic activity of several azo dyes chemically related to trypan blue. *Anat. Rec.* **123**, 313.

Wilson, J. G. (1960). Experimental production of congenital cardiac defects. *In* "Congenital Heart Disease" (A. D. Bass and G. K. Moe, eds.), p. 65. Publication No. 63 of the American Association for the Advancement of Science, Washington, D.C.

Wilson, J. G., and Karr, J. W. (1951). Effects of irradiation on embryonic development. I. X-rays on the 10th day of gestation in a rat. *Amer. J. Anat.* **88**, 1.

Wilson, J. G., Brent, R. L., and Jordan, H. C. (1953a). Differentiation as a determinant of the reaction of rat embryos to X-irradiation. *Proc. Soc. Exp. Biol. Med.* **82**, 67.

Wilson, J. G., Jordan, H. C., and Brent, R. L. (1953b). Effects of irradiation on embryonic development. II. X-rays on the ninth day of gestation in the rat. *Amer. J. Anat.* **92**, 153.

Wilson, J. G., Roth, C. B., and Warkany, J. (1953c). An analysis of the syndrome of malformations induced by maternal vitamin A deficiency. Effects of restoration of vitamin A at various times during gestation. *Amer. J. Anat.* **92**, 189.

Wilson, J. G., and Warkany, J. (1949). Aortic arch and cardiac anomalies in the offspring of vitamin A deficient rats. *Amer. J. Anat.* **85**, 113.

Chapter 9

EMBRYOGENESIS OF TRANSPOSITION

At the level of the 6th or most posterior of the aortic arches (cephalic end of the truncus) the pulmonary artery lies in a sinistrodorsal position and the aorta occupies a dextroventral position. In complete transposition of the great arteries, the aorta and the pulmonary artery descend without twisting around each other, so that at the caudal end of the truncus, the pulmonary artery occupies a sinistrodorsal position and arises from the left ventricle, while the aorta occupies a dextroventral position and arises from the right ventricle. Theories of the embryogenesis of transposition of the great arteries could be classified as phylogenetic, ontogenetic, or hemodynamic. An excellent presentation and discussion of the earlier theories on transposition of the great arteries are found in the works of Lev and Saphir (1937, 1945) and Harris and Farber (1939).

Phylogenetic Theories

In 1812, Meckel noted the resemblance of the malformed heart to that of the lower vertebrates, and suggested that transposition of the great arteries is due to failure of development at an early stage. A similar observation on the resemblance of hearts with congenital heart disease to those of lower vertebrates was made by Keith (1909) and Robertson (1913). On the basis of a comparative study of the heart in phylogenesis and ontogenesis, Spitzer (1919, 1921, 1923) evolved a phylogenetic theory of the normal development of the heart as well as of the abnormal development in transposition. This theory has been translated into English by Lev and Vass and the following is a summary of this translation (Lev and Vass, 1951).*

---

* From Lev, M. and Vass, A. (1951). "The Architecture of Normal and Malformed Hearts." Courtesy of Charles C. Thomas, Springfield, Illinois.

With the substitution of the lung type of respiration for the gill type, the pulmonary circulation gradually assumes a relatively greater importance. This is manifested in the degree of heart septation which presents an ascending series from the amphibia upward in the scale of phylogenesis, correlated with the development of the pulmonary circulation. Thus, the development of pulmonary respiration and heart septation are intimately related phylogenetically. Pulmonary respiration is essentially the primary and cardiac septation the secondary mechanism. In the fish the gill circulation is connected directly with the heart and the propulsive force of the latter mainly benefits this circulation. Since animals living on land require more energy and, therefore, a more efficient circulation, the mechanical disadvantage of the gill circulation is gradually overcome by placing the pulmonary circulation in parallel. The simple placement of the two circulations adjacent to each other, however, still does not produce the desired effect for an exchange of blood between the two circuits, and separation of the two blood streams must be affected. This is obtained by torsion of the arterial end of the loop in a clockwise direction and by extension of the dividing spur between the aorta and the pulmonary artery into the lumen of the truncus down to the heart. Since the tube is fixed at both ends, torsion at one end must result in detorsion (countertorsion) at the other end. In order to prevent the nullification of the effects of torsion on the arterial end by the countertorsion at the venous end, detorsion occurs at a point peripheral to the point of division between the pulmonary and the systemic veins. This would affect only the systemic venous channels. If we postulate a spiral septum anlage as confined to the cavae, then both atria would originally be connected in series, the right atrium being the distal one, and only secondarily would they become parallel. The atrial septum would thus develop originally as a transverse septum, and secondarily it would be transformed into a longitudinal septum. Similarly, the ventricular septum would develop originally as a transverse septum and later would be transformed into a longitudinal septum. Those postulated stages in phylogenesis actually occur in ontogenesis. Thus, the original heart tube becomes elongated and bowed to the right. Four areas of dilatations situated behind each other could be recognized: sinus venosus, atrium, ventricle, and bulbus. The most acute kink in the heart tube is found in the middle of the ventricular portion. In this kinked area a fold is formed perpendicular to the axis of the tube representing the plane of the future ventricular septum. The site of this kind divides the tube into venous and arterial limbs in each of which a separate septum develops. The arterial and venous septa unite in the ventricular region to form a single longitudinal septum.

The mechanical forces which are available to pulmonary respiration to phylogenetically carry out these processes are the pressure forces of the blood stream. These are (1) the continuous lateral pressure of the blood, (2) the intermittent pulse pressure, and (3) the collision force of the blood stream acting in a longitudinal direction upon the wall. All these forces commence to operate before the establishment of pulmonary respiration but become especially prominent with the increase in blood volume concomitant with the development of pulmonary respiration. These mechanical forces act locally to produce local dilatations and generally produce generalized dilatation and lengthening of the heart tube. Local changes on the arterial side take the form of shortening and dilatation of the truncus and centripetal growth of the truncus septum. On the venous end they take the form of septum formation and bringing both venous ostia close to the heart. Similarly lateral pressure and longitudinal traction result in lateral distension and longitudinal stretching of the four heart compartments. The narrow segments between these compartments are pulled in opposite directions, in this way longitudinal folds, because of the stretching of the endocardium, make their appearance in narrow regions. These folds are the distal and proximal bulbar swellings, the endocardial cushions of the atrioventricular canal and the sinoatrial folds. Diffuse dilatation and lengthening of the heart tube will result in the following (1) The production of the sharp kink in the ventricular loop, approximation of both limbs of the tube, and the protrusion of the bulboauricular spur into the lumen at the point of maximal kinking. (2) Torsion, since a torsioned tube requires less space than a straight one. To be able to accommodate the increased amount of blood, torsion of the limbs of the tube occurs and the heart bow turns to the right. On the arterial side, clockwise torsion takes the form of the spiral descent of the truncus septum, and the distal and proximal bulbar swellings and septa. (3) Formation of septa. As a result of torsion these ridges assume an oblique position and accordingly become subjected to a hydrodynamic pressure superimposed on the previous single lateral pressure. They are stimulated to grow both in length and height, and in this way septa are formed. (4) Countertorsion. Evidence of countertorsion would be found in the series of folds restricted to the right atrium of the human embryo. These folds, as seen on the septal wall of the right atrium, are curved in a direction opposite to the folds in the arterial end, i.e., in a counterclockwise direction. Spitzer pointed out that the fact that these folds are restricted to a region peripheral to the entry of the pulmonary veins proves that the atria were situated originally in series. (5) Arrangement of the atria originally in series and subsequently in parallel. This arrangement of the atria could be explained as a mechanical consequence of pulmonary respiration in phylogenesis. With the development of pulmonary circulation, the proximal portions of both pulmonary and systemic veins enlarge and form venous sinuses which are later incorporated into the venous end of the heart tube. The dividing portion between these venous areas protrudes in the lumen in the form of a ridge (septum primum) and is situated at first on the left lateral wall. Because the blood from the cavae meets this septum at right angles, the stream is deviated to the right with consequent dilatation of the right wall of the tube and placement of the atria in parallel. The originally transverse septum primum is now a longitudinal septum situated on the posterior wall. The atrial septum is completed later when the countertorsion septal folds in the peripheral vena caval sac, and together with the left valve of the sinus venosus are pressed against it and fused with it by means of the blood stream. (6) The arrangement of the ventricles originally in series and subsequently in parallel. Originally, the ventricular septum is transverse, but later it is transformed into a longitudinal septum. This is related to the mechanical conditions produced by pulmonary respiration which increase the tortuosity of the heart tube. Ontogenetically the ventricular septum consists of a ridge arising from the apical wall of the ventricular region directed against the bulboauricular spur. Accordingly, it lies in a plane transverse to the longitudinal axis of the heart tube. With displacement of the atrial canal to the right behind the bulbus and beyond the plane of the ventricular septum, the atrial septum becomes situated in the midline of the atrioventricular ostium. This divides the blood stream into two currents passing on each side of the ventricular septum. Accordingly the upper basal portion of the ventricular septum is converted into a longitudinal septum and each ventricle acquires an inflow tract. Meanwhile, the bulbus shifts anteriorly and to the left and the lower margin of the bulbus septum approaches the plane of the upper anterior free margin of the ventricular septum. When these two margins fuse together each ventricle acquires an outflow region. In this way the anterior half of the ventricular septum is converted also into a longitudinal septum. Phylogenetically speaking, a transverse septum is formed at the sharp bend in the ventricular region. This becomes a place of septum formation because of the abrupt change in the direction of blood flow in this region produced by the greater outpouching of the ventricular region as compared to the amphibia. The parallel longitudinal axes of both limbs are almost in the same plane as the transverse septum. The latter comes to lie in the longitudinal axes of both limbs after a slight deviation of the posterior half of the upper septum margin to the left by the atrial flow septation force, and

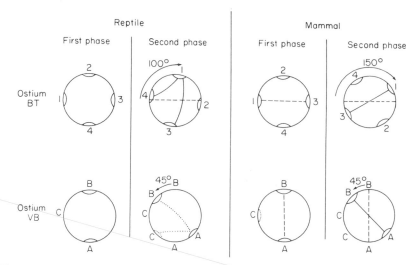

Fig. 9.1. Comparison between the bulbus of the reptile and that of the mammal. Note that the number and the location of the bulbar cushions are the same. The difference lies in the number of ridges extending through the bulbus, connecting the distal and proximal cushions. There are three ridges in the reptile—ridges 1A, 4B, and 3C. In the mammal there are only two ridges—1A and 3B. Therefore, two septa are formed in the reptilian bulbus, but only one septum is formed in the mammalian bulbus. BT, bulbotruncare; VB, ventriculobulbare. From Lev and Saphir (1945), by permission of *Arch. Pathol.*

the anterior half of the upper margin to the right by the septum formation force coming from the arterial end of the tube. The posterior portion of the septum comes in line with the atrial canal and becomes a venous septum, while the anterior portion comes in line with the bulbus and becomes the arterial septum.

The reptilian circulation is peculiar in presenting a right aorta and a pulmonary artery connected to the right venous ventricle, and a left aorta connected to the left arterial ventricle. There are four swellings in the distal bulbus of reptiles, birds, and mammals (1, 2, 3, and 4). The proximal bulbar region of both reptiles, and birds contains three swellings (A, B, and C), whereas in mammals it contains two swellings only (A and B) (Fig. 9.1). In birds and mammals fusion of opposite swellings 1 and 3 produces only one septum (septum aorticopulmonale), which divides the bulbus into aorta and pulmonary artery. In reptiles, fusion of swellings 1, 3, and 4 produces two perpendicular septa; septum aorticopulmonale and septum aorticum, which divide the bulbus into one pulmonary artery and two aortae. In reptiles septum aorticopulmonale separates the systemic from the pulmonary circulation, while septum aorticum extends downward into the ventricles separating the arterial from venous blood. Septum aorticopulmonale of mammals is situated, on the one hand, between the aorta and the pulmonary artery, like the septum aorticopulmonale of reptiles, and, on the other hand, extends downward into the ventricular septum like septum aorticum of the crocodiles. Since it behaves like a derivative of fusion of both reptilian septa, it should be called the secondary septum aorticopulmonale. While the ventricular extension of septum aorticum in the highest reptiles separates both ventricles, septum aorticopulmonale ends unattached to the right ventricle appearing there as a muscle ridge. This ridge has two extensions to the superior and inferior ventricular walls, thus demarcating the two outflow tracts of the right ventricle. In man, the crista supraventricularis and the trabecula septomarginalis (moderator band) are present on the superior and inferior right ventricular walls, respectively. These two muscle bands are morphologically similar to the two muscular ridges derived from septum aorticopulmonale in the reptilian heart. The crista supraventricularis and the trabecula septomarginalis, therefore, do not demarcate the inflow regions of the right ventricle, but separate the pulmonary outflow portion from the blind end of the rudimentary right ventricular aorta. The inflow region is separated from the remainder of the right ventricle by the anterior tricuspid ledge. This is a slightly elevated muscular ridge which originates apically in the trabecula and proceeds backward and is marked by a rim of papillary muscles and chordae. It demarcates the inflow region of the right ventricle from the rudimentary outflow portion of the right ventricular aorta which exists in the form of a crevicelike excavation between the ledge and the crista supraventricularis. The most median part of the crevice is excavated in the form of a cupula representing the aortic conus of the right ventricle. If birds, mammals, and reptiles are traced to a common hypothetical progenitor, in which the pulmonary circulation is as yet not well developed and the pulmonary artery is small, ontogenetic clues indicate that in this form the primary septum aorticopulmonale was stretched between distal bulbar swelling 1 and 2, and the septum aorticum between swellings 1 and 4. Similarly the bulbar septa were formed from swellings 1, 2, and 4. The semilunar cusps of the aorta and the pulmonary artery develop from all distal bulbar swellings. Consequently each of swellings 1, 2, and 4 consisted of a valve-forming component (1v, 2v, and 4v) and a septum-forming component (1s, 2s, and 4s). Only swelling 3 was a purely valvular ridge (3v). During phylogenesis and concomitant with the increase in the pulmonary blood flow, lateral migration of septa occurred. The divergent legs of the two, bulbar septa emigrate toward each other, and against the valvular ridge 3v and fuse together giving rise to a single septum aorticopulmonale. In this way the right ventricular aorta disappeared leaving the left ventricular aorta and the pulmonary artery as the two vessels emerging from the heart. In reptiles this process is incomplete and the valvular ridge is left entirely in the field of the right ventricular aorta. Since, in reptiles, the primary septa do not reach the valvular ridge, 3v, the valvular components of 2, 3, and 4 remain with the pulmonary artery, the right ventricular aorta, and the left ventricular aorta, respectively. The valvular component of swelling 1 is common to all three vessels. In homeothermic animals both primary septa fuse in the plane of the valvular components of swellings 1 and 3 to form a single septum which divides each of the two swellings into two parts. This explains the fact that in reptiles each of the three vessels contains two cusps whereas in mammals each vessel contains three cusps. In phylogenesis there is a tendency toward the concentration of anlage material of the two primary septa at opposite poles. This process has already started in reptiles, and is complete in mammals. In mammals the primary septum aorticopulmonale extends from the truncus spur 5/6 downward to the base of the ventricle where its free margin forms the crista supraventricularis. The septum aorticum extends from the ostium venosum below, up to, and ending with its free margin at the distal bulbus border. Thus, only in the central portion of the truncus-bulbus-ventricle tube, is there a double septum, the fused leaves of which have obliterated the right ventricular aorta. Consequent to the separation of the two septa in the proximal region, the rudimentary conus of the right ventricular aorta was preserved. As a result of the disappearance of septum aorticum distally, both right and left aortas fused into a common ascending aorta and both aortic arches remained patent. In reptiles both aortas remained open and because of moderate torsion, the left ventricular aorta became connected with the right aortic arch, and the right ventricular aorta with the left arch. In mammals, because of further increased torsion, the entire arch became situated in the direction of the left ventricular blood stream now flowing in a more oblique direction and thus became transformed into the definitive aortic arch. The right aortic arch could not be closed because of the absence of septum aorticum. In birds, the left 4th arterial arch which was originally continuous with the right ventricular aorta is obliterated. The single aorta of birds must therefore empty into the right 4th arch as it actually does. The process of reduction of septum aorticum begins in reptiles but here it is so minimal and the primary peripheral growth center of septum aorticum at the truncus spur is preserved and is even more potent than the septum-forming force working from the ventricular region. In crocodiles, the presence of two centers of septum formation and the beginning stronger development of the proximal anlage manifest themselves in a zone of perforation in the fusion of the two formation foci (foramen of Panizza).

Spitzer's Phylogenetic Theory of Abnormal Cardiac Development in Transposition

Spitzer explained his four types of transposition as described below.

Type 1. Riding Aorta

In this type the aortic orifice straddles the ventricular septum over a defect, thus emerging from both ventricles. Since torsion is essential for normal development of the ventricular septum, the ventricular septal defect is the immediate result of incomplete torsion. The defect is situated in the upper part of the ventricular septum beneath the aorta, i.e., the posterior half of the arterial ventricular septum, exactly at the site of the proximal part of the septum aorticum which disappears first with incomplete torsion. Torsion produces fusion of septum aorticopulmonale and septum aorticum which results in closure of the right ventricular aorta by means of the proximal portion of the septum aorticum. In detorsion this portion of septum aorticum is lifted up, therefore, reopening the right ventricular aortic conus which fuses with the left ventricular one, thus giving the appearance of a riding aorta. In ontogeny the flow of blood through the right ventricular aorta is increased while that through the pulmonary artery is diminished. Moreover, the crista now dividing the two main streams, is subject to the same forces which normally cause the development of the ventricular septum. Its potentialities as a septum become evident and it hypertrophies. The pulmonary artery becomes smaller as a consequence of the smaller volume of blood which passes through it and because it is compressed between the hypertrophied crista and the anterior ventricular septum. Detorsion prevents the complete migration of septum aorticopulmonale which does not reach the valvular component of swelling 3, and the latter is not divided between the pulmonary artery and aorta but is given completely to the aorta. The pulmonary artery remains small and its valve receives two cusps only and a stenotic and bicuspid valve artery results. Manifestation of detorsion is seen also in deficient twisting of the aorta and pulmonary artery about each other, the aorta arising more to the right rather than posterior to the pulmonary artery. The position of the semilunar cusps is altered, so that the anterior pulmonary cusp is more to the left, and the posterior aortic cusp is more to the right. The crista supraventricularis proceeds from the ventricular septum over the base of the ventricle to the right and anteriorly in a less transverse and more oblique direction than it normally does. It thus approaches the sagittal plane, and the angle between it and the anterior septum becomes more acute than normal.

Type 2. Simple Transposition

An increase in the amount of detorsion has taken place as shown by the fact that a larger ventricular septal defect is present and both aorta and pulmonary artery emerge from the right ventricle. The aorta is situated to the right of the pulmonary artery. Between both arterial ostia, at the base of the right ventricle, there is the hypertrophied crista which is directed more sagittally. The pulmonary valve is stenotic and bicuspid. Detorsion removes the left aorta from its connection with the left ventricle, but blood flow through it ceases and it is obliterated. In contrast, the right ventricular aorta reopens. In this way both aorta and pulmonary artery arise from the right ventricle and an apparent transposition of the aorta has taken place. The semilunar cusps are more rotated to the left, and are responsible for abnormalities of the coronary arteries found in all more pronounced cases of detorsion. These abnormalities take the form of either a single branch of one coronary artery becoming fused with the stem of the other, or the complete coronary artery arising from the opposite valve sinus. The anterior descending coronary artery arises from the right aortic sinus, instead of the left, the former being frequently rotated to the left anterior, or even to the left posterior position. Likewise, the posterior descending coronary artery often arises abnormally from the left aortic sinus which is rotated to the right position, or even to the right and posterior position. The primary normal right circumflex artery arising from the right aortic sinus is rudimentary. The anomalies of these coronary arteries could be explained by the detorsion portion of the semilunar cusps, and rotation of the sinus of one artery to the district of the other.

Type 3. Transposition (Crossed or Complete)

Detorsion of the aorta and pulmonary artery is more pronounced as indicated by the aortic ostium being situated anteriorly and to the right of the pulmonary artery ostium. Each of the two vessels emerges from the wrong ventricle. The semilunar cusps are rotated more counterclockwise; the posterior aortic cusp is more anterior and slightly to the right. Since in this type of transposition the aorta is also a right ventricular aorta, the part of the ventricular septum lying anterior to the septal defect, i.e., between the two vessels, cannot be identical with the true anterior septum in Type 2 since the latter lies to the left of the pulmonary artery. The anterior ventricular septum in Type 3 must be a hypertrophied crista, which appears to be a true ventricular septum because it has been rotated into the plane of the preserved true posterior septum due to increased torsion. At the same time, because of an advanced degree of torsion, the true anterior septum, to the left of the pulmonary artery, has completely disappeared. The ventricular septum is therefore composed posteriorly of the true ventricular septum and anteriorly of the hypertrophied crista supraventricularis. Transposition of the pulmonary artery is therefore only apparent. The reasons for the marked reduction in the anterior septum, and the largely intact posterior septum, are both phylogenetic and ontogenetic and are basically due to detorsion. Since the posterior septum is situated between the venous ostia and the anterior septum between the arterial ostia, and since because of detorsion the septum-forming force being strongest at the venous end and weakest at the arterial end, the anterior septum is suppressed. In addition, displacement of the dividing plane of both blood streams primarily affects the arterial limb, where the crista takes over the role of the anterior septum, while the posterior septum remains in its original dividing plane. Normally the septum forming folds A and B grow from the arterial limb toward the venous limb. The inhibition of their formation in the bulbus limb must also injure their ventricular growth, thus disturbing the formation of the posterior septum and causing its regression. As long as the crista meets the ventricular septum at an angle (as in marked detorsion) a slight atrophy of the posterior septum will accompany the main atrophy of the anterior septum. When the detorsion becomes more marked, the crista becomes lined up with the posterior septum. This exposes the crista to the full effect of the plane of diversion of the two circulations. The enlargement of the septal defect is inhibited. Reduction of the posterior septum is stopped and actual regeneration may occur. The constriction of the pulmonary ostium between the rudimentary left ventricular aortic conus and the true anterior septal remnants, on the one hand, and between the hypertrophied crista and the right ventricular aortic ostium, on the other, explains the bicuspid pulmonary valve and pulmonary stenosis. There are two variants of this type of transposition; Type 3A with absent ventricular septum, and Type 3B with an intact ventricular septum. The difference between these is that in Type 3A the balance of forces favors the production of a defect while in Type 3B septum formation is favored. As long as the crista is situated at an angle to the ventricular septum, the reducing factors predominate. If the crista occupies the plane of the posterior septum, then both come under the full septum-building force of the divided blood streams. Complete closure of the ventricular septum forces the left ventricular blood into the pulmonary artery, which dilates and its valve restores the three cusps. The coronary arteries reveal transposition of their ostia so that the right coronary artery originates from the left aortic sinus which is now situated posteriorly, while the left coronary artery originates from the right aortic sinus which is now situated to the left.

Type 4. Mixed Atrioventricular Transposition

In this type of transposition not only the pulmonary artery but also the right atrioventricular valve open into the wrong ventricle, so that the right ventricle contains the aortic ostium only. The position of the semilunar cusps presents more detorsion so that the posterior cusp lies anteriorly and somewhat to the left, while the anterior pulmonary cusp lies posteriorly. This position of the semilunar cusps as well as the position of the aortic ostium being far anterior, and of the pulmonary artery being far posterior and somewhat to the left of the aorta, indicates that the detorsion has already passed beyond the stage reached in Type 3. The crista, as it turns further counterclockwise, leaves the plane of the posterior septum and is now past the tricuspid orifice and in the plane of the anterior tricuspid ledge. In this position the crista lies between two blood streams and is stimulated to hypertrophy. The inhibition which previously affected the anterior septum, now involves the posterior septum as well so that the entire septum disappears. The muscular structure appearing to be a true septum is formed anteriorly by the crista and posteriorly by the anterior tricuspid ledge. If the crista in its detorsion has passed the plane of the posterior septum but has not yet reached the plane of the anterior tricuspid ledge, then the plane of the crista is situated between these two structures and it fuses with both apically. Both ridges hypertrophy and compress the tricuspid orifice between them which becomes narrow and possesses rudimentary cusps. If the detorsion of the crista occurs slowly then the triscupid orifice is completely obliterated. Since the two atrioventricular valves open into the left ventricle, while the right ventricle possesses only the outflow region of the right ventricular aorta, filling of this ventricle becomes more difficult particularly as the septal defect becomes smaller. As a result the pulmonary artery becomes dilated, while stenosis of the aorta results from diminished blood flow.

Although other writers (Meckel, 1812; Keith, 1909; Robertson, 1913) had preceded Spitzer in noting the resemblance between congenitally malformed hearts and the hearts of lower vertebrates, it was Spitzer who applied the theory of recapitulation to the development of the human heart. Since the publication of Spitzer's theory in 1923, most papers on the embryology of transposition referred to Spitzer's work in one way or another. Other papers include those by Mautner and Lowy (1921), Homma (1923), Monckeberg (1924), Fuchs (1925), Pernkopf (1926), Wurm (1927), Graevinghoff (1927), Freudenthal (1927), Aschoff (1929), Gertsmann (1929), Schramm (1929), Shapiro (1930), Kung (1931), Humphreys (1932), Jensen (1932), Hoffmann (1933), Lev and Saphir (1937, 1945), Abbott (1937), Harris and Farber (1939), Liebow and McFarland (1941), Brown (1950), Bremer (1957), Grant (1962), de Vries and Saunders (1962), Van Mierop and Wiglesworth (1963), Van Praagh (1967), and others. It is also significant that Monckeberg (1924) who wrote a chapter of 183 pages on congenital heart disease in Volume 2 of "Handbuch der Speziellen Pathologischen Anatomie und Histologie" without mentioning Spitzer's theory, had to supplement a chapter of 23 pages at the end of this volume which he devoted completely to Spitzer's theory. Moreover, Lev and Vass translated it into English and published it in 1951 "to provide a broader concept of the underlying malformations and to unfold Spitzer's phylogenetic theory for those who diagnose, those who cure and those who study morphologically malformations of the heart." In the introduction to this translation Saphir said "Twenty-seven years have elapsed since Spitzer's publication. The more one studies congenital malformations of the heart, the greater one's respect for Spitzer's genius."

Although it was generally agreed that Spitzer's main contribution was a theory of normal cardiac development, Spitzer, because of criticism of his explanations of congenital malformations, had to reexplain his theory in 1927, 1928, and 1929. In 1921, Mautner and Lowy produced evidence in support of Spitzer's theory. The authors reported a case of a single ventricle in which the aorta arose anteriorly and to the right while the narrow bicuspid pulmonary artery was situated behind it. Between the pulmonary artery and the anterior leaflet of the mitral valve, the rudimentary conus of the obliterated left aorta was thought to be present. Fuchs (1925) studied the development of the heart in Vanellus Cristatus and supported Spitzer's theory concerning the formation of the ventricles, the formation of the ventricular septum, migration of septum aorticopulmonale, and homology of the crista supraventricularis and trabecula septomarginalis to the two muscle ridges derived from septum aorticopulmonale in the reptilian heart. Harris and Farber (1939) pointed out that Spitzer's main contribution was a theory of normal cardiac development since its fundamental postulate is the orderly development of the organ as a unit, in response to the varying conditions, forces, and demands in a series rising from fishes to birds and mammals. In addition, it admits of no fortuitous variations which disregard the phylogenetic interrelationships of these groups and is capable of explaining, on mechanical grounds, some of the shortcuts in the ontogenetic recapitulations of these events. In 1941, Liebow and McFarland reported a case of corrected transposition and persistent rudimentary right aorta and summarized Spitzer's main contribution as follows.

1. Emphasis on the part played by the advent of a pulmonary circulation during the transition from an aquatic to a terrestrial habitat in causing torsion.

2. The principle of torsion in septation of the heart so that crossing of the pulmonary and systemic circulation results. This is more effective than the tandem arrangement in the gill circulation of fishes.

3. The recognition of a rudimentary right aorta homologous to that of reptiles, the crista supraventricularis acting as a guide to the position of this rudiment.

4. Certain septa may be the result of hypertrophy of structures such as the crista supraventricularis, tricuspid ledge, or bulboatrial ledge with regression of the true interventricular septum because of hemodynamic changes.

5. Detorsion with reopening of the right reptilian aorta.

6. Establishment of four types of transposition dependent upon the degree of torsion.

7. Emphasis on the fact that in no case is there true transposition of any great vessel arising from the right side of the heart to the left, if the position of the true interventricular septum is used as the plane of reference.

On the other hand, Monckeberg (1924), with whom Pernkopf (1926) agreed, emphasized that he could not find a remnant of the ventricular septum to the left of the pulmonary artery in his cases, and accordingly the septum between the aorta and the pulmonary artery must be the true ventricular septum. Pernkopf (1926) pointed out that Spitzer's theory should be regarded as strongly hypothetical as long as no proof could be found for latency of the phylogenetic factors. Moreover, the signs of detorsion which Spitzer saw in the position of the aortic sinuses and the coronary arteries are irrelevant if one considers that one artery can communicate with the descending branch of the other. Similarily, Pernkopf and Wirtinger (1933) could not find any evidence of a reptilian stage in human development or of any homology between the reptilian right aorta and the niche designated by Spitzer in human hearts. Referring to Spitzer's work, Abbott (1937) said "fascinating and ingenious as this theory is and based, as it is, upon an accurate and meticulous investigation of a large series of type specimens in the light of his profound knowledge of comparative embryology, it cannot as yet be said to have covered all the points at issue. It therefore represents a stride forward in the clearer understanding of this complex problem, rather than its full solution." Lev and Saphir (1937) thought that while Spitzer's theory explained the anatomical facts beautifully, it was difficult to accept it in its form, for (1) as proved by Pernkopf and Wirtinger (1933), torsion at the ostium ventriculobulbare (proximal bulbar ostium) is not responsible for the spiral twisting of the vessels. The latter is related to the shortening and absorption of the bulbus into the ventricle. (2) The formation of the heart loop with torsion, and the bayonetlike kinking of the bulbus have already occurred in dypnoë. There is no proof that there is an ascending series in torsion of the bulboventricular loop and that there has been less torsion in reptiles than in mammals. They thought that the right aorta is not obliterated in mammals and that the mammalian aorta probably represents fusion of the two. Harris and Farber (1939) pointed out that a great amount of criticism had been directed against the complexity and apparent improbability of Spitzer's explanation of the malformations. For example, in Type 3 (crossed or complete) the entire architecture of the heart may appear normal except for the interchanging aorta and pulmonary artery. It would be difficult to accept the opinion that the ventricular septum is any other than the normal one. The changes postulated by Spitzer seem too radical even to construct a cardiac architecture which conforms to the normal so closely as it does in this type of case. Moreover, the authors cited Sato (1914) and Kung (1931) as having demonstrated a normal course of the atrioventricular bundle in these cases which must be a proof against the presence of a false septum. In addition, no case had been reported in which two definite aortae were present, and the atrial portions of the heart may be normal in cases of transposition in which the postulated detorsions should affect the venous as well as the arterial ends of the primitive loop. Recently Grant (1962) criticized Spitzer's theory and pointed out that in Spitzer's days the idea that congenital anomalies were instances of species-reversal was still popular in the lay mind, although biologists had discredited it. Today the notion is in even less repute, and it is not thought to play a significant role in teratology or mutation. Furthermore, Spitzer leaned heavily upon teleology in his explanations, as if one part of the heart might somehow "know" what the functional requirements of another part of the heart might be at some later day or in some later evolutionary state. Grant concluded that while phylogeny provides fascinating glimpses into the intricate network of evolution it can shed light only indirectly, if at all, on problems in teratology. de Vries and Saunders (1962) rejected all phylogenetic theories and said "The rather rigid phylogenetic concepts based on the theory of recapitulations, which are inherent in the views of Keith (1906, 1909, 1924), Robertson (1913–1914), and Spitzer (1923), are not acceptable substitutes for serial observations of the changes in structure and function of the developing human heart. Most of the hypothesis based on recapitulation theory are inadequate as explanations for anomalous condition, lack confirmation in static morphology, and preclude direct proof of the causitive factors involved . . . Spitzer's improbable theory and questionable interpretations of morphology cannot be accepted by us in their entirety." Shaner (1962a) described the development of the great vessels and bulbus in normal embryos of the frog, pig, alligator, and bird. He pointed out that the mammalian bulbus is an adopted and specialized form of the amphibian bulbus with only a general resemblance to the reptilian bulbus. He pointed out that the embryological evidence fails to support Spitzer's theory, that the anomalous transposed aorta of the human heart is an atavistic revival of the reptilian right ventricular aorta. Finally, Van Praagh (1967) wrote "Spitzer's atavistic hypothesis which has often been doubted but never disproved—is considered to be invalidated by the completely left ventricular morphological characteristics of the chamber from which the transposed pulmonary artery classically arises."

Pernkoff and Wirtinger's Theory of Partial Inversion

In 1933, Pernkopf and Wirtinger reported a study of normal cardiac development, assuming that the dorsal mesocardium marks the longitudinal axis of the primitive cardiac tube. This fixed position serves as a guide to torsions which occur during cardiac development. Pernkof and Wirtinger pointed out that the septal anlage arises in a spiral form. Thus, there is −180° rotation (counterclockwise) of this septum in the atrial region, +180° rotation (clockwise) in the ventricular region, and another +180° rotation in the bulbar region. The total spiral of the septal anlage is +180° which results in crossing of the pulmonary and systemic circulations. At 4–5 mm of fetal length the auricular, ventricular proximal bulbar ridges A and B and distal bulbar ridges 1, 2, 3, and 4 begin to form. During development, the cardiac tube moves in two phases. The first phase consists of +90° at the atrial portion reaching its maximum at the atrioventricular junction. Similarly there is a −90° rotation at the bulbar portion reaching its maximum at the bulboventricular junction. Since the tube is fixed at both ends, at the termination of this phase the position of the atrial septum is −90°, the ventricular septum 0°, the bulbar septum +270°, and the truncal septum 0°. After the first torsion is completed, the endocardial ridge 1, at first running along the left side of the bulbotruncus orifice, will start high up on the right side, then descend along the posterior bulbar wall to the left, crossing it toward the anterior side, and continue down the frontal wall to end anteriorly at the central bulbar orifice. Ridge 3, at first running along the right side of the bulbar orifice, will start, after torsion, from the top of the left side then cross the frontal wall of the bulbus, turn backward and follow the dorsal wall until it ends posteriorly and to the right just behind the terminal point of ridge 1. In these two central end points, endocardial cushions A and B, respectively, will be formed. Ridges 2 and 4 will run parallel to the others as far as they reach. The second phase of cardiac development takes place from the 5th to the 8th week of fetal life and is concerned mainly with the absorption of the bulbus, a process that occurs only in amniotes (reptiles, birds, and mammals), but is incomplete in reptiles. In mammals a torsion of −150° occurs at the bulbotruncal end, and a torsion of +45° occurs at the bulboventricular ostium. The final form of the truncal septum will be +150°, the bulbar septum +75°, the ventricular septum +45°, and the atrial septum −90°. The bulbus shifts ventrally and to the left while the auricular canal shifts to the right. Expansion of the tricuspid orifice and of the dorsal wall of the distal portion of the primitive ventricle, and shrinkage of the proximal portion of the ventricle and of the dorsal wall of the proximal bulbus occur. In this way the bulbus is absorbed into the ventricles, its aortic portion disappearing, and its ventral portion assuming the role of the conus of the right ventricle.

On these foundations Pernkopf and Wirtinger (1935) evolved their theory of partial inversion as a cause of transposition. They pointed out that since each segment contains a spiral septum rotating 180°, complete inversion of any segment will not alter the course of the pulmonary or systemic circuits. On the other hand, if the septum in any segment fails to spiral, then complete separation of the two circuits will result. They pointed out that partial inversion could affect any segment, and explained complete transposition of the great arteries (crossed transposition) on the basis of partial inversion of the septal anlage in the bulbar region. They assumed that in transposition the proximal portion of the bulbar anlage rotates +90° (clockwise) while the distal portion rotates −90° (counterclockwise) and the total spiral in this segment would be zero. Since the atrial and ventricular septa are normal, the total spiral of the entire septum is also zero. The pulmonary and systemic circulations will not cross. Partial inversion of the atrial of ventricular septa may also occur, and according to the segment or segments involved other types of transposition may result.

Lev and Saphir's Ontogenetic–Phylogenetic Theory

Lev and Saphir (1937) criticized the theory of Pernkopf and Wirtinger on the grounds that it is difficult to conceive of cardiac development without the influence of irritative hydrodynamic factors. They discarded the idea of inherent spiraled nature of the septum formation but retained the concept of movements of the cardiac tube. They pointed out that the process of shrinkage of the bulbus is linked with the process of untwisting of the bulbar ridges, and shifting of the twist to the truncus ridges. This is obtained by a torsion of 150° at the ostium bulbotruncare, and is complete by ventral deviation of the bulbus and back torsion of 45° at the ostium ventriculobulbare. The bulboauricular spur (bulboventricular of some authors) constitutes a fixed point about which the bulbus rotates and backtorsion takes place. Ridge A is fused early with the main ridge of the ventricular septum, and this likewise represents a stabilizing unit making possible torsion at the ostium bulbotruncare and backtorsion at the ostium ventriculobulbare. If the bulboauricular spur is abnormal from any cause, it prevents the bulbus from embedding itself in the auricular furrow and fixed point is not obtained. This leaves the ostium ventriculobulbare free to rotate about the relatively fixed point, i.e., the point of fusion of ridge A with the ventricular septum, or less commonly about its center as an axis. Untwisting of the bulbar ridges is achieved by backtorsion at the proximal bulbar orifice in excess of that which usually takes place. The more detorsion at this site, the less at the distal bulbar orifice, so that in extreme degrees of backtorsion there is no torsion at the distal orifice. No twist is given to the truncus ridges and the picture of transposition results.

In 1945, Lev and Saphir pointed out that all types of transposition may be considered to be due to a phylogenetic abnormality complicated by further ontogenetic abnormalities as postulated by Spitzer. In their opinion the phylogenetic abnormality is an abnormal formation of ridge 3B (the normal mammalian bulbus presents two ridges, 1A and 3B). This ridge is a new formation not present below mammals and apparently results from fusion of ridges 3C and 4B by the hydrodynamic principles. In the embryo, whose parent will present the anomaly of transposition, this new ridge 3B is not produced, but one or other or neither of its com-

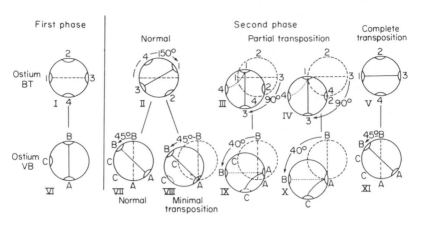

Fig. 9.2. Normal and abnormal absorption of the bulbus. In transposiiton there is an abnormality in the formation of the ridge 3B, whereby it is poorly formed or replaced by ridge 4B or 3C. This results in decreased torsion at the distal ostium. In addition, this torsion occurs either around cushion 1 as a center or close to cushion 1. At the proximal ostium backtorsion occurs around cushion A as a center or close to cushion A. This backtorsion may be 45°, or it may be 90° as normally observed in an earlier stage. 1, 2, 3, and 4, Distal bulbar cushions; A, B, and C, proximal bulbar cushions; BT, ostium bulbotruncare; VB, ostium ventriculobulbare. I, VI, distal and proximal bulbar ostia, respectively, at the end of the first phase (normal and in transposition); II, VII, distal and proximal bulbar ostia during the second phase in normal absorption of the bulbus; II, VIII, bulbar ostia in transposition with congenital aneurysm of the membranous septum during the absorption of the bulbus; III, IX, bulbar ostia in partial transposition during the absorption of the bulbus when torsions occur close to cushions 1 and A as centers; IV, X, bulbar ostia in partial transposition during the absorption of the bulbus when torsions occur about cushions 1 and A as centers; V, XI, bulbar ostia in complete transposition in which no torsion occurs at the distal ostium while mild backtorsion occurs at the proximal ostium. From Lev and Saphir (1945) , by permission of *Arch. Pathol.*

ponents 4B and 3C are. Yet the hydrodynamic forces for the absorption of the bulbus are there. The absorption of such a bulbus, with a well formed ridge 1A but abnormal ridges 4B and 3C or a poorly developed ridge 3B or with only ridge 1A, proceeds abnormally. In the first place, torsion at the distal and proximal ostia cannot occur around the center of the tube as an axis, therefore, the center of rotation will be at a point somewhere between the center of the tube and cushion 1 and A, or on the periphery at cushion 1 and cushion A. In addition, there will be less torsion at the distal ostium. Since torsion is produced by the action of the centripetal force on the spiral ridges, the presence of only one ridge with or without an opposite ridge with a lesser twist will lessen the torsion. Torsion of the proximal ostium may remain the same but will be eccentric with its center close to A or at A. Thus the coni of the aorta and the pulmonary artery will take up the abnormal positions after the absorption of the bulbus. Hence, the ontogenetic complication of phylogenetically abnormally formed bulbar ridges is the abnormal absorption of the bulbus (Fig. 9.2).

Ontogenetic Theories

In 1837, Kurschner stated that transposition of the great arteries occurs because of failure in the spiraling of the great vessels and faulty fusion of the septum of the ventricles and the truncus. Meyer (1857) explained transposition as due to an arrested development at a stage before the vessels have assumed their spiral course. Peacock (1866) thought that transposition of the great arteries is caused by faulty development of the aorta and pulmonary artery from the primitive truncus. He pointed out that the production of this form of malformation is due to irregular division of the arterial trunk, so that the branchial arches ordinarily associated with the portion which becomes the aorta, are in connection with the pulmonary artery. This deviation from the natural development may take place either after the septum of the ventricle is completed, or while the growth of the septum is in progress, so that transposition may involve the ventricles as well as the vessels. In 1872, Pye-Smith pointed out that transposition of the great arteries must have begun at a period in fetal life when the truncus was still undivided, but the septa of the auricles and ventricles had already commenced. The ventricular septum growing up from the apex to base does not continue between the future conus of each side. The division of the bulbus arteriosus is made by another septum, which grows downward from between the 4th and 5th arches of the left side, and first dividing the truncus arteriosus into the pulmonary artery and aorta, is then continued so as to divide the bulbus arteriosus into the conus venosus and conus arteriosus. This septum begins at the back of the truncus arteriosus and having its faces at first directed laterally, twists as it grows downward, so that the left hand one comes to look almost directly forward and the right hand one backward. He suggested that if the septum were to preserve its anteroposterior position with its faces looking right and left, without twisting it would separate the aorta on the right from the pulmonary artery on the left.

Von Rokitansky's Ontogenetic Theory

In 1875, von Rokitansky considered that every type of transposition could be explained on the basis of an abnormal development of the truncus septum. He assumed that the normal truncus septum begins as a swelling in the left posterior portion of the primitive truncus and grows toward the right anterior portion in a curved manner with its convexity normally directed anteriorly (Fig. 3.1, p. 32). The aorta is situated on the concave side while the pulmonary artery is situated on the convex side. Since the ventricular septum originates to the left of the truncus arteriosus the aorta and the pulmonary artery open first into the right ventricle. A defect in the anterior interventricular septum effects connection between the left ventricle and the aorta. The aorta is transferred into the left ventricle as a result of the growth of the right side of the ventricular septum around the truncus septum, and fuses with the right side of the endocardial cushions of the atrioventricular canal. The ventricle on that side from which the ventricular septum originates will be the normal left ventricle with a bicuspid atrioventricular valve, while the other will be the normal right ventricle with a tricuspid atrioventricular valve. von Rokitansky postulated that the truncus septum may assume any position in the lower truncus. The ventricular septum may therefore vary in its inception either from the right or from the left. This gives rise to eight possible variations in the position of the aorta and the pulmonary artery, doubled by the assumption that the truncal septum may have the concavity reversed (see Fig. 3.1, p. 32). Referring to the work of von Rokitansky, Abbott (1937) said "subsequent investigations and the advances in comparative embryology have in part superceded, and to a certain extent invalidated, his conclusions, but his exact anatomic observations, extraordinary insight into the mechanical principles at work and brilliant deductions therefore constitute a real landmark in the eludication of this subject and contribution to it of immense and lasting value." Similarly Brown (1950) thought that the work of von Rokitansky was a landmark in the history of congenital heart disease, and it was more remarkable because it allowed von Rokitansky to foresee anomalies that he had not already observed.

In 1909, Keith concluded that von Rokitansky's theory does not help in understanding the problem of transposition, and that the clue is found in a study of the transformation of the mammalian heart. Normally the part of the bulbus cordis connected to the aorta atrophies while the part connected to the pulmonary artery expands. In transposition of the great vessels abnormal absorption of the bulbus cordis occurs and the processes are reversed. The aorta instead of being the dorsal vessel becomes the ventral one and is situated toward the greater instead of toward the lesser curvature of the ventricle. With atrophy of the lesser curvature of the ventricle and the pulmonary artery portion of the bulbus, the pulmonary artery in place of the aorta comes in contact with the auricles. In effect the origin of the great vessels is reversed in regard to the auricular canal.

Robertson (1913) after studying the comparative anatomy of the bulbus cordis, was mainly in accord with von Rokitansky's theory. She suggested that if the bulbus cordis develops as a short straight tube without any disparity in the length of the walls of its middle segment, no torsion of the vessels will take place. The septum in the distal part of the bulbus (truncus arteriosus) situated across it right to left, will grow down toward the proximal segment and will meet there the two proximal bulbar ridges. These two proximal ridges are usually situated left posteriorly and right anteriorly. Theoretically, the left posterior ridge may come to occupy any position from directly posterior to directly anterior along the left side of the bulbus, while the right ridge will move through a more or less corresponding semicircle on the right. As the distal septum does not twist, its right side joins with the right and its left with the left proximal bulbar ridge. Any degree of lateral displacement of the pulmonary artery to the left that may occur at the proximal end of the great vessels will be determined by the exact positions of the proximal bulbar ridges. If various positions of the proximal bulbar swellings were possible, a series of positions may occur where the pulmonary artery and aorta are placed dorsoventrally at their distal extremities, while proximally they may occupy any position from the pulmonary artery on the right and the aorta on the left, to aorta on the right and pulmonary artery on the left. Throughout these series the vessels will be transposed and will open out of the wrong ventricles. Because of the nonrotation of the great vessels, the posterior vessel in these cases will be the pulmonary artery.

In 1915, Lewis and Abbott advanced the theory that the embryonic cardiac tube in transposition of the great arteries bends in the reverse direction to that which is normal, so that the aortic limb turns upward on the left side of the common ventricle instead of the right. This brings the great arteries into an apparently reversed relationship with the vessels of the arch. If, however, the reversal is complete and development proceeds on this basis, no pathological results would ensue since the relationship of all parts concerned would be entirely in reverse. The aorta although placed anteriorly, would continue to drain the left ventricle and the pulmonary artery although placed posteriorly would continue to drain the right ventricle. The displacement of the orifices relative to the pulmonary and aortic trunks and to the atrioventricular orifices would take effect only when the reversal is incomplete. Such partial reversal would have the effect of throwing the aorta into communication with the right ventricle and the pulmonary artery with the left ventricle.

Bremer (1942, 1957) pointed out that embryologically the various types of transposition indicate increasing degrees of detorsion of the normal dextral spiral in the ascending limb of the heart loop. The inner ridges are an inherent part of the tube and their spiral course is inherent in the spiral torsion of the tube as a whole. He rejected the theory that their course may be reversed within the still normally rotated tube and suggested that one should look for a cause for the failure or partial failure of the normal dextral rotation of the truncus and conus, or for the reduction of that rotation after it has been established. The primary cause for the dextral spiral within the heart tube is the ring form of the heart, acquired as a means of accommodating greater length within a confined space. If there is no deviation of the bulbus to the right and the whole heart lies in one sagittal plane, no ring will form and no dextral torsion will occur in the conus and truncus. Theoretically, this form of heart might result in crossed (complete) transposition. The now transverse bulboventricular ridge might be absorbed as in normal development throwing the ventricular and bulbar limbs into one large ventricle, entered from behind by both tricuspid and mitral passages. The septum within the conus, now without spiral course, might be continued downward invading the common ventricle, dividing it sagittally into right and left parts. The aorta would arise from the right ventricle and the pulmonary artery from the left ventricle. Another cause which might lead to detorsion of the conotruncal region was suggested by Bremer. As the bulbar region becomes the right ventricle there is an outgrowth of the endothelial sinusoids which takes place chiefly at the sharpest convexity of the tube, i.e., caudally, laterally, and ventrally. The dorsal wall in contrast remains relatively smooth and flat. The deep sinusoidal invasion causes the corresponding walls of the bulb to bulge and assume the shape of the right ventricle. The expanding chest wall readily accommodates the enlarging ventricle, so that the torsion of the bulbar limb is in no way affected. During early development the caudal wall of the common atrium, the atrioventricular canal, and the left ventricle become fixed in position. If taking advantage of its free and unattached condition, the bulb should turn so that its sharpest convexity points dorsally instead of ventrally, the deepest growth of the sinusoids would be dorsal and the ventricular wall would bulge in that direction. This would encounter the pulsating right atrium and the septum transversum which at this period of development is almost vertically disposed, backed by the relatively solid liver. Meeting this, the heart itself as it expands must tend to be lifted forward. Only the freely movable bulbar portion responds by a ventral rolling motion. The lateral or right wall will be rolled forward carrying with it the crista supraventricularis, and this rotary motion in a sinistral direction will be transmitted upward to the common aortic-pulmonary trunk, thus tending to unwind the normal dextral spiral of that portion.

Shaner (1951, 1962b) suggested that complete transposition of the great arteries could be explained on the basis of a delayed descent of the aorticopulmonary septum. In the heart of a normal 7 mm pig embryo two longitudinal spiral ridges labeled 1 and 3 are found in the bulbus. Ridge 1 begins proximally in front of the interventricular septum, and ridge 3 begins opposite it in the endocardial tissue around the atrioventricular canal. Each ridge spirals distally so that ridge 1 begins on the left side of the proximal bulbus and ends on the right side of the distal bulbus and aortic sac. As the bulbus leaves the pericardial sac two small ridges labeled 2 and 4 appear and mark the site of the future semilunar valves. The aorticopulmonary septum pushes down between the 4th and 6th arterial arches in the frontal plane and joins the tips of ridges 1 and 3 and follows them as far as the semilunar valves. The aorta and pulmonary artery so created must be twisted and lengthened by a clockwise movement of the distal end of the bulbus about 180° and by shrinkage and absorption of the bulbus into the right ventricle. If the aorticopulmonary septum delayed its descent and waited until the distal bulbar cushions have rotated, its left tip would meet, not the usual ridge 3, but ridge 1. The aorta would thus be connected with the semilunar valves and inlet of the pulmonary artery. In the same way the pulmonary artery would be connected to the left ventricle. With subsequent shrinkage of the bulbus, the two great vessels would be drawn out into nearly parallel vessels.

de la Cruz and da Rocha (1956) thought that most theories explaining congenital conotruncal malformations, were not always supported by consistent embryological or phylogenetic data. They suggested an ontogenetic theory based upon Davis (1927), Kramer (1942), and Streeter's (1948) "modern school of human embryology," as well as on a study of pathological specimens of patients dying with congenital heart disease. In their view, conotruncal malformations of the heart are those produced by an abnormal development of the following embryological components, isolated or combined: (1) the conoventricular flange, (2) the conotruncal ridges, and (3) the aortic and pulmonary semilunar primordia. If the conotruncal ridges develop without rotation, the conotruncal septum will also present no rotation. The pulmonary artery, lying in a sinistrodorsal position at the cephalic end of the truncus conus, will continue in the same position until it reaches the caudal end of the bulbus and thus will arise from the left ventricle. The aorta, on the other hand, which occupies a dextroventral position at the cephalic end of the truncusconus, will remain in the position until it reaches the caudal end, thus arising from the right ventricle in front of the crista supraventricularis. The caudal end of the conotruncal septum remains at the normal position in relation to the free border of the muscular ventricular septum, and it will fuse with the right side of this septum without the occurrence of an interventricular septal defect. The occurrence of a ventricular septal defect must, therefore, be explained by a different mechanism. de Vries and Saunders (1962) rejected this theory and said "Our reservations about the acceptance of de la Cruz work coincide with those we have expressed in regard to the embryology she cited."

Van Mierop and Wiglesworth (1963) pointed out that the midtruncus is divided by a pair of opposing mesenchymal swellings; the dextrosuperior truncus swelling which grows distally and to the left, and the sinistroinferior truncus swelling which grows distally and to the right. When these fuse together, the truncus septum is formed and extends distally as well as proximally. Similarly the bulbus cordis is divided by a dextrodorsal swelling and sinistroventral swelling which fuse together and proceed distally to meet the truncus septum. The dextrosuperior truncus swelling meets the dextrodorsal bulbus swelling, and the sinistroinferior truncus swelling joins the sinistroventral conus swelling. Each truncus swelling carries a pair of tubercles, the primordia of the semilunar valves, on each extremity of its distal surface; one of each pair will be assigned to the pulmonary artery and to the aorta. Opposite the fused truncus swellings, two intercalated valve swellings appear. These are situated dextroinferiorly and sinistrosuperiorly and form the third tubercle of the aortic and pulmonary valve primordia, respectively. Starting at the tubercles, the semilunar valves and sinuses of Valsalva are formed by a process of excavation of the truncus and intercalated valve swellings in a proximal direction. The arterial valves, therefore, at first lie far distally, compared to a much more proximal position in the fully developed heart. The developmental error of the truncus responsible for complete transposition of the great arteries is the result of a reversal of the roles played by the truncus swellings and of the intercalated valve swellings. The latter develop slightly later but at about the same level as the truncus swellings. If the intercalated valve swellings appear earlier than the truncus swellings, they become the major structure and divide the truncus. Thus the pulmonary intercalated valve swelling forms a sinistrosuperior truncus swelling and becomes continuous with the sinistroanterior conus swelling. Similarly the aortic intercalated valve swelling develops into a dextroinferior truncus swelling and becomes continuous with the dextrodorsal bulbus swelling. Meanwhile, the true truncus swelling acts as the intercalated valve swellings. The final result is that the aorta arises anteriorly from the right ventricle, and the pulmonary artery posteriorly from the left ventricle.

Van Praagh (1967) pointed out that normally the subpulmonary infundibulum develops while the subaortic infundibulum does not. The subpulmonary infundibulum is believed to be posterior to the subaortic infundibulum, just as pulmonary arch 6 is posterior to aortic arch 4. When the subpulmonary infundibulum undergoes expansile growth, it must protrude anteriorly since it is the only direction in which there is room for expansion. It is this emergence of the subpulmonary infundibulum from posterior to anterior which normally twists the developing great arteries, because they are fixed distally by the arterial arches. The emergence from posterior to anterior of the subpulmonary conus and artery appears to result from two factors: (1) cardiac looping, and (2) development of the subpulmonary conus without development of the subaortic conus. In transposition the aortic infundibulum develops, and typically the pulmonary infundibulum does not. Since the aortic infundibulum initially is anterior, its expansile growth requires no emergence. It begins anteriorly and it stays anteriorly. Its development causes no twist because the proximal aorticopulmonary relationship remains the same as the distal aorticopulmonary relationship. To apply this theory to four heart specimens with "transposition and posterior aorta," Van Praagh *et al.* (1971) pointed out that normally *d*-loop formation results in a side by side semilunar relation. The developing pulmonary and mitral valves are relatively left-sided, whereas the future aortic and tricuspid valves are relatively right-sided. To cross the circulations the left-sided subpulmonary conus lifts the pulmonary valve away from the mitral valve and left ventricle, protruding the pulmonary artery anteriorly so that it overrides the anterior right ventricle. This movement has a reciprocal effect on the aortic part of the truncus with posterior and inferior tilting of the aortic valve toward the posterior left ventricle and mitral valve. Normal aortic–mitral approximation is facilitated by failure of development of right-sided subaortic conal musculature. In cases with "transposition and posterior aorta" the left-sided subpulmonary conus develops but remains much shorter than normal. This elevates the pulmonary valve but to a degree which is not sufficient to bring the pulmonary artery above the anterior right ventricle. Accordingly, the aortic valve will be depressed inferiorly and posteriorly toward the mitral valve and left ventricle but remains above the right ventricle and muscular ventricular septum. Deficient development of subaortic conal musculature permits tenuous aortic–mitral valve continuity.

The possible relationship between anomalies of the conotruncus, and the atrioventricular canal has been discussed by several authors. Shaner (1949) examined pig embryos with a defective fusion of the dorsal and ventral atrioventricular endocardial cushions. Each one showed some external or internal malformation of the conotruncus which took the form of overriding aorta, double outlet right ventricle, pulmonary stenosis, aortic stenosis or ventricular septal defect. He pointed out that two internal modifications are required for the migration of the conus. First, the conoventricular flange is flattened out of existence, and, second, after the dorsal and ventricular atrioventricular canal cushions have fused, the ventral cushion is deeply excavated in its middle so that only its two tubercles remain. The aortic orifice now can utilize the excavation in the ventral cushion and drain the left ventricle. In addition, the proximal part of the aorticopulmonary septum can now reach the free edge of the interventricular septum and participate in the closure of the interventricular foramen. An arrest in the growth or in the secondary resorption of the atrioventricular cushions may, therefore, be expected to affect the migration and the normal evolution of the conus. Doerr (1952) also accepted the possibility that malformed atrioventricular canal cushions might interfere with proper torsion of the conus. McCullough and Wilbur (1944) thought that transposition of the great arteries could be explained on the basis of abnormal development of the ventral atrioventricular cushion. In their view transposition of the great arteries is the result of spiraling of the bulbar septum in a direction the reverse of that which is normal. This reversal is conceivable if one assumes that, during the fourth week, the dorsal endocardial atrioventricular cushion appeared but no ventral one grew out to meet it. This unusual condition sufficiently affects the flow of the coursing fetal blood that, though the bulbar ridges and eventually the bulbar septum are stimulated to develop, their direction is the reverse of the normal. In the absence of a ventral cushion, the pillar of tissue which divides the primitive atrioventricular communication may be provided entirely by the dorsal cushion or the ventral cushion may appear, but too late to assume its normal significance. Once established, the reversed bulbar septum seeks its normal union with the interventricular septum. In the absence (or inadequacy) of what is normally supplied by the ventral cushion, such union cannot be complete, hence, an anterior ventricular septal defect. Ivemark (1955) pointed out that the conotruncus and the atrioventricular region have one tissue component in common which is the gelatinous reticulum. This substance is vital for the division of the atrioventricular canal and for septation of the conotruncus. Hypothetically an arrest of the growth rate of this substance, would seriously interfere with the normal evolution of these structures. Grant (1962) assumed that in transposition of the great vessels there is a shift in the orientation of the fibroblastic continuum which lines the primitive cardiac tube. This continuum extends from the atrioventricular canal to the truncus arteriosus. Normally it holds the aortic part of the truncus in fibrous continuity with the mitral part of the atrioventricular canal. He suggested that in transposition, truncal septation proceeds normally and the aorta and pulmonary artery are normally elaborated from the truncus, but the pulmonary part of the truncus is held in continuity with the mitral ring. The aorta is simply, in effect, pushed anteriorly by the strong fibrous attachment between the mitral and pulmonary rings and comes to lie in a position where normally musculature of the crista supraventricularis lies. Such an abnormality in the ventricular skeleton should be accompanied by predictable changes in the ventricular architecture and in the position of the coronary ostia. These predictable abnormalities include changes in the planes of the outflow tracts of both ventricles, narrowing of the crista supraventricularis, presence of the coronary ostia on each side of the tendon connecting the aorta and the pulmonary artery, irregular transillumination of the pars membranacea separating the left ventricle from the right ventricle, and shortening of the aortic–pulmonary ligament which results in the loss of the left ventricular muscle shoulder and probably also responsible for the occurrence of a ventricular septal defect.

The Hemodynamic Theory of Transposition

One of the oldest theories suggests that the normal position of the aorta and the pulmonary artery is due to the mechanical effects of the spiraling flow of blood through the bend primitive cardiac tube. Transposition of the great arteries, therefore, could be due to an abnormality in the spiral course of the blood flow. Goerttler (1956) thought that the shape of the myoepicardium of the primitive heart tube and the position of the blood streams are due to asymmetrical growth of the various components of the heart. The shape of the myoepicardium and the hemodynamic factors are the basis for the formation of cardiac valves, the occlusion of the ventricular septum, and the correct separation of the aorta and the pulmonary artery. He also pointed out that if damage affects certain parts of the myoepicardium, other growing parts are forced into abnormal torsions, and through this, blood streams alter their course and abnormal septation may result. Again if the growth of a heart section is retarded by relative or absolute diminution of cell number, there is an increase of the less damaged cells which originally had less metabolic activity. In general, the quickest growing parts expand to the side and front, where most space is available, since the vertebral column and later the differentiated atria are present dorsally. During the fifth week the growth of the proampoule from which the left ventricle develops is predominant. If growth of the proampoule is slowed down, the metaampoule (right ventricle) comes to the front. Goerttler used glass models representing this stage of heart development and found that the streams alter their course the more the metaampoule comes to the front. At first there was little change in the course of the two blood streams, but later part of the aortic stream joined the pulmonary stream or vice versa. Further diminution in the left ventricular part pushed the aortic stream anteriorly and to the right and the pulmonary stream posteriorly and to the left. Goerttler thought that these changes were characteristic of dextroposition of the aorta, and transposition of the great arteries, respectively. At strong angulation of the proampoule against the metaampoule, where the latter is far in front, streams characteristic of mitral stenosis or atresia, and aortic atresia are produced. He pointed out that all these malformations have in common hyperplasia of the right ventricle and hypoplasia of the left ventricle, often associated with a relative mitral stenosis or atresia. The right ventricle often forms the anterior wall of the heart, while sometimes the left ventricle is displaced dorsally as a rudimentary annex. Rychter and Lemez (1957, 1958) applied a rhombic clamp at the bulboventricular sulcus of the hearts of developing chick embryos at the third day of incubation. This resulted in origin of the aorta and the pulmonary artery from the right ventricle. The two vessels lay side by side with the aortic ostium to the right of the pulmonary artery ostium. A channel-like defect in the ventricular septum was usually present. In some cases, a rounded ledge extended from the ventricular septum to the pulmonary artery ostium and directed the blood stream from the left ventricle to the aorta "so that the transposition was hemodynamically corrected." When the clamp was applied on the fourth day of incubation, i.e., at a stage when the heart and bulbus septation were already advanced, transposition of the aorta did not always occur. In some instances the right edge of the atrioventricular cushions failed to fuse with the ventricular septum resulting in an unusually large ventricular septal defect. In others the right atrioventricular ostium had the appearance of the mitral valve. In a few isolated cases complete transposition of the aorta and the pulmonary artery was observed, but the mechanism of its production in these experiments remained ungoverned. Grant (1962) pointed out, however, that the hemodynamic factors may be due to the energy source responsible for the anomaly, and that such a theory does not identify the growth abnormality that takes place. Furthermore, the architectural changes in transposition are much more constant and systemic from case to case than would be expected from the vagaries of blood flow alone.

The Author's View on the Embryogenesis of Transposition

Two events occur during early cardiac development which will bring about normal alignment of the great arteries. (1) Torsion or twisting of the bulbus cordis, and (2) shift of the bulbus cordis to the midline. Abnormalities of the torsion mechanism will give rise to a spectrum of abnormalities in the anteroposterior relationship between the aorta and the pulmonary artery. Transposition of the great arteries, i.e., the aorta anterior to the pulmonary artery results from lack of torsion of the bulbus cordis. If the bulbus also fails to shift to the midline, the transposed great arteries will arise from the right ventricle. On the other hand, if the bulbus shifts to the midline the anterior aorta will arise from the right ventricle in front of the crista supraventricularis, and the posterior pulmonary artery will arise from the left ventricle. Much like the normal heart, a fibrous continuity develops between the mitral valve and the posterior semilunar valve, in this case the pulmonary.

Of the other theories, very few authors believe in the phylogenetic theories because of the apparent improbability and complexity of these theories. As pointed out by Van Praagh the hemodynamic theory did not demonstrate that the junctioning of the right and left ventricular streams in hearts with transposition is in fact different than when the great arteries are normally related. Of the ontogenetic theories, only two authors took into account the anatomy of the coronary arteries in transposition: Grant (1962) and Van Praagh (1967, 1971). Grant's hypothesis fails to explain what makes the pulmonary, rather than the aortic, part of the truncus held in continuity with the mitral ring thus giving rise to transposition. Van Praagh's original theory and its modification suggest that a slight deviation from the normal development of the subpulmonary conus gives rise to an extremely rare condition "transposition with posterior aorta," whereas a severe deviation gives rise to a common condition, "transposition with anterior aorta." Commenting on this theory Van Mierop (1971) said that it displays an amazing degree of flexibility to say the least.

References

Abbott, M. E. (1937). Congenital heart disease. *Nelson's Loose-Leaf Med.* 4, 207.
Aschoff, L. (1929). *Arch. Entwicklungsmech. Organismen* 116, 267. (Cited by Harris and Farber.)

Bremer, J. L. (1942). Transposition of the aorta and the pulmonary artery: an embryologic study of its cause. *Arch. Pathol.* **34**, 1016.

Bremer, J. L. (1957). "Congenital Anomalies of the Viscera, Their Embryological Basis." Harvard University Press, Cambridge, Massachusetts.

Brown, J. W. (1950). "Congenital Heart Disease," 2nd Ed. Staples Press, London.

Davis, C. L. (1927). Development of the human heart from its first appearance to the stage found in embryos of 20 paired somites. *Contrib. Embryol.* **19**, 245.

de la Cruz, M. V., and da Rocha, J. P. (1956). An ontogenetic theory for the explanation of congenital malformation involving the truncus and conus. *Amer. Heart J.* **51**, 782.

de Vries, P. A., and Saunders, J. B. D. M. (1962). Development of the ventricles and spiral outflow tract in the human heart. A contribution to the development of the human heart from age group IX to age group XV. *Contrib. Embryol.* **37**, 89.

Doerr, W. (1952). Pathologische Anatomie typischer Grundformen angeborener Herzfehler. *Monatsschr. Kinderheilk.* **100**, 107.

Freudenthal, P. (1927). *Virch. Arch. Pathol. Anat. Physiol.* **266**, 640. (Cited by Harris and Farber.)

Fuchs, F. (1925) . *Z. Anat. Entwicklungsgesch.* **75**, 1. (Cited by Harris and Farber.)

Gertsmann, H. (1929). *Virch. Arch. Pathol. Anat. Physiol.* **271**, 1. (Cited by Harris and Farber.)

Goerttler, K. (1956). Hämodynamische Untersuchun Über die Entstehung der Missbidungen des arteriellen Herzendes. *Virch. Arch.* **328**, 391.

Graevinghoff, W. (1927). *Monatsschr. Kinderheilk.* **35**, 273. (Cited by Harris and Farber.)

Grant, R. P. (1962). The morphogenesis of transposition of the great vessels. *Circulation* **26**, 819.

Harris, J. S., and Farber, S. (1939). Transposition of the great cardiac vessels with special reference to the phylogenetic theory of Spitzer. *Arch. Pathol.* **28**, 427.

Hoffmann, H. (1933) . *Zentralbl. Allg. Pathol. Pathol. Anat.* **56**, 321. (Cited by Harris and Farber.)

Homma, H. (1923). *Wien. Klin. Wochenschr.* **36**, 810. (Cited by Harris and Farber.)

Humphreys, E. M. (1932). *Arch. Pathol.* **14**, 671. (Cited by Harris and Farber.)

Ivemark, B. I. (1955). Implications of agenesis of the spleen on the pathogenesis of cono-truncus anomalies in childhood; analysis of heart malformations in splenic agenesis syndrome, with 14 new cases. *Acta Paediat. Scand.* **44**, (Suppl. 104) 1.

Jensen, G. (1932) . *Frankfurt. Z. Pathol.* **43**, 545. (Cited by Harris and Farber.)

Keith, A. (1906). Malformation of the bulbus cordis. *In* "Studies in Pathology" (William Bullock, ed.), Vol. 21, p. 57. Aberdeen University Studies, Aberdeen.

Keith, A. (1909). The Huntarian lectures on malformations of the heart. *Lancet* **2**, 359, 453, 519.

Keith, A. (1924). Schorstein lecture on the fate of the bulbus cordis in the human heart. *Lancet* **2**, 1267.

Kramer, T. C. (1942). The partioning of the truncus and conus and the formation of the membranous portion of the interventricular septum in the human heart. *Amer. J. Anat.* **71**, 343.

Kung, S. K. (1931). Trifft die Spitzer' sche Theorie fur die Fälle von Transposition der grossen Gefässe zu? *Beitr. Pathol. Anat. Allg. Pathol.* **88**, 127.

Kurschner, T. (1837). Commentatio de corde cuius ventricule inter se communicant. (Cited by J. W. Brown, "Congenital Heart Disease." Staples Press, London, 1950.)

Lev, M., and Vass, A. (1951). "The Architecture of Normal and Malformed Hearts." Thomas, Springfield, Illinois.

Lev, M., and Saphir, O. (1937). Transposition of the large vessels. *J. Tech. Methods* 17, 126.

Lev, M., and Saphir, O. (1945). A theory of transposition of the arterial trunks based on the phylogenetic and ontogenetic development of the heart. *Arch. Pathol.* 39, 172.

Lewis, F. T., and Abbott, M. (1915). Reversed torsion of the human heart. *Anat. Rec.* 9, 103.

Liebow, A. A., and McFarland (1941). "Corrected transposition" and persistent rudimentary "right aorta" as evidence in support of Spitzer's theory. *Arch. Pathol.* 32, 356.

McCullough, A. W., and Wilbur, E. L. (1944). Defect of endocardial cushion development as a source of cardiac anomaly. A presentation of four cases from autopsy reports. *Amer. J. Pathol.* 20, 321.

Mautner, H., and Lowy, M. (1921). *Virch. Arch. Pathol. Anat. Physiol.* 229, 337. (Cited by Harris and Farber.)

Meckel, J. (1812). "Handbuch Path. Anatomie," Band I. Leipsig. (Cited by J. W. Brown, "Congenital Heart Disease." Staples Press, London.)

Meyer, H. (1857). *Virch. Arch. Pathol. Anat. Physiol.* 12, 364. (Cited by Harris and Farber, 1939.)

Monckeberg, J. G. (1924). Die Missbildungen des Herzes. *In* "Handbuch der Speziellen Pathologischen Anatomie und Histologie" (F. Henke and O. Lubarsch, eds.), Vol. 2, pp. 1–183. Springer, Berlin.

Peacock, T. B. (1866). "On Malformation of the Human Heart," 2nd Ed. Churchill, London.

Pernkopf, E. (1926). Der partielle situs inversus der Eingeweide beim Menchen. *Z. Anat. Entwicklungsgesch.* 79, 577.

Pernkopf, E., and Wirtinger, W. (1933). Die transposition der Herzostien—ein Versuch der Erklärung dieser Erscheinung. *Z. Anat.* 100, 563.

Pernkopf, E., and Wirtinger, W. (1935). Das Wesen der transposition im Gebiete des Herzens. *Virch. Arch.* 295, 143.

Pye-Smith, P. H. (1872). Transposition of the aorta and pulmonary artery. *Trans. Pathol. Soc. London* 23, 80.

Robertson, J. I. (1913). The comparative anatomy of the bulbus cordis with special reference to abnormal positions of the great vessels in the human heart. *J. Pathol. Bacteriol.* 18, 191.

Rychter, Z., and Lemez, L. (1957). Experimentelle Untersuchung über die Entstehung sowie über die Lage und Grösse von Kammerseptum defekten am Herzen von Hühnerembryonen. *Verhandl. Anat. Ges.* 54, 97.

Rychter, Z., and Lemez, L. (1958). Experimenteller Beitrag zur Entstehung der Transposition von Aorta in die rechte Herzkammer der Huhnerembryonen. *Verhandl. Anat. Ges.* 55, 310.

Sato, S. (1914). Über die Entwickelung der Atrioventrikularklappen. *Anat. Hefte* 50, 193.

Schramm, H. G. (1929). *Beit. Z. Pathol. Anat. Allg. Pathol.* 82, 153. (Cited by Harris and Farber.)

Shaner, R. F. (1949). Malformation of the atrio-ventricular cushions of the embryo pig and its relation to defects of the conus and truncus arteriosus. *Amer. J. Anat.* 84, 431.

Shaner, R. F. (1951). Complete and corrected transposition of the aorta, pulmonary artery and ventricles in pig embryos, and a case of corrected transposition in a child. *Amer. J. Anat.* **88**, 35.

Shaner, R. F. (1962a). Comparative development of the bulbus and ventricles of the vertebrate heart with special reference to Spitzer's theory of heart malformations. *Anat. Rec.* **142**, 519.

Shaner, R. F. (1962b). Anomalies of the heart bulbus. *J. Pediat.* **61**, 233.

Shapiro, P. F. (1930). Detorsion defects in congenital cardiac anomalies. Report of three cases, with an analysis of the mechanism of their formation. *Arch. Pathol.* **9**, 54.

Spitzer, A. (1919). Uber die Urasachen und den Mechanismus der Zweiteilung des Wirbeltienherzens. *Arch. Entwicklungsmech. Organismen* **45**, 686.

Spitzer, A. (1921). Uber die Urasachen und den Mechanismus der Zweiteilung des wirbeltienherzens. *Arch. Entwicklungsmech. Organismen* **47**, 510.

Spitzer, A. (1923). Uber den Bauplan des normalen und missbildeten Herzens. *Virch. Arch. Path. Anat. Physiol.* **243**, 81. (Translated by M. Lev and A. Vass, Thomas, Springfield, Illinois, 1951.)

Spitzer, A. (1927). Zur Kritik der phylogenetischen Theorie der normalen und missbildeten Herzarchitektur. *Z. Anat. Entwicklungsgesch.* **84**, 30.

Spitzer, A. (1929). *Virchows Arch. Pathol. Anat. Physiol.* **271**, 226. (Cited by Harris and Farber.)

Streeter, G. L. (1948). Developmental horizons in human embryos. Description of age groups XV, XVI, XVII and XVIII, being the third issue of a servey of the Carnegie Collection. *Contrib. Embryol.* **32**, 133.

Van Mierop, L. H. S. (1971). Transposition of the great arteries. I. Clarification or further confusion. *Amer. J. Cardiol.* **28**, 735.

Van Mierop, L. H. S., and Wiglesworth, F. W. (1963). Pathogenesis of transposition complexes. II. Anomalies due to faulty transfer of the posterior great artery. *Amer. J. Cardiol.* **12**, 226.

Van Praagh, R. (1967). Complete transposition of the great arteries. *In* "Heart Disease in Infancy and Childhood" (J. D. Keith, R. D. Rowe, and P. Vlad., eds.), 2nd Ed. MacMillan, New York.

Van Praagh, R. (1971). Transposition of the great arteries. II. Transposition clarified. *Amer. J. Cardiol.* **28**, 739.

Van Praagh, R., Perez-Trevino, C., Lopez-Cuellar, M., Baker, F. W., Zuberbuhler, J. R., Quero, M., Perez, V. M., Moreno, F., and Van Praagh, S. (1971). Transposition of the great arteries with posterior aorta, anterior pulmonary artery, subpulmonary conus, and fibrous continuity between aortic and atrio-ventricular valves. *Amer. J. Cardiol.* **28**, 621.

von Rokitansky, C. F. (1875). "Die Defecte der Scheidewande des Herzens." Braumuller, Vienna.

Wurm, H. (1927). Angeborener Herzfehler mit "korrigierter" transposition der grossen Gefässe. *Virch. Arch. Pathol. Anat. Physiol.* **263**, 123.

Chapter 10

CARDIAC PATHOLOGY

One hundred and seventy-eight specimens with complete transposition of the great arteries were examined by the author. In each specimen the aorta arose from the right ventricle and the pulmonary artery from the left ventricle. Excluded from this study were specimens with mitral, tricuspid, or pulmonary atresia, or common ventricle. The identity of 166 specimens was known, and whenever applicable, associated lesions were studied in relationship to the age at death as follows: 0 to 2 weeks; 2 weeks to 3 months; 3 months to 1 year; and above 1 year.

In almost all specimens the heart and lungs were attached and thus the position of the cardiac apex was determined. In a few specimens the lungs were not attached to the heart and the position of the cardiac apex was obtained from the clinical records of the patient. Depending on the presence or absence of a ventricular septal defect or left ventricular outflow tract obstruction, specimens were classified into four groups.

Group I   With an intact ventricular septum—105 specimens
Group II   With an intact ventricular septum and left ventricular outflow tract obstruction—13 specimens
Group III With a ventricular septal defect—48 specimens
Group IV   With a ventricular septal defect and left ventricular outflow tract obstruction—12 specimens

Atria, Ventricles, and Great Arteries

THE SITUS OF THE HEART AND THE FORMATION OF THE CARDIAC APEX

In 175 specimens the heart was normally situated. Dextrocardia with solitus atria was present in 1, and with inversus atria in 2. In these 3 specimens the ventricular septum was intact. Table 10.1 shows the for-

TABLE 10.1

APEX FORMATION

Group	Age [a]	LV [b]	RV [b]	Both	Total
Group I	0–2w	32	3	23	58
(105 cases)	2w–3m	21	—	6	27
	3m–1y	6	—	2	8
	Above 1y	7	—	—	7
	Unknown	4	—	1	5
Total		70	3	32	105
Group II	0–2w	1	—	—	1
(13 cases)	2w–3m	—	—	2	2
	3m–1y	1	—	1	2
	Above 1y	3	—	2	5
	Unknown	2	—	1	3
Total		7	—	6	13
Group III	0–2w	5	—	1	6
(48 cases)	2w–3m	18	—	2	20
	3m–1y	9	—	1	10
	Above 1y	4	—	4	8
	Unknown	3	—	1	4
Total		39	—	9	48
Group IV	0–2w	—	1	—	1
(12 cases)	2w–3m	1	—	1	2
	3m–1y	—	—	1	1
	Above 1y	5	—	3	8
	Unknown	—	—	—	—
Total		6	1	5	12

[a] w, weeks; m, months; y, years.
[b] LV, left ventricle. RV, right ventricle.

mation of the cardiac apex in the four groups. Regardless of the anatomy of the associated defects or the age group, the apex of the heart was formed by the left ventricle in the majority of cases. Of the 178 specimens in this series the apex was formed by the left ventricle in 122, by the right ventricle in 4, and by both ventricles in 52.

The occurrence of complete transposition of the great arteries in situs inversus is extremely rare. Keith *et al.* (1958) encountered it among their material with dextrocardia. Jue *et al.* (1966) reported the anatomical and clinical features of such a case. Complete transposition with situs inversus was present in 2 patients of Deverall *et al.* (1969) and 1 patient of Indeglia *et al.* (1970). The present series and published reports suggest that situs inversus occurs in about 0.5% of the patients with complete transposition of the great arteries.

There is only one reference in the literature on the formation of the cardiac apex in transposition. Wilkinson *et al.* (1960) studied the formation of the apex of the heart in autopsied cases of complete transposition. They found that in cases with or without a ventricular septal defect, the apex is usually equally formed by both ventricles; occasionally the right or left ventricles predominated. In cases with a ventricular septal defect and pulmonary stenosis the apex is totally formed by the left ventricle but occasionally the right ventricle contributed partially. There is no explanation for the discrepancy between the present findings and those of Wilkinson and associates. Hemodynamic data, however, tend to support the present findings since most patients with transposition have increased pulmonary blood flow.

TABLE 10.2

SIZE OF VENTRICLES

Group	Age [a]	LV [a] larger	RV [a] larger	Equal	Total
Group I	0–2w	28	12	18	58
(84 cases)	2w–3m	18	4	5	27
	3m–1y	6	2	—	8
	Above 1y	6	1	—	7
	Unknown	3	1	1	5
Total		61	20	24	105
Group II	0–2w	1	—	—	1
(13 cases)	2w–3m	—	2	—	2
	3m–1y	1	1	—	2
	Above 1y	3	2	—	5
	Unknown	2	1	—	3
Total		7	6	—	13
Group III	0–2w	3	1	2	6
(36 cases)	2w–3m	16	—	4	20
	3m–1y	9	—	1	10
	Above 1y	3	1	4	8
	Unknown	2	—	2	4
Total		33	2	13	48
Group IV	0–2w	—	1	—	1
(12 cases)	2w–3m	—	—	2	2
	3m–1y	—	1	—	1
	Above 1y	4	2	2	8
	Unknown	—	—	—	—
Total		4	4	4	12

[a] Abbreviations as in Table 10.1.

SIZE OF THE VENTRICLES

The comparative size of the ventricles in relationship to each other is shown in Table 10.2. It is worth noting that the left ventricle appeared larger than the right ventricle in the majority of the specimens in the two groups without left ventricular outflow tract obstruction (Groups I and III) (Fig. 10.1). On the other hand, in the two groups with left ventricular outflow tract obstruction (Groups II and IV) the right ventricle was larger than the left in 36% of the secimens, the left larger than the right in 45%, and the two ventricles of equal size in 19%. In 10 specimens an unusually small right ventricle was present; 3 in Group I, 1 in Group II, and 6 in Group III (Fig. 10.2). Preductal coarctation of the aorta was present in 3 of these 10 specimens; 1 in Group I, and 2 in Group III. An unusually small left ventricle was observed in 2 specimens (Fig. 10.3). In 1 of these 2 specimens, left ventricular outflow tract obstruction, ventricular septal defect, and double mitral orifice were associated. In the other, the ventricular septum was intact and the small left ventricular cavity was caused by massive hypertrophy of the walls of this ventricle.

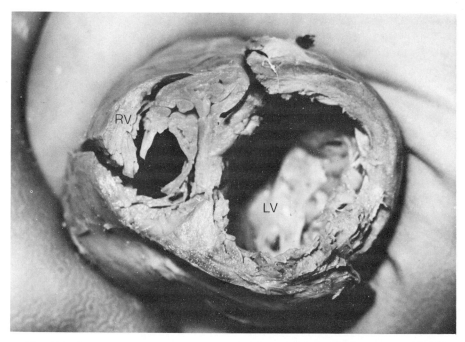

Fig. 10.1. Cross section of a heart with transposition and ventricular septal defect viewed from the apex showing left ventricle (LV) larger than right ventricle (RV).

The occurrence of hypoplastic right ventricle in some patients with transposition is well recognized. Smyth (1955) reported such a case associated with a ventricular septal defect and hypoplasia of the ascending aorta and preductal coarctation. Kessler and Adams (1957) reported the autopsy and clinical findings in a patient with transposition and hypoplasia of the right ventricle. Shaher *et al.* (1967) reported another case associated with left ventricular outflow tract obstruction, and pointed out that hypoplastic ventricles could pose a problem in the postoperative management of this condition. Riemschneider *et al.* (1968) reported 8 other cases with a small right ventricle; in 7 cases, a ventricular septal defect was present. Other lesions included hypoplasia of the aortic arch and patent ductus in 1, subaortic stenosis in 2, and subpulmonary stenosis in 2. As far as I can tell, hypoplasia of the left ventricle has not been described in transposition before.

THICKNESS OF THE VENTRICLES

The ventricular free walls and septum were measured at the point of maximum thickness, which was usually located at the midportion of the

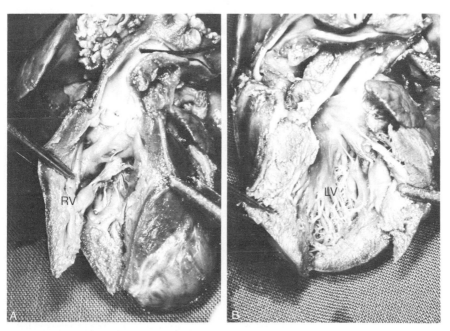

Fig. 10.2. Difference in size of the two ventricles. (A) The right ventricle (RV) is unusually small; (B) the left ventricle (LV) is larger.

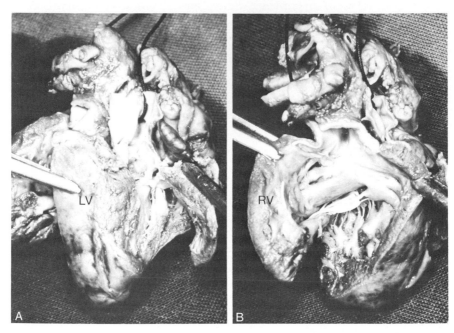

Fig. 10.3. Difference in size of the two ventricles. (A) Left ventricle (LV) with a ventricular septal defect is unusually small; (B) right ventricle (RV) is much larger.

free wall and the lower portion of the septum. The findings in the four groups are shown in Table 10.3. No attempt was made to quantitate the findings against normal controls since the left ventricle in complete transposition is a pulmonary ventricle and the right ventricle is a systemic ventricle. Fifty-two percent of all specimens had equal ventricular wall thickness. The majority of those with a predominant right ventricle had an intact ventricular septum. When the left ventricle was predominate, a ventricular septal defect was present in about 50%.

Calleja and Hosier (1960) measured the thickness of the ventricular walls in 25 patients with transposition of the great arteries. Isolated right ventricular hypertrophy occurred in 36%, isolated left ventricular hypertrophy in 8%, combined ventricular hypertrophy in 52%, and no ventricular hypertrophy in 4%. The anatomy of the ventricular septum in these cases was not described. In 1964, Calleja *et al.* reported that isolated right ventricular hypertrophy is produced either by a single shunt due to an atrial septal defect or by a shunt combination of a patent ductus and a ventricular septal defect. Left ventricular hypertrophy, isolated or com-

TABLE 10.3

THICKNESS OF VENTRICLES

Group	Age [a]	Dominant LV [a]	Dominant RV [a]	Equal	Total
Group I	0–2w	11	7	40	58
(105 cases)	2w–3m	11	8	8	27
	3m–1y	—	4	4	8
	Above 1y	—	7	—	7
	Unknown	—	1	4	5
Total		22	27	56	105
Group II	0–2w	1	—	—	1
(13 cases)	2w–3m	—	2	—	2
	3m–1y	—	1	1	2
	Above 1y	—	4	1	5
	Unknown	1	—	2	3
Total		2	7	4	13
Group III	0–2w	2	—	4	6
(48 cases)	2w–3m	10	—	10	20
	3m–1y	4	1	5	10
	Above 1y	2	4	2	8
	Unknown	1	—	3	4
Total		19	5	24	48
Group IV	0–2w	1	—	—	1
(12 cases)	2w–3m	—	—	2	2
	3m–1y	1	—	—	1
	Above 1y	2	2	4	8
	Unknown	—	—	—	—
Total		4	2	6	12

[a] Abbreviations as in Table 10.1.

bined with mild right ventricular hypertrophy, is produced exclusively by a patent ductus. Biventricular hypertrophy results from ventricular septal defect as a single shunt or from multiple shunts. On the other hand, Lev *et al.* (1969) quantitated 103 hearts with transposition of the great arteries against the normal controls of Rowlatt *et al.* (1963). They pointed out that in complete transposition with an atrial septal defect and patent ductus, there is pressure and volume hypertrophy of the right atrium and ventricle, and, in some cases, pressure hypertrophy of the left atrium and left ventricle. When there is a ventricular septal defect, in addition, there is greater hypertrophy and enlargement of the left ventricle. When there is pulmonary stenosis in addition to the ventricular septal defect, then the left ventricle reveals only pressure hypertrophy and its size is distinctly smaller than in cases without pulmonary stenosis.

THE ATRIOVENTRICULAR VALVES AND PAPILLARY MUSCLES

Anomalies of the atrioventricular valves and papillary muscles were observed in 14 specimens. Table 10.4 enumerates these anomalies in the four groups. Of the 3 in Group I, a parachute mitral valve (Shone *et al.,* (1963) and a small tricuspid valve were observed in 1, a small mitral valve in 1, and a small tricuspid valve in 1. Of the 3 in Group II, a parachute mitral valve was present in 1, and small tricuspid valve in 1, and a cleft anterior leaflet of the mitral valve in 1 with a common atrium. Of the 5 in Group III, a parachute mitral valve was observed in 2, a small mitral valve in 1, congenital mitral stenosis in 1, and a small tricuspid valve in 1. Of the 3 in Group IV a small mitral valve was present in 1, a cleft anterior leaflet of the mitral valve in 1, and double mitral orifice in 1 (both orifices appeared narrowed) (Fig. 10.4). In the last 2 specimens the ventricular septal defect was of the atrioventricular canal type.

TABLE 10.4

ANOMALIES OF THE ATRIOVENTRICULAR VALVES AND PAPILLARY MUSCLES

	Group I	Group II	Group III	Group IV
Parachute mitral	1	1	2	—
Small mitral	1	—	1	1
Mitral stenosis	—	—	1	—
Small tricuspid	2	1	1	—
Cleft mitral	—	1	—	1
Double mitral orifice	—	—	—	1
Number of specimens	3	3	5	3

The earliest reference on abnormalities of the atrioventricular in patients with intact ventricular septum is quoted by Cockle (1863) who reported a patient with transposition and two tricuspid atrioventricular valves. Among cases with an intact ventricular septum reported by Elliott *et al.* (1963a), a cleft in the septal leaflet of the tricuspid valve was observed in one. In another, the basal aspect of the medial portion of each of the two cusps of the mitral valve was attached to the ventricular wall in a manner similar to that observed in cases of Ebstein's malformation of the tricuspid valve. In addition, the ventricular aspect of the anterior cusp was adherent to the septal wall of the outflow tract of the left ventricle in such a way that the effective channel of the outflow tract of this ventricle was reduced to a width of a few millimeters. Evidence of incompetence of the mitral valve was found in the form of a rolling of its edges and in enlargement of the left atrium. In a study on anomalies of the valves in transposition, Layman and Edwards (1967) reported abnormalities of the semilunar or atrioventricular valves in 23 of 88 specimens with complete transposition of the great arteries. Of the group with an intact ventricular septum, a cleft anterior leaflet of the mitral valve with an accessory orifice was seen in 1, a parachute mitral in 2, and a cleft between the anterior and septal leaflets of the tricuspid valve in 1.

The earliest reference on abnormalities of the atrioventricular valves in patients with a ventricular septal defect is given by King (1844). This author reported a patient with transposition of the great arteries, ventri-

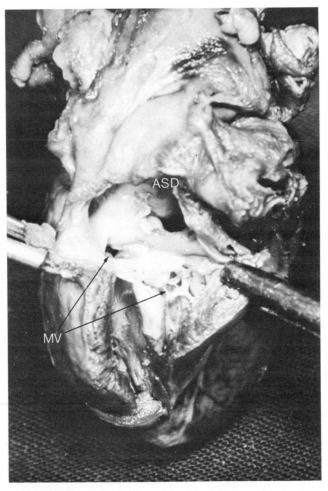

Fig. 10.4. Left ventricle and atrium. Arrows point to double mitral orifice. **MV,** mitral valve; ASD, atrial septal defect.

cular septal defect, and two tricuspid atrioventricular valves. Ashby (1881) reported a patient in whom one of the cusps of the tricuspid valve herniated through a ventricular septal defect into the left ventricle. In Case 8 of Harris and Farber (1939) the medial cusp of the right atrioventricular valve was not attached to a papillary muscle, but was attached directly to the ventricular septum. In Weiss's patient (1947) each of the two atrioventricular valves presented two large leaflets and a third smaller one, the demarcation of these leaflets being more distinct in the left valve. Case 123 of Andersen and Kelly (1956) had a bicuspid right atrioventricular valve and a tricuspid left atrioventricular valve. One of the 12 patients of Emerson and Green (1942) and 2 of the 75 of Baffes *et al.* (1957) had mitral stenosis. Slight stenosis of the mitral valve was present in Case 6, Group 2B of Noonan *et al.* (1960). In the group of 95 cases of complete transposition of the great arteries associated with a ventricular septal defect or a single ventricle studied morphologically by Lev *et al.* (1961), tricuspid atresia or stenosis were present in 11, and a common atrioventricular orifice in 8. Of the 22 cases with a ventricular septal defect reported by Elliott *et al.* (1963), 3 had a cleft in the septal leaflet of the tricuspid valve and a communication between the left ventricle and the right atrium. Layman and Edwards (1967) reported that among their specimens with complete transposition and a ventricular septal defect a cleft between the anterior and septal leaflets of the tricuspid valve with a left ventricular–right atrial communication occurred in 1, a cleft anterior leaflet of the mitral valve in 2 (one with an accessory orifice), a parachute mitral valve in 1, and a partial atrioventricularis communis in 1. In 5 other specimens, in which the presence or absence of a ventricular septal defect was not stated, the anterior leaflet of the mitral valve was adherent to the ventricular septum. Riemenschneider *et al.* (1969) described 2 patients with transposition of the great arteries and a ventricular septal defect. In each case, redundant tricuspid valve tissue protruded through the ventricular septal defect into the left ventricular outflow tract, producing severe obstruction to the outflow of blood from the left ventricle. Rastelli *et al.* (1969a) emphasized the frequent association between complete transposition of the great arteries with left ventricular outflow tract obstruction and anomalies of the mitral valve. Of their 8 autopsied cases, abnormalities of the mitral valve were observed in 3. One patient had a parachutelike mitral valve with two orifices and an anterior leaflet with a large aneurysmlike formation that bulged and partially obstructed the left ventricular outflow tract. One patient had valvular tissue that extended from the mitral valve to the right ventricle where it attached through the ventricular septal defect.

One patient had a fibrous attachment of the anterior leaflet of the mitral valve to the anterior aspect of the left ventricular outflow tract giving rise to subvalvular pulmonary stenosis.

MITRAL VALVE–PULMONARY VALVE CONTINUITY

A continuity between the anterior leaflet of the mitral valve and the posterior cusp of the pulmonary valve and the pulmonary valve ring occurred in all but 6 specimens; 1 in Group I, 3 in Group II, and 2 in Group III. In these 6 specimens, mitral–pulmonary valve discontinuity was present and a muscular subpulmonary conus existed.

In all specimens there was no fibrous continuity between the aortic valve and either the mitral or tricuspid valves.

TABLE 10.5

SIZE OF ATRIA

Group	Age [a]	RA>LA [b]	LA>RA	Equal	Damage
Group I	0–2w	36	1	15	6
(105 cases)	2w–3m	14	—	12	1
	3m–1y	4	—	4	—
	Above 1y	3	—	1	3
	Unknown	4	1	—	—
Total		61	2	32	10
Group II	0–2w	—	—	1	—
(13 cases)	2w–3m	2	—	—	—
	3m–1y	2	—	—	—
	Above 1y	1	—	3	1
	Unknown	3	—	—	—
Total		8	0	4	1
Group III	0–2w	5	1	—	—
(48 cases)	2w–3m	8	3	8	1
	3m–1y	4	2	2	2
	Above 1y	3	1	1	3
	Unknown	3	—	1	—
Total		23	7	12	6
Group IV	0–2w	1	—	—	—
(12 cases)	2w–3m	2	—	—	—
	3m–1y	1	—	—	—
	Above 1y	6	—	1	1
	Unknown	—	—	—	—
Total		10	0	1	1

[a] Abbreviations as in Table 10.1.
[b] LA, left atrium; RA, right atrium.

SIZE OF THE ATRIA

As shown in Table 10.5 the right atrium was larger than the left atrium in 102 specimens, the left atrium was larger than the right atrium in 9, while the two atria were of equal size in 49. Of the remaining 18 specimens, a common atrium was present in 1, and the comparative size of the atria could not be assessed because of surgical procedures involvig the atrial septum in 17.

POSITION OF THE ATRIAL APPENDAGES

In five specimens there was left juxtaposition of the atrial appendages; 2 in Group I, 1 in Group II, and 2 in Group IV. In these 5 specimens the heart was normally situated and the two atrial appendages were placed side by side to the left of the great arteries.

The term left or right juxtaposition of the atrial appendages has been suggested by Dixon (1954) to describe the condition where both atrial appendages lie side by side to the left or to the right of the great arteries, respectively. Left juxtaposition of the atrial appendages was present in necropsied cases of complete transposition of the great arteries reported by Miskall and Fraser (1948), Smyth (1955), Stuart and Flint (1957), Edwards (1960), Roberts et al. (1962), Snllen et al. (1962); 4 cases, Elliott et al. (1963a); 2 cases, Puech et al. (1966), Melhuish and Van Praagh (1968); 3 cases with subaortic conus, Rastelli et al. (1969b), Daicoff et al. (1969), and Wagner et al. (1970). Case 117 of Andersen and Kelly (1956) had malposition of the right auricular appendage.

POSITION OF THE AORTA AND THE PULMONARY ARTERY

The external relationship of the aorta and the pulmonary artery to each other when the specimen is held so that the ventricular septum

TABLE 10.6

POSITION OF THE AORTA AND THE PULMONARY ARTERY

Group	Side to side	Anterior and right	Anterior	Anterior and left
Group I (105 cases)	35	67	1	2 (situs inversus)
Group II (13 cases)	4	9	—	—
Group III (48 cases)	21	27	—	—
Group IV (12 cases)	—	12	—	—
Total	60	115	1	2

forms the median plane is given Table 10.6. The most common pattern is that in which the aorta lies anteriorly and to the right of the pulmonary artery. Less frequently is that in which the two vessels lie side by side with the aorta to the right of the pulmonary artery. In only one specimen the aorta was directly in front of the pulmonary artery, while in two others with situs inversus, the aorta was anterior and to the left of the pulmonary artery. As pointed out by Elliott *et al.* (1963) when the aorta is anterior and to the right of the pulmonary artery the left aortic sinus is situated along the left aspect of the aorta. With a side to side relationship between the aorta and the pulmonary artery, the left aortic sinus is situated in the left anterior position.

According to Lev *et al.* (1961), the aorta is usually situated anteriorly and to the right and the pulmonary artery posteriorly and to the left. Occasionally the aorta is situated anteriorly and the pulmonary artery posteriorly, or the aorta is to the right and the pulmonary artery to the left. In

TABLE 10.7

SIZE OF AORTA AND PULMONARY ARTERY

Group	Age	PA>Ao [a]	Ao>PA	Equal	Total
Group I	0–2w	21	1	36	58
(105 cases)	2w–3m	14	—	13	27
	3m–1y	3	—	5	8
	Above 1y	6	—	1	7
	Unknown	3	—	2	5
Total		47	1	57	105
Group II	0–2w	—	—	1	1
(13 cases)	2w–3m	1	—	1	2
	3m–1y	2	—	—	2
	Above 1y	2	1	2	5
	Unknown	2	1	—	3
Total		7	2	4	13
Group III	0–2w	4	—	2	6
(48 cases)	2w–3m	18	1	1	20
	3m–1y	10	—	—	10
	Above 1y	8	—	—	8
	Unknown	3	—	1	4
Total		43	1	4	48
Group IV	0–2w	—	1	—	1
(12 cases)	2w–3m	—	2	—	2
	3m–1y	—	1	—	1
	Above 1y	—	8	—	8
	Unknown	—	—	—	—
Total		—	12	—	12

[a] Ao, aorta; PA, pulmonary artery. Other abbreviations the same as in Table 10.1.

one of their cases with an intact ventricular septum, the aorta was anterior and to the left, and the pulmonary artery posterior and to the right. Elliott *et al.* (1963) classified the relationship of the aorta and the pulmonary artery in their 60 cases as follows: (1) oblique relationship (39 cases), where the aorta was situated obliquely with respect to the pulmonary artery, and more anterior than the latter vessel; and (2) side to side relationship (19 cases), where the ascending aorta was situated to the right of the pulmonary artery.

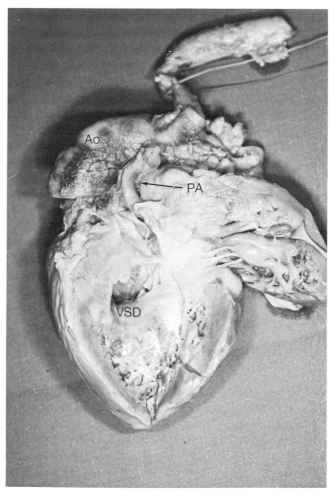

Fig. 10.5. Ventricular septal defect and pulmonary infundibular stenosis. Pulmonary artery (PA) much smaller than aorta (Ao). Ventricular septal defect (VSD) of the A-V canal type.

Size of the Aorta and the Pulmonary Artery

Table 10.7 shows the size of the aorta and pulmonary artery in the four groups. In cases with an intact ventricular septum the aorta and the pulmonary artery were of equal size in slightly more than 50% of the specimens. When a ventricular septal defect was associated, the pulmonary artery was almost always larger than the aorta. In all specimens with a ventricular septal defect and pulmonary stenosis, the aorta was larger than the pulmonary artery (Fig. 10.5). On the other hand, in the group

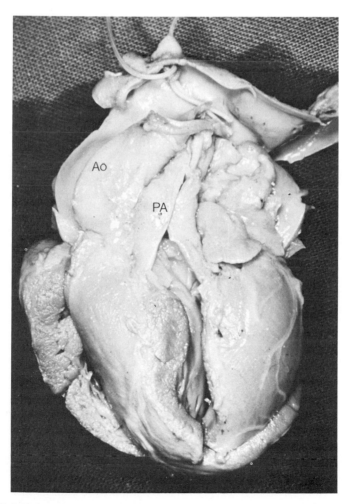

Fig. 10.6. External view of a heart with muscular obstruction of the outflow tract of the left ventricle. Note the small pulmonary artery (PA) compared to aorta (Ao).

of an intact ventricular septum and left ventricular outflow tract obstruction, the pulmonary artery was larger than the aorta in 7, the two vessels were of equal size in 4, and the aorta was larger than the pulmonary artery in 2 (Fig. 10.6).

In the group of patients studied by Mustard *et al.* (1954), 60% had equal sized aorta and pulmonary artery. In most of the remainder, the pulmonary artery was greater than the aorta in diameter, while in a small minority the aorta was larger than the pulmonary artery. Lev *et al.* (1961) reported that the pulmonary artery was larger than, equal to, or smaller than the aorta in those with an intact ventricular septum. In most of their cases with a ventricular septal defect without pulmonary stenosis, the pulmonary artery was larger than the aorta. When pulmonary stenosis was associated with a ventricular septal defect, the pulmonary artery was smaller than the aorta or they were the same size, being related to the poststenotic dilatation. Among 60 cases reported by Elliott *et al.* (1963a), the pulmonary artery was equal in size or larger than the aorta in 58, while in the remaining 2, the aorta was of normal size and the diameter of the pulmonary artery was half the diameter of the aorta. Both of these cases had pulmonary stenosis.

POSITION OF THE AORTIC ARCH

In only two specimens with dextrocardia with situs inversus the aortic arch was right sided.

The occurrence of a right aortic arch in transposition is very uncommon. Review of the literature shows that in 1 of the 8 cases reported by Ash *et al.* (1939), 2 of the 9 cases of Abrams (1951), and 2 of the 60 cases of Elliott *et al.* (1963a), the aortic arch was situated on the side opposite to that of the cardiac apex.

THE AORTIC AND PULMONARY VALVES

In all specimens the aortic valve was normal. The pulmonary valve appeared normal in almost all specimens in Groups I and III. A bicuspid pulmonary valve was observed in only 3 specimens in Group III. On the other hand, the pulmonary valve was abnormal in a significant number of the specimens in Groups II and IV. This finding will be discussed in the section on left ventricular outflow tract obstruction.

It would seem that abnormalities of the aortic valve are extremely rare in transposition. A bicuspid aortic valve was present in 2 of the 60 specimens reported by Elliott *et al.* (1963a). Of the 88 specimens examined by Layman and Edwards (1967), a bicuspid aortic valve was present in 1, and a unicuspid stenotic aortic valve in 1.

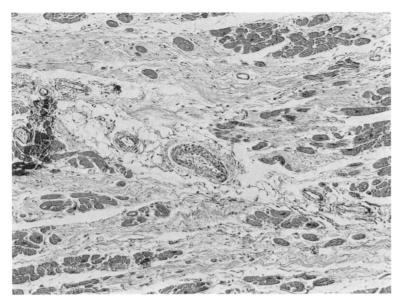

Fig. 10.7. Section from the right ventricle showing diffuse myocardial fibrosis (x100).

THE MYOCARDIUM

Microscopic examination of the myocardium of 8 patients in this series (Shaher, 1963) demonstrated myocardial hypertrophy of the right ventricle in 7 and of the left ventricle in 4. Focal or diffuse fibrosis of the right ventricular myocardium occurred in 6, and of the left ventricle in 3 (Fig. 10.7). Patchy subendocardial fibrosis of the right ventricle was observed in 3 patients.

The occurrence of myocardial fibrosis and infarction in some patients with transposition is recognized. Thus, Abbott (1936) reported a case of complete transposition with extensive fibrosis of the myocardium of the conus of the right ventricle which caused occlusion of the aortic orifice. Case 8 of Harris and Farber (1939) showed moderate interstitial edema and slight degenerative changes in the subendocardial myocardium, while their Case 11 showed marked congestion, mild scattered vacuolation, and a coarse granular appearance of the muscle fibers. Astley and Parsons (1952) found that microscopic examination of the myocardium in transposition always shows necrobiotic changes in the heart muscle with loss of striations, nuclear degeneration, and hyaline changes; destruction of muscle fibers is often severe. Bernreiter (1958) reported in a case of a 7-week-old baby with transposition of the great arteries, an intact ventricular septum, patent foramen ovale, and patent ductus arteriosus. Before death the electrocardiogram showed the pattern of myocardial infarction and at postmortem small areas of ischemic necrosis associated with interstitial hemorrhages in the ventricular septum were found. In a group of babies who cried as though they were in pain, reported by Noonan *et al.* (1960), the electrocardiogram of one showed the signs of myocardial ischemia and histological evidence of subacute myocardial necrosis was found at postmortem. Three additional infants were also found to have myocardial necrosis. The occurrence of myocardial infarcts in transposition has also been emphasized by Franciosi and Blanc (1968).

The etiology of myocardial fibrosis and infarction in some cases of complete transposition of the great arteries is probably related to the degree of coronary arterial blood desaturation, and the amount of pressure or volume work performed by the ventricles. It is significant that coronary arterial thrombosis was not a feature of reported cases in which myocardial infarction had occurred.

THE ENDOCARDIUM

Localized thickening of the endocardium of the left side of the ventricular septum was observed in 6 specimens with an intact ventricular septum and muscular subvalvular pulmonary stenosis. In each specimen the endocardial thickening was present above the side of muscular obstruction. In an additional specimen with ventricular septal defect and pulmonary stenosis, fibroelastosis of the left atrium was found.

Endocardial fibrosis has been reported in some cases of transposition. The case described by Pung *et al.* (1955) showed slight thickening and fibrosis of the lining of the two sides of the heart. Andersen and Kelly (1956) pointed out that in transposition localized fibrosis (jet effect) occurs on the right ventricular wall in the region of the conus which lies opposite the ventricular septal defect. Thickening of the endocardium of the left surface of the septum was often seen in older infants. In older cases moderate fibrosis was observed throughout both right atrium and ventricle. Endocardial fibrosis was observed in 1 of the cases of Keith *et al.* (1958), and in 6 of the 21 autopsied cases described by Noonan *et al.* (1960).

The Coronary Arteries

The main coronary arteries and their branches were dissected free of epicardial tissue or superficial myocardium in all specimens. The main

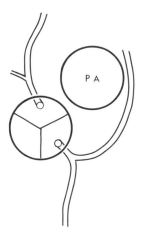

Fig. 10.8. Origin of the left coronary artery from left sinus and right artery from posterior sinus. PA, pulmonary artery. From Shaher and Puddu (1966), by permission of *Amer. J. Cardiol.*

branches were identified. The aortic sinuses were designated right, left, and posterior. Nine coronary arterial patterns could be recognized (Shaher and Puddu, 1966). These patterns are illustrated in Fig. 10.8–10.16 and are correlated to the associated defects in Table 10.8.

ORIGIN OF THE LEFT CORONARY ARTERY FROM LEFT SINUS AND RIGHT ARTERY FROM POSTERIOR SINUS—SINGLE OSTIUM ABOVE LEFT SINUS AND SINGLE OSTIUM ABOVE POSTERIOR OSTIUM (111 SPECIMENS; FIG. 10.8)

A single coronary ostium above the left sinus gave rise to the left coronary artery, while a single coronary ostium above the posterior sinus gave rise to the right coronary artery. The left artery emerged between the root of the aorta and that of the pulmonary artery and divided almost at once into one or more anterior descending arteries and the left circumflex artery. The anterior descending artery ran in the anterior interventricular sulcus toward the apex of the heart. It supplied branches to the anterior surface of both ventricles and to the ventricular septum. The left circumflex artery coursed to the left either immediately in front of the root of the pulmonary artery or a few millimeters below it and was embedded in the superficial epicardium or myocardium. After giving branches to the left atrium and lateral wall of the left ventricle, it continued its course in the left atrioventricular sulcus to end as small branches on the posterior surface of the heart.

TABLE 10.8

CORONARY ARTERIAL ANATOMY IN THE FOUR GROUPS STUDIED

Coronary arterial anatomy	Intact ventricular septum	Intact ventricular septum and PS	Ventricular septal defect	Ventricular septal defect and pulmonary stenosis
1. Right artery from posterior sinus Left artery from left sinus	71	7	26	7
2. Left circumflex branch of right coronary artery				
a. Single posterior ostium	14	1	5	3
b. Double posterior ostium	6	1	3	0
3. Single coronary artery				
a. From left sinus	1	2	0	0
b. From posterior sinus, left artery behind pulmonary artery	4	0	1	0
c. From posterior sinus, left artery in front of aorta	0	0	1	0
d. From posterior sinus, common origin of right coronary and left circumflex	0	0	1	0
e. From right sinus	0	0	1	0
4. Anterior descending artery branch of right coronary artery	2	0	4	0
5. Common origin of right and left arteries				
a. Above posterior sinus, left circumflex in front of pulmonary artery	3	0	1	0
b. Above posterior sinus, left circumflex behind pulmonary artery	1	0	0	0
c. Above posterior sinus, anterior descending branch of right artery	0	1	0	0
d. Above right sinus	0	0	0	1
6. Absent left circumflex	1	0	3	0
7. Single artery and additional small branch				
a. Single artery above posterior sinus, small branch above left sinus				
i. Left circumflex branch of right artery	0	0	0	1
ii. Common origin of left circumflex and anterior descending artery	0	0	1	0
b. Single artery above left sinus, small branch above posterior sinus	0	0	1	0

TABLE 10.8 Cont'd.

8. Two left circumflex arteries	2	0	0	0
9. Origin of right coronary artery from left sinus and left coronary artery from posterior sinus	0	1	0	0
Total	105	13	48	12

The right coronary artery emerged from the posterior coronary sinus. The first branch was usually the sinoatrial artery which ran on the anterior wall of the right atrium. Occasionally, however, the right conal artery was the first branch. It continued its course in the right atrioventricular sulcus as the right circumflex artery and supplied branches to the right atrium and the lateral wall of the right ventricle then proceeded in the posterior atrioventricular sulcus. After giving off branches to the posterior atrial and ventricular walls, it ended in the posterior interventricular groove as the posterior descending artery.

Left Circumflex Artery as a Branch of Right Coronary Artery (33 Specimens)

Single Ostium above Left Sinus and Single Ostium above Posterior Sinus (23 Specimens; Fig. 10.9A)

A single ostium above the left sinus gave rise to the anterior descending artery only and a single ostium above the posterior sinus gave rise to an artery which divided at once into the left circumflex artery and the

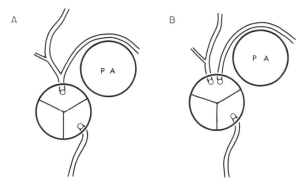

Fig. 10.9. Left circumflex artery as a branch of right coronary artery. (A) Single ostium above left sinus and single ostium above posterior sinus. (B) Single ostium above left sinus. Double posterior ostia. From Shaher and Puddu (1966), by permission of *Amer. J. Cardiol.*

right coronary artery. The left circumflex artery coursed behind the pulmonary artery to appear in the left anterior atrioventricular sulcus immediately lateral to the pulmonary artery. The right coronary artery coursed in the right anterior atrioventricular sulcus to the posterior surface of the heart.

Single Ostium above Left Sinus and Double Ostia above Posterior Sinus (11 Specimens; Fig. 10.9B)

A single ostium above the left sinus gave origin to the anterior descending artery. A right and left ostia above the posterior sinus gave origin to the right coronary artery and the left circumflex branch, respectively. The left circumflex branch coursed behind the pulmonary artery.

SINGLE CORONARY ARTERY (11 SPECIMENS)

Single Ostium above Left Sinus (3 Specimens; Fig. 10.10A)

A single ostium above the left sinus gave rise to a single coronary artery. This artery divided at once into a right coronary artery, anterior descending artery, and a left circumflex artery. The left circumflex artery coursed in front of the pulmonary artery.

Single Ostium above Posterior Sinus (7 Specimens; Fig. 10.10B,C,D)

In 7 specimens a single ostium above the posterior sinus gave origin to a single artery which pursued three different courses. In 5, the artery divided at once into right and left branches. The left branch ran to the left behind the pulmonary artery. At the angle between the pulmonary artery and the left atrial appendage it appeared on the anterior surface of the heart and divided into the anterior descending artery and the left circumflex artery. The right artery pursued its normal course (Fig. 10.10B).

In one specimen the single artery divided at once into two branches (Fig. 10.10C); the first branch gave two branches to the right atrium and continued in the right atrioventricular sulcus to end as the posterior descending artery. The second branch gave off right marginal branches and turned to the left in front of the aortic root. At the level of the ventricular septum it gave off the anterior descending artery and continued in front of the pulmonary artery and in the left anterior atrioventricular groove as the left circumflex artery. In one specimen the single artery divided into two branches (Fig. 10.10D). One branch gave rise to the right coronary artery and the left circumflex artery which coursed behind the pulmonary artery, while the other branch turned to the right to partially encircle the root of the aorta and continued as the anterior descending artery.

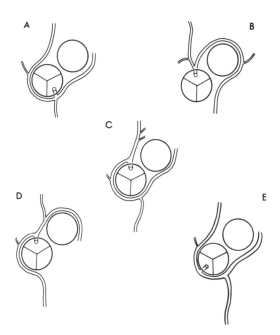

Fig. 10.10. Single coronary artery. (A) Single ostium above left sinus. (B) Single ostium above posterior sinus. The left coronary artery courses behind the pulmonary artery. (C) Single ostium above posterior sinus. The left coronary artery courses in front of the root of aorta. (D) Single ostium above posterior sinus, the left circumflex branch of right artery. The anterior descending artery courses in front of the aortic root. (E) Single ostium above right sinus. The left coronary artery courses in front of the aortic root. Shaher and Puddu (1966), by permission of *Amer. J. Cardiol.*

Single Ostium above Right Sinus (1 Specimen; Fig. 10.10E)

In one specimen a single ostium above the right sinus gave origin to a single artery which divided at once into right and left branches. The right branch continued as the normal right coronary artery. The left branches gave off the anterior descending coronary artery and pursued anterior to the pulmonary artery as the left circumflex artery.

ORIGIN OF THE RIGHT CORONARY ARTERY AND THE ANTERIOR DESCENDING ARTERY FROM THE LEFT SINUS, ORIGIN OF THE LEFT CIRCUMFLEX ARTERY FROM THE POSTERIOR SINUS (6 SPECIMENS; FIG. 10.11)

A single ostium above the left sinus gave rise to the anterior descending artery and the right coronary artery. A single ostium above the pos-

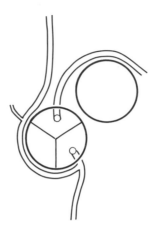

Fig. 10.11. Anterior descending artery and right coronary artery from left sinus. The left circumflex artery arises from the posterior sinus. From Shaher and Puddu (1966), by permission of *Amer. J. Cardiol.*

terior sinus gave rise to the left circumflex artery. This artery coursed to the left behind the pulmonary artery and terminated in the left atrioventricular groove by supplying branches to the left atrium and anterior and lateral walls of the left ventricle. The ostium above the left sinus gave rise to an artery which divided into one or more anterior descending arteries and then coursed to the right in front of the aortic root in the right anterior atrioventricular groove. It gave off marginal branches and terminated as the posterior descending artery.

TWO OSTIA ABOVE ONE SINUS (ONE OSTIUM GIVES RISE TO THE RIGHT CORONARY ARTERY AND THE OTHER OSTIUM GIVES RISE TO THE LEFT CORONARY ARTERY (7 SPECIMENS; FIG. 10.12A,B,C,D)

Two Ostia above Posterior Sinus (6 Specimens)

Three different patterns were encountered. In 4 specimens the left artery arose from the left ostium, appeared on the anterior surface of the heart between the aorta and the pulmonary artery, and then divided into the anterior descending and the left circumflex arteries (Fig. 10.12A). The right artery arose from the right ostium and took a normal course.

In one specimen the left artery coursed behind the pulmonary artery and appeared on the anterior surface of the heart lateral to the pulmonary artery in the anterior left atrioventricular sulcus. It divided into an anterior descending and left circumflex arteries (Fig. 10.12B). The right artery arose from the right ostium and pursued a normal course. In one specimen the right ostium gave rise to the left circumflex artery, which coursed behind the pulmonary artery, while the left ostium gave rise to an artery which appeared on the anterior surface of the heart between the pulmonary artery and the aorta (Fig. 10.12C). It divided into the anterior descending artery and the right coronary artery.

Two Ostia above the Right Sinus (1 Specimen)

Two ostia were situated above the right anterior sinus (Fig. 10.12D). The right ostium gave off the right coronary artery while the left ostium gave rise to the left coronary artery. The left artery divided into the anterior descending and the left circumflex arteries. The left circumflex artery coursed to the left in front of the root of the aorta and that of the pulmonary artery to the left atrioventricular sulcus.

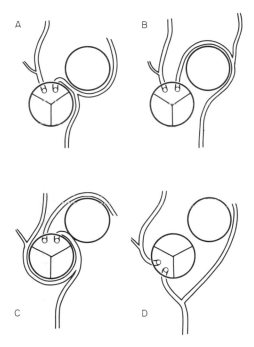

Fig. 10.12. (A) Two ostia above posterior sinus. The right ostium gives right coronary artery. The left ostium gives left artery which reaches the anterior surface of the heart between the aorta and the pulmonary artery. (B) Two ostia above posterior sinus. The left ostium gives rise to left coronary artery which courses behind the pulmonary artery. (C) Two ostia above posterior sinus. The left ostium gives anterior descending and right coronary artery. The right ostium gives the left circumflex artery. (D) Two ostia above right sinus. The right ostium gives right coronary artery. The left ostium gives left coronary artery. From Shaher and Puddu (1966), by permission of *Amer. J. Cardiol.*

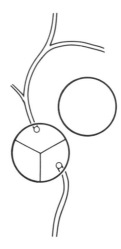

Fig. 10.13. Absent left circumflex artery. From Shaher and Puddu (1966), by permission of *Amer. J. Cardiol.*

ABSENT LEFT CIRCUMFLEX ARTERY (4 SPECIMENS; FIG. 10.13)

A single ostium above the posterior sinus gave origin to the right coronary artery and a single ostium above the left sinus gave origin to the anterior descending artery only. The right coronary artery gave off marginal branches, the posterior descending artery and continued in the left posterior atrioventricular sulcus giving branches to the lateral wall of the left ventricle.

SINGLE OSTIUM GIVING RISE TO THE RIGHT AND LEFT CORONARY ARTERIES AND SINGLE OSTIUM GIVES RISE TO A SMALL ADDITIONAL BRANCH (3 SPECIMENS; FIG. 10.14A, B, C)

Single Ostium above Posterior Sinus Gives Rise to a Single Artery. Single Ostium above Left Sinus Gives Small Additional Branch (2 Specimens)

In one case, the posterior ostium gave rise to a single artery which appeared on the anterior surface of the heart behind the right border of the aorta. It divided almost at once into two large branches. The right branch gave rise to several branches to the anterior surface of the right ventricle, continued in front of the base of the aorta, and terminated as the anterior descending artery (Fig. 10.14A). The left artery divided into two branches. The first was the left circumflex artery which coursed to the left behind the pulmonary artery. The second branch was the right coronary artery. The single ostium above the left sinus gave off a small artery which supplied the anterior surface of the right ventricle. In the other specimen a single ostium above the posterior sinus gave rise to the right and left coronary arteries. The left coronary artery coursed behind the pulmonary artery. A small ostium above the left sinus gave rise to a small additional branch (Fig. 10.14B).

Single Ostium above Left Sinus Gives Rise to a Single Artery. Single Ostium above Posterior Sinus Gives Rise to Additional Branch (1 Specimen)

A single ostium above the left sinus gave origin to a single artery and a single ostium above the posterior sinus gave off an additional small branch (Fig. 10.14C). The single artery divided into four branches of

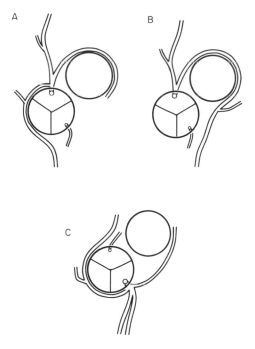

Fig. 10.14. (A) Single ostium above posterior sinus gives single artery. A small additional branch above left sinus. Left circumflex artery branch of right coronary artery. (B) Single ostium above posterior sinus. Small additional branch above left sinus. The left artery courses behind the pulmonary artery. (C) Single ostium above right sinus gives the single artery. Single ostium above posterior sinus gives an additional branch. From Shaher and Puddu (1966), by permission of *Amer. J. Cardiol.*

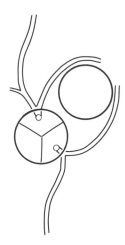

Fig. 10.15. Two left circumflex arteries. From Shaher and Puddu (1966), by permission of *Amer. J. Cardiol.*

equal size—a left circumflex, which coursed in front of the root of the pulmonary artery, two anterior descending arteries, and a right coronary artery. The right artery passed in front of the root of the aorta to the lateral border of the heart where it turned in the right atrioventricular sulcus and continued as the posterior descending artery. The single ostium above the posterior sinus gave origin to a small branch which supplied the right atrium and the right ventricle.

TWO LEFT CIRCUMFLEX ARTERIES (2 SPECIMENS; FIG. 10.15)

In two specimens a single ostium above the left sinus gave origin to the left coronary artery and a single ostium above the posterior sinus gave origin to the right coronary artery and an additional small left circumflex artery. The additional circumflex artery ran behind the pulmonary artery to terminate in the left atrioventricular sulcus.

ORIGIN OF THE RIGHT CORONARY ARTERY FROM LEFT SINUS AND LEFT ARTERY FROM POSTERIOR SINUS—NORMAL PERIPHERAL DISTRIBUTION (1 SPECIMEN; FIG. 10.16)

The right coronary artery arose from the left sinus and the left artery from the posterior sinus. The left artery coursed behind the pulmonary artery to appear on the anterior surface of the heart lateral to the pulmonary artery. It divided into anterior descending and left circumflex arteries. The right artery coursed in front of the root of the aorta to the right anterior atrioventricular sulcus.

The anatomy of the coronary arteries in complete transposition of the great arteries has been discussed by several writers. Spitzer (1923) recognized partial and complete transposition of the coronary arteries, and explained their occurrence on a phylogenetic basis. Harris and Farber (1939) gave detailed anatomy of the coronary arterial pattern in 17 cases of variable grades and types of transposition of the aorta and the pulmonary artery. Keith *et al.* (1953) dissected the coronary arteries in 37 cases of transposition of the great arteries and in 1958, Keith *et al.* reviewed the anatomy in 80 specimens of variable types of transposition differentiating them into four types. In 1962, Rowlatt described the anatomy of the coronary arteries in 135 hearts with transposition. In 46, tricuspid atresia, mitral atresia, common ventricle, corrected transposition, or common atrioventricular valve were present. Elliott *et al.* (1963a) divided the coronary atrial pattern in 60 specimens of complete transposition into two major groups and correlated them with the position of the aorta and of the pulmonary artery. Shaher and Puddu (1966) reported 9 coronary arterial patterns in 141 specimens with transposition.

It is generally agreed (Keith *et al.,* 1958; Rowlatt, 1962; Elliott *et al.,* 1963a) that the two most common coronary arterial patterns in complete transposition are (1) origin of the left coronary artery from the left aortic sinus and the right coronary artery from the posterior sinus, and (2) origin of the right coronary artery and the left circumflex artery from the posterior sinus and the anterior descending coronary artery from the left sinus.

No definite coronary arterial pattern could be correlated to the presence or absence of a ventricular septal defect or left ventricular outflow tract obstruction. In all groups the most common coronary arterial pat-

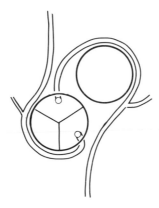

Fig. 10.16. Right coronary artery from left sinus, and left artery from posterior sinus. From Shaher and Puddu (1966), by permission of *Amer. J. Cardiol.*

TABLE 10.9

INCIDENCE OF CORONARY ARTERIAL PATTERNS

Coronary arterial anatomy	This series	Rowlatt (1962)	Elliott et al. (1963a)
1. Right artery from posterior sinus Left artery from left sinus	111	67	39
2. Left circumflex artery branch of right coronary artery	33	14	16
3. Single coronary artery	11	1	0
4. Anterior descending branch of right coronary artery	6	2	0
5. Common origin of right and left arteries	7	0	2
6. Absent left circumflex	4	0	0
7. Single artery and a small additional branch	3	1	0
8. Two left circumflex arteries	2	0	2
9. Right artery from left sinus and left artery from posterior sinus	1	4	0
10. Right artery from right sinus and left artery from posterior sinus	0	0	1
Total	178	89	60

tern was the origin of the left coronary artery from the left sinus and the right coronary artery from the posterior sinus. The second most common pattern was the origin of the left circumflex artery from the right coronary artery. These figures are supported by those of Rowlatt (1962), and Elliott et al. (1963a).

The following three patterns, which have been encountered in the present study and have not been described before are as follows: (1) single coronary artery from the posterior sinus or from left sinus; (2) common origin of the right and left arteries with the two ostia above the right sinus, and (3) absent left circumflex artery. On the other hand, the one pattern, which has been reported by other workers, but has not been observed in the present study is the right coronary artery from right sinus and left coronary artery from posterior sinus (1 specimen, Elliott et al., 1963a). The incidence of the various coronary arterial patterns in this series as well as in 89 of Rowlatt, and 60 of Elliott, is tabulated in Table 10.9.

Elliott and associates (1963a) pointed out that the coronary arterial pattern in which the left circumflex and the anterior descending arteries have a common stem, occurs most often when the great arteries show an oblique relationship to one another. When the left circumflex artery arises as a branch of the right coronary artery, the prevailing tendency for the great arteries is to show a side to side relationship. No attempt has been made in this study to test the validity of this observation. When a heart specimen is examined the external relationship of the great vessels depends to a considerable extent on the plane of the ventricular septum. If the ventricular septum is made to lie in the median plane, the great arteries may lie side by side or the aorta slightly anterior and to the right of the pulmonary artery. This position of the ventricular septum, however, is artifactual since during life the right ventricle in complete transposition of the great arteries lies anteriorly and the left ventricle lies posteriorly, though slight overlap of the ventricles may occur, while the ventricular septum lies in the frontal plane. Under such circumstances the aorta is almost always anterior to the pulmonary artery.

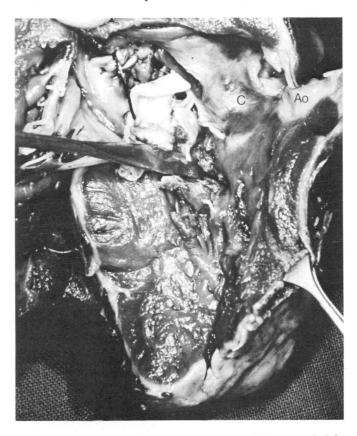

Fig. 10.17. Right ventricle. A probe points to a ventricular septal defect posterior and inferior to the crista (C) . Ao, aorta.

Associated Defects

VENTRICULAR SEPTAL DEFECTS

Position

Becu *et al.* (1956) divided isolated ventricular septal defects into two groups: (1) defects involving ventricular outflow tracts, divided into (a) defects posteroinferior to the crista supraventricularis, (b) defects anterosuperior to the crista supraventricularis, and (2) defects not related to ventricular outflow tracts, divided into (a) defects related to the atrioven-

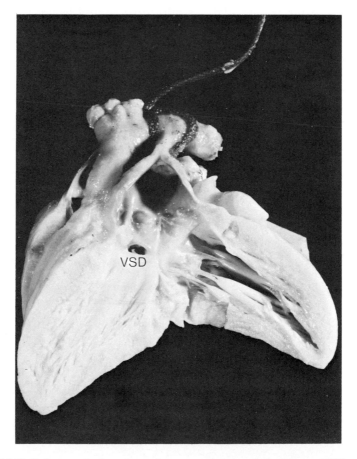

Fig. 10.18. Left ventricular view of a ventricular septal defect (VSD) posterior and inferior to the crista.

tricular valves, and (b) defects involving the apical portion of the ventricular septum. The outflow tract of the right ventricle, as defined by Becu *et al.* (1956), is that part which lies between the pulmonary valve above and the nearest portion of the tricuspid valve below. The portion of the ventricular septum related to the left ventricular outflow tract extends from the point where the anterior mitral leaflet joins the ventricular septum posteriorly to a point located below the midportion of the left aortic cusp anteriorly. Along its entire upper border, the left ventricular aspect of the outflow portion of the ventricular septum is related to the aortic valve. The crista supraventricularis divides the ventricular septum in the outflow tract of the right ventricle into two regions: one posterior and inferior to it extending between the crista supraventricularis and the tricuspid ring, and the other superior and anterior to it and extending to the annulus fibrosus of the pulmonary valve. The pars membranacea lies posterior and inferior to the crista. The right ventricular side of the ventricular septum lying posterior and inferior to the crista supraventricularis is

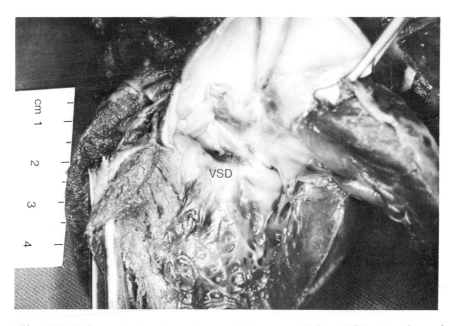

Fig. 10.19. Left ventricular view of a ventricular septal defect (VSD) posterior and inferior to the crista. Defect situated beneath the right posterior cusp of the pulmonary valve.

overhung by the left half of the anterior leaflet, and the anterior half of the septal leaflet of the tricuspid valve.

Utilizing the criteria of Becu *et al.*, ventricular septal defects in this series have been divided into the following groups: (1) posterior defects, 33, of which one was closed by fibrous tissue; (2) anterior defects, 7; (3) defects related to the atrioventricular valves, 8; (4) muscular defects, 8; and (5) multiple defects, 4.

Posterior Defects. In 33 specimens the defect was posterior and inferior to the crista. Pulmonary stenosis was present in 3 of these 33 speci-

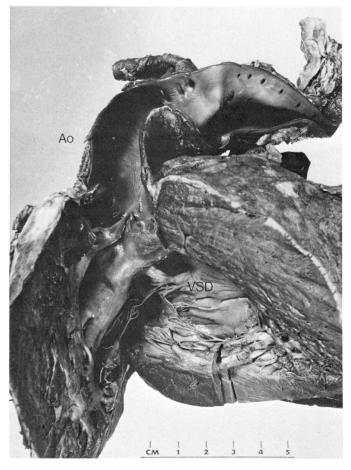

Fig. 10.20. Right ventricle shows a ventricular septal defect (VSD) among the muscle bundles of the septal limb of the crista. The defect extends anteriorly to be in direct relation with the aorta (Ao).

mens. When viewed from the right ventricle, these defects occupied the position of the membranous septum in the normal heart (Fig. 10.17). They were partly or completely covered by the left half of the anterior leaflet and the anterior half of the septal leaflet of the tricuspid valve. Anteriorly, they were separated from the aortic valve by the crista supraventricularis. Of the 31 defects in which the relationship of the papillary muscle of the conus could be determined, this muscle was inserted in the anterior edge of the defect in 15, inferior edge in 11, and posterior edge

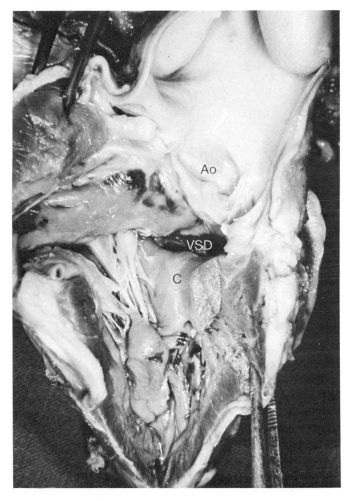

Fig. 10.21. Right ventricle shows an anterior ventricular septal defect (VSD) directly related to the aorta (Ao). C, Crista.

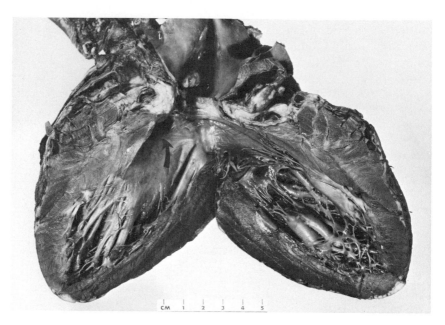

Fig. 10.22. Left ventricular view of anterior ventricular septal defect. Arrow points to defect.

in 5. From the left ventricular side, these defects were situated in the out-flow tract of the left ventricle in the area between the pulmonary valve superiorly and the anterior leaflet of the mitral valve laterally (Fig. 10.18). In a few instances, the defect was situated immediately beneath the right posterior cusp of the pulmonary valve (Fig. 10.19). In the majority, the edges of the defects were completely muscular, and a ridge of muscle tissue separated them from the pulmonary valve.

Anterior Defects. In 7 specimens (4 with pulmonary stenosis) the defect was situated among the muscle bundle of the septal limb of the crista (Fig. 10.20). In two with pulmonary stenosis, the defect lay immediately beneath the junction between the left and posterior cusps of the aortic valve (Fig. 10.21). From the left ventricular side these defects were more anterior than those in the last group. They were separated by a small ridge of muscle tissue from the junction between the anterior and the right posterior cusps of the pulmonary valve (Fig. 10.22).

Defects Related to the Atrioventricular Valves. In 8 specimens (5 with pulmonary stenosis) the defect extended posteriorly so that the junction between the tricuspid and mitral valve rings formed its superior boundary. Continuity between tricuspid and mitral valve leaflets occurred across the septal defect (Fig. 10.23). Anomalies of the atrioventricular valves were noted in 3 of these 8 specimens. In 2 with pulmonary stenosis, double mitral orifice occurred in 1, and a cleft anterior mitral leaflet in 1. In 1 without pulmonary stenosis, the mitral valve ring appeared small and stenotic. The valve leaflets were thickened and rolled in and the papillary muscles were rudimentary.

Muscular Defects. Muscular defects occurred in 8 specimens without pulmonary stenosis. These defects were unrelated to ventricular outflow tracts and occurred in the muscular portion of the ventricular septum (Fig. 10.24).

Multiple Defects. In each of 4 specimens without pulmonary stenosis, multiple defects were found. In two specimens one defect was muscular and the other was posterior (Fig. 10.25). In 1 specimen, one defect was muscular and the other was related to the atrioventricular valves. In the remaining specimen both defects were muscular. The mitral valve ring appeared small in the specimen with an atrioventricular canal defect.

Among patients with complete transposition of the great arteries asso-

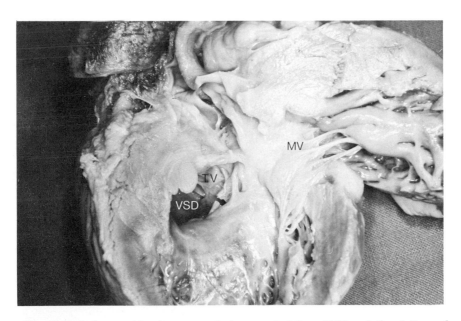

Fig. 10.23. Left ventricle shows ventricular septal defect (VSD) of the A-V canal type that has extended posteriorly to the junction between mitral (MV) and tricuspid (TV) valve rings.

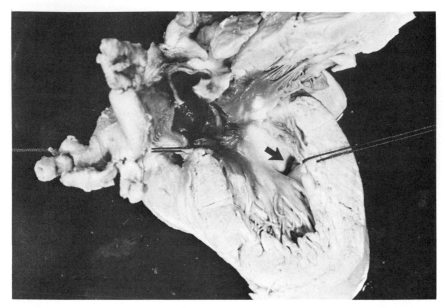

Fig. 10.24. Left ventricle shows a muscular ventricular septal defect. Arrow points to defect.

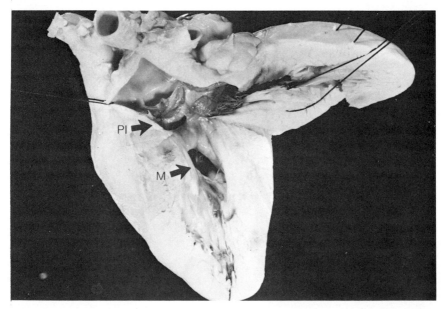

Fig. 10.25. Left ventricle shows two defects; one muscular (M), and one posterior and inferior defect (PI).

ciated with a ventricular septal defect, Lev *et al.* (1961) found that the defect may be situated in the anterior septum at the base, at the junction of the anterior and posterior septa at the base, in the pars membranacea, or in the posterior septum at the base. Uncommonly, the defect was situated in a more apical portion in the septum. Multiple defects were present in a few cases. Of the 22 cases with a ventricular septal defect reported by Elliott *et al.* (1963a), posterior–inferior septal defects were present in 13. In 10 of these, the septal defect communicated the right ventricle to the left ventricle, while in the remaining

TABLE 10.10
SIZE OF VENTRICULAR SEPTAL DEFECT [a]

	Age [b]	A. Size in mm²									
		1 mm	2 mm	3 mm	4 mm	5 mm	6 mm	7 mm	8 mm	9 mm	10 mm
VSD	0–2w	—	1	2	1	—	—	1	—	—	
(48 cases) [b]	2w–3m	1	6	6	2	2	2	—	1	—	2
	3m–1y	—	2	—	—	2	—	—	2	—	3
	Above 1y	—	—	1	—	1	—	—	2	—	3
	Unknown	—	1	3	—	—	—	—	—	—	—
Total		1	10	12	3	5	2	1	5	—	8
VSD and PS	0–2w	—	—	1	—	—	—	—	—	—	—
(12 cases)	2w–3m	—	—	—	—	1	—	1	—	—	—
	3m–1y	—	—	—	—	—	—	—	—	—	—
	Above 1y	—	—	—	1	—	1	—	2	—	5
	Unknown	—	—	—	—	—	—	—	—	—	—
Total		—	—	1	1	1	1	1	2	—	5

	Age [b]	B. Size of mm/m²						
		5–10 mm	11–15 mm	16–20 mm	21–25 mm	26–30 mm	31–35 mm	36–40 mm
VSD	0–2w	1	2	1	—	—	1	—
(41 cases)	2w–3m	6	6	3	2	2	—	2
	3m–1y	2	1	1	—	—	1	4
	Above 1y	2	2	1	—	—	1	—
Total		11	11	6	2	2	3	6
VSD and PS	0–2w	—	1	—	—	—	—	—
(8 cases)	2w–3m	—	—	1	—	1	—	—
	3m–1y	—	—	—	—	—	—	—
	Above 1y	1	1	1	1	1	—	—
Total		1	2	2	1	2	—	—

[a] Not counted is one case with fibrous occlusion of ventricular septal defect.
[b] Abbreviations as in Table 10.1.

TABLE 10.11

TYPE OF INTERATRIAL COMMUNICATION [a]

Group	PFO	Surgical ASD	PFO and ASD	ASD	Surg. ASD and PFO	Common atrium	Septum damaged	No comm.	Total
Group I	56	34	1	1	3	0	10	0	105
Group II	3	4	1	3	0	1	1	0	13
Group III	29	8	1	1	2	0	4	3	48
Group IV	2	2	1	2	0	0	3	2	12
Total	90	48	4	7	5	1	18	5	178

[a] ASD, atrial septal defect; Comm., communication; PFO, patent foramen ovale.

3 this communication was between the left ventricle and the right atrium. In these 3 specimens the defect opened into a space formed by a cleft in the tricuspid valve at the junction of the septal and the anterior leaflets. In each case, adhesions of the edges of the valve to the ventricular septum resulted in a direct communication between the left ventricle and the right atrium (Elliott *et al.*, 1963b). Defects anterosuperior to the crista supraventricularis were present in 3 of their cases. Isolated muscular defects were present in 2 cases, while 4 others had multiple defects. Of the 32 specimens reported by Imamura *et al.* (1971), an anterior defect was present in 2, a posterior defect in 26, and muscular or isolated defects in 4.

Size of the Ventricular Septal Defects

The diameter of the ventricular septal defects in the 60 specimens varied from 1.0 to 22.5 mm (Table 10.10A). When 49 defects were correlated to body surface area, 11 were 10 mm/m^2 or less while 38 were more than 10 mm/m^2 (Table 10.10B).

Partial Occlusion of Ventricular Septal Defects

In 5 specimens a papillomatous mass of endocardium protruded into the ventricular septal defect, almost completely occluding it. The diameter of each of these defects varied between 2 to 3 mm. In these specimens the papillomatous mass appeared to have originated from the endocardium surrounding the defect. In 2, the mass was connected by chordae tendineae to the edges of the defect as well as to the papillary muscles of the tricuspid valve.

Spontaneous Closure of Ventricular Septal Defects

Spontaneous closure of a ventricular septal defect was observed in 1 specimen in this series. The defect, which was posterior and inferior to the crista, was obliterated by fibrous tissue. This finding has been reported separately by Li *et al.* (1969).

Interatrial Communication

The types of interatrial communication and the size of the foramen ovale are shown in Tables 10.11 and 10.12. In the whole series of 178,

TABLE 10.12
SIZE OF THE FORAMEN OVALE [a]

Group	Age [b]	1 mm	2 mm	3 mm	4 mm	5 mm	6 mm	7 mm	8 mm	9 mm	10 mm or more
Group I	0–2w	—	8	6	7	8	—	—	—	—	—
(56 cases)	2w–3m	1	5	5	1	3	—	—	—	—	—
	3m 1y	—	2	2	1	—	—	—	1	—	—
	Above 1y	—	—	—	—	—	—	—	—	—	1
	Unknown	—	2	1	—	1	—	1	—	—	—
Total		1	17	14	9	12	—	1	1	—	1
Group II	0–2w	—	—	—	—	—	—	—	—	—	—
(3 cases)	2w–3m	—	—	—	—	—	—	—	—	—	—
	3m–1y	—	—	—	1	—	—	—	—	—	—
	Above 1y	—	—	—	—	—	—	—	—	—	—
	Unknown	—	1	—	—	1	—	—	—	—	—
Total		—	1	—	1	1	—	—	—	—	—
Group III	0–2w	—	2	1	1	—	—	—	—	—	—
(29 cases)	2w–3m	1	6	3	1	—	2	—	—	—	—
	3m–1y	2	1	1	2	1	1	—	—	—	—
	Above 1y	—	1	—	—	—	—	—	—	—	—
	Unknown	—	2	1	—	—	—	—	—	—	—
Total		3	12	6	4	1	3	—	—	—	—
Group IV	0–2w	—	—	—	—	—	—	—	—	—	—
(2 cases)	2w–3m	—	—	1	—	—	—	—	—	—	—
	3m–1y	—	—	—	—	—	—	—	—	—	—
	Above 1y	—	1	—	—	—	—	—	—	—	—
	Unknown	—	—	—	—	—	—	—	—	—	—
Total		—	1	1	—	—	—	—	—	—	—

[a] Size in mm².
[b] Abbreviations as in Table 10.1.

no communication at the atrial level occurred in 5. Most specimens had a foramen ovale which varied between 2 to 5 mm in diameter. In 4 specimens a pinpoint foramen was present (1 mm in diameter) while in 1 the size of the foramen ovale was 10 mm in diameter. An atrial septal defect was observed in 11 specimens. In 10 specimens the atrial septal defect was of the ostium secundum variety. In one specimen with a ventricular septal defect of the atrioventricular canal type and pulmonary stenosis, there was an ostium primum defect. In the whole group of 178 specimens an interatrial defect, as the only communication between the two circuits, existed in 13. A surgical atrial septal defect had been created earlier in life in 3 of these 13.

TABLE 10.13

STATE AND INTERNAL SIZE OF THE PATENT DUCTUS [a]

Group	Age [b]	Damaged	Closed	1 mm	2 mm	3 mm	4 mm	5 mm or more	Total
Group I	0–2w	4	2	12	22	9	1	8	58
(105 cases)	2w–3m	3	1	11	7	4	0	1	27
	3m–1y	0	4	1	2	1	0	0	8
	Above 1y	0	5	2	0	0	0	0	7
	Unknown	0	3	0	1	1	0	0	5
Total		7	15	26	32	15	1	9	105
Group II	0–2w	0	0	0	0	1	0	0	1
(13 cases)	2w–3m	0	0	2	0	0	0	0	2
	3m–1y	1	0	1	0	0	0	0	2
	Above 1y	0	5	0	0	0	0	0	5
	Unknown	0	1	1	1	0	0	0	3
Total		1	6	4	1	1	0	0	13
Group III	0–2w	0	2	1	3	0	0	0	6
(48 cases)	2w–3m	0	2	10	7	0	1	0	20
	3m–1y	0	5	1	3	1	0	0	10
	Above 1y	0	5	2	1	0	0	0	8
	Unknown	1	1	1	1	0	0	0	4
Total		1	15	15	15	1	1	0	48
Group IV	0–2w	0	0	1	0	0	0	0	1
(12 cases)	2w–3m	1	1	0	0	0	0	0	2
	3m–1y	0	0	0	0	1	0	0	1
	Above 1y	0	5	2	0	1	0	0	8
	Unknown	0	0	0	0	0	0	0	0
Total		1	6	3	0	2	0	0	12

[a] Measurements in **mm**.
[b] Abbreviations as in Table 10.1.

TABLE 10.14

VENTRICULAR DOMINANCE IN GROUP I

	Thicker right ventricle	Thicker left ventricle	Equal
A. In relationship to size of patent ductus arteriosus			
1mm			
26 Specimens	11	3	12
2 mm			
32 Specimens	4	8	20
3 mm			
15 Specimens	1	5	9
4 mm			
1 Specimen	0	1	0
5 mm or more			
9 Specimens	0	6	3
Total: 83 Specimens	16	23	44
B. In cases with a closed ductus			
15 Specimens	8	0	7

It is generally agreed that an interatrial communication exists in the majority of cases of transposition (Lev *et al.,* 1961; Elliott *et al.,* 1963a). Elliott reported that in their 60 necropsied cases the communication consisted of a valvular component foramen ovale in half of the cases and of a small atrial septal defect of the fossa ovalis in the other half.

THE DUCTUS ARTERIOSUS

The state and size of the ductus in the different age groups are shown in Table 10.13. A patent ductus was present in 84% of cases with an intact septum, 68% with a ventricular septal defect, 50% with an intact septum and left ventricle outflow tract obstruction, and 45% with ventricular septal defect and left ventricle outflow tract obstruction. A large patent ductus arteriosus (3 mm or more) was found in 25 cases with an intact septum, in two of each of Groups III and IV, and in 1 in Group II. Most of these 30 patients were in the age group 0–3 months. The highest incidence of the ductus was also found in this age group. Thus, of the 117 who died in this age period, a patent ductus was found in 101. On the other hand, of the 28 who survived the first year of life, the ductus was closed in 20. In 76 of the 117 who died in the age group 0–3 months, the ductus was 2 mm in diameter or less. It would seem that the high incidence of patent ductus in this age group is probably due to either of two factors. First, a closing ductus has a detrimental effect on the

TABLE 10.15

REPORTED CASES WITH AN ISOLATED PATENT DUCTUS ARTERIOSUS

Age of patient	Authors
10 weeks	Langstaff (1811)
5 days	Duges (1827)
18 days	Ward (1850–1851)
96 days	Ogston (1873)
2 days	Theremin (1895), Case 37
3 weeks	Ingham and Willius (1938), Case 1
4 weeks	Harris and Farber (1939), Case 11
2 weeks	Walker and Dardiniski (1945)
41 days	Elyan and Ruffle (1952), Case 1
2 months	Kirklin et al. (1961), 1 case

course of these patients. Second, these patients die at a stage when the ductus is still patent.

Table 10.14A shows the ventricular hypertrophy pattern in Group I correlated to the size of the ductus. When the ductus was 1 mm in diameter most specimens showed equal ventricular wall thickness or a right ventricular wall thicker than the left ventricular wall. Between 2 and 3 mm most specimens showed equal wall thickness or left ventricular wall thicker than right ventricular wall. When the ductus was more than 3 mm in diameter the left ventricle was thicker than the right ventricle in the majority. Table 10.14B shows the ventricular wall thickness in 15 specimens in Group I with a closed ductus. The right ventricle was thicker than the left in the majority.

Although a ductus arteriosus as the only communication between the two circuits was not seen in this series, review of the literature shows that there are at least 26 reported cases displaying the combination of complete transposition of the great arteries and an isolated patent ductus arteriosus. Cases with this combination in whom the age of the patients were recorded are listed in Table 10.15. Other cases in whom the age was not recorded were reported by Simmonds (1900); Philpott (1936), 3 cases; Gibson and Clifton (1938), 1 case; Abrams et al. (1951), 1 case; and Calleja et al. (1964), 4 cases.

LEFT VENTRICULAR OUTFLOW TRACT OBSTRUCTION

In 25 specimens there was obstruction of the outflow tract of the left ventricle. The ventricular septum was intact in 13, while a ventricular septal defect existed in 12. Two types of outflow tract obstruction of the left ventricle were observed: valvular and subvalvular pulmonary stenosis.

Pulmonary Valvular Stenosis

In all specimens but 2 with this type of obstruction, the pulmonary valve was essentially bicuspid with varying degrees of commissural fusion. In addition, the pulmonary valve ring was narrowed. In 2 specimens the pulmonary valve was tricuspid and the cusps were nodular and thickened and the commissures partly fused (Fig. 10.26).

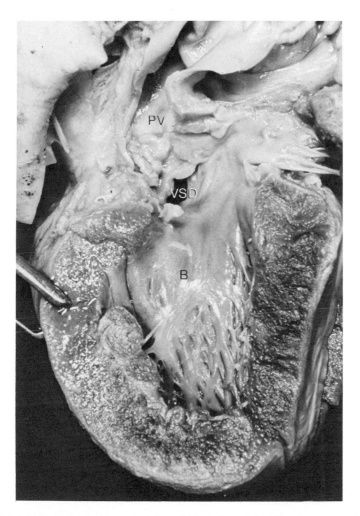

Fig. 10.26. Left ventricle shows nodular, thickened, and fused pulmonary valve cusps (PV) and bulging of the ventricular septum (B) into the cavity of the left ventricle. The ventricular septal defect (VSD) is above the bulging septum and 5 mm below the pulmonary valve.

Subvalvular Pulmonary Stenosis

Three different types were identified:

1. Subvalvular muscular obstruction caused by bulging of the ventricular septum in the cavity of the left ventricle. In the majority there was a

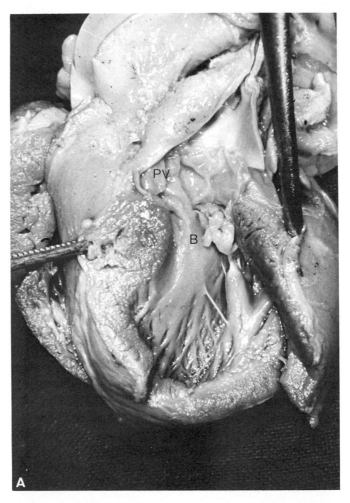

Fig. 10.27. (A) Left ventricle with an intact ventricular septum shows marked bulging of the septum (B) into the cavity of the left ventricle.. The pulmonary valve (PV) is normal. Note lack of continuity between mitral and pulmonary valves. (B) Left ventricle with a intact ventricular septum. The septum (B) bulges into the cavity of the ventricle, and the endocardium is thickened above site of obstruction.

thickened fibroelastic patch of endocardium above the site of the muscular obstruction (Fig. 10.27A,B).

2. Subvalvular fibromuscular stenosis. In this type the fundamental anomaly is formed by a narrow tunnel of fibromuscular tissue lined by fibroelastic tissue leading to a stenosed pulmonary valve (Fig. 10.28).

3. Subvalvular ring or diaphragm with or without a coexisting anomaly of the pulmonary valve (Fig. 10.29A,B).

Specimens with an intact ventricular septum were classified into three subgroups depending on the type of left ventricular outflow tract obstruc-

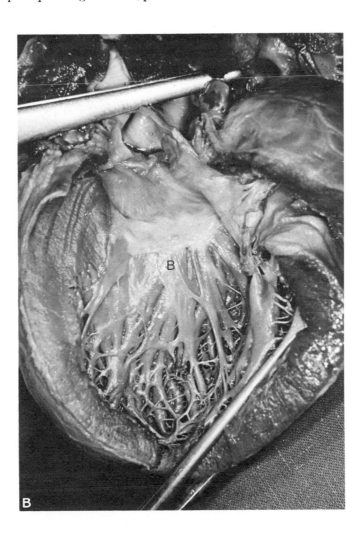

tion (Table 10.16). The first subgroup comprised 4 specimens with pulmonary valve stenosis. The third specimen in this subgroup had an additional subvalvular ring, while the fourth had bulging of the ventricular septum in the cavity of the left ventricles. The second subgroup comprises 2 specimens with subvalvular fibrous ring, or ridge. In both specimens the pulmonary valve was tricuspid. The third subgroup comprises 7 spec-

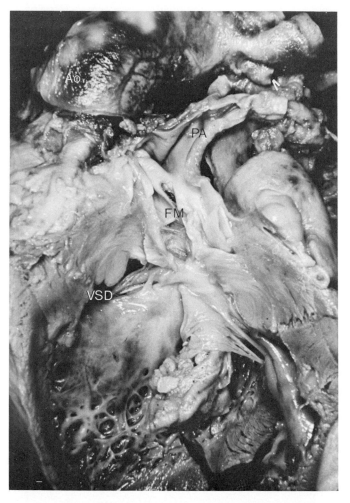

Fig. 10.28. Left ventricle shows severe fibromuscular obstruction (FM) of the outflow tract of this ventricle. The obstruction extends from the pulmonary artery (PA) above to a distant ventricular septal defect (VSD) below. Note very small pulmonary artery. Fibromuscular obstruction intervenes between mitral and pulmonary valves. Ao, Aorta.

imens with mild to severe obstruction of the left ventricular outflow tract caused by a bulging ventricular septum. In all specimens the pulmonary valve was tricuspid. In 6 of these 7 specimens the endocardium between the pulmonary valve and the site of the muscular obstruction was thickened.

Similarly, specimens with a ventricular septal defect were classified into three subgroups according to the type of left ventricular outflow tract obstruction (Table 10.17). Isolated pulmonary valvular stenosis was observed in 2 specimens only. Combined valvular and subvalvular muscular obstruction was observed in the second subgroup which comprises 6 specimens. The last subgroup comprises 4 specimens with pulmonary valvular stenosis. Of these 4 specimens, 3 had additional severe fibromuscular obstruction, while 1 had a subvalvular fibrous diaphragm. Additional muscular obstruction in the form of bulging of the ventricular septum in the cavity of the left ventricle below the distal obstruction was found in 2.

The incidence of left ventricular outflow tract obstruction in autopsied cases in this series is 12.9%. The incidence of left ventricular outflow tract obstruction in the literature varies between 6 to 33%. According to Becker and Brill (1948) pulmonary stenosis occurs in more than one-third of the cases of transposition of the great vessels, while in the experi-

TABLE 10.16

THIRTEEN PATIENTS WITH AN INTACT VENTRICULAR SEPTUM AND LEFT VENTRICULAR OUTFLOW TRACT OBSTRUCTION

Case no.	Age	No. of cusps	Valvular	Subvalvular muscular	Subvalvular fibro-muscular	Subvalvular ring	Size of great arteries[a]
1	11 Days	2	+	−	−	−	Equal
2	3 Months	3 Nodular	+	−	−	−	Equal
3	3 Years	2	+	−	−	+	Ao>PA
4	12 Years	2	+	+	−	−	PA>Ao
5	9 Months	3	−	−	−	Partial	PA>Ao
6	—	3	−	−	−	+	PA>Ao
7	2 Months	3	−	+	−	−	PA>Ao
8	9 Months	3	−	+	−	−	PA>Ao
9	14 Months	3	−	+	−	−	Ao>PA
10	3 Years	3	−	+	−	−	PA>Ao
11	3½ Years	3	−	+	−	−	Equal
12	—	3	−	+	−	−	Ao>PA
13	—	3	−	+	−	−	PA>Ao

[a] Ao, aorta; PA, pulmonary artery.

ence of Edwards (1960) pulmonary stenosis is not so commonly associated. Among the 75 patients of Baffes *et al.* (1957), 12 had pulmonary valvular stenosis. Of the 23 autopsied cases of Noonan *et al.* (1960),
3 had pulmonary stenosis. In the group of 112 cases of complete transpo-

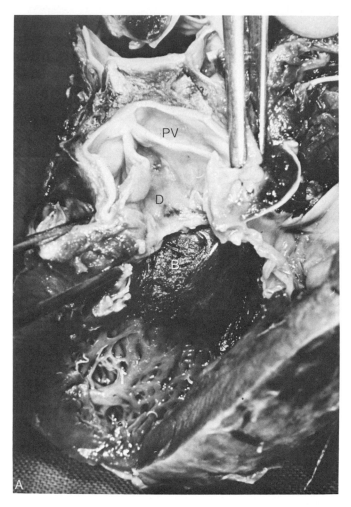

Fig. 10.29. (A) Left ventricle shows a bicuspid pulmonary valve (PV), subvalvular
diaphragm (D), and bulging of the ventricular septum (B) into the cavity of this
ventricle. The ventricular septal defect is not shown in this picture. (B) Left ventricle
with an intact ventricular septum. Note the subvalvular ring (SR), and considerable
thickening of the wall of the left ventricle and a thick band of muscle between the
mitral and pulmonary valves.

sition without mitral or tricuspid atresia or common ventricle reported by Lev *et al.* (1961) 6 had pulmonary stenosis. Of the 60 autopsied cases of Elliott *et al.* (1963a) 4 had left ventricular outflow tract obstruction.

The occurrence of pulmonary stenosis in cases of transposition and ventricular septal defect is well recognized (Becker and Brill, 1948; Edwards, 1960; Noonan *et al.*, 1960; Lev *et al.*, 1961; Mehrizi *et al.*, 1966). Subpulmonary stenosis produced by redundant tricuspid valve protruding through a ventricular septal defect in 2 patients was reported by Riemenschneider *et al.* (1969). Few reported cases showed the com-

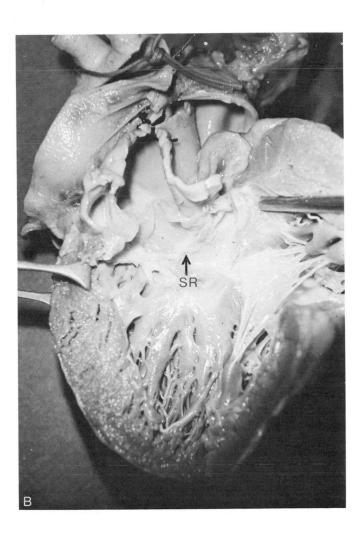

bination of transposition of the great arteries, intact ventricular septum, and pulmonary valvular or subvalvular stenosis of the diaphragm type. Such cases have been reported by Pung *et al.* (1955), Cleland *et al.* (1957), Noonan *et al.* (1960), Lev *et al.* (1961), Gerbode *et al.*

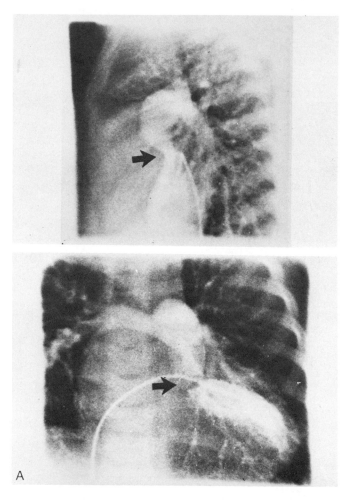

Fig. 10.30. (A) Left ventricular angiogram. Top, lateral projection shows moderate narrowing of the outflow tract caused by bulging of the septum, indicated by arrow. Bottom, anteroposterior projection. The bulging septum produces a radiolucent filling defect (arrow) in the outflow tract. (B) Specimen of left ventricle shows mild bulging of the septum (B) into the cavity of this ventricle. Note thickening of the endocardium above the bulge.

(1967), and Daicoff *et al.* (1969). In 1 of the 38 cases with an intact septum reported by Elliott *et al.* (1963a), the mitral valve was deformed and adhering abnormally to the ventricular septum constituting a barrier to the egress of blood from the left ventricle.

Shaher *et al.* (1967) emphasized the occurrence of muscular obstruction of the outflow tract of the left ventricle in cases with or without a ventricular septal defect. Muscular obstruction of the outflow tract of the left ventricle was observed in 16 specimens in this series; 8 with a ventricular septal defect and 8 with an intact ventricular septum. Pulmonary

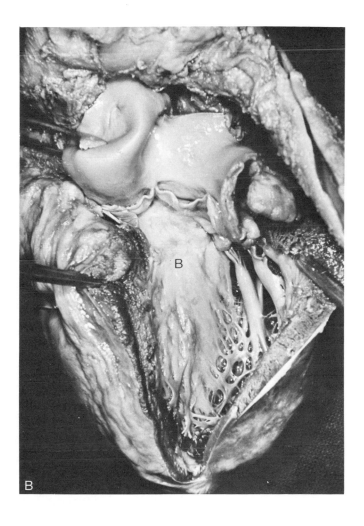

TABLE 10.17

TWELVE PATIENTS WITH A VENTRICULAR SEPTAL DEFECT AND LEFT VENTRICULAR OUTFLOW
TRACT OBSTRUCTION

Case no.	Age	No. of cusps	Valvular	Subvalvular muscular	Subvalvular fibro- muscular	Subvalvular ring	Size of great arteries[a]
1	6 Days	2	+	−	−	−	Ao>PA
2	10 Months	2	+	−	−	−	Ao>PA
3	1 Month	2	+	+	−	−	Ao>PA
4	1 Month	2	+	+	−	−	Ao>PA
5	20 Months	3 Nodular	+	+	−	−	Ao>PA
6	24 Months	2	+	+	−	−	Ao>PA
7	3 Years	Destroyed	+	+	−	−	Ao>PA
8	3 Years	2	+	+	−	−	Ao>PA
9	3 Years	Destroyed	+	−	+	−	Ao>PA
10	4 Years	Destroyed	+	+	+	−	Ao>PA
11	4¼ Years	2	+	+	−	+	Ao>PA
12	9½ Years	2	+	−	+	−	Ao>PA

[a] Ao, aorta; PA, pulmonary artery.

valvular stenosis was an associated finding in all specimens with a ventricular septal defect and in 1 with an intact ventricular septum. Of the remaining 7 specimens with an intact ventricular septum and isolated muscular subpulmonary stenosis, this obstruction appeared severe in 1, moderate in 3, and mild in 3. The left ventricular angiogram of one of these patients suggested that the obstruction during life was more pronounced during life than the appearance suggested at autopsy (Fig. 10.30). As pointed out by Shaher *et al.* (1967) muscular obstruction of the outflow tract of the left ventricle seems to occur as a result of the following:

1. Pulmonary valvular stenosis and diminished pulmonary blood flow. This is suggested by the fact that it was observed in 8 of our 12 cases with a ventricular septal defect and pulmonary valvular stenosis.
2. Septal hypertrophy secondary to right ventricular hypertrophy. This was the probable underlying mechanism in 4 of 7 specimens with an intact septum and isolated muscular obstruction. In these 4, the right ventricle appeared larger and thicker than the left ventricle.
3. Excessive pulmonary blood flow. This was the probable underlying mechanism in 3 specimens with an intact ventricular septum and isolated

muscular subpulmonary stenosis. In these 3 specimens the two ventricles had an equal wall thickness and in 2 the left ventricular cavity appeared larger than the right ventricular cavity.

Although sufficient hemodynamic and autopsy data are not available, the present findings as well as recent reports (Shaher *et al.* 1967; Tynan *et al.,* 1969; Plauth *et al.,* 1970) suggest that subvalvular muscular obstruction in cases with or without a ventricular septal defect could be acquired and progressive. This is substantiated by the fact that younger patients in this series tended to have valvular and muscular septal hypertrophy, whereas older patients tended to have valvular and severe fibromuscular stenosis. Lev *et al.* (1961) suggested that the subvalvular stenosis in transposition may be acquired due to the distance of the ventricular septal defect from the pulmonary valve, and that the fibroelastic reaction may be attributed to the turbulent blood flow.

PERIPHERAL STENOSIS OF THE PULMONARY ARTERIES

Peripheral stenosis of the pulmonary arteries was not observed in the autopsied cases in this series. As far as I can tell only 3 cases have been reported in the literature. These have been reported by Rothlin and Senning (1965), Mehrizi *et al.* (1966), and Waldhausen *et al.* (1971).

RIGHT VENTRICULAR OUTFLOW TRACT OBSTRUCTION

Anatomical obstruction of the outflow tract of the right ventricle by massive hypertrophy of the crista supraventricularis was observed in one patient with a ventricular septal defect. The ascending aorta appeared much smaller than the pulmonary artery. The aortic valve was tricuspid and not stenotic.

Anatomical obstruction of the outflow tract of the right ventricle in complete transposition of the great arteries is rare. In a case with an intact ventricular septum reported by Abbott (1936, Fig. 3, p. 54) the outflow tract of the right ventricle was occluded by extensive fibrosis and the aortic valve cusps were rudimentary. A massive crista resulted in an anatomical obstruction of the outflow tract of the right ventricle of Case 9 of Harris and Farber (1939). One of the patients of Baffes *et al.* (1957) had aortic valvular stenosis. Of the 60 specimens reported by Elliott *et al.* (1963a), obstruction of the outflow of the right ventricle by a hypertrophied crista was observed in 4 with an intact ventricular septum and in 2 with a ventricular septal defect. One of the cases reported by Mehrizi *et al.* (1966) had subaortic obstruction produced by asymmetrical hypertrophy of the septum.

TABLE 10.18

REPORTED AUTOPSIED CASES OF COMPLETE TRANSPOSITION OF THE GREAT ARTERIES AND COARCTATION OF THE AORTA

Preductal	Postductal	Unspecified
Lees, 1879–1880	Baffes *et al.*, 1957; 1 case	Rolleston, 1887
Dreyfuss, 1925		Harding, 1934
Read and Krumbhaar, 1932; Case 5		Leech 1935; Case 59
McCullough and Wilbur, 1944; Case 2		Harris and Farber, 1939; Case 11
Weiss, 1947		Andersen and Kelly, 1956; Case 114
Smyth, 1955		
Baffes *et al.*, 1957; 10 cases		
Noonan *et al.*, 1960; 3 cases		
Elliott *et al.*, 1963a; 6 cases		
Layman and Edwards, 1967; 1 case		

MALFORMATION OF THE AORTIC ARCH

Coarctation of the Aorta

Preductal coarctation of the aorta was observed in 11 specimens, and postductal coarctation in 2.

Of the 11 with preductal coarctation, the obstruction was in the form of a long segment of hypoplasia of the aorta in 8. The left subclavian artery originated from the lower, middle, or upper part of this segment. In 1 case the left vertebral artery arose from the hypoplastic segment. The ventricular septum was intact in 1 and a ventricular septal defect was present in 7. In the remaining 3 specimens with preductal coarctation, the obstruction took the form of a ring of constriction of the lumen of the aorta above the ductus. Two were in Group I and 1 in Group II. Postductal coarctation was present in 2 specimens; 1 with an intact septum and 1 with a ventricular septal defect. In both the obstruction took the form of a ring of constriction of the descending aorta immediately below the ductus. Of the 13 specimens with coarctation, the ductus was closed in 4, 1 × 1 mm in 4, 2 × 2 mm in 4, and 5 × 5 mm in 1.

The findings in this series and in published reports suggest that in the majority of cases of coarctation and transposition, a ventricular septal defect is present, and that the coarctation is of the preductal long segment type. Pulmonary stenosis, valvular or subvalvular, rarely occurs in association with coarctation and transposition. Reported autopsied cases of complete transposition of the great arteries and coarctation are shown in Table 10.18.

Interruption of the Aortic Arch

Complete interruption of the aortic arch was not seen among autopsied cases in this series. Of the whole group of 409 patients, this diagnosis was confirmed by angiography in 2.

The earliest reference to complete interruption of the aortic arch is reported by Rannels and Propst (1937) in the case of a 10-day-old female with a ventricular septal defect. The aorta arose from the right ventricle and supplied the innominate, subclavian, and the carotid arteries. The pulmonary artery arose from the left ventricle and was continuous with the abdominal aorta with a constriction where the ductus arteriosus should have been. There was no apparent continuity between the ascending aorta and the abdominal aorta. In 1937, Hamburger reported a case of a 3-week-old baby in whom cyanosis, which was more pronounced in the upper half of the body, was sharply demarcated at a line just beneath the level of the umbilicus, below which the blood supply to the skin seemed fairly well aerated. At autospy the aorta arose from the right ventricle and the pulmonary artery from the left ventricle. There was a patent foramen ovale, a small ventricular septal defect, and complete interruption of the aortic arch beyond the left subclavian artery. The descending aorta was supplied with blood from the pulmonary artery through a patent ductus arteriosus. Based on Hamburger's case, Taussig (1947) described the syndrome "transposition of the great vessels and interruption of the aortic arch." She stated that she was consulted on the case and that although she was familiar with cases with complete interruption of the aortic arch with more cyanosis of the lower part of the body, she failed to deduce that the presence of transposition in addition to the interrupted arch would give an opposite distribution of cyanosis.

At least 17 cases of transposition with complete interruption of the aortic arch have been reported. These cases are tabulated in Table 10.19. Of these 17 cases the interruption occurred distal to the left subclavian artery in 10 and between the left common carotid and left subclavian arteries in 6. In one the site of the interruption was not specified. A ventricular septal defect and patent ductus arteriosus occurred in all. Castellanos et al. (1959) reported a patient who had a patent ductus and differential cyanosis at the age of 6 years. When he died at 9 years, the ductus had closed and considerable collateral circulation was found around the atretic aorta.

TABLE 10.19

REPORTED CASES OF COMPLETE TRANSPOSITION OF THE GREAT ARTERIES WITH COMPLETE INTERRUPTION OF THE AORTIC ARCH

Type	Author	Sex	Age
Distal to left sub-	Rannels and Propst, 1937	F	10 days
clavian artery	Hamburger, 1937	M	3 weeks
	Castellanos *et al.,* 1959	M	9 years
	Blake *et al.,* 1962	F	4 months
	Buckley *et al.,* 1965	F	7 years
	Bowers *et al.,* 1965	M	5 months
	Moller and Edwards, 1965	—	—
	Layman and Edwards, 1967	—	—
	Tawes *et al.,* 1969	M	10 weeks
	Norton *et al.,* 1970	M	4 days
Between left common	Coles and Holesh, 1957	—	8½ weeks
carotid and left sub-	Coles and Holesh, 1957	—	5 days
clavian arteries	Elliott *et al.,* 1963a	M	2 months
	Elliott *et al.,* 1963a	M	3 months
	Moller and Edwards, 1965	—	—
	Waldhausen *et al.,* 1969	—	11 months
Unspecified	Venables, 1966	—	Infant

Vascular Abnormalities

In one specimen with an intact ventricular septum the ascending aorta coursed from right to left behind the trachea. The left common carotid artery originated on the right of the trachea and the left subclavian artery on its left. There was a large and long patent ductus arteriosus that coursed to the left of the trachea and connected the aortic arch at the origin of the left subclavian artery, with the pulmonary artery.

As far as I can tell vascular abnormalities in association with complete transposition have been reported in only 5 cases. Miller *et al.* (1958) briefly mentioned that one of their cases with transposition had a vascular ring surrounding the trachea. A double aortic arch associated with complete transposition of the great arteries was reported by Noonan *et al.* (1960), and Higashino and Ruttenberg (1968). The latter authors quoted von Siebold (1837) as having reported 2 cases of complete transposition with double aortic arch.

Anomalous Pulmonary Venous Drainage

In one specimen in this series the left upper pulmonary vein drained into the left superior vena cava via the left innominate vein. The other pulmonary veins drained normally into the left atrium. The ventricular septum was intact.

Partial or total anomalous pulmonary venous drainage rarely occurs in complete transposition of the great arteries. Total anomalous pulmonary venous drainage into the right atrium was observed in the case reported by Feldman and Chalmers (1933). In a case reported by Abbott (1936), the inferior vena cava, which was greatly enlarged, received one of the pulmonary veins. One of the cases of Emerson and Green (1942) had anomalous drainage of two pulmonary veins into the right atrium. Cases 13, 17, and 22 of Friedlich *et al.* (1950) were believed to have anomalous pulmonary venous drainage into the right atrium, superior vena cava, and inferior vena cava, respectively. This diagnosis however, was established by cardiac catheterization alone. In the case reported by Messeloff and Weaver (1951) two aberrant pulmonary veins from the right lower and middle lobes of the lung entered the right atrium. The case described by Ostund (1959) showed partial anomalous pulmonary venous drainage into the right atrium. Whitaker *et al.* (1964) reported a case of complete transposition of the great arteries with total anomalous pulmonary venous drainage into the superior vena cava. The diagnosis was confirmed by angiocardiography. Partial anomalous pulmonary venous drainage of the right upper lobe into the right atrium was observed in the patient of Gerbode *et al.* (1967). Two of the 69 patients of Danielson *et al.* (1969) had anomalous pulmonary venous connection of the right lung to the superior vena cava or right atrium. Sapsford *et al.* (1972) successfully corrected a case of complete transposition of the great arteries associated with total anomalous pulmonary venous drainage into the left innominate vein.

Anomalous Systemic Venous Drainage

In 4 specimens a persistent left superior vena cava was present. In 3 it drained into the coronary sinus, while in 1 it connected directly with the left atrium.

There are two reported cases of complete transposition in which a systemic vein connected with the left atrium. An anomalous systemic vein connected the right internal jugular vein with the left atrium in the case reported by Harris *et al.* (1927). In Case 5 of Read and Krumbhaar (1932) a systemic vein apparently entered the roof of the left atrium.

Cor Triatriatum

There are two reported cases of complete transposition of the great arteries and cor triatriatum. One case is mentioned by Keith *et al.* (1967)

and documented by Van Praagh and Corsini (1969). Senning (1966) mentioned briefly that in one of his cases with a ventricular septal defect there were three atria and two superior venae cavae.

References

Abbott, M. E. (1936). "Atlas of Congenital Cardiac Disease." American Heart Association, New York.

Abrams, H. L., Kaplan, H. S., and Purdy, A. (1951). Diagnosis of complete transposition of the great vessels. *Radiology* **57**, 500.

Andersen, D. H., and Kelly, J. (1956). Endocardial fibro-elastosis. 1. Endocardial fibro-elastosis associated with congenital malformations of the heart. *Pediatrics* **18**, 513.

Ash, R., Wolman, I. J., and Bromer, R. S. (1939). Diagnosis of congenital cardiac defects in infancy. *Amer. J. Dis. Child.* **58**, 8.

Ashby, H. (1881). A case of transposition of the aorta and pulmonary artery in a child of seven months. *J. Anat. Physiol.* **16**, 90.

Astley, R., and Parsons, S. (1952). Complete transposition of the great vessels. *Brit. Heart J.* **14**, 13.

Baffes, T. G., Ricker, W. L., DeBoer, A., and Potts, W. J. (1957). Surgical correction of transposition of the aorta and the pulmonary artery. *J. Thorac. Surg.* **34**, 469.

Becker, M. C., and Brill, R. M. (1948). Complete transposition of the great vessels. *Arch. Pediat.* **65**, 249.

Becu, L. M., Fontana, R. S., DuShane, J. W., Kirklin, J. W., Burchell, H. B., and Edwards, J. E. (1956). Anatomic and pathologic studies in ventricular septal defect. *Circulation* **14**, 349.

Bernreiter, M. (1958). Myocardial infarction in an infant with transposition of the great vessels. *J. Amer. Med. Ass.* **167**, 459.

Blake, H. A., Manion, W. C., and Spencer, F. C. (1962). Atresia or absence of the aortic isthmus. *J. Thorac. Cardiov. Surg.* **43**, 607.

Bowers, D. E., Schiebler, G. L., and Krovetz, L. J. (1965). Interruption of the aortic arch with complete transposition of the great vessels. Hemodynamic and angiocardiographic data of a case diagnosed during life. *Amer. J. Cardiol.* **16**, 442.

Buckley, M. J., Mason, D. T., Ross, J., Jr., and Braunwald, E. (1965). Reversed differential cyanosis with equal desaturation of the upper limbs. Syndrome of complete transposition of the great vessels with complete interruption of the aortic arch. *Amer. J. Cardiol.* **15**, 111.

Calleja, H. B., and Hosier, D. M. (1960). Complete transposition of the great vessels: An electrocardiographic and anatomic correlation. *Circulation* **22**, 730.

Calleja, H. B., Hosier, D. M., and Grajo, M. Z. (1964). The natural course of complete transposition of the great vessels. I. The malformation. *St. Thomas J. Med.* **19**, 237.

Castellanos, A., Garcia, O., and Gonzalez, E. (1959). Complete interruption of the aortic arch with transposition of the great vessels. (Report of a case diagnosed *in vivo*). *Cardiologia* **34**, 53.

Cleland, W. P., Goodwin, J. F., Steiner, R. E., and Zoob, M. (1957). Transposition of aorta and pulmonary artery with pulmonary stenosis. *Amer. Heart J.* **54**, 10.

Cockle, J. (1863). A case of transposition of the great vessels of the heart. *Med. Chir. Trans.* **46**, 193.

Coles, H. M. T., and Holesh, S. (1957). Transposition of the great vessels with absence of the aortic arch. *J. Fac. Radiol.* 8, 355.

Diacoff, G. R., Schiebler, G. L., Elliott, L. P., Van Mierop, L. H. S., Bartley, T. D., Gessner, I. H., and Wheat M. W. (1969). Surgical repair of complete transposition of the great arteries with pulmonary stenosis. *Ann Thorac. Surg.* 7, 529.

Danielson, G. K., Mair, D. D., Ongley, P. A., Wallace, R. B., and McGoon, D. C. (1971). Repair of the transposition of the great arteries by transposition of venous return. Surgical considerations and results of operation. *J. Thorac. Cardiov. Surg.* 61, 96.

Deverall, P. B., Tynan, M. J., Carr, I., Panagopoulos, P., Aberdeen, E., Bonham-Carter, R. E., and Waterston, D. J. (1969). Palliative surgery in children with complete transposition of the great arteries. *J. Thorac. Cardiov. Surg.* 58, 721.

Dixon, A. (1954). Juxtaposition of atrial appendages; two cases of unusual congenital cardiac deformity. *Brit. Heart J.* 16, 153.

Dreyfuss, M. (1925). Complete transposition of arterial trunks with stenosis of aortic arch, patent ductus Botallo, open foramen ovale, and defect of interventricular septum. *Proc. N. Y. Pathol. Soc.* 25, 114.

Duges (1827). *J. Gen. de Med.,* p. 88. (Cited by K. Kato, *Amer. J. Dis. Child.* 39, 363, 1930.)

Edwards, J. E. (1960). Congenital malformations of the heart and great vessels. *In* "Pathology of the Heart" (S. E. Gould, ed.) , 2nd Ed. P. 356. Thomas, Springfield, Illinois.

Elliott, L. P., Neufeld, H. N., Anderson, R. C., Adams, P., Jr., and Edwards, J. E. (1963a). Complete transposition of the great vessels. I. An anatomic study of sixty cases. *Circulation* 27, 1105.

Elliott, L. P., Carey, L. S., Adams, P., Jr., and Edwards, J. E. (1963b). Left ventricular—right atrial communication in complete transposition of the great vessels. *Amer. Heart J.* 66, 29.

Elyan, M., and Ruffle, F. C. (1952). Two cases of complete transposition of the great vessels of the heart. *Med. Aust.* 2, 91.

Emerson, P. W., and Green, H. (1942). Transposition of the great cardiac vessels. *J. Pediat.* 21, 1.

Feldman, W. M., and Chalmers, A. (1933). A case of complete transposition of the great vessels of the heart with a patent foramen ovale. *Brit. J. Child. Dis.* 30, 27.

Franciosi, R. A., and Blanc, W. A. (1968). Myocardial infarcts in infants and children. I. A necropsy study in congenital heart disease. *J. Pediat.* 73, 309.

Friedlich, A., Bing, R. J., and Blount, S. G., Jr. (1950). Physiological studies in congenital heart disease. IX. Circulatory dynamics in the anomalies of venous return to the heart including pulmonary arteriovenous fistula. *Bull. Johns Hopkins Hosp.* 86, 20.

Gerbode, F., Selzer, A., Hill, J. D., and Åberg, T. (1967) . Transposition of the great arteries: surgical repair of a complicated case in a 36 year old woman. *Ann. Surg.* 166, 1016.

Gibson, S., and Clifton, W. M. (1938). Congenital heart disease. A clinical and post mortem study of one hundred and five cases. *Amer. J. Dis. Child.* 55, 761.

Hamburger, L. P., Jr. (1937). Congenital cardiac malformation presenting complete interruption of the isthmus aortae with transposition of the great vessels. *Bull. Johns Hopkins Hosp.* 61, 421.

Harding, H. E. (1934). An uncommon malformation of the heart. *Brit. Med. J.* 2, 306.

Harris, J. S., and Farber, S. (1939). Transposition of the great cardiac vessels with special reference to the phylogenetic theory of Spitzer. *Arch. Pathol.* 28, 427.

Harris, H. A., Gray, S. H., and Whitney, C. (1927). The heart of a child aged twenty-two months presenting an anomalous vein from the pulmonary auricle to the right internal jugular vein, transposition of the great vessels and left superior vena cava. *Anat. Rec.* **36**, 31.

Higashino, S. M., and Ruttenberg, H. D. (1968). Double aortic arch associated with complete transposition of the great vessels. *Brit. Heart. J.* **30**, 579–581.

Imamura, E. S., Morikawa, T., Tatsuno, K., Konno, S., Arai, T., and Sakakibara, S. (1971). Surgical considerations of ventricular septal defects associated with complete transposition of the great arteries and pulmonary stenosis. *Circulation* **44**, 914.

Indeglia, R. A., Moller, J. H., Lucas, R. V., Jr., and Castaneda, A. R. (1970). Treatment of transposition of the great vessels with an intraatrial baffle (Mustard procedure). *Arch. Surg.* **101**, 797–805.

Ingham, D. W., and Willius, F. A. (1938). Congenital transposition of the great arterial trunks. *Amer. Heart J.* **15**, 482.

Jue, K. L., Adams, P., Jr., Pryor, R., Blount, S. G., Jr., and Edwards, J. E. (1966). Complete transposition of the great vessels in total situs inversus. Anatomic, electrocardiographic and radiologic observations. *Amer. J. Cardiol.* **17**, 389.

Keith, J. D., Neill, C. A., Vlad, P., Rowe, R. D., and Chute, A. L. (1953). Transposition of the great vessels. *Circulation* **7**, 830.

Keith, J. D., Rowe, R. D., and Vlad, P. (1958). "Heart Disease in Infancy and Childhood," 1st Ed. MacMillan, New York.

Keith, J. D., Rowe, R. D., and Vlad, P. (1967). "Heart Disease in Infancy and Childhood," 2nd Ed. MacMillan, New York.

Kessler, A., and Adams, P. (1957). Association of transposition of the great vessels and rudimentary right ventricle with and without tricuspid atresia. *Pediatrics* **19**, 851.

King, T. W. (1844). Case of transposition of the aorta and pulmonary artery with remarks on the causes of communication between the two sides of the heart. *London Edinburgh Monthly J. Med. Sci.* **4**, 32.

Kirklin, J. W., Devloo, R. A., and Weidman, W. H. (1961). Open intracardiac repair for transposition of the great vessels: 11 cases. *Surgery* **50**, 58.

Langstaff (1811). Case of a singular malformation of the heart. *London Med. Rev.* **4**, 88.

Layman, T. E., and Edwards, J. E. (1967). Anomalies of the cardiac valves associated with complete transposition of the great vessels. *Amer. J. Cardiol.* **19**, 247.

Leech, C. B. (1935). Congenital heart disease. Clinical analysis of seventy-five cases from the Johns Hopkins Hospital. *J. Pediat.* **7**, 802.

Lees, D. B. (1879–1880). Case of malformation of the heart with transposition of the aorta and pulmonary artery. *Trans. Pathol. Soc. London* **31**, 58.

Lev, M., Alcalde, V. M., and Baffes, T. G. (1961). Pathologic anatomy of complete transposition of the arterial trunks. *Pediatrics* **28**, 293.

Lev, M., Rimoldi, H. J. A., Paiva, R., and Arcilla, R. A. (1969). The quantitative anatomy of simple complete transposition. *Amer. J. Cardiol.* **23**, 409.

Li, M. D., Collins, G., Disenhouse, R., and Keith, J. D. (1969). Spontaneous closure of ventricular septal defect. *Can. Med. Ass. J.* **100**, 737.

McCullough, A. W., and Wilbur, E. L. (1944). Defect of endocardial cushion development as a source of cardiac anomaly. A presentation of four cases from autopsy reports. *Amer. J. Pathol.* **20**, 321.

Mehrizi, A., Rowe, R. D., Hutchins, G. M., and Folger, G. M., Jr. (1966). Transposition of the great vessels with pulmonary stenosis and ventricular septal defect. *Bull. Johns Hopkins Hosp.* **119**, 200.

Melhuish, B. P. P., and Van Praagh, R. (1968). Juxtaposition of the atrial appendages. A sign of severe cyanotic heart disease. *Brit. Heart J.* **30**, 269.

Messeloff, C. R., and Weaver, J. C. (1951). A case of transposition of the large vessels in an adult who lived to the age of 38 years. *Amer. Heart J.* **42**, 467.

Miller, R. A., Baffes, T. G., and Wilkinson, A. A. (1958). Transposition of the great vessels. Diagnostic considerations and surgical therapy. *Pediat. Clin. N. Amer.* **5**, 1109.

Miskall, E. W., and Fraser, J. A. (1948). Complete transposition of the great vessels. *Ohio State Med. J.* **44**, 709.

Moller, J. H., and Edwards, J. E. (1965). Interruption of aortic arch. Anatomic patterns and associated cardiac malformations. *Amer. J. Roentgenol. Radium Ther. Nucl. Med.* **95**, 557.

Mustard, W. T., Chute, A. L., Keith, J. D., Sirek, A., Rowe, R. D., and Vlad, P. (1954). A surgical approach to transposition of the great vessels with extracorporeal circuit. *Surgery* **36**, 39.

Noonan, A., Nadas, A. S., Rudolph, A. M., and Harris, G. B. C. (1960). Transposition of the great arteries. A correlation of clinical, physiologic and autopsy data. *N. Engl. J. Med.* **263**, 592.

Norton, J. B., Ullyot, D. J., Stewart, E. T., Rudolph, A. M., and Edmunds, L. H. (1970). Aortic arch atresia with transposition of the great vessels. Physiologic considerations and surgical management. *Surgery* **67**, 1011.

Ogston, A. (1873). *Oesterr. Jahrb. Paediat.* **4**, 169. (Cited by K. Kato, *Amer. J. Dis. Child.* **39**, 363, 1930.)

Ostund, E. (1959). The syndrome of transposition of the great arteries. *Arch. Pediat.* **76**, 427.

Philpott, N. W. (1936). Relative incidence of congenital cardiac anomalies in Montreal hospitals. *J. Tech. Methods* **15**, 96.

Plauth, W. H., Jr., Nadas, A. S., Bernhard, W. F., and Fyler, D. C. (1970.) Changing hemodynamics in patients with transposition of the great arteries. *Circulation* **42**, 131.

Puech, P., Latour, H., Hertault, J., Grolleau, R., and Robert. M. (1966). La juxtaposition des auricules. *Arch. Mal. Coeur. Vaiss.* **59**, 239.

Pung, S., Gottstein, W. K., and Hirsch, E. F. (1955). Complete transposition of the great vessels in a male aged 18 years. *Amer. J. Med.* **18**, 155.

Rannels, H. W., and Propst, J. H. (1937). Incidence of congenital cardiac anomalies found at autopsies performed in Hospital of the University of Pennsylvania. *J. Tech. Methods* **17**, 113.

Rastelli, G. C., Wallace, R. B., and Ongley, P. A. (1969a). Complete repair of transposition of the great arteries with pulmonary stenosis. A review and report of a case corrected by using a new surgical technique. *Circulation* **39**, 83.

Rastelli, G. C., McGoon, D. C., and Wallace, R. B. (1969b). Anatomic correction of transposition of the great vessels with ventricular septal defect and pulmonary stenosis. *J. Thorac. Cardiov. Surg.* **58**, 545.

Read, W. T., Jr., and Krunbhaar, E. B. (1932). Eight cases of congenital heart disease (three cases of Fallot's tetralogy; two cases of complete transposition of the great vessels; two anomalies of the semilunar cusps, one with coarctation of the aorta, one case of premature closure of the foramen ovale). *Med. Clin. N. Amer.* **16**, 229.

Riemenschneider, T. A., Goldberg, S. J., Ruttenberg, H. D., and Gyepes, M. T. (1969). Subpulmonic obstruction in complete (d) transposition produced by redundant tricuspid tissue. *Circulation* **39**, 603–609.

Riemenschneider, T. A., Vincent, W. R., Ruttenberg, H. D., and Desilets, D. T. (1968). Transposition of the great vessels with hypoplasia of the right ventricle. *Circulation* 38, 386.

Roberts, W. C., Mason, D. T., and Braunwald, E. (1962) . Survival to adulthood in a patient with complete transposition of the great vessels. Including a note on the association of endocrine tumors with heart disease. *Ann. Intern. Med.* 57, 834.

Rolleston, H. D. (1897). Malformation of heart. Transposition of aorta and pulmonary artery. *Pediatrics* 4, 108.

Rothlin, M., and Senning, A. (1965). Zur chirurgischen Behandlung der transposition der grossen arterien. *Deut. Med. Wochenschr.* 90, 417.

Rowlatt, U. F. (1962). Coronary artery distribution in complete transposition. *J. Amer. Med. Ass.* 179, 269.

Rowlatt, U. F., Rimoldi, H. J. A., and Lev, M. (1963). The quantitative anatomy of the normal child's heart. *Pediat. Clin. N. Amer.* 10, 499.

Sapsford, R. N., Aberdeen, E., Watson, D. A., and Crew, A. D. (1972). Transposed great arteries combined with totally anomalous pulmonary veins: A report of a successful correction. *J. Thorac. Cardiov. Surg.* 63, 360.

Senning, A. (1966) . Surgical correction of transposition of the great vessels. *Surgery* 59, 334.

Shaher, R M. (1963). The coronary circulation in complete transposition of the great vessels. *Brit. Heart J.* 25, 481.

Shaher, R. M., and Puddu, G. C. (1966) . Coronary arterial anatomy in complete transposition of the great vessels. *Amer. J. Cardiol.* 17, 355.

Shaher, R. M., Puddu, G. C., Khoury, G., Moes, C. A. F., and Mustard, W. T. (1967). Complete transposition of the great vessels with anatomic obstruction of the outflow tract of the left ventricle. Surgical implications of anatomic findings. *Amer. J. Cardiol.* 19, 658.

Shone, J. D., Sellers, R. D., Anderson, R. C., Adams, P., Jr., Lillehei, C. W., and Edwards, J. E. (1963). The developmental complex of "parachute mitral valve," supravalvular ring of left atrium, subaortic stenosis and coarctation of aorta. *Amer. J. Cardiol.* 11, 714.

Simmonds (1900) . *Deut. Med. Wochenschr.* 26, 81. 1900. (Cited by K. Kato, *Amer. J. Dis. Child.* 39, 363, 1930.)

Smyth, N. P. D. (1955). Lateroposition of the atrial appendages. *Arch. Pathol.* 60, 259.

Snllen, H. A., Dankmeijer, J., Dekker, A., and van Ingen, H. C. (1962). Embryonic development and congenital cardiovascular anomalies. Memorias Del IV Congreso Mundial de Cardiologia. Tomo 1-A, Mexico, p. 132.

Spitzer, A. (1923) . Uber den Bauplan des normalen und missbildeten Herzens. *Virch. Arch. Pathol. Anat. Physiol.* 243, 81, 1923. (Translated by M. Lev and A. Vass, Thomas, Springfield, Illinois 1951.)

Stuart, K. L., and Flint, H. E. (1957) . Transposition of the ventricles and arterial stems with cerebral abscess. *Postgrad. Med. J.* 33, 131.

Taussig, H. (1947). "Congenital Malformation of the Heart," 1st Ed. The Commonwealth Fund, New York.

Tawes, R. L., Panagopoulos, P., Aberdeen, E., Waterston, D. J., and Bonham-Carter, R. E. (1969). Aortic arch atresia and interruption of the aortic arch. Experience in 11 cases of operation. *J. Thorac. Cardiov. Surg.* 58, 492.

Theremin, E. (1895) . "Édudes sur les Affections Congénitales du Coeur." Asselin and Houzeau, Paris.

Tynan, M., Carr, I., Graham, G., and Bonham-Carter, R. E. (1969). Subvalvular pulmonary obstruction complicating the postoperative course of balloon atrial septostomy in transposition of the great arteries. *Circulation* **39**, 223.

Van Praagh, R. V., and Corsini, I. (1969). Cor triatriatum. Pathologic anatomy and a consideration of morphogenesis based on 13 post mortem cases and a study of normal development of the pulmonary vein and atrial septum in 83 human embryos. *Amer. Heart J.* **78**, 379.

Venables, A. W. (1966). Complete transposition of the great vessels in infancy with reference to palliative surgery. *Brit. Heart J.* **28**, 335.

Von Siebold (1837). Cited by Higashino and Ruttenberg, 1968.

Wagner, H. R., Alday, L. E., and Vlad, P. (1970). Juxtaposition of the atrial appendages. A report of six necropsied cases. *Circulation* **42**, 157.

Waldhausen, J. A., Boruchow, I., Miller, W., and Rashkind, W. J. (1969). Transposition of the great arteries with ventricular septal defect. Palliation by atrial septostomy and pulmonary artery banding. *Circulation* **39** and **40** (Suppl. 1), 215.

Waldhausen, W., Pierce, W. S., Park, C. D., Rashkind, W. J., and Friedman, S. (1971). Physiologic correction of transposition of the great arteries. *Circulation* **43**, 738.

Walker, J. W., and Dardiniski, V. J. (1945). Complete uncorrected transposition of the vessels; report of a case. *Arch. Pediat.* **62**, 209.

Ward, O. 1850–1851) . Transposition of the aorta and pulmonary artery. *Trans. Pathol. Soc. London* **3**, 63.

Weiss, W. (1947). Complete transposition of the great vessels with coarctation of the aorta. *Bull. Int. Ass. Med. Mus.* **27**, 187.

Whitaker, W., Watson, D. A., and Keates, P. G. (1964). Total anomalous pulmonary venous drainage into the left innominate vein associated with transposition of the great vessels. *Circulation* **30**, 918.

Wilkinson, A. H., Potts, W. J., and Lev, M. (1960). The post mortem external appearance of congenitally malformed hearts as an aid to surgical diagnosis. *J. Thorac. Cardiov. Surg.* **39**, 363.

Chapter 11

EXTRACARDIAC PATHOLOGY

The Pulmonary Vasculature

A microscopic study of the lungs of 218 patients in this series was undertaken. Lung tissue was obtained at autopsy in 216 instances and by biopsy in 2. In each autopsied case one or two blocks of lungs were available. Sections were stained with hematoxylin and eosin and with Verhoeff's elastic tissue stain counterstained with van Giessen's stain. Of the 218 lung sections, 128 were in Group I, 13 in Group II, 69 in Group III, and 8 in Group IV.

The findings in the pulmonary arterial tree which have been classified according to the criteria of Heath and Edwards (1958) are in Table 11.1. As pointed out by Ferencz (1966) in young infants in whom the small pulmonary arteries have a thick muscular media and a narrow lumen, a clear-cut line cannot be drawn between the degree of muscular hypertrophy, normally present in the fetal state, and one which is abnormal. As she suggested, all patients were classified, regardless of the age as showing medial hypertrophy (Grade 1) if in the majority of muscular arteries the thickness of the media exceeded 15–20% of the external diameter of the vessel.

The pulmonary arteries appeared normal in 51 patients. Of these 51 patients 36 had an intact ventricular septum, 5 had an intact ventricular septum and pulmonary stenosis, and 9 had a ventricular septal defect. A thick muscular media was present in 167 patients. In 103 cases this was the only finding (Grade 1) (Fig. 11.1) and in 64 patients it was associated with intimal changes. Mild to moderate fibrosis in the small elastic and in the muscular pulmonary arteries (Grade 2) was observed in 42 patients (Fig. 11.2). Occlusive intimal fibrosis (Grade 3) was found in 17 instances (Fig. 11.3). Plexiform lesions (Grade 4) were observed in 5 patients (Fig. 11.4). The pulmonary veins appeared normal in all sec-

TABLE 11.1

PULMONARY VASCULATURE IN 218 CASES

Group	Age	Normal	Grade 1	Grade 2	Grade 3	Grade 4
Group I	0–1 months	28	52	4	0	0
(128 Cases)	1–6 months	6	13	12	1	0
	6–12 months	1	2	1	0	1
	1 year or more	1	1	3	2	0
Group II	0–1 month	1	1	0	0	0
(13 Cases)	1–6 months	1	1	0	0	0
	6–12 months	1	1	0	0	0
	1 year or more	2	2	1	1	1
Group III	0–1 month	5	8	1	0	0
(69 Cases)	1–6 months	4	15	12	1	0
	6–12 months	1	4	2	0	0
	1 year or more	0	1	2	11	2
Group IV	0–1 month	0	0	0	0	0
(8 Cases)	1–6 months	0	1	0	0	0
	6–12 months	0	0	0	0	0
	1 year or more	0	1	4	1	1
Total		51	103	42	17	5

tions. Thrombotic lesions were found in 4 patients with a ventricular septal defect and pulmonary stenosis.

The presence of hypertensive changes in the small pulmonary arteries of patients with transposition has been noted by Ferguson *et al.* (1960). Ferencz (1966) examined the lung sections of 106 patients with transposition of the great arteries and concluded that a state of high pulmonary vascular resistance exists in these individuals. Among her patients, intimal fibrosis appeared within the first month of life and progressed so rapidly that destruction of the normal pulmonary arterial architecture was almost the rule in patients over 2 years of age. Wagenvoort *et al.* (1968) examined the pulmonary vasculature of the lungs taken for biopsy from 80 patients with complete transpositions. Of their 31 cases with an intact ventricular septum the media of the muscular pulmonary arteries was normal in 12, slightly hypertrophied in 3, and atrophic in 16. Slight intimal fibrosis was observed in 7. Of their group with a ventricular septal defect the media was normal in 2 and hypertrophied in 26 (slight in 9, moderate in 13, and severe in 4.) Cellular proliferation and fibrosis of the intima were prominent features in this group being slight in 2, moderate in 13, and severe in 4. Occasional thrombi in the process of organization were seen in 8. Plexiform lesions were seen in 1 patient only. In the group with pulmonary stenosis with or without a ventricular septal defect, the media of the pulmonary arteries was usually atrophic. Thrombotic lesions were numerous in the group with a ventricular septal defect and pulmonary stenosis. The authors thought that the difference in material could explain in part the discrepancy between their observation and those of Ferguson, and Ferencz in the group with an intact ventricular septum.

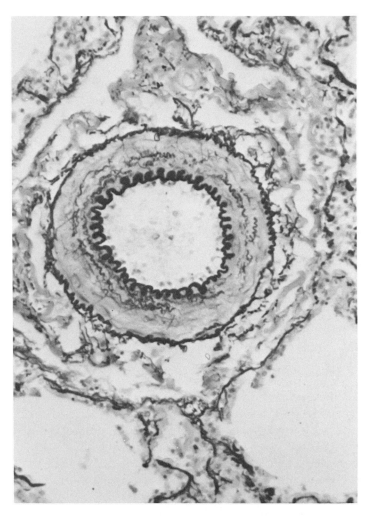

Fig. 11.1. Grade 1 pulmonary vascular changes. A small muscular artery showing hypertrophy of the media and slight constriction of the lumen as indicated by wrinklng of the internal elastic lamina. × 380.

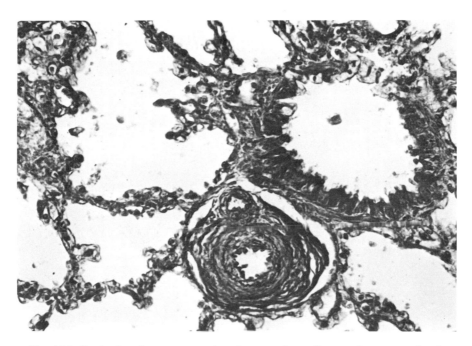

Fig. 11.2. Grade 2 pulmonary vascular changes. A small muscular artery showing medial hypertrophy and cellular internal proliferation. × 380.

In addition, they pointed out that in the first 2 weeks of life when the pulmonary arterial media is normally very thick the distinction between normal media and medial hypertrophy may be extremely difficult to ascertain. Viles *et al.* (1969) examined the lung sections taken at autopsy in 53 patients with complete transposition of the great arteries. Twenty-three had intact ventricular septa, and 30 had ventricular septal defects. They pointed out that children of similar age and associated defects had widely differing degrees of pulmonary vascular disease. The presence of pulmonic stenosis (congenital or acquired by pulmonary artery banding in infancy), a small ventricular septal defect, or a large atrial septal defect did not always protect against the development of pulmonary vascular disease. Newfeld *et al.* (1972) studied the pulmonary vessels in 198 patients with complete transposition of the great arteries, 95 having hemodynamic measurements. There were 14 interoperative lung biopsy specimens. Ninty-nine patients had hemodynamically significant ventricular septal defect. Patients with normal pulmonary artery pressure had either normal vessels, Grade 1 or at most by Grade 2 changes. With an intact ventricular septum, only 8 patients showed pulmonary vessel changes

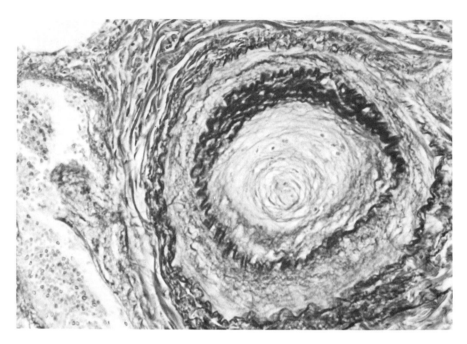

Fig. 11.3. Grade 3 pulmonary vascular changes. A small muscular artery showing medial hypertrophy. The lumen is obliterated by organizing fibrous tissue with reduplication of the internal elastic lamina. × 380.

greater than Grade 2, 2 showed Grade 3, and 6 showed Grade 4. In contrast, with a large ventricular septal defect, Grade 3 and 4 changes were found as early as 6 months of age and were the rule over 1 year. Of 36 infants under 6 months of age with a large ventricular septal defect, only 1 had Grade 4 and 5 had Grade 3 changes. The findings in this present study confirm the conclusions of Ferguson *et al.* (1960), Ferencz (1966), Wagenvoort *et al.* (1968), and Viles *et al.* (1969) that significant pulmonary vascular disease occurs in the majority of patients with transposition after the age of 6 months. The presence of a large ventricular septal defect accelerates the development of severe vascular damage to the pulmonary arterioles. However, as pointed

Fig. 11.4. Grade 4 pulmonary vascular changes. (A) A small muscular artery whose lumen is partially obliterated by organizing fibrous tissue with a dilated vascular channel in the adventitia forming an early plexiform lesion. (B) Origin of the dilated arteriolar channel from the parent artery and containing organized thrombus and fibrous tissue.

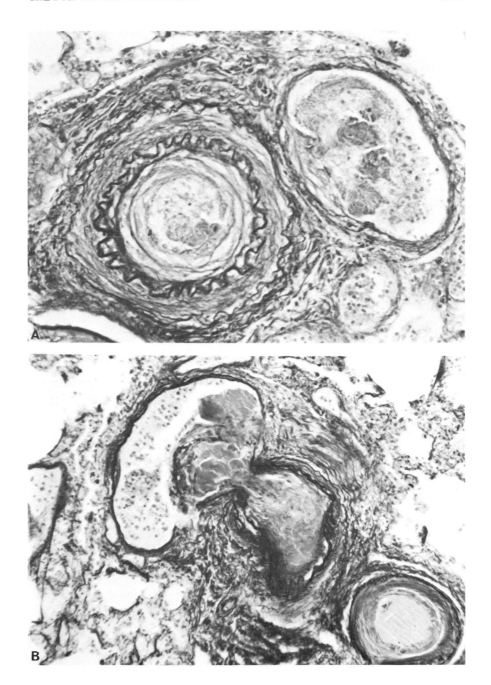

out by Viles *et al.* (1969) neither the presence of pulmonary stenosis nor an intact ventricular septum protects against the development of pulmonary vascular disease.

The Bronchial Arteries

In only one patient in Group IV in this series autopsy examination demonstrated bronchial arteries around the lung hilar and the base of the pericardium.

The earliest reference to the bronchial vessels in transposition is by Cockle (1863) who reported a patient with transposition of the great vessels who died at the age of 2 years and 8 months. At necropsy there was an intact ventricular septum and a patent foramen ovale. The aorta just beyond the arch gave off five small arteries of which were thought to be bronchial, esophageal, or thymic. Abbott (1937) suggested that dilated bronchial arteries may have a role in the exchange of blood between the two circuits in transposition of the great arteries. In Case 1 of transposition and pulmonary stenosis reported by Cleland *et al.* (1957), the bronchial arteries were greatly enlarged, the supply to the left lung being more profuse than that of the right lung. In a case of transposition with pulmonary hypertension, Folse *et al.* (1961) demonstrated large bronchial arteries entering the hila of the lungs. Microscopically many dilated thick-walled bronchial arteries surrounding the bronchi were seen, and there was proliferation of the intima of these arteries. Collateral bronchial arterial circulation was observed in a case associated with pulmonary stenosis, reported by Roberts *et al.* (1962). Gross bronchial collaterals were observed in one of the patients with an intact ventricular septum reported by Aberdeen *et al.* (1965). In a case of complete transposition without pulmonary stenosis, Cudkowicz and Armstrong (1952) demonstrated by injection technique an extensive bronchial collateral circulation. They found no evidence, however, of direct communication between the bronchial and pulmonary arteries. A network of very fine arterioles, which coursed across the adventitia of the pulmonary arteries, filled with the injection medium. These vessels were thought to be dilated vasa vasorum which are normally derived from the bronchial arteries. They concluded that these small branches of the bronchial arteries which do not normally communicate directly with the pulmonary arteries can, in the presence of diminished pulmonary blood flow or pulmonary occlusion, anastomose directly with the lumina of these vessels. Robertson (1965) combined microangiographical and histological studies on 6 cases of transposition, varying in ages between 1 day and 7 weeks. An intact ventricular septum was present in all. The contrast medium was injected into the pulmonary artery in 5, and into the bronchial arteries via the aorta in 1. In all the bronchial arteries were well visualized in the microangiograms. They were wider and more tortuous than normal and gave off abnormal branches which left the bronchial wall to ramify in the adjacent pulmonary parenchyma. In this way many alveolar groups displayed a double arterial vascularization and there seemed to be widespread capillary anastomosis between branches of the pulmonary and bronchial arteries. Some vessels with the structure and course of bronchial arteries were found to be branches of the pulmonary artery, originating near the hilum.

In 1968, Robertson reported the results of microangiographical and histological studies of the pulmonary and bronchial arterial systems on 52 normal human fetuses, infants, and children and on a series of 17 infants with transposition of the great arteries. An abnormal pattern of the pulmonary arterial system, including abnormal bronchopulmonary arteries, was a prominent feature in isolated transposition, though less so in transposition with a ventricular septal defect. In isolated transposition there was a considerable increase in the bronchial arterial supply of the pulmonary parenchyma via bronchopulmonary arteries. In transposition associated with a ventricular septal defect, the pulmonary parenchyma had a normal or moderately increased bronchial arterial supply.

Thromboembolic Manifestations.

Thromboembolic manifestations were found at autopsy in 21 patients and involved the central nervous system, the gastrointestinal tract, the kidneys, the lungs, and the aorta. Table 11.2 shows these manifestations in each of the 21 patients. Table 11.3 summarizes the type and frequency of the thromboembolic manifestations in the organs involved. These findings suggest that the brain is the most common site of these manifestations and that, in some cases, more than one system is involved.

Review of the literature also suggests that the central nervous system is the most common site for these complications. Case 9 of Harris and Farber (1939) had thromophlebitis of the longitudinal and left sigmoid sinus and infarction of the right cerebral hemisphere. Berthrong and Sabiston (1951) described 6 cases with complete transposition of the great arteries. Recent and old encephalomalacia were found in 2, recent infarction in 2, diffuse microscopic perivascular hemorrhage in 1, and subarachnoid hemorrhage in 1. Five of these patients died after an interval that varied from a few hours to 20 days after surgical interference. Ma-

TABLE 11.2

THROMBOEMBOLIC MANIFESTATIONS (21 PATIENTS)

Group I	
1; 3 days	Moderate subarachnoid hemorrhage surrounding base of the brain
2; 7 days	Small area of subarachnoid hemorrhage over the right uncus
3; 16 days	Extensive subarachnoid hemorrhage around the base of the brain coming from 4th ventricle. Hemorrhage in 4th and lateral ventricles
4; 7 weeks	Thrombosis of sagittal, transverse, and sigmoid sinuses. Large infarct (4 x 7 cm) in right hemisphere. Calcified mass in bifurcation of aorta (probable old saddle embolus). Hemorrhage in both kidneys
5; 3 months	Died of hematemesis and melena. Whole large bowel from coecum contained a moderate amount of changed blood
6; 3 months	Large hemorrhage in the right middle cerebral fossa, which arose from a grossly dilated cerebral vein. Thrombosis of veins over left hemisphere. Infarction of the spleen
7; 4 months	Thrombus occupying aorta from renal to iliac arteries. Superior longitudinal sinus and cerebral veins thrombosis. Left parietal lobe infarction. Bilateral kidney infarction
8; 5 months	Thrombosis of superior longitudinal sinus and cerebral veins. Cerebral infarction
Group III	
9; 5 days	Slight intraventricular hemorrhage of the left side
10; 2 weeks	Thrombosis in the left middle cerebral artery. Large infarcts of left hemisphere. Snbarachnoid hemorrhage around cerebellum and cord. Small infarcts in the lungs. Thrombosis of renal veins and inferior vena cava. Multiple infarcts of the kidneys
11; 22 days	Hemorrhage in the 4th and lateral ventricles
12; 3½ months	Thrombosis of superior mesenteric artery. Small thrombus at bifurcation of aorta. Gangrene of bowel from jejunum to sigmoid colon. Infarct left kidney
13; 5½ months	Bilateral pontine and thalamic hemorrhages
14; 6 months	Infarction of kidneys and adherent thrombus in abdominal aorta
15; 7 months	Thrombosis of intercranial venous sinuses. Softening of left parietal region
16; 7 months	Right lateral sinus thrombosis, left internal carotid thrombosis, cerebral edema
17; 18 years	Large areas of hemorrhagic consolidation and brown induration in the lungs
Group IV	
18; 9 months	Atrophy of left cerebral cortex
19; 2 years	Bilateral frontoparietal infarction with cystic changes
20; 3 years	Old cerebral cortical infarcts in left frontal and parietal lobes
21; 21 years	Died of gastrointestinal hemorrhage. Mucosal hemorrhages in stomach, duodenum, small and large intestines

TABLE 11.3

Frequency and Type of Thromboembolic Manifestations in Various Organs (21 Patients)

1. Central nervous system
   a. Infarction of the cerebral hemispheres; 6
   b. Thrombosis of cerebral sinuses; 5
   c. Hemorrhage in the ventricles; 5
   d. Subarachnoid hemorrhage; 4
   e. Thrombosis of cerebral veins; 3
   f. Thrombosis middle cerebral artery; 1
   g. Thrombosis internal carotid artery; 1
   h. Hemorrhage in cerebral hemispheres; 1

2. Gastrointestinal tract
   a. Hemorrhage; 2
   b. Infarct of spleen; 1
   c. Superior mesenteric artery thrombosis; 1
   d. Gangrene of bowel; 1
   e. Thrombosis of inferior vena cava; 1

3. Kidneys
   a. Infarcts; 4
   b. Hemorrhage; 1
   c. Renal vein thrombosis; 1

4. Lungs
   a. Hemorrhage; 1
   b. Infarction; 1

5. Aorta
   a. Saddle embolus or thrombus; 4

ronde (1958) reported a patient with transposition of the great arteries
who died at the age of 7 years with subarachnoid hemorrhage. In Case 4,
Group I of Noonan *et al.* (1960) there was thrombosis of the sagittal sinus. In the patient of Roberts *et al.* (1962) old and recent thrombi occluded the superior sagittal sinus and the middle cerebral artery.

Of the other thromboembolic phenomena, the patient of Janeway
(1877) with complete transposition of the great arteries had a fatal intestinal hemorrhage. At necropsy no embolus was found in the superior
mesenteric artery but there was intense congestion of the ilium and slight-
er congestion of the colon. Berthrong and Sabiston (1951) pointed out
that all their patients with transposition who had cerebral lesions, had
pulmonary vascular thrombi in spite of what would have been considered
a very adequate blood flow. One of their patients had a focal scar in the
renal cortex. Case 3, Group I of Noonan *et al.* (1960) had renal infarction while their Case 5 in the same group had thromboembolism of the

inferior mesenteric artery and massive gastrointestinal bleeding. The patient of Roberts *et al.* (1962) had thrombi in the mesenteric arteries and in the iliac, femoral, and splenic veins. Multiple infarcts were present in the liver, spleen, and left lung. Balboni and Nammack (1964) reported 2 cases of complete transposition of the great vessels in each of which necrosis of the small intestines complicated thrombosis of the superior mesenteric artery. Of the 180 autopsied cases of transposition of the great arteries seen at the Johns Hopkins Hospital and reported by Oppenheimer (1969), thrombosis was noted in 37 cases. Venous and arterial thrombosis were simultaneously present in 13 cases; thrombosis of the ductus arteriosus and pulmonary artery in 1 case, and arterial occlusion occurred in the absence of demonstrated venous thrombosis in 6 instances. There were 11 cases with thrombosis in only the venous system and 6 additional instances of thrombosis of a surgical pulmonary–subclavian anastomosis. The venous thrombi were the source of the arterial thrombi in the 13 patients with both lesions. In addition, the ductus arteriosus was the source of pulmonary emboli in the patient with thrombosis of the ductus and the pulmonary artery. The highest incidence of arterial thrombosis occurred in the neonates and infants 1 month of age or younger. Shunting surgical procedures did not appear to have caused any alteration in the probable route transversed by visceral emboli. On the other hand, iatrogenic atrial septal defects provided passage for emboli to the lungs. In three cases mesenteric artery thrombosis was the probable cause of death and widespread cerebral infarction caused death in 11 children. Parsons *et al.* (1971) reported the case of a 6-week-old baby with transposition who developed cerebral venous thrombosis with hemiparesis. This was followed by intestinal obstruction and urinary suppression. Necropsy showed organized clot on the atrial wall near the septostomy scar and large clots in the descending aorta and at the aortic bifurcation.

The Glomerulus in Transposition

In 1953, Meessen and Litton drew our attention to the occurrence of glomerular enlargement in patients with cyanotic congenital heart disease. The degree of glomerular enlargement was proportionate to the degree of cyanosis. Widening of the vasa afferentia was often observed while, in contrast, the vasa efferentia were seldom affected. The glomerular counts of patients with cyanotic heart disease and those of control patients showed no essential difference. The authors believed that chronic hypoxia and carbon dioxide retension gave rise to dilatation of the glomerular arterioles and widening of the vasa afferentia which facilitates the glomerular circulation. The adaptation to chronic hypoxia is thus accomplished by capillary loop ectasia which, in turn, results in glomerular enlargement. The tubular epithelium was intact in their cases. Spear (1960) also commented upon glomerular enlargement in 17 of 288 cases of cyanotic congenital heart disease. Of these 17 patients, 8 had complete transposition of the great arteries. The glomeruli were prominent in these 17 cases with congestion and extreme dilatation of the capillaries along the peripheral margins of the glomerular tufts. In the intercapillary tissue, particularly in the central stalk of the mesangium, a fibrillar or granular eosinophilic material positive in periodic acid-Schiff were present. An increase in the number of cells in the central stalk and thickening of the basement membrane were present in all cases. Venous thrombosis was present in 3, and in 2 of these only a single small vein was affected. Arterial thrombi were seen in 2 cases and renal infarcts in 4. Bauer and Rosenberg (1960) examined the kidneys of 29 patients with Fallot's tetralogy and provided objective and quantitative confirmation of glomerular enlargement in cyanotic congenital heart disease.

In 1964, Spear summarized the glomerular abnormalities that may occur in some patients with cyanotic congenital heart disease apart from the effects of thromboembolism or bacterial endocarditis. There may be enlargement, congestion or capillary dilatation; an increased number of capillary loops; hypercellularity and deposition of granulofibrillar eosinophilic material in the mesangium; generalized hypercellularity; focal sclerosis; thickening or destruction of capillary walls; dilatation of afferent arterioles; and prominence of juxta-glomerular apparatus. In 1966, Spear and Vitsky described hyalinization of the afferent and efferent glomerular arterioles in 3 patients with congenital heart disease. Their Patient 3, who died at 8 years of age, was a case of complete transposition of the great arteries with a ventricular septal defect. Ingelfinger *et al.* (1970) pointed out that proteinuria is usually the clinical manifestation of glomerulomegaly in cyanotic heart disease and that its course is usually benign but it should be investigated to rule out primary renal disease.

In the present series, sections of the kidneys were available in one patient. These showed an enormous increase in the size of the glomeruli. Several fibrosed glomeruli were present and calcium salts were deposited immediately external to the outer layer of the epithelium of Bowman's capsule, i.e., in the connective tissue. Calcification, however, was not confined to the region of the glomeruli, others were situated in relation to the tubules or in the interstitial tissue between two blood vessels. Some large pale foam cells which have taken up lipid deposits were also seen. There were no striking mesangial changes but a minority of the glomeruli with increased fibrous tissue were observed.

Bone Lesions in Transposition

Ascenzi and Marinozzi (1958) were the first to recognize thickening of the skull associated with cyanotic congenital heart disease. Mariani and Bosman (1962) reported radiographs of the skull, sternum, and spine of 26 cyanotic patients with congenital heart disease. Diploic thickening of the skull was present in 3, thickening of the upper and lower margins of the vertebral bodies in 6, and the sternum was affected in 1. Caffey (1961) and Mosley (1963) also mentioned the occurrence of bone lesions in cyanotic heart disease. Nice et al. (1964) reported 6 patients with congenital heart disease and central cyanosis. Of their 6 patients, Cases 1 and 2, aged 10 years and 7 years, respectively, had complete transposition of the great arteries with a ventricular septal defect. In both patients roentgenograms of the skull showed moderate thickening of the diploe in the frontal region and considerable thickening in the parietal region. Roentgenograms of the distal ends of the long bones revealed widening of the medullary cavities, cortical thickening, and coarsening of the trabecular pattern. Similar changes were present in the lumbosacral spine, pelvis, and upper portion of the femoral bone. The authors pointed out that these bony lesions could be divided into two categories on the basis of their similarity to other lesions. Thus "pulmonary osteoarthropathy" with thickening of the mid or distal shafts of the long bones due to periosteal deposition may occur. This entity is frequently associated with digital clubbing and occasionally with arthralgia with or without effusions in the joints. A neurovascular mechanism is probably responsible for this phenomenon (Diner, 1962). The second category is that which generally occurs with chronic anemias, e.g., Cooley's anemia and congenital hemolytic anemia. These abnormalities include: skull—widening of the diploe, thickening of the tables, and the "hair-end-on" striations; long bones—endosteal cortical defects, widening of the medullary canals, loss of diaphyseal tapering, loss of trabeculations in some areas, and coarsening in other areas; pelvis, spine, and ribs—mottled areas of sclerosis and/or alterations in trabecular pattern. The hyperplastic bone marrow that may result from constant stimulation by anoxia causes endosteal cortical erosions, widens medullary cavities and obliterates trabeculae producing the radiolucent roentgenographical findings. The sclerotic changes are the result of deposition of new bone on existing bone or osseous metaplasia in the marrow spaces. Bone infarction may play some role in producing bone sclerosis.

Endocrine Tumors and Transposition

Bartler *et al.,* in 1960, reported a cyanotic 25-year-old man who died with congenital heart disease and an endocrine tumor. The patient presented with the clinical picture of Cushing's syndrome and had total anomalous pulmonary venous drainage into the right atrium pituitary adenoma and bilateral cortical hyperplasia. Roberts *et al.* (1962) reported 4 autopsied cases with congenital heart disease and an endocrine tumor. Two of these patients had aortic stenosis and unilateral cortical adenomas which were not apparent clinically. The third patient, who died at 21 years of age, had complete transposition of the great arteries, pulmonary stenosis, and a ventricular septal defect. At necropsy there was a left adrenal cortical carcinoma which had invaded the capsule. The fourth patient, with total anomalous pulmonary venous drainage, had an islet cell tumor of the pancreas which had metastasized to the pancreatic lymph nodes. Folger *et al.* (1964) reported the clinical and pathological features of 5 patients with pheochromocytoma associated with cyanotic congenital cardiac malformations. Two of their cases had Fallot's tetralogy, 1 had double outlet right ventricle, 1 had Ebstein's anomaly of the tricuspid valve, and 1 had transposition of the great arteries. In 3 of these (including the patient with transposition) the diagnosis was made during life, and was confirmed at surgery in 2, and at autopsy in 2. Clinical manifestations of the tumor did not appear until 12 to 41 years after birth. Their patient with transposition was a 14-year-old girl, who, years before death, began having attacks of nervousness, recurrent frontal headaches, profuse sweating, insomnia, periodic vomiting, and tachycardia. The blood pressure varied from 98/100 to 150/110 mm Hg. Shortly before death a phentolamine test was positive. Autopsy confirmed the diagnosis of transposition of the great arteries and a pheochromocytoma was present in the left adrenal gland with metastasis in a regional lymph node and in the liver.

Roberts *et al.* (1962) pointed out that the association between heart disease, particularly of the cyanotic variety, and endocrine tumors appears to be more than mere coincidence, and conceivably could be related to the stress produced by prolonged hypoxemia. Folger *et al.* (1964) confirmed this view and added that the tumors in their cases were unlikely to be congenital since their clinical manifestations appeared a long time after birth. They pointed out that persistent hypoxia could produce adrenal medullary hyperplasia and finally an autonomously functioning medullary tumor.

Extracardiac Congenital Malformations

In this series extracardiac congenital malformations occurred in 25 patients (Table 11.4). Table 11.5 shows the anomalies encountered in the various systems. Origin of a vertebral artery from the aorta appeared to be the most common single congenital abnormality in this series.

Review of the literature suggests that extracardiac abnormalities in transposition are uncommon. Wiland (1956) found no extracardiac anomalies in his 24 cases of transposition of the great vessels. Case 2 of Jacobson (1921) had 2 accessory spleens, while Harris and Farber (1939) cite an example of spastic paraplegia and undescended testicles

TABLE 11.4

EXTRACARDIAC CONGENITAL MALFORMATIONS (25 PATIENTS)

Group I

1	Meningocele, Arnold-Chiari malformation, hydrocephalus
2	Left vertebral artery from aorta
3	Bifid rib
4	Stricture of urethra, hydroureters
5	Aberrant renal vessels to the upper poles of both kidneys. Annular pancreas
6	Rubella syndrome, microphthalmia, malformed left ear
7	Left vertebral artery from aorta
8	Accessory spleen
9	Hydroureters

Group III

10	Two small pedunculated papillomata left side of the face
11	Double left ureter and pelvis
12	Right cryptorchism
13	Duodenal atresia
14	Infantile caecum and incomplete absorption of the paracolic gutter. Chronic duodenal ulcer invading pancreas. Oxyntic cells in second and third parts of duodenum
15	Left vertebral artery from aorta
16	Agenesis of right subclavian artery
17	Congenital hypoplastic kidneys
18	Right subclavian and right common carotid; no innominate artery
19	Vertebral artery from aorta, perforated duodenal ulcer
20	Cystic dilatation of distal convoluted tubules
21	Vertebral artery from aorta
22	Vertebral artery from aorta

Group IV

23	Left cryptorchism
24	Meckel's diverticulum
25	External carotid from innominate

(Case 9). Emerson and Green (1942) pointed out that 4 of their cases had deformities elsewhere than the heart. Case 1 of Becker and Brill (1948) had congenital hydroureters and congenital hydronephrosis, while their Case 3 had 2 left renal arteries, hemivertebrate C7, T1, and L1, and synostosis of the second and third right ribs. The patient of Miskall and Fraser (1948) had a bifid 8th thoracic vertebra and through it a meningocele protruded. Brown (1950) reported a spina bifida in a case of complete transposition of the great arteries. Of the cases of congenital

TABLE 11.5

EXTRACARDIAC CONGENITAL MALFORMATIONS (25 PATIENTS)

1. Vascular system
    a. Vertebral artery from aorta; 6
    b. Aberrant renal arteries
    c. External carotid from innominate
    d. Agenesis of right subclavian
    e. Four brachiocephalic branches from aorta
    f. Vascular ring

2. Genitourinary system
    a. Undescended testicle; 2
    b. Cystic dilation of convoluted tubules
    c. Congenital hypoplastic kidney
    d. Stricture urethra and hydroureter
    e. Double ureter and pelvis
    f. Stenosis pelvic junction of left ureter
    g. Hydroureters

3. Central nervous system
    a. Meningocele
    b. Arnold-Chiari malformation
    c. Hydrocephalies

4. Skeletal
    a. Bifid rib

5. Gastrointestinal
    a. Meckel's diverticulum
    b. Annular pancreas
    c. Accessory spleen
    d. Duodenal atresia
    e. Chronic duodenal ulcer; 2

6. Skin
    a. Papilloma

7. Others
    a. Microphthalmia
    b. Malformed ear

heart disease with endocardial fibroelastosis reported by Andersen and Kelly (1956), 14 had complete transposition of the great arteries of which 5 had extracardiac congenital malformations. Their Case 113 had congenital cystic kidney, Case 116 double pelvis in the right kidney, Case 117 hemangioma of the liver sinusoids and anomalous origin of the vertebral artery, Case 118 anomalous lobulation of the left lung with an accessory lobe, and Case 120 atresia of the rectum and imperforate anus. Among the 22 autopsied cases of Noonan *et al.* (1960), Case 7, Group 2B, had a hypoplastic left main bronchus and a porencephalic cyst of the right cerebral hemisphere. Of the 167 autopsied cases of transposition reported by Boesen *et al.* (1963) 7 had extracardiac malformations. Harelip and/or cleft palate were present in 2, gastrointestinal malformations in 3, urogenital malformations in 1, malformations of bones and joints in 3, while nonclassified malformations occurred in 2. In the case reported by Sterns *et al.* (1964) the right subclavian artery arose as the fourth branch of the aortic arch. Mellins and Blumenthal (1964) reported 2 cases of complete transposition associated with esophageal atresia. One of these two cases also had congenital absence of the right radius. A polycystic kidney was observed in one of the 28 patients reported by Mehrizi *et al.* (1964). Of the 400 cases with congenital heart disease reported by Humphry and Munn (1966), 22 had renal abnormalities. Of these 22, transposition of the great vessels occurred in 2.

References

Abbott, M. E. (1937). Congenital heart disease. *Nelson's Loose-Leaf Med.* 4, 207.

Aberdeen, E., Waterston, D. J., Carr, I., Graham, G., Bonham-Carter, R. E., and Subramarian, S. (1965). Successful 'correction' of transposed great arteries by Mustard's operation. *Lancet* i, 1233.

Andersen, D. H., and Kelly, J. (1956). Endocardial fibro-elastosis. I. Endocardial fibro-elastosis associated with congenital malformations of the heart. *Pediatrics* 18, 513.

Ascenzi, A., and Marinozzi, V. (1958). Sur le crane en bosse au cours de polyglobules secondaires a l'hypoxemie chronique. *Acta Haematol.* 19, 253.

Balboni, F. A., and Nammack, G. P. D. (1964). Mesenteric vascular occlusion and complete transposition of the great vessels. A report of two cases. *Heart Cent. Bull. St. Francis Hosp. (Roslyn, N. Y.)* 19, 2.

Bartler, F. C., Liddle, G. W., Bell, N. H., Braunwald, E., Hilbish, T. G., Cornell, W., and Hicklin, M. (1960). Problem in differential diagnosis; clinical pathological conference at the National Institutes of Health. *Ann. Intern. Med.* 52, 1289.

Bauer, W. C., and Rosenberg, B. F. (1960). A quantitative study of glomerular enlargement in children with tetralogy of Fallot. *Amer. J. Pathol.* 37, 695.

Becker, M. C., and Brill, R. M. (1948). Complete transposition of the great vessels. *Arch. Pediat.* 65, 249.

Berthrong, M., and Sabiston, D. C., Jr. (1951). Cerebral lesions in congenital heart disease. A review of autopsies on one hundred and sixty-two cases. *Bull. Johns Hopkins Hosp.* **89**, 384.

Boesen, I., Melchior, J. C., Tersley, E., and Vendel, S. (1963). Extracardiac congenital malformations in children with congenital heart diseases. *Acta Pediat. Suppl.* **146**, 28.

Brown, J. W. (1950). "Congenital Heart Disease," 2nd Ed. Staples Press, London.

Caffey, J. (1961). "Pediatric X-Ray Diagnosis," p. 1125. Yearbook Medical, Chicago, Illinois.

Cleland, W. P., Goodwin, J. F., Steiner, R. E., and Zoob, M. (1957). Transposition of aorta and pulmonary artery with pulmonary stenosis. *Amer. Heart J.* **54**, 10.

Cockle, J. (1863). A case of transposition of the great vessels of the heart. *Med. Chir. Trans.* **46**, 193.

Cudkowicz, L., and Armstrong, J. B. (1952). Injection of the bronchial circulation in a case of transposition. *Brit. Heart J.* **14**, 374.

Diner, W. C. (1962). Hypertrophic osteoarthropathy. *J. Amer. Med. Ass.* **181**, 555.

Emerson, P. W., and Green, H. (1942). Transposition of the great cardiac vessels. *J. Pediat.* **21**, 1.

Ferencz, C. (1966). Transposition of the great vessels. Pathophysiologic considerations based upon a study of the lungs. *Circulation* **33**, 232.

Ferguson, D. J., Adams, P., and Watson, D. (1960). Pulmonary arteriosclerosis in transposition of great vessels. *Amer. J. Dis. Child* **99**, 653.

Folger, G. M., Jr., Roberts, W. C., Mehrizi, A., Shah, K. D., Glancy, D. L., Carpenter, C. C. J., and Esterly, J. R. (1964). Cyanotic malformations of the heart with pheo-chromocytema. A report of five cases. *Circulation* **29**, 750.

Folse, R., Roberts, W. C., and Cornell, W. P. (1961). Increased bronchial collateral circulation in a patient with transposition of the great vessels and pulmonary hypertension. *Amer. J. Cardiol.* **8**, 282.

Harris, J. S., and Farber, S. (1939). Transposition of the great cardiac vessels with special reference to the phylogenetic theory of Spitzer. *Arch. Pathol.* **28**, 427.

Heath, D., and Edwards, J. E. (1958). The pathology of hypertensive pulmonary vascular disease. *Circulation* **18**, 533.

Humphry, A., and Munn, J. D. (1966). Abnormalites of the urinary tract in association with congenital cardiovascular disease. *Can. Med. Ass. J.* **95**, 143.

Ingelfinger, J. R., Kissane, J. M., and Robson, A. M. (1970). Glomerulomegaly in a patient with cyanotic congenital heart disease. *Amer. J. Dis. Child* **120**, 69–71.

Jacobson, V. C. (1921). Deviation of the aortic septum: complete transposition of great vessels, with report of two cases in infants. *Amer. J. Dis. Child.* **21**, 176.

Janeway, E. G. (1877). Malposition of aorta and pulmonary artery—thrombus in heart and cerebral embolism, death from intestinal hemorrhage. *Med. Rec.* **12**, 811.

Mariani, M., and Bosman, C. (1962). Über skelettveranderungen bei kongenitalen herznissbildungen mit zyanose. *Beitr. Pathol. Anat. Allg. Pathol.* **126**, 145.

Maronde, R. F. (1958). Cause of death in persons with congenital heart disease. *Amer. J. Med. Sci.* **236**, 41.

Meessen, H., and Litton, M. A. (1953). Morphology of the kidney in morbus caeruleus. *Arch. Pathol.* **56**, 480.

Mehrizi, A., Hirsch, M. S., and Taussig, H. B. (1964). Congenital heart disease in the neonatal period. Autopsy study of 170 cases. *J. Pediat.* **65**, 721.

Mellins, R. B., and Blumenthal, S. (1964). Cardiovascular anomalies and esophageal atresia. *Amer. J. Dis. Child.* **107**, 160.

Miskall, E. W., and Fraser, J. A. (1948). Complete transposition of the great vessels. *Ohio State Med. J.* **44**, 709.

Mosley, J. E. (1963). "Bone Changes in Hematologic Disorders." Grune and Stratton, New York.

Newfeld, E. A., Muster, A. J., and Paul, M. (1972). The pulmonary vascular bed in complete transposition. Hemodynamic–pathologic correlations. *Circulation* **46**, Suppl. 2, 97.

Nice, C. M., Jr., Daves, M. L., and Wood, G. H. (1964). Changes in bone associated with cyanotic congenital cardiac disease. *Amer. Heart J.* **68**, 25.

Noonan, A., Nadas, A. S., Rudolph, A. M., and Harris, G. D. C. (1960). Transposition of the great arteries. A correlation of clinical, physiologic and autopsy data. *N. Engl. J. Med.* **263**, 592.

Oppenheimer, E. H. (1969). Arterial thrombosis (? paradoxical embolism) in association with transposition of the great vessels. *Johns Hopkins Med. J.* **124**, 202.

Parsons, C. G., Astley, R., Burrows, F. G. O., and Singh, S. P. (1971). Transposition of the great arteries. A study of 65 infants followed for 1 to 4 years after balloon septostomy. *Brit. Heart J.* **33**, 725.

Roberts, W. C., Mason, D. T., and Braunwald, E. (1962). Survival to adulthood in a patient with complete transposition of the great vessels. Including a note on the association of endocrine tumors with heart disease. *Ann. Intern. Med.* **57**, 834.

Robertson, B. (1965). Microangiographic studies of the lung in transposition of the great arteries. *Acta Paediat. Scand.* **159**, 84.

Robertson, B. (1968). The intrapulmonary arterial pattern in normal infancy and in transposition of the great vessels. *Acta Paediat. Scand. Suppl* **184**, 7.

Spear, G. S. (1960). Glomerular alterations in cyanotic congenital heart disease. *Bull. John's Hopkins Hosp.* **106**, 347.

Spear, G. S. (1964). The glomerulus in cyanotic congenital heart disease and primary pulmonary hypertension. *Nephron* **1**, 238.

Spear, G. S., and Vitsky, B. H. (1966). Hyalinization of afferent and efferent glomerular arterioles in cyanotic congenital heart disease. *Amer. J. Med.* **41**, 309.

Sterns, L. P., Baker, R. M., and Edwards, J. E. (1964). Complete transposition of the great vessels. Unusual longevity in a case with subpulmonary stenosis. *Circulation* **29**, 610.

Viles, P. H., Ongley, P. A., and Titus, J. L. (1969). The spectrum of pulmonary vascular disease in transposition of the great arteries. *Circulation* **40**, 31.

Wagenvoort, C. A., Nauta, J., van der Schaar, P. J., Weeda, H. W. H., and Wagenvoort, N. (1968). The pulmonary vasculature in complete transposition of the great vessels, judged from lung biopsies. *Circulation* **38**, 746.

Wiland, O. K. (1956). Extracardiac anomalies in association with congenital heart disease. *Lab. Invest.* **5**, 380.

Chapter 12

CLINICAL FEATURES

Symptoms

CYANOSIS

All 409 patients in this series were cyanotic. Cyanosis was detected at birth or during the first or second day of life in 375 patients. Delayed onset of cyanosis was observed in 34 patients; 4 in Group I, 1 in Group II, 25 in Group III, and 4 in Group IV (Table 12.1). Differential cyanosis with the upper half of the body more cyanotic than the lower half, described by Taussig (1960) as a sure sign of transposition, was not seen in this series.

In most reported cases, cyanosis was observed at birth. In a few cases the onset of cyanosis was delayed. Thus, one of the 12 cases of Emerson and Green (1942) was acyanotic. Abrams *et al.* (1951) reviewed the literature and found that cyanosis was present at birth in 58 cases, but its onset was delayed in 26. Of those with a delayed onset of cyanosis, it developed hours to days in 6 and after weeks or months in 15 cases; in 5 the interval between birth and the onset of cyanosis was not noted. Among the 50 patients with transposition reported by Noonan *et al.* (1960), cyanosis was present from birth in 36 cases and in 10 others was noted within the first 4 months of life. In 3 infants cyanosis was not noted until about 1 year of age, and in 1 child cyanosis was first described at 3 years and 8 months. These authors, however, have included cases with single ventricle and origin of both great vessels from the right ventricle in their material. Mehrizi and Taussig (1963) reported two cases of "acyanotic transposition." In each of these 2 cases, however, the aorta and pulmonary artery overrode the ventricular septum. Differential cyanosis with the upper half of the body more cyanotic than the lower half of the body was observed by Astley and Parsons (1952) in one of their patients with transposition, but the authors had to omit the case from their series

TABLE 12.1

CLINICAL FEATURES

Group	Cyanosis	Breathlessness	Cyanotic spells	Respiratory infections	Squatting
Group I Intact septum (209)	All at birth except: 3rd Week in 1 4th Week in 1 6th Week in 1 5th Month in 1	121	38	26	0
Group II Intact septum and pulmonary stenosis (16)	All at birth except: 1st Week in 1	11	4	6	0
Group III Ventricular septal defect (138)	All at birth except: 1st Week in 7 1st Month in 7 2nd Month in 3 3rd Month in 4 4th Month in 1 5th Month in 1 6th Month in 1 3rd Year in 1	75	26	40	3
Group IV Ventricular septal defect and pulmonary stenosis (46)	All at birth except: 3rd Week in 1 1st Month in 3	22	8	10	2

as it was impossible to obtain adequate particulars at necropsy. Fowler and Ordway (1952) admitted that they had never seen the clinical picture of differential cyanosis among their patients with transposition. Review of the literature shows that there are at least 9 reported cases of transposition associated with differential cyanosis. These cases were reported by Lees (1879), Hecko (1948) 2 cases; Jimenez (1956); Elyan and Ruffle (1952) case 1, Noonan *et al.* (1960), and Toole *et al.* (1960) 3 cases.

When complete interruption of the aortic arch is associated with complete transposition of the great arteries, the lower half of the body is perfused with blood which contains more oxygen than that perfusing the upper part of the body. Taussig (1960) points out that the clinical diagnosis of this condition is based on the findings of an infant with intense cyanosis and severe dyspnea whose feet and lower extremities are almost of normal color. The line of demarcation of the cyanosis is usually at the brim of the pelvis. This sign in patients with transposition and complete interruption of the aortic arch was reported by Hamburger (1937), Castellanos *et al.* (1959), and Buckley *et al.* (1965). On the other hand, it was not observed in the 2 patients with complete interruption of the aortic arch in this series, the 2 cases of Coles and Holesh (1957), or the 1 case of Norton *et al.* (1970). In the case described by Rannels and Propst (1937) in which there was no apparent continuity between the ascending and descending aorta, the authors made no comment on the presence or absence of differential cyanosis.

HEART FAILURE

Of the whole group of 409 patients, 200 developed congestive heart failure during the course of the disease. Table 12.2 shows the number and age of the patients who developed heart failure in each group. The incidence of heart failure was 51% in Group I, 68% in Group II, 53% in Group III, and 22% in Group IV. In the whole series heart failure tended to have three peaks. The first and largest occurred during the first 2 weeks of life when a significant number of patients with an intact ventricular septum develop heart failure. The second peak occurred during the second and third months of life when a significant number of patients with a ventricular septal defect develop heart failure. The third and smallest peak occurred in the second and third years of life when some survivors develop complications or undergo heart surgery. Pericardial effusion complicated heart failure in 2 patients in this series (Fig. 12.1).

McCue and Young (1961) found that the mean age of onset of symptoms of heart failure in 11 patients with transposition was 1½ months.

TABLE 12.2

CONGESTIVE HEART FAILURE [a]

Group	Weeks				Months											Years										
	1	2	3	4	2	3	4	5	6	7	8	9	10	11	12	2	3	4	5	6	7	8	9	10	11	12
Group I Intact septum (106)	56	12	5	5	9	6	1	4	0	0	1	0	1	1	0	0	3	0	0	1	0	0	1	0	0	0
Group II Intact septum and pulmonary stenosis (11)	2	3	0	0	0	1	0	0	0	0	0	0	0	0	0	2	1	1	0	1	0	0	0	0	0	0
Group III Ventricular septal defect (73)	9	13	4	5	18	10	1	3	4	0	0	0	0	0	0	1	2	1	0	0	1	0	0	0	0	1
Group IV Ventricular septal defect and pulmonary stenosis (10)	2	1	0	3	1	0	0	0	0	0	0	1	0	0	0	1	0	0	1	0	0	0	0	0	0	0
Total	69	29	9	13	28	17	2	7	4	0	1	1	1	1	0	4	6	2	0	3	1	1	1	0	0	1

[a] Data for 200 cases.

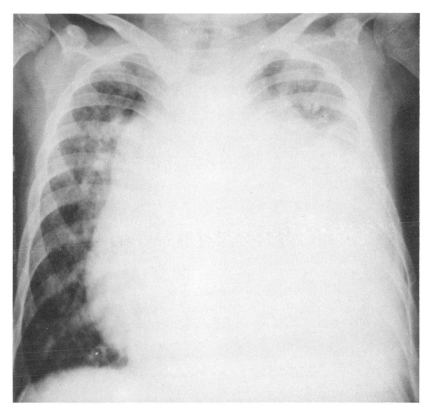

Fig. 12.1. Chest roentgenogram of a 10-year-old child with transposition and ventricular septal defect showing massive cardiac enlargement caused by pericardial effusion.

Keith *et al.* (1958) found that in 60% of cases of complete transposition of the great arteries heart failure becomes manifest between 1 and 4 months. Seventeen percent of their cases were under 14 days when seen with a full-blown picture of decompensation. Among Noonan's *et al.* (1960) 50 patients, a history of congestive heart failure was present in 37. Of these, 24 were 4 months of age or younger, 4 between 5 and 18 months, and 9 over 18 months. In 3 patients, each more than 18 months of age, heart failure resulted from a shunt procedure for pulmonary stenosis. Of the 28 who developed heart failure below the age of 18 months, 10 had an intact ventricular septum, and 18 had a ventricular septal defect without pulmonary stenosis.

BREATHLESSNESS

Breathlessness on exertion was observed in 229 patients with a fairly uniform distribution in the four groups (Table 12.1). Among the few patients who survived more than 5 years, 1 patient in Group IV could not walk more than 20 yards. On the other hand, another patient in the same group could walk several miles. One patient in Group III used to go swimming, while another in the same group used to go to "Rock and Roll" classes until he died following an appendectomy operation. Although paroxysmal dyspnea was not observed in any patient in the series, it was noted in the patients reported by Langstaff (1811), Walshe (1842), and in 3 of the 16 patients of Astley and Parsons (1952).

CYANOTIC SPELLS

Table 12.1 shows that 76 patients in the whole series developed cyanotic spells. The highest incidence of cyanotic spells occurred in the first few weeks or months of life. This phenomenon tended to occur less frequently in older patients than in younger ones.

Whereas blue spells were not observed among the 10 patients of Abrams *et al.* (1951) 9 of the 12 patients reported by Emerson and Green (1942), slightly less than half of the patients of Nadas (1957), and 13 of the 50 patients of Noonan *et al.* (1960) did report such symptoms.

RESPIRATORY INFECTIONS

In the whole series a history of recurrent cough and respiratory infections occurred in 82 patients (Table 12.1). Of these 82 patients 26 were in Group I, 6 in Group II, 40 in Group III, and 10 in Group IV. Recurrent lung infections were not a feature of transposition in infancy but tended to be a frequent complication in older children and sometimes they precipitated congestive heart failure.

SQUATTING

Only 5 patients in this series squatted. In 3 there was a ventricular septal defect, and in 2 there was a ventricular septal defect and left ventricular outflow tract obstruction.

While squatting occurred in 20% of the cases reported by Campbell and Suzman (1951) and in 2 of the 16 patients reported by Astley and Parsons (1952), it was not seen in patients of walking age studied by Keith *et al.* (1958) and was present in 1 of the 18 patients in the same age group reported by Noonan *et al.* (1960). Mehrizi *et al.* (1966) pointed out that unlike tetralogy of Fallot, squatting is unusual in transposition with a ventricular septal defect and pulmonary stenosis.

ANGINA

Only one patient in Group I had a history of recurrent attacks of midsternal pain related to effort. One child in Astley and Parson's series (1952) had angina, while in the group of 18 patients old enough to talk reported by Noonan *et al.* (1960), 5 complained of chest pain related to effort.

Signs

GROWTH AND DEVELOPMENT

Retardation of growth was almost invariable and generally appeared in all patients after the first few months of life. Criteria for mental retardation were difficult to select, since motor development is often delayed so that the physical milestones of early childhood lose much of their significance. Since speech does not seem to be affected by cyanotic heart disease alone, as pointed out by Tyler and Clark (1957a), any child who did not talk by the age of 3 years was considered mentally retarded. Utilizing this criterion, 3 patients in Group III were considered mentally retarded.

Although several writers have commented on the near-normal intellectual functions of patients with congenital heart disease (Campbell and Reynolds, 1949; Chazan *et al.*, 1951) and of those with transposition (Noonan *et al.*, 1960), Tyler and Clark (1957a) found that 17.7% of their patients with transposition without pulmonary stenosis and 1 of their 13 patients with transposition and pulmonary stenosis had mental retardation.

THE ARTERIAL PULSES AND EVIDENCE OF INCREASED SYSTEMIC BLOOD FLOW

In most patients the arterial pulses were unremarkable. Heart failure was often associated with small volume pulses. Bounding pulses, distended finger and arm veins, and warm extremities were noted in some of the older patients in this series. These signs were attributed to increased systemic blood flow and hyperkinetic systemic circulation by Shaher (1964). Increased systemic blood flow producing distension of the veins of the fingers in some of the very cyanotic children with transposition was also reported by Campbell and Suzman (1951). Case 4 of Hemsath *et al.* (1936), and Case 9 of Harris and Farber (1939) had prominent scalp veins. One patient reported by Dorning (1890), another by Harris *et al.* (1927), and 5 of the 12 patients reported by Emerson and Green (1942) had dilatation of the superficial skin veins. In 8 severely cyanosed patients with complete transposition associated with pulmonary stenosis, Cleland *et al.* (1957) noticed that the peripheral pulses had a remarkable full volume and in 1 case there was visible pulsation of the dorsalis pedis and posterior tibial vessels. Noonan *et al.* (1960) noticed that infants with transposition and marked cyanosis had varicostities of the extremities and scalp.

CLUBBING OF THE FINGERS

Clubbing of the fingers was present in almost all patients between the age of 3 to 6 months. Keith *et al.* (1958) pointed out that clubbing is

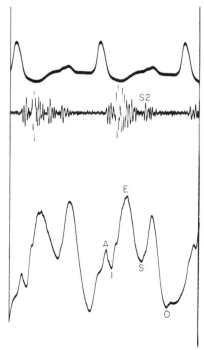

Fig. 12.2. Upper tracing, electrocardiogram; middle tracing, phonocardiogram; lower tracing, precordial pulsations recorded in the left fourth space in the midclavicular line. All data from a 10-year-old child with transposition and ventricular septal defect. A, I, E, S, O are the waves of the apex cardiogram. Note the early diastolic vibration between S and O probably caused by pulmonary incompetence.

rare in transposition since the early death of the patient prevents its development. Among their patients, it was noticed as early as 5 months. Clubbing was present and was proportionate to the degree of cyanosis in all patients except the very young infants reported by Noonan *et al.* (1960).

CHEST DEFORMITY

Precordial bulging, as early as the age of 6 months, was observed in 58 patients, 18 in Group I, 3 in Group II, 28 in Group III, and 9 in Group IV.

Noonan *et al.* (1960) pointed out that chest deformity was relatively common among older infants and children with transposition. Twenty-two of their 50 patients had a generalized increase in the anterioposterior chest diameter, whereas 18 showed an advanced prominence of the left half of the chest. A right-sided chest deformity was present in 2.

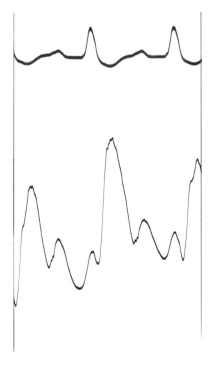

Fig. 12.3. Precordial pulsations (lower tracing) recorded from the second left space of a child 10 years of age with transposition and ventricular septal defect and aorta occupying the left heart border in the position of the normal main pulmonary artery. Note the arterial pulse wave recorded. Upper tracing is the electrocardiogram.

PRECORDIAL MOVEMENT AND PALPATION

According to Perloff (1970), in complete transposition in the new-born period the right ventricular impulse may be indistinguishable from normal. Later, the right ventricular impulse persists and becomes more pronounced. The right ventricular pulsation is especially prominent in the presence of a hyperkinetic systemic circulation with marked increase in the systemic blood flow (Fig. 12.2). A pulmonary arterial impulse is absent since that vessel lies in a posterior position. When the aorta occupies a position at the left cardiac border an aortic impulse may be recorded in the second left space (Fig. 12.3). A left ventricular impulse is especially prominent when a ventricular septal defect occurs with increased pulmonary blood flow and pressure. When the pulmonary blood flow is diminished due to pulmonary stenosis or pulmonary vascular obstruction, the impulse of the left ventricle is less apparent or absent altogether.

THRILLS

A systolic thrill occurred in 45 cases in this series (Table 12.3). The lowest incidence of a systolic thrill occurred in patients with an intact ventricular septum, while the highest incidence occurred in patients with a ventricular septal defect and left ventricular outflow tract obstruction.

Of the 50 patients reported by Noonan *et al.* (1960) a systolic thrill was felt in 14 and occurred with approximately equal frequency in all their groups.

TABLE 12.3

THRILLS AND HEART SOUNDS

Group	Thrill	Split second sound	Single second sound	Ejection sound	Third sound
Group I Intact septum	5	64	101	13	10
Group II Intact septum and pulmonary stenosis	3	2	15	2	0
Group III Ventricular septal defect	16	43	36	10	14
Group IV Ventricular septal defect and pulmonary stenosis	21	3	28	4	0
Total	45	112	180	29	24

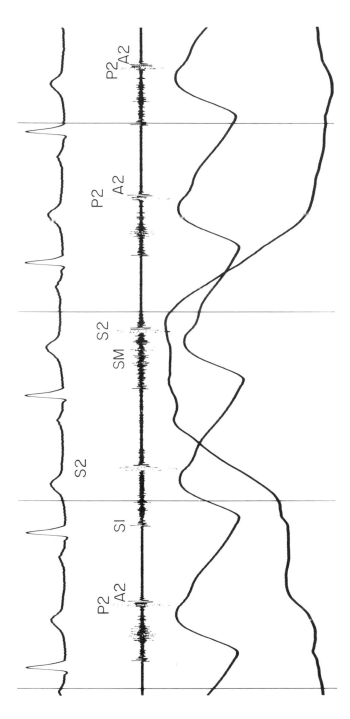

Fig. 12.4. Phonocardiogram after the Mustard procedure demonstrating paradoxical splitting of the second heart sound. Upper tracing, electrocardiogram; second tracing, phonocardiogram; third tracing, aortic pressure pulse; fourth tracing, respiration. A₂, aortic valve closure; P₂, pulmonary valve closure; S₁, first heart sound; S₂, second heart sound; SM, systolic murmur.

HEART SOUNDS

The first heart sound was described as normal in all patients. Of 292 patients in whom the second heart sound was described in the hospital chart, it was recorded as split in 112, and single in 180. Paradoxical splitting of the second heart sound was recorded in 1 patient after Mustard's procedure (Fig. 12.4). An ejection sound was recorded on 29 occasions and a third heart sound on 24. Table 12.3 shows the incidence of thrills, split second heart sound, ejection click, and a third heart sound in the four groups.

Perloff (1970) pointed out that in transposition the first heart sound is usually normal. A pulmonary ejection sound usually means that the pulmonary vascular resistance is elevated and the pulmonary artery dilated. The ejection sound is maximal in the vicinity of the second or third left intercostal space but is sometimes well heard at the apex because the pulmonary artery takes origin from the left ventricle, which usually forms the cardiac apex. According to Perloff (1970) ejection sound could originate from a dilated aorta in patients with a ventricular septal defect and pulmonary stenosis. Of the 13 cases with an intact ventricular septum, reported by Wells (1963), the phonocardiogram showed variable splitting of the second heart sound in 7, a narrow fixed split in 2, and a single sound in 4. The intensity of the second sound was increased in 3 and normal in 10. Of the 10 with a ventricular septal defect, the phonocardiogram did not differ in pattern from those with an intact septum in 8. Of the remaining 2 the second was single in 1, and occasionally split in 1. Of the 3 with a ventricular septal defect and pulmonary stenosis, the second sound was single in 2, and widely split with faint pulmonary valve closure in 1. Perloff (1970) explained the frequent occurrence of a single second heart sound in transposition. Aortic closure is louder than normal because of the anterior position of the aortic valve. Even when the pulmonary component is increased by pulmonary hypertension, splitting is usually absent because the pressures in the great vessels tend to be equal so that there is synchronous closure of the semilunar valves. Splitting is not heard in pulmonary stenosis because an already soft pulmonic component is further altered by the posterior position of the pulmonary artery. According to Campbell and Suzman (1951) a booming second sound is a most important physical sign in transposition and by itself may be enough to exclude the diagnosis of tetralogy of Fallot. Paradoxical splitting of the second heart sound in a patient with transposition, a small ventricular septal defect, and right bundle branch block was recorded by Zuberbuhler *et al.* (1967).

TABLE 12.4

HEART MURMURS

Group	Number with murmurs	Murmurs[a]					Onset of murmur				
		Ejection	Pansys-tolic	Mid. diastolic	Early diastolic	Contin-uous	1st week	1st month	2–6 months	7–12 months	More than 1 year
Group I Intact septum	133	127	3	2	1	3	59	12	5	1	0
Group II Intact septum and pulmonary stenosis	15	15	0	1	0	0	8	1	2	0	1
Group III Ventricular septal defect	130	115	16	5	6	4	59	30	16	1	1
Group IV Ventricular septal defect and pulmonary stenosis	46	46	0	1	1	4	18	2	1	0	1

HEART MURMURS

Table 12.4 shows the type and, if known, age at onset of heart murmurs in the four groups. Of the whole group of 409 patients heart murmur were present in 325. Patients without heart murmurs were mainly those who died during the first few days of life, hence, the high incidence of 31.5% of patients without murmurs in the group with an intact ventricular septum. The age at onset of the heart murmur was recorded, and in the majority of 218 instances appeared by the age of 1 week. A murmur was first discovered between 1 and 4 weeks in 55, between 2 and 6 months in 24, between 7 and 12 months in 2 and above the age of 1 year in 3. Ejection systolic murmurs were most commonly heard in all groups. A pansystolic murmur was most frequently auscultated in the group with a ventricular septal defect. A continuous murmur was heard on 11 instances; with a patent ductus in 5, and with a surgical aorta-pulmonary artery shunt in 6. Early diastolic murmurs almost always meant pulmonary hypertension with pulmonary incompetence. In one patient with pulmonary stenosis, this murmur developed after pulmonary valvotomy. Mid-diastolic murmurs were most frequently auscultated in the group with a ventricular septal defect.

Of the 49 cases of complete transposition of the great arteries studied by Abbott (1937), an intact ventricular septum was present in 32, and a ventricular septal defect in 17. Heart murmurs were present in 8 of the 32 cases with an intact ventricular septum, and in 10 of the 17 with a ventricular septal defect. Taussig (1938) pointed out that although the quality and intensity of murmurs and thrills in transposition vary according to the nature of the concomitant malformation, the mechanism of their production depends primarily upon the relative pressure in the systemic and pulmonary circuits. These factors permit such wide diversity of physical findings that the murmurs and thrills are of no diagnostic aid. Of the 10 cases studied by Abrams et al. (1951) murmurs were present in 6, while the remaining 4 had no murmurs throughout their lives. In one patient there was no murmur at birth but a harsh systolic murmur developed at 2 weeks of age. Among 77 cases collected by the authors from the literature, 23 had no murmurs, 2 had systolic and diastolic murmurs, while the remainder had a systolic murmur alone. The authors pointed out that no definite correlation could be established between the type of murmur and the associated findings at autopsy. Of the 25 patients with transposition of the great arteries reported by Campbell and Suzman (1951), 8 had no murmurs, while one-fourth had a diastolic murmur. Among the 18 with a ventricular septal defect reported by Keith et al.

(1953), 13 had a systolic murmur, while of the 26 without a ventricular septal defect 8 had a systolic murmur. Of their 14 cases with no systolic murmur, 2 had a ventricular septal defect. Anderson and Adams (1955) pointed out that whereas cases with a ventricular septal defect are frequently associated with a loud murmur, cases with an intact ventricular septum are often associated with a soft murmur. Keith *et al.* (1958) found that one-third of all transpositions had no murmurs. When present, murmurs were faint, short systolic of variable locations in half the cases and loud and rather harsh in the other half. Of their cases with harsh murmurs 60% had a ventricular septal defect, 23% pulmonary stenosis, and 17% an intact ventricular septum. Significant murmurs were most often absent with an intact ventricular septum. Significant murmurs located low at the left sternal border were present in 52% of their cases with a ventricular septal defect. Pulmonary stenosis was associated with a murmur high up in the second or third left space. The authors concluded that in transposition the murmurs are inconsistent and only rarely significant. On the other hand, all 50 patients with or without a ventricular septal defect reported by Noonan *et al.* (1960) had systolic murmurs. Diastolic murmurs were noted in 28 patients and were of two types, a mid-diastolic rumble, and an early diastolic insufficiency flow. A flow rumble was heard in 31% of their cases with an intact ventricular septum and in 61% of their cases with a ventricular septal defect. An early insufficiency murmur was most common among those with a ventricular septal defect and pulmonary vascular obstruction, and was not heard in those with an intact ventricular septum. Of the 13 cases with an intact ventricular septum studied by Wells (1963), a systolic ejection murmur with a peak intensity at or before mid-systole was present in all. The vibrations were not of the coarse variety commonly found in organic murmurs. A presystolic murmur was also present in all. The findings in his 10 cases with a ventricular septal defect without pulmonary stenosis were identical except in one where the systolic murmur was louder and later than the others. Among his 3 cases with a ventricular septal defect and pulmonary stenosis, a long ejection murmur was present in 2, while the third had no murmurs. Perloff (1970) pointed out that a variety of murmurs or none at all, occur in transposition. A right-to-left systolic shunt across a ventricular septal defect is responsible for a murmur whose timing, length, and loudness vary with the size of the defect and the pressure difference across the septum. When there is severe pulmonary stenosis or high pulmonary vascular resistance, there is a left-to-right systolic shunt through the ventricular septal defect, but the shunt does not generate a murmur. Patent ductus may be associated with systolic murmurs of varying lengths. Pulmonic stenosis is accompanied by mid-systolic murmurs that vary considerably in length and loudness. When the pulmonary blood flow is increased, mid-systolic murmurs are caused by the ejection of a large left ventricular volume into a dilated pulmonary artery. Short mid-diastolic–presystolic apical murmurs are related to increased mitral valve flow in patients with low pulmonary vascular resistance and volume overload of the left heart.

Complications

THROMBOEMBOLISM

Cerebrovascular Accidents

In the entire group of 409 patients cerebrovascular accidents gave rise to symptoms in 12. Table 12.5 summarizes the clinical findings and the age at onset of these complications. In 1 of these 12 patients central ner-

TABLE 12.5

CLINICAL CEREBROVASCULAR ACCIDENTS (12 PATIENTS) [a]

	Clinical features	Age at complication
Group I	1. Convulsive disorders at 2 months, grand mal fits involving right arm and leg; later all four limbs. CSF: Xanthochromia, 450 cells, R.B.Cs. Recovered.	3 months
	2. Right hemiplegia. Recovered.	3 months
	3. Hemiparesis. Recovered.	15 years
Group II	4. Left hemiplegia, severe melena on the 7th day after surgical creation of an atrial septal defect. Improved.	2 years
Group III	5. Right hemiplegia. Died.	7 months
	6. Left hemiparesis. Recovered.	5 years
	7. Facial palsy, aphasia, double vision left hemiplegia. Recovered.	10 years
	8. Right retinal artery embolism. Recovered.	20 years
Group IV	9. Right hemiplegia. Died after 2 months.	8 months
	10. Left hemiparesis. Died at surgery 6 months afterward.	2 years
	11. Left hemiplegia secondary to subacute bacterial endocarditis. Died.	3 years
	12. Left hemiparesis and fits. EEG: focal lesion right frontal lobe. Recovered.	4 years

[a] Data of 12 patients.

vous system symptoms were secondary to embolic manifestations of subacute bacterial endocarditis.

The occurrence of cerebrovascular accidents in transposition of the great arteries is well recognized. Tyler and Clark (1957a,b) found that the incidence of cerebrovascular accidents was significantly greater in patients with transposition or tricuspid atresia than in other forms of congenital heart disease. Among their 125 patients with transposition, 14 had cerebrovascular accidents. The authors pointed out that the incidence of cerebrovascular accidents was highest in those forms of congenital heart disease that produced the severest cyanosis and hypoxia in the first 2 years of life. Of their 14 patients with cyanotic heart disease and cerebrovascular accidents who came to necropsy all showed large infarction in the distribution of the middle cerebral artery. Additional venous thrombosis was observed in one. Maronde (1958) reported a patient with transposition of the great arteries who died at the age of 7 years with subarachnoid hemorrhage. Of the 38 infants with transposition palliated by balloon atrial septostomy by Singh *et al.* (1969), 2 died of cerebral thrombosis. According to Parsons *et al.* (1971) cerebrovascular disturbances in transposition have a characteristically slow onset followed by one of two different syndromes, the hemiplegic and the hydrocephalic. In the hemiplegic syndrome, restlessness, screaming attacks, irritability, loss of appetite, fits, or weakness of a limb, is followed after several days by hemiparesis. In the hydrocephalic syndrome, characteristically, a haunting look of terror was the prelude to sudden deterioration, lethargy, and coma. Signs of increasing intracranial pressure with a tense bulging anterior fontanelle and congested scalp and intraocular veins, are followed by papilledema, periorbital edema, and sometimes squint. The cerebrospinal fluid protein level is usually elevated. Their 9 patients who died were found to have a dilated cerebral ventricular system with extensive infarction and softening of the brain. Venous sinus thrombosis was usual, but arterial thrombosis was also seen and 2 children had occlusion of the internal carotid arteries only. Of the 43 patients with transposition palliated by balloon atrial septostomy by Baker *et al.* (1971), 5 developed cerebrovascular accidents and 7 others showed seizure activity during the follow-up. Of the 60 patients with transposition reported by Rashkind (1971), 8 developed strokes with 3 deaths occurring. Half of the strokes occurred in children under 1 year of age and 6 were preceded by severe infections.

Berthrong and Sabiston (1951) pointed out that since the majority of cerebral infarcts were produced by specific vascular occlusions, the polycythemia present in most patients with cyanotic heart disease must be recognized as the most important cause responsible for these occlusions. These may develop as an *in situ* thrombosis or as cerebral emboli from thrombosis in other locations. Polycythemia increases the viscosity of the blood which, in turn, leads to sluggishness of the blood flow which predisposes to thrombosis. They found, however, that in cyanotic heart disease the degree of polycythemia was the same in those with or without thrombosis and suggested that transient elevations of polycythemia as in dehydration may play an important role in initiating thrombus formation. Similarly, in a cyanotic attack there is a decrease in the cardiac output and in the cerebral blood flow which encourages thrombus formation. Surgical operation may also encourage thrombus formation by giving rise to dehydration and anoxia. The number of circulating platelets is also known to increase after surgical operations. Tyler and Clark (1957b) thought that in the younger age group hypoxia seemed to play as important a role as polycythemia in the causation of thrombosis, while in the older age group polycythemia seemed to be the major precipitating factor. Cohen (1960) suggested that brain infarcts occur because of the inability of the circulation to deliver oxygen and adequate nutrients to the brain and specific occlusions rarely occur. Cottrill and Kaplan (1971) studied 29 patients with cerebral vascular accidents complicating cyanotic congenital heart disease. All patients were 4 years of age or less, 14 had transposition of the great arteries, and 12 had tetralogy of Fallot. The dominant vascular lesion was thrombosis of dural sinuses and intracranial veins (19 patients). Arterial thrombosis was rare and was seen in only 3 instances. They speculated that since intracranial thrombosis in these children was not necessarily related to high hemoglobin and hematocrit levels, changes in blood viscosity as a function of abnormal red cell deformability is a major factor in the development of intravascular thrombosis.

Other Thromboembolic Complications

A history of hemoptysis was obtained in 6 patients; 5 with a ventricular septal defect, and 1 with a ventricular septal defect and pulmonary stenosis. The youngest patient in this group was 8 years of age when the complication occurred. One of these 6 patients developed a cold 10 days prior to admission to the hospital. This was followed by wheezing with blood-stained sputum. He died 2 days afterward and at autopsy large areas of hemorrhagic consolidation and brown induration were found in both lungs. Another patient died of severe gastrointestinal hemorrhage and at necropsy mucosal hemorrhages were found in the stomach, and small and large intestines.

Brain Abscess

Four patients in this series developed a brain abscess. Table 12.6 gives the pertinent clinical information on these 4 patients. A detailed account on the clinical course of 3 of these patients has been published elsewhere (Shaher and Deuchar, 1972). A hematogenous origin of the abscess was thought to be definite in Patients 1, 3, and 4. In patient 2 otorrhea and pain in the right ear occurred 4 months before the brain abscess. At autopsy there were no signs of dural involvement and the abscess was in the occipital lobe. The origin of the brain abscess in this case was thought to be hematogenous rather than secondary to a direct spread of infection from the right ear.

The first case of brain abscess in association with congenital heart disease was reported by Farre (1814) who described the clinical and pathological findings in a 9-year-old boy who died as a result of a cerebral

TABLE 12.6

Brain Abscess

Patient	Clinical characteristics	Age at complication (years)
1	Ventricular septal defect, and complete interruption of the aortic arch. Fever, convulsions, and left hemiparesis. Abscess right fronto-parietal lobe, drained three times. Bacitracin and penicillin in abscess. Recovery after 2 months.	4
2	Ventricular septal defect. Otorrhea. Four months later severe headache. Drowsy, confused and febrile. Neck rigidity and papilledema. Lumbar puncture turbid fluid under tension. Autopsy: pus in subarachnoid space, large abscess right occipital lobe. Right middle ear contained viscid mucus and mucosa was inflamed. No dural involvement.	4½
3	Ventricular septal defect. Dental extraction followed by headache, fever, neck rigidity, and papilledema. Lumbar puncture turbid fluid. Autopsy: chronic otitis media of right ear, basal cisterns contained purulent fluid, cerebellar cone, abscess in right temporal lobe. Dura mater intact.	25
4	Ventricular septal defect, pulmonary stenosis. Blalock's anastomosis at 15 years. Headache, left hemiplegia. 15ml of pus aspirated from right temporal lobe. Recovered.	3

abscess and a defect of the ventricular septum. Ballet (1880) was the first to emphasize the relationship between brain abscess and congenital heart disease. He collected 4 cases previously published and added 1 of his own, and noted that apart from congenital heart disease there were no other factors to explain the abscess. Stone (1881), Peacock (1881), and Northrup (1894) reported similar cases, and Peacock remarked that in "the malformation of the heart in which the pulmonary artery is constricted and the septum of the ventricles defective so that the aorta communicates with both ventricles . . . the death of the patient is, in the largest proportion of these cases, as in the present instance, caused by cerebral disease."

Abbott et al. (1923) collected from the literature 12 cases of paradoxical cerebral embolism, and added 2 of their own. Of these 14 cases, 6 were proved at necropsy to be cerebral abscesses. In a later paper, Baumgartner and Abbott (1929) reported a case of cerebral abscess associated with Eisenmenger's complex and further comment was made on the 6 cases reported by Abbott et al. (1923). They pointed out that the age ranged between 6 and 26 years and that men were predominately affected. Rabinowitz et al. (1932) reviewed the literature and brought the number up to 10 cases and added 1 of their own in which at autopsy the abscess was found in the cerebellum. Seven cases of paradoxical embolism were reported by Ingham (1938) in all of which the condition was associated with a patent foramen ovale and preceded by pulmonary embolism. His case 7, showed sufficient localizing signs to warrant exploration of the left temporoparietal lobe for a cerebral abscess. Death followed on the thirteenth postoperative day. This was probably the first recorded case in which there was a brain abscess and an embolus of the pulmonary artery, and probably also the first one in which an attempt was made to drain the cerebral abscess. Wechsler and Kaplan (1940) reported 2 further cases in association with congenital heart disease. The diagnosis of the abscess was correctly made before death and surgical treatment carried out. Hanna (1941) reviewed the literature, collected 17 cases and added 6 of his own. In these 23 cases the cardiac lesions were as follows: Fallot's tetralogy in 11, patent foramen ovale in 6, ventricular septal defect in 4, ventricular septal defect and patent foramen ovale in 1, and Eisenmenger's complex in 1. Robbins (1945) reported 3 cases of brain abscess in association with Fallot's tetralogy and confirmed that among congenital heart disease, Fallot's tetralogy is the most common cause of a hematogenous brain abscess. Gates et al. (1947) described 5 new cases and coined the name "the syndrome of cerebral abscess and congenital cardiac disease." Sancetta and Zimmerman (1950) collected from the literature 42 cases of hematogenous brain abscess and added 2 of their own. The most common lesion was Fallot's tetralogy which occurred in 8 cases. The age ranged from 3 to 57 years with an average of 16.6 years. Clark and Clarke (1952) reported 26 new cases of which 19 had Fallot's tetralogy, 6 had other cyanotic heart lesions (type not specified), and 1 was acyanotic and had an atrial septal defect. The ages ranged from 2½ to 23 years with an average of 8½ years. Sixteen were males and 10 were females. Newton (1956) reviewed 72 reported cases and added 7 of his own, while Campbell (1957) reported 15 new cases.

As far as I can tell only 12 cases of hematogenous brain abscess in association with complete transposition of the great arteries have been reported. Acker (1895) reported a 6-year-old girl who had an attack of influenza, then was subject to convulsions of an epileptiform nature. At necropsy there was complete transposition of the great arteries, pulmonary atresia, and an abscess of a cerebral hemisphere (side not mentioned). Deneke (1907) reported a boy aged 18 years whose cyanosis and clubbing of the fingers dated from early life. Ten days before his death there was a sudden onset of severe headache, and left-sided hemiplegia developed. At autopsy there was transposition of the great arteries, a ventricular septal defect, a narrow patent ductus arteriosus, and pulmonary stenosis. A streptococcal abscess of the right cerebral hemisphere was found. Case 3 of Broager and Hertz (1952) was a 5-year-old boy who developed fever and right hemiparesis. At necropsy there was complete transposition of the great arteries, a ventricular septal defect, and pulmonary valvular stenosis. There was a multiocular brain abscess of the central part of the left hemisphere reaching from the surface of the cortex to the third ventricle with perforation into the ventricle. Case 2 of Gluck *et al.* (1952) was a boy aged 7 years. At necropsy there was complete transposition of the great arteries, interatrial and interventricular septal defects, and pulmonary valvular and subvalvular stenosis. There was an abscess in the left temporal lobe which extended from the posterior horn of the left lateral ventricle almost to the surface of the brain but without rupturing into the ventricle. In the Case Records of the Massachusetts General Hospital (1953) a post mortem examination of a 16-year-old girl showed complete transposition of the great arteries, a ventricular septal defect, a patent foramen ovale, a small patent ductus arteriosus, and pulmonary stenosis. A brain abscess was found in the left occipital lobe. Tyler and Clark (1957a) mentioned 2 cases of brain abscess among their 76 cases of complete transposition with or without pulmonary stenosis above the age of 2 years. Under the title of "transposition of the ventricles and arterial stems with cerebral abscess," Stuart and Flint (1957) cited another example of complete transposition of the great arteries with a closed ventricular septum and a brain abscess. González *et al.* (1963) described a case of complete transposition of the great arteries which exhibited a large atrial septal defect. The patient lived 5½ years and died of a cerebral abscess of the right hemisphere. Plauth *et al.* (1968), Azzolina *et al.* (1972), and Clarkson *et al.* (1972) briefly mentioned that one of their parents died with a brain abscess at 5, 3, and 7 years of age, respectively.

Fontana and Edwards (1962) explained the fact that Fallot's tetralogy is the most common congenital anomaly encountered among patients with cardiac disease in whom cerebral abscess develops, while transposition of the great arteries is not as common on the following grounds. Fallot's tetralogy is the most common type of cardiac malformation characterized by a large right-to-left shunt in which the patient has a good chance of surviving 3 years or more. Polycythemia and cerebral hypoxia are likely to be encountered and cerebrovascular complications may occur also. On the other hand, the majority of patients with complete transposition of the great arteries do not live long enough for the complications of cerebral abscess to develop.

There is no special problem related to the development of brain abscess secondary to otitis media in transposition of the great arteries; the infection reaches the brain by a direct spread from the middle ear. Such a case has been reported by Emanuel (1906) in a boy 11 years of age. On the other hand, the etiology of hematogenous brain abscess in transposition, as well as in cyanotic congenital heart disease, presents several problems.

Abbott *et al.* (1923) thought that cerebral abscess is especially liable to occur when there is a defect in the ventricular septum as well as dextroposition of the aorta. This combination seems to favor a direct path for the transmission of a crossed infected embolus to the brain. Gates *et al.* (1947), Edwards (1960), and Fontana and Edwards (1962) suggested that in the presence of a right-to-left shunt, the natural process of clearance of bacteria from the blood stream by the lungs is defective. Bacteremia may develop in every person from time to time. It may arise as a result of infective process, dental extraction, or a surgical procedure. In patients with a right-to-left shunt, the bacteria entering the peripheral venous blood may bypass the lungs and be carried directly into the systemic circulation. Newton (1956) quoted Wright (1927) as finding a considerable proportion of blood-borne bacteria filtered out of the circulation in the lungs. Moreover, Tyler and Clark (1957a) and Wood *et al.* (1951) have emphasized the effective and protective role of the pulmonary and the systemic capillary bed, as well as the reticuloendothelial cells of the splenic and hepatic sinusoids in removing bacteria from the blood. On the other hand, Robbins (1945) pointed out that the work of Malinovski (1891) and others showed that direct implantation of organisms into the brains of animals either by infection of the blood stream or by direct inoculation will not give rise to brain abscess and that the technique used by Graff (1934), Markley (1941), Thomas (1942), and Falconar et al. (1943) to produce these abscesses all depend upon using various agents to produce an initial brain injury with subsequent implantation of organisms at the site of the lesion.

A special susceptibility of the brain to infection in morbus caeruleus has been suggested by Maronde (1950) and Cohen et al. (1951). Rabinowitz et al. (1932), Wechsler and Kaplan (1940), and Robbins (1945) suggested that vascular disease of the brain together with consequent encephalomalacia prepares a focus which is receptive to infection, and if, by chance, organisms circulate in the blood they may cause the formation of a brain abscess. Hanna (1941) believed that an infarcted area in the brain, secondary to a paradoxical embolism, may be secondarily infected giving rise to a brain abscess. Among the 135 patients with cyanotic congenital heart disease studied by Berthrong and Sabiston (1951) cerebral infarction occurred in 25. The authors emphasized the important role of polycythemia in the production of intravascular thrombosis as a cause of the infarct. Whether the thrombosis develops in a peripheral vein and reaches the cerebral arteries as a paradoxical embolism through a cardiac defect, or from the cardiac chambers to embolize the brain, or develops in situ in the cerebral arteries was not known to them. They thought, however, that all three mechanisms may occur. The work of Berthrong and Sabiston (1951) has been confirmed by Tyler and Clarke (1957b). They studied 75 patients with cyanotic congenital heart disease in whom a cerebrovascular accident occurred, and concluded that the two factors of polycythemia and anoxia may act either singly or in combination to give rise to cerebral infarction.

The work of Rich (1948) has shown that progressive thrombosis of a special type occurring in the pulmonary vessels of microscopic size, is a frequent occurrence in patients with Fallot's tetralogy. He suggested that the predisposing factors are the increased viscosity of the blood resulting from compensatory polycythemia, and the reduced rate of flow in the pulmonary vascular system. These findings suggested to Gluck et al. (1952) that in cases of brain abscess secondary to congenital heart disease, the lungs could be another source of emboli entering the arterial circulation through the pulmonary veins, left atrium, and left ventricle. Similarly, Best and Heath (1958) thought that embolization from the lungs a possible cause of brain abscess. Newton (1956), however, thought that there was little clinical or pathological support for this theory, since it is difficult to show from clinical or postmortem study that infarction is an essential pathogenic process in the majority of the cases. He believed that defective elimination of bacteria from the blood is the most important factor in pathogenesis. From a study of the central nervous system lesions in congenital heart disease, Cohen (1960) concluded that the inability of the circulation to deliver oxygen and adequate nutrients to the brain is responsible for the infarction, and that specific occlusions rarely occur. This author as well as Matson and Salam (1961) pointed out that under these circumstances a brain abscess may result from bacteria which are intermittently present in the venous blood, but which, as a result of the right-to-left shunt, may enter the cerebral circulation directly. When there is a diminishd oxygen tension or actual brain infarction already present, then the arrival of such shunted blood containing virulent organisms may well be followed by focal infection.

BACTERIAL ENDOCARDITIS

Two patients in this series developed the clinical features of bacterial endocarditis during the course of the disease. Both had a ventricular septal defect, pulmonary stenosis, and a Blalock-Taussig's anastomosis. The pertinent data on each of these 2 patients is in Table 12.7. It is of interest that autopsy examination of Patient 1 showed that the vegetations were on the mitral and pulmonary valves, and the ventricular septal defect. The site of the Blalock's anastomosis was spared.

Bacterial endocarditis supervening on transposition of the great arteries is rare. Abbott (1926) found that bacterial endocarditis supervened

TABLE 12.7
BACTERIAL ENDOCARDITIS

Patient	Clinical features	Age at complication (years)
1	Ventricular septal defect and pulmonary stenosis; Blalock's anastomosis at 1 year. Fever 2 weeks prior to death. Autopsy: vegetation on mitral valve, pulmonary valve, and ventricular septal defect.	3
2	Ventricular septal defect and pulmonary stenosis. Blalock's anastomosis at 15 years. Fever and loss of weight of 2 months duration, positive blood culture for streptococcus. Recovered on penicillin. This patient is also Case 4 in Table 12.6.	24

98 times among 555 collected cases of congenital heart disease. Of these 555 cases, 59 had transposition of the great vessels of which 6 had bacterial endocarditis. On the other hand, in her analysis of 1000 cases of congenital heart disease in 1937, 49 had complete transposition of the great arteries, but bacterial endocarditis as a cause of death was not encountered. Complete transposition of the great arteries was not present among other types of congenital heart disease complicated by bacterial endocarditis reported by Jacobius and Moore (1938), Gelfman and Levine (1942), White et al. (1945), Donzelot et al. (1953), Kerr (1955), Cutler et al. (1958), Blumenthal et al. (1960), and Vogler and Dorney (1962). An authenticated case was reported by Froment et al. (1960) of a male aged 26 years who died in congestive heart failure. At necropsy there was bacterial endocarditis of the tricuspid valve and complete transposition of the great arteries. A questionable history of bacterial endocarditis was elicited in 3 of the 50 cases studied by Noonan et al. (1960. Several writers found that bacterial endocarditis rarely develops in infants and young children (Thayer, 1931; Clawson, 1941; Gelfman and Levine, 1942; White, 1944; Fontana and Edwards, 1962). The rarity of bacterial endocarditis supervening on transposition has been explained by Robinson (1905), Abbott (1926), and Fontana and Edwards (1962). Patients with transposition are liable to die before the age at which the acute infective process is likely to occur. It is significant that Patient 2 in this series and the patient of Froment et al. (1960) were 20 years of age at the time of the bacterial infection.

GOUT

One patient in Group III developed gouty arthritis at the age of 23 years. The heels and fingers were affected and later tophi developed on the right ear and right and left index fingers. The blood uric acid was 15 mg. At autopsy gouty lesions were found in the effected joints. The kidneys had a finely granular external surface and were markedly congested. Sections showed well-developed arteriosclerosis as well as occasional small areas of infarction. Urate deposits, however, were not found in the pyramids. This patient was reported earlier by Somerville (1961).

It is generally agreed that the incidence of gout in cyanotic congenital heart disease is higher than in the general population (Whitby and Britton, 1953; Lewis, 1961; Somerville, 1961). Somerville (1961) reported an incidence of 2% as compared to 0.2 to 0.5% in the general population. Weiss and Segaloff (1959) listed the conditions associated with secondary gout. These range from polycythemia and leukemia to lymphadenoma and other lumphatic dysplasia. In secondary gout there is no metabolic error, but there is increased formation and destruction of red and white cells present in excess. This results in increased nucleic acid metabolism and hyperuricemia (Yu *et al.* 1953). When the elevation of the blood uric acid persists over a long period of time precipitation into joints may occur and lead to gout (Talbot, 1957). Somerville (1961) points out that the development of gout in cyanotic congenital heart disease is related to the degree of elevation of the hemoglobin and the age of the patient, and that the presence of renal disease may be responsible for its occurrence particularly in patients under 25 years. In each of her 9 patients the hemoglobin was over 130% and the serum uric acid more than 6 mg at the time of the first attack. Lewis (1961) suggested that the combination of secondary polycythemia and renal disease and diuretic therapy, is a favorable one to cause gout whether the patient is predisposed to familial gout or not.

References

Abbott, M. E. (1926). On the incidence of bacterial inflammatory process in cardiovascular defects and on malformed semilunar cusps. *Ann. Clin. Med.* 4, 189.

Abbott, M. E. (1937). Causes and types of heart disease. I. Congenital heart disease. *Nelson's Loose-Leaf Med.* 4, 207.

Abbott, M. E., Lewis, D. S., and Beattie, W. W. (1923). Differential study of a case of pulmonary stenosis of inflammatory origin (ventricular septum closed) and two cases of (a) pulmonary stenosis and (b) pulmonary atresia of developmental origin with associated ventricular septal defect and death from paradoxical cerebral embolism. *Amer. J. Med. Sci.* 165, 636.

Abrams, H. L., Kaplan, H. S., and Purdy, A. (1951). Diagnosis of complete transposition of the great vessels. *Radiology* 57, 500.

Acker, G. N. (1895). A case of cardiac anomaly. *Arch. Pediat.* 12, 828.

Anderson, R. C., and Adams, P., Jr. (1955). Differentiation of associated cardiac defects in transposition of the great vessels. *Lancet* 75, 60.

Astley, R., and Parsons, S. (1952). Complete transposition of the great vessels. *Brit. Heart J.* 14, 13.

Azzolina, G., Eufrate, S. A., and Pensa, P. M. (1972). Closed interatrial septostomy: modified technique and results. *Ann. Thorac, Surg.* 13, 338.

Baker, F., Baker, L., Zoltun, R., and Zuberbuhler, J. R. (1971). Effectiveness of the Rashkind procedure in transposition of the great arteries in infants. *Circulation* 43 (Suppl. 1), 1.

Ballet, G. (1880). Des abscès du cerveau consecutifs à certaines malformations cardiaques. *Arch. Gen. Med.* 5, 659.

Baumgartner, E. A., and Abbott, M. E. (1929). Interventricular septal defect with dextroposition of aorta and dilatation of the pulmonary artery ("Eisenmenger Complex") terminating by cerebral abscess. *Amer. J. Med. Sci.* 177, 639.

Berthrong, M., and Sabiston, D. C., Jr. (1951). Cerebral lesions in congenital heart disease. A review of autopsies on one hundred and sixty-two cases. *Bull. Johns Hopkins Hosp.* 89, 384.

Best, P. V., and Heath, D. (1958). Pulmonary thrombosis in cyanotic heart disease without pulmonary hypertension. *J. Pathol. Bacteriol.* **75**, 281.

Blumenthal, S., Griffiths, S. P., and Morgan, B. C. (1960). Bacterial endocarditis in children with heart disease. *Pediatrics* **26**, 993.

Broager, B., and Hertz, J. (1952). Cerebral complications in congenital heart disease. *Acta Med. Scand. Suppl.* **266**, 293.

Buckley, M. J., Mason, D. T., Ross, J., Jr., and Braunwald, E. (1965). Reversed differential cyanosis with equal desaturation of the upper limbs. Syndrome of complete transposition of the great vessels with complete interruption of the aortic arch. *Amer. J. Cardiol.* **15**, 111.

Campbell, M. (1957). Cerebral abscess in cyanotic congenital heart disease. *Lancet* i, 111.

Campbell, M., and Reynolds, G. (1949). The physical and mental development of children with congenital heart disease. *Arch. Dis. Childhood* **24**, 294.

Campbell, M., and Suzman, S. (1951). Transposition of the aorta and pulmonary artery. *Circulation* **4**, 329.

Castellanos, A., Garcia, O., and Gonzalez, F. (1959). Complete interruption of the aortic arch with transposition of the great vessels. (Report of a case diagnosed *in-vivo*). *Cardiologia* **34**, 53.

Chazan, M., Harris, T., O'Neill, D., and Campbell, M. (1951). The intellectual and emotional development of children with congenital heart disease. *Guy's Hosp. Rep.* **100**, 331.

Clark, D. B., and Clarke, E. S. (1952). Brain abscess as complication of congenital cardiac malformation. *Trans. Amer. Neurol. Ass.* **77**, 73.

Clarkson, P. M., Barratt-Boyes, B. G., Neutze, J. M., and Lowe, J. B. (1972). Results over a ten year period of palliation followed by corrective surgery for complete transposition of the great arteries. *Circulation* **45**, 1251.

Clawson, B. J. (1941). Incidence of types of heart disease among 30,265 autopsies, with special reference to age and sex. *Amer. Heart J.* **22**, 607.

Cleland, W. P., Goodwin, J. F., Steiner, R. E., and Zoob, M. (1957). Transposition of aorta and pulmonary artery with pulmonary stenosis. *Amer. Heart J.* **54**, 10.

Cohen, I., Bergman, P. S., and Malis, L. (1951). Paradoxic brain abscess in congenital heart disease. *J. Neurosurg.* **8**, 225.

Cohen, M. M. (1960). The central nervous system in congenital heart disease. *Neurology* **10**, 452.

Coles, H. M. T., and Holesh, S. (1957). Transposition of the great vessels with absence of the aortic arch. *J. Fac. Radiol.* **8**, 355.

Cottrill, C. M., and Kaplan, S. (1971). Cerebral vascular accidents in cyanotic congenital heart disease. *Circulation Suppl.* II **43**, 44, 95.

Cutler, J. G., Ongley, P. A., Schwachman, H., Massell, B. F., and Nadas, A. S. (1958). Bacterial endocarditis in children with heart disease. *Pediatrics* **22**, 706.

Deneke, T. (1907). Zur Rontgendiagnostik Seltenerer Herzleiden. *Deut. Arch. Klin. Med.* **89**, 39.

Donzelot, E., LeBozec, J. M., Kaufmann, H., and Escalle, J. E. (1953). Le pronostic de l'endocardite infectieuse subaigüe traitée par les antibiotiques resultats du traitement de 202 cas. *Arch. Mal. Coeur Vaiss.* **46**, 97.

Dorning, J. (1890). A case of transposition of the aorta and pulmonary artery with patent foramen ovale; death at 10 years of age. *Trans. Amer. Pediat. Soc.* **2**, 46.

Edwards, J. E. (1960). Congenital malformations of the heart and great vessels. *In* "Pathology of the Heart" (S. E. Gould, Ed.), 2nd Ed. Thomas, Springfield, Illinois.

Elyan, M., and Ruffle, F. C. (1952). Two cases of complete transposition of the great vessels of the heart. *Med. J. Aust.* **2**, 91.

Emanuel, J. G. (1906). Three specimens of congenital deformity of the heart. *Rep. Soc. Stud. Dis. Child.* **6**, 240.

Emerson, P. W., and Green, H. (1942). Transposition of the great cardiac vessels. *J. Pediat.* **21**, 1.

Falconer, M. A., McFarlan, A. M., and Russell, D. S. (1943). Experimental brain abscess in the rabbit. *Brit. J. Surg.* **30**, 245.

Farre, J. R. (1814). Pathological Researches. Essay No. 1. Malformations of the Human Heart. p. 29. London.

Fontana, R. S., and Edwards, J. E. (1962). "Congenital Cardiac Disease: A Review of 357 Cases Studied Pathologically." Saunders, Philadelphia, Pennsylvania.

Fowler, R. E. L., and Ordway, N. K. (1952). Circulatory dynamics in complete transposition of the great vessels. Physiologic considerations with report of four cases. *Amer. J. Dis. Child.* **83**, 414.

Froment, R., Perrin, A., and Brun, F. (1960). Transposition complète des gros vaisseaux de la base chex un adulte avec dolicho-mega-coronaires. *Arch. Mal. Coeur* **53**, 449.

Gates, E., Rogers, H. M., and Edwards, J. E. (1947). The syndrome of cerebral abscess and congenital heart disease. *Proc. Staff Meet. Mayo Clin.* **22**, 401.

Gelfman, R., and Levine, S. A. (1942). The incidence of acute and subacute endocarditis in congenital heart disease. *Amer. J. Med. Sci.* **204**, 324.

Gluck, R., Hall, J. W., and Stevenson, L. D. (1952). Brain abscess associated with congenital heart disease. *Pediatrics* **9**, 192.

González, L. A., Estrada, C., Oriol, A., and Espino Vela, J. (1963). Transposición completa de los grandes vasos. *Arch. Inst. Cardiol. Mex.* **33**, 239.

Graff, R. A. (1934). Experimental production of abscess of the brain in cats. *Arch. Neurol. Psychiat.* **31**, 199.

Hamburger, L. P., Jr. (1937). Congenital cardiac malformation presenting complete interruption of the isthmus aortae with transposition of the great vessels. *Bull. Johns Hopkins Hosp.* **61**, 421.

Hanna, R. (1941). Cerebral abscess and paradoxic embolism associated with congenital heart disease. Report of seven cases with review of literature. *Amer. J. Dis. Child.* **62**, 555.

Harris, H. A., Gray, S. H., and Whitney, C. (1927). The heart of a child aged twenty-two months presenting an anomalous vein from the pulmonary auricle to the right internal jugular vein, transposition of the great vessels and left superior vena cava. *Anat. Rec.* **36**, 31.

Harris, J. S., and Farber, S. (1939). Transposition of the great cardiac vessels with special reference to the phylogenetic theory of Spitzer. *Arch. Pathol.* **28**, 427.

Hecko, I. (1948). Fifth International Congress of Pediatrics. *Acta Paediat.* **36**, 684.

Hemsath, F. A., Greenberg, M., and Shain, J. H. (1936). Congenital cardiac anomalies in infants. Report of five cases (1) accessory ventricle, (2) tetralogy of Fallot with right aortic arch and redundant left ductus arteriosus, (3) tetralogy of Fallot with anomalous band in right auricle, (4) complete transposition of arterial trunks, and (5) double defects of ventricular septum. *Amer. J. Dis. Child.* **51**, 1336.

Ingham, D. W. (1938). Paradoxical embolism. *Amer. J. Med. Sci.* **196**, 201.

Jacobius, H. L., and Moore, R. A. (1938). Incidence of congenital cardiac anomalies in the autopsies of the New York Hospital. *J. Tech. Methods* **18**, 133.

Jimenez, J. F. (1956). Transposition of the great vessels with patent ductus arteriosus. *Clin. Proc. Child. Hosp.* (Wash) **12**, 207.

Keith, J. D., Neill, C. A., Vlad, P., Rowe, R. D., and Chute, A. L. (1953) . Transposition of the great vessels. *Circulation* 7, 830.

Keith, J. D., Rowe, R. D., and Vlad, P. (1958). "Heart Disease in Infancy and Childhood," 1st Ed. MacMillan, New York.

Kerr, A., Jr. "Subacute Bacterial Endocarditis." Thomas, Springfield, Illinois.

Langstaff (1811). Case of a singular malformation of the heart. *London Med. Rev.* 4, 88.

Lees, D. B. (1879–1880). Case of malformation of the heart, with transposition of the aorta and pulmonary artery. *Trans. Pathol. Soc. London* 31, 58.

Lewis, J. G. (1961). Gout and the haemoglobin level in patients with cardiac and respiratory disease. *Brit. Med. J.* 1, 24.

McCue, C. M., and Young, R. B. (1961) . Cardiac failure in infancy. *J. Pediat.* 58, 330.

Malinovski, N. (1891) . Ueber Kunstlich erzeugte Gehirn-abscesse. *Zentralbl. Med. Wiss.* 29, 162.

Markley, G. M. (1941). A method for the experimental production of brain abscesses. *Proc. Soc. Exp. Biol. Med.* 47, 171.

Maronde, R. F. (1950). Brain abscess and congenital heart disease. *Ann. Intern. Med.* 33, 602.

Maronde, R. F. (1958). Cause of death in persons with congenital heart disease. *Amer. J. Med. Sci.* 236, 41.

Massachusetts General Hospital Case Records. Weekly Clinicopathological Exercises: Case 39351. (1953). *N. Engl. J. Med.* 249, 371.

Matson, D. D., and Salam, M. (1961). Brain abscess in congenital heart disease. *Pediatrics* 27, 772.

Mehrizi, A., and Taussig, H. B. (1963). Acyanotic transposition of the great vessels. *Bull. Johns Hopkins Hosp.* 112, 239.

Mehrizi, A., Rowe, R. D., Hutchins, G. M., and Folger, G. M., Jr. (1966) . Transposition of the great vessels with pulmonary stenosis and ventricular septal defect. *Bull. Johns Hopkins Hosp.* 119, 200.

Nadas, A. S. (1957). "Pediatric Cardiology," 1st Ed. Saunders, Philadelphia, Pennsylvania.

Newton, E. J. (1956). Haematogenous brain abscess in cyanotic congenital heart disease. *Quart. J. Med.* 25, 201.

Noonan, A., Nadas, A. S., Rudolph, A. M., and Harris, G. B. C. (1960). Transposition of the great arteries. A correlation of clinical, physiologic and autopsy data. *N. Engl. J. Med.* 263, 592.

Norton, J. B., Ullyott, D. J., Stewart, E. T., Randolph, A. M., and Edmunds, L. H. (1970) . Aortic arch atresia with transposition of the great vessels: physiologic considerations and surgical management. *Surgery* 67, 1011.

Northrup, W. P. (1894). Congenital pulmonary stenosis (conus arteriosus): Incompleteness of septum ventriculorum—cyanosis—abscess of the brain—death at four and a half years (specimen shown). *Arch. Pediat.* 11, 673.

Parsons, C. G., Astley, R., Burrows, F. G. O., and Singh, S. P. (1971). Transposition of the great arteries. A study of 65 infants followed for 1 to 4 years after balloon septostomy. *Brit. Heart J.* 33, 725.

Peacock, T. B. (1881). Malformation of heart; great obstruction of orifice of pulmonary artery; aorta arising from both ventricles. *Trans. Pathol. Soc.* London 32, 35.

Perloff, J. (1970). "Clinical Recognition of Congenital Heart Disease." Saunders, Philadelphia, Pennsylvania.

Plauth, W. H., Jr., Nadas, A. S., Bernhard, W. F., and Gross, R. E. (1968). Transposition of the great arteries. Clinical and physiological observations on 74 patients treated by palliative surgery. *Circulation* **37**, 316.

Rabinowitz, M. A., Weinstein, J., and Marcus, I. H. (1932). Brain abscess (paradoxical) in congenital heart disease. *Amer. Heart J.* **7**, 790.

Rannels, H. W., and Propst, J. H. (1937). Incidence of congenital cardiac anomalies found at autopsies performed in Hospital of University of Pennsylvania. *J. Tech. Methods* **17**, 113.

Rashkind, W. J. (1971). Transposition of the great arteries. *Pediat. Clin. N. Amer.* **18**, 1075.

Rich, A. R. (1948). Hitherto unrecognized tendency to development of widespread vascular obstruction in patients with congenital pulmonary stenosis (tetralogy of Fallot). *Bull. Johns Hopkins Hosp.* **82**, 389.

Robbins, S. L. (1945). Brain abscess associated with congenital heart disease. *Arch. Intern. Med.* **75**, 279.

Robinson, G. C. (1905). The relation between congenital malformations of the heart and acute endocarditis, with report of two cases. *Bull. Ayer. Clin. Lab Penn. Hosp.* **2**, 45.

Sancetta, S. M., and Zimmerman, H. A. (1950). Congenital heart disease with septal defects in which paradoxical brain abscess caused death. A review of the literature and report of 2 cases. *Circulation* **1**, 593.

Shaher, R. M. (1964). The hemodynamics of complete transposition of the great vessels. *Brit. Heart J.* **26**, 343.

Shaher, R. M., and Deuchar, D. C. (1972). Hematogenous brain abscess in cyanotic congenital heart disease. Report of three cases, with complete transposition of the great vessels. *Amer. J. Med.* **52**, 349.

Singh, S. P., Astley, R, and Burrows, F. G. D. (1969). Balloon septostomy for transposition of the great arteries. *Brit. Heart J.* **31**, 722.

Somerville, J. (1961). Gout in cyanotic congenital heart disease. *Brit. Heart J.* **23**, 31.

Stone, W. H. (1881). A case of tricaelian heart with insufficiency of the ventricular septum. *St. Thomas Hosp. Rep.* **11**, 57.

Stuart, K. L., and Flint, H. E. (1957). Transposition of the ventricles and arterial stems with cerebral abscess. *Postgrad. Med. J.* **33**, 131.

Talbot, J. H. (1957). "Gout." Grune & Stratton, New York. (Cited by Somerville, 1961.)

Taussig, H. B. (1938). Complete transposition of the great vessels. Clinical and pathologic features. *Amer. Heart J.* **16**, 728.

Taussig, H. (1960). "Congenital Malformation of the Heart," 2nd Ed. The Commonwealth Fund, New York.

Thayer, W. S. (1931). Cited by Fontana and Edwards, 1962.

Thomas, L. (1942). A single stage method to produce brain abscess in cats. *Arch. Pathol.* **33**, 472.

Toole, A. L., Glenn, W. W. L., Fisher, W. H., Whittemore, R., Ordway, N. K., and Vidone, R. A. (1960). Operative approach to transposition of the great vessels. *Surgery* **48**, 43.

Tyler, H. R., and Clark, D. B. (1957a). Incidence of neurological complications in congenital heart disease. *Arch. Neurol. Psychiat.* **77**, 17.

Tyler, H. R., and Clark, D. B. (1957b). Cerebrovascular accidents in patients with congenital heart disease. *Arch. Neurol. Psychiat.* **77**, 483.

Vogler, W. R., and Dorney, E. R. (1963). Bacterial endocarditis in congenital heart disease. *Amer. Heart J.* **64**, 198.

Walshe, W. H. (1842). Case of cyanosis, depending upon transposition of the aorta and pulmonary artery. *Med. Chir. Trans.* **25**, 1.

Wechsler, I. S., and Kaplan, A. (1940). Cerebral abscess (paradoxic) accompanying congenital heart disease. *Arch. Intern. Med.* **66**, 1282.

Weiss, T. E., and Segaloff, A. (1969). "Gouty Arthritis and Gout." Thomas, Springfield, Illinois.

Wells, B. (1963). The sounds and murmurs in transposition of the great vessels. *Brit. Heart J.* **25**, 748.

Whitby, L. E. H., and Britton, C. J. C. (1953). "Disorders of the Blood; Diagnosis, Pathology, Treatment and Technique," 7th Ed. Grune and Stratton, New York.

White, P. D. (1944). "Heart Disease," 3rd Ed. p. 1025. MacMillan, New York.

White, P. D., Mathews, M. W., and Evans, E. (1945). Notes on the treatment of subacute bacterial endocarditis encountered in 88 cases at the Massachusetts General Hospital during the six year period 1939 to 1944 (inclusive). *Ann. Intern. Med.* **22**, 61.

Wood, W. B., Smith, M. R., Perry, W. D., and Berry, J. W. (1951). Studies on the "Cellular Immunology of Acute Bacteremia." *J. Exp. Med.* **94**, 521.

Wright, H. D. (1927). *J. Pathol. Bacteriol.* **30**, 185. (Cited by Newton.)

Yu, T. F., Wasserman, L. R., Benedict, J. R., Bien, E. J., Gutman, A. B, and Stetten, D. (1953). A stimulaneous study of glycine-N^{15}, incorporation into uric acid and heme, and of Fe^{59} utilization, in case of gout associated with polycythemia, secondary to congenital heart disease. *Amer. J. Med.* **15**, 845.

Zuberbuhler, J. R., Bauersfeld, S. R., and Pontius, R. G. (1967). Paradoxic splitting of the second sound with transposition of the great vessels. *Amer. Heart J.* **74**, 816.

Chapter 13

THE ELECTROCARDIOGRAM

The electrocardiograms of 332 patients in this series were studied. Five hundred eighty-one tracings were available, each consisting of 3 standard, 3 unipolar, and 6 precordial leads. Patients were classified into 4 groups as follows:

Group I   With an intact ventricular septum; 162 patients, 259 tracings.
Group II   With an intact ventricular septum and left ventricular outflow tract obstruction; 14 patients, 27 tracings
Group III   With a ventricular septal defect; 113 patients, 203 tracings.
Group IV   With a ventricular septal defect and left ventricular outflow tract obstruction; 43 patients, 92 tracings.

In each group, the electrocardiograms were studied in relationship to the following age groups: (1) Age in days in the first week of life; (2) from the 8 to 14 days; (3) from 15 days to 3 months; (4) from 4 to 6 months; (5) from 7 months to 1 year; (6) from 1 to 3 years; (7) from 3 to 10 years; and (8) above 10 years.

Criteria

Various criteria were used for the diagnosis of abnormalities in the electrocardiogram. These criteria are listed below.

THE ELECTRICAL AXIS

Normal axis deviation was considered present in the age group 0 hours to 16 years if this varied within plus or minus 30° from the following average normal values of Ziegler (1951) tabulated below.

Age	Degrees	Age	Degrees
0–24 hours	+137	1–3 years	+62
1 day–1 week	+128	3–5 years	+64
1 week–1 month	+105	5–8 years	+69
1–3 months	+ 76	8–12 years	+64
3–6 months	+ 67	12–16 years	+66
6 months–1 year	+ 64		

In adults above the age of 16 years a normal axis was considered present if it ranged between 0 to +60°.

In all age groups the limit between extreme right axis deviation and extreme left axis deviation is considered to be 270°.

THE P WAVES

According to Martins de Oliveira and Zimmerman (1959), the normal P wave in the limb leads should not exceed 0.10 seconds in duration and 2.5 millimeters in amplitude. A normal atrial wave should not show notching or peaking in its morphology. The normal P vector is between +30° and +75°.

THE P–R INTERVAL

Ziegler's (1951) average normal figures for this interval are tabulated as shown below.

Age	Seconds	Age	Seconds
0–24 hours	0.099	1–3 years	0.110
1 day–1 week	0.097	3–5 years	0.125
1 week–1 month	0.092	5–8 years	0.134
1–3 months	0.102	8–12 years	0.139
3–6 months	0.096	12–16 years	0.149
6 months–1 year	0.103		

In adults the P–R interval varies from 0.12 to 0.20 seconds (Wood, 1956). In interpreting the P–R interval the heart rate was taken into consideration, since the interval varies inversely to the sinus rate. According to Sodi-Pallares *et al.* (1958a) the heart rate at different ages is as follows:

Newborn	May be as high as 200 beats per minute
1 month–1 year	125–150 per minute
1–3 years	115–130 per minute
3–5 years	90–105 per minute
5–8 years	90–100 per minute
8–12 years	85–90 per minute
12–16 years	80–85 per minute

QRS DURATION

According to Ziegler (1951) and Sodi-Pallares *et al.* (1958a) the QRS duration is slightly shorter in early childhood than in adults. The values range between 0.06 and 0.07 seconds up to the third year of age, and from the third to the sixteenth year the duration varies between 0.07 and 0.08 seconds. In adults the whole QRS complex rarely exceeds 0.08 seconds in duration (Wood, 1956).

THE T WAVES

According to Sodi-Pallares *et al.* (1958a) at birth the T waves are upright in the right precordial leads and frequently inverted in the left precordium. Afterward the waves gradually become negative in the right and positive in the left precordial leads. Before the age of 1 year the T waves are negative from V_1 to V_3. The T waves recorded in subsequent precordial leads are positive and may show a deep notching with a double hump in its morphology. After the age of 12 years the precordial leads show positive T waves in the majority of cases.

VENTRICULAR HYPERTROPHY

The criteria employed for signs of right, left, and biventricular hypertrophy are those suggested by Vince and Keith (1961) using the normal values of Ziegler (1951) for patients above 1 year up to an including 16 years, of Scott and Franklin (1963) for infants below the age of 1 year, and of Kossman and Johnston (1935) for patients above the age of 16 years.

A. Right Ventricular Hypertrophy
   1. Voltage of R in V_1 greater than maximal normal for age
   2. Voltage of S in V_6 greater than maximum normal for age
   3. R/S ratio in V_1 greater than maximum normal for age
   4. Positive T in V_1 after third day of life when R/S ratio greater than 1.0
   5. qR pattern in V_1

B. Left Ventricular Hypertrophy
   1. Voltage of R in V_6 greater than maximum normal for age
   2. Voltage of S in V_1 greater than maximum normal for age
   3. R/S ratio in V_1 less than minimum normal for age
   4. Secondary T inversion in V_5 and/or V_6
   5. Deep Q over the left precordium—4 mm or greater
C. Biventricular Hypertrophy
   1. Direct signs of right plus direct signs of left ventricular hypertrophy
   2. Direct signs of right ventricular hypertrophy in association with the following:
      a. Q of 2 mm or more in V_6.
      b. Tall biphasic complexes in midprecordial leads over 50 mm in height (Katz-Wachtel sign).

THE KATZ–WACHTEL SIGN

Katz and Wachtel (1937) suggested that the presence of diphasic QRS complexes in the standard limb leads confirms a diagnosis of congenital heart disease, and that when the two phases of the complex are large and of equal extent the finding is pathognomonic. Katz *et al.* (1952) discussed large diphasic QRS complexes in the electrocardiogram of an infant with congenital heart disease and thought that these complexes represented biventricular hypertrophy or alternatively were caused by abnormal intraventricular conduction. Sodi-Pallares and Calder (1956) referred to this phenomenon as the Katz-Wachtel sign and defined it as consisting of diphasic complexes of great voltage in leads V_2, V_3, and V_4 as well as in the standard leads. They pointed out that complexes of this morphology are seen mainly in ventricular septal defect, but also occasionally in atrial septal defect and in patent ductus arteriosus. Dack (1960) thought that the presence of large diphasic QRS complexes in the precordial leads V_2–V_4 as well as in the extremity leads suggests biventricular hypertrophy in ventricular septal defect, and pointed out that these are generally observed in infancy and are less common in older patients. Elliott *et al.* (1963b) accepted tall equiphasic complexes in the midprecordial leads over 50 mm in height as being suggestive of combined ventricular hypertrophy, while Elliott *et al.* (1963a) and Shaher and Deuchar (1966) utilized this sign in assessing biventricular hypertrophy in their cases of complete transposition of the great arteries. In this series, the Katz-Wachtel sign has been used to indicate enlargement of both ventricles.

Findings

RHYTHM

Abnormalities in the cardiac rhythm were observed in 21 patients. The arrhythmia occurred in the immediate postoperative course in 20, and 9 months after surgical creation of an atrial septal defect in 1. The surgical procedure was a Mustard's operation in 16, and creation of an atrial septal defect in 5. Of the 16 patients who underwent the Mustard procedure, nodal rhythm was observed in 6 (Fig. 13.1), atrial flutter in 7 (Fig. 13.2), nodal tachycardia in 2 (Fig. 13.3), and complete heart block in 1 (Fig. 13.4). Of the 5 patients who underwent surgical creation of an atrial septal defect, nodal rhythm occurred in 3 (Fig. 13.5), atrial flutter 9 months after surgery in 1, and nodal tachycardia in 1 (Fig. 13.6).

Chronic abnormalities of rhythm and conduction not related to heart surgery, rarely occur in transposition. Gerbode *et al.* (1967) reported the case of a 36-year-old woman with complete transposition and atrial fibrillation. One of the patients reported by Corvacho (1968) had complete heart block. Of the 6 patients with transposition and pulmonary stenosis

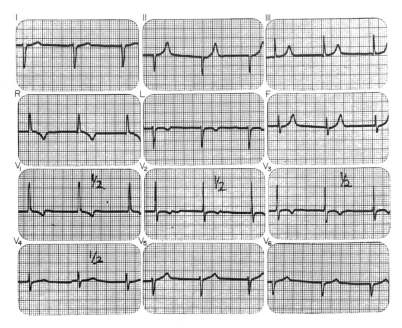

Fig. 13.1. The electrocardiogram of a 7-year-old patient with transposition and intact ventricular septum after total repair with the Mustard procedure, showing nodal rhythm.

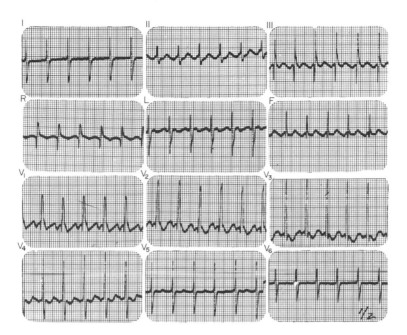

Fig. 13.2. The electrocardiogram of a 6-year-old patient with transposition and intact ventricular septum after total repair with the Mustard procedure showing atrial flutter.

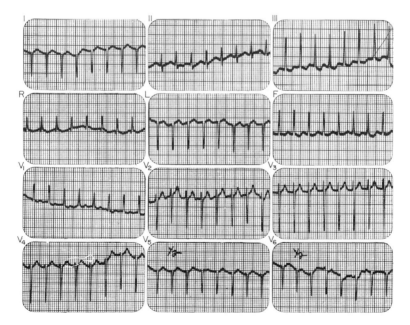

Fig. 13.3. The electrocardiogram of a 2-year-old patient with transposition and intact ventricular septum after the Mustard procedure showing nodal tachycardia.

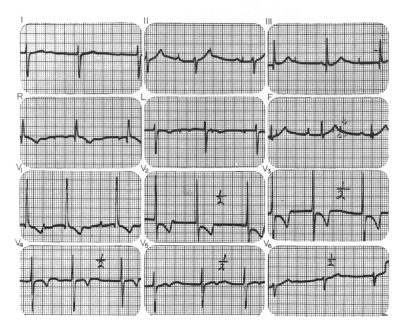

Fig. 13.4. Complete heart block after the Mustard procedure in a 9-year-old child with transposition and a small ventricular septal defect. The atrial rate is slower than the ideoventricular rate.

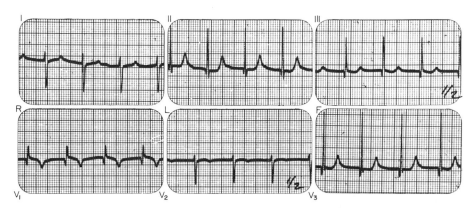

Fig. 13.5. The electrocardiogram of a 1-year-old child with transposition and ventricular septal defect after the Blalock-Hanlon procedure showing nodal rhythm.

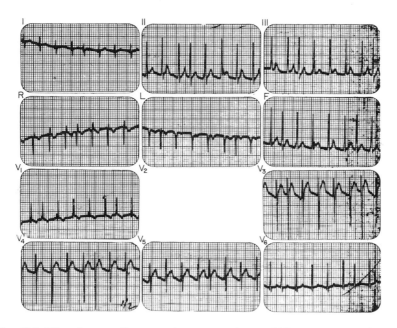

Fig. 13.6. The electrocardiogram of a 10-month-old child with transposition and ventricular septal defect after the Blalock-Hanlon procedure showing nodal tachycardia.

reported by Daicoff *et al.* (1969), the electrocardiogram of an 18-year-old girl showed persistent atrial tachycardia with variable block. According to Khoury *et al.* (1966) atrial flutter frequently occurs in the post-operative course of the Mustard procedure, while nodal rhythm may complicate surgical creation of an atrial septal defect. Aberdeen *et al.* (1965) described 9 patients operated on by the Mustard technique, 7 of which were successful. Of these, 5 patients had supraventricular arrhythmia in the first weeks after the operation. Three of these patients were discharged in atrial flutter with 2:1 atrioventricular block. Zuberbuhler and Bauersfeld (1967) reported 2 patients who had been successfully surgically treated by the Mustard procedure. In the postoperative course, variable degrees of sinoatrial nodal block occurred in 1, and two levels of atrioventricular block occurred in the other. Of the 26 patients with transposition of the great vessels who underwent a Blalock-Hanlon's procedure reported by Hamilton *et al.* (1968), 16 developed disturbances in atrial conduction or rhythm. Aberrations of the P wave occurred in 10, atrioventricular rhythm in 9, atrioventricular dissociation in 5, sinus bradycardia in 2, escape-capture bigeminy in 1, atrial premature beats in 1, and atrial flutter in 1. The first onset of these disturbances occurred from immediately to 3 years postoperatively. Some of these changes were transient and occurred within 2 weeks after surgery. The authors pointed out that tissue trauma produced by the clamp and resection of the atrial septum may be the genesis of the early postoperative disturbances. Later changes may be attributed to changes in atrial size secondary to postoperative pathophysiology although digitalis intoxication and congestive heart failure could not be excluded as contributory factors in either early or late disturbances. Of the 112 patients totally corrected by the Mustard procedure by Aberdeen (1971), nodal rhythm occurred in 22, second-degree heart block in 4, complete atrioventricular dissociation in 17, and atrial flutter in 15. The author pointed out that the incidence of postoperative arrhythmia had diminished since attempts were made to avoid damage to either the sinus or the atrioventricular nodes or to the interatrial conduction pathways. El-Said *et al.* (1972) studied dysrhythmias after the Mustard procedure in 60 patients who survived the operation. Three types of dysrhythmias were observed. Those due to failure of initiation or failure of propagation of the sinus impulse were designated passive dysrhythmias. Rhythm disturbances characterized by rapid ectopic atrial or A-V junctional impulses (paroxysmal atrial tachycardia and atrial flutter) were termed active dysrhythmias. A-V conduction defects made up the third group. Only 3 patients consistently had sinus rhythm after the operation. The incidence of passive dysrhythmias remained nearly the same at about 50% during the follow-up period. These dysrhythmias consisted of sinoatrial block, wandering pacemaker, A-V junctional rhythm, and A-V dissociation by default. Eight patients showed at various times junctional rhythm with right inferior P wave axis. The P wave axis was directed inferiorly to the right and anteriorly, occurring either before or after the QRS complex with fixed P-R or R-P intervals. The characteristics of the junctional rhythm with right inferior P axis remained during subsequent attacks of supraventricular tachycardia. Whereas the incidence of sinus rhythm gradually decreased from about 30% until the end of the first year to 13% after 3 years, the incidence of active dysrhythmias gradually increased from 9% in the first week after surgery to 36% after 3 years. The incidence of A-V conduction defects was low and occurred mainly as Grade 1 A-V block. There were no instances of second or third degree atrioventricular block. Wolff–Parkinson–White syndrome, type A, developed and persisted in 1 patient. Isaacson *et al.* (1972) correlated postoperative arrhythmias after the Senning operation, the Mustard procedure or the creation of an atrial septal defect with interruption of the atrial conduction (internodal) pathways in the hearts of 49 patients with transposition of the great arteries. Eight of the 49 patients had no postoperative dysrhythmias. Seven of the 8 underwent a Blalock–Hanlon procedure, and in all 7 the areas of the anterior and middle pathways were intact, although the region of the posterior pathway was interrupted. After a Senning procedure, 1 patient had apparent disruption of all 3 pathways but did not manifest dysrhythmia. Twenty-two of the 23 patients who underwent a Senning operation had postoperative dysrhythmias. Nodal rhythm occurred in 11 patients, and in 10 of them there was apparent interruption of all 3 pathways; in the eleventh, the region of the posterior pathway was intact. Atrioventricular dissociation occurred in 6 patients, and the areas of all 3 pathways were disrupted in each. Atrial fibrillation was present in 2 patients, 1 with disruption of the region of all pathways and 1 with apparent preservation of the posterior pathway. Complete heart block existed in 2 patients, a ventricular septal defect also had been closed. One patient had ventricular tachycardia and disruption of all atrial pathways. One of the 23 patients had disruption of all 3 pathways but no apparent dysrhythmia. After the Mustard procedure, dysrhythmias were recorded in all 14 patients whose hearts were studied. Of the 7 with nodal rhythm, 5 had apparent destruction of all 3 pathways; in the other 2, the region of the anterior pathway was intact. All pathway areas were disturbed in the 3 with atrioventricular dissociation, the 2 with ventricular tachycardia, and the 2 with atrial fibrillation or flutter. Of the 12 patients who underwent the Blalock–Hanlon procedure, 7 had no postoperative dysrhythmia, and the areas of the anterior and middle pathways were intact; however, the region of the posterior pathway was disturbed in all 7. Five patients in whom a central part of the atrial septum was excised had nodal rhythm. The region of the middle pathway had been excised in all 5; in addition there was apparent injury to the anterior pathway in 2 and to the posterior pathway in 1. The authors concluded that (1) extensive disturbance of the atrial septal connections between the sinus and atrioventricular nodes frequently is associated with serious dysrhythmia, and (2) disruption of the region of the middle atrial conduction pathway, especially when coupled with damage to another pathway, is frequently associated with dysrhythmia, most commonly nodal rhythm.

In contrast to the relatively frequent occurrence of complete heart block in congenitally corrected transposition (Anderson *et al.* 1957; Schiebler *et al.* 1961; and others), this conduction disturbance has been documented in one reported case with complete transposition of the great arteries (Corvacho, 1968). Paul *et al.* (1951) and Sodi-Pallares and Calder (1956) state that complete heart block has been reported in complete transposition of the great arteries, but review of the cases which have been described in the literature as having this combination shows that Case 2 of Abbott (1936, p. 56) and the patient of Aitchison *et al.* (1955) had a single ventricle. The case reported by Dickson and Jones (1948) is an example of complete transposition with a single ventricle with a rudimentary chamber and tricuspid atresia. In Case 2 of Ingham and Willius (1938) there was corrected transposition of the great vessels in a situs inversus heart.

THE P WAVE

Apart from the 21 tracings which showed postoperative atrial arrhythmia, the P vector was between 30° and 90° in all but 2. Of these two, a superior orientation of the vector was observed in 1 patient with a common atrium, and right axis deviation was seen in 1 patient with dextrocardia with situs inversus. Both patients were in Group 1.

In Group I normal P waves were observed in 56% of the tracings and tall and pointed waves in 44% (Table 13.1). In Group II normal P waves were observed in 50% and right atrial hypertrophy in 50% (Table 13.2). In Group III a normal atrial pattern was seen in 44%, right atrial hypertrophy in 52%, and combined ventricular hypertrophy in 4% (Table 13.3). In Group IV normal atrial hypertrophy pattern was present in 33%, right atrial hypertrophy in 65% (Fig. 13.7), and combined atrial hypertrophy in 2% (Table 13.4).

Abnormalities of the shape of the P waves were noted in the immediate postoperative course after surgical creation of an atrial septal defect in 26 patients. The P wave became notched, its amplitude diminished, and its duration was prolonged to an average of 0.085 seconds, an increase of 0.035 seconds from the preoperative values. After the Mustard operation the P wave appeared flat in 9, and dome-shaped in 2.

The present series confirms the earlier observation of Martins de Oliveira and Zimmerman (1959), and of Elliott *et al.* (1963a) that the frontal projection of the P vector is usually within normal limits in most cases. On the other hand, abnormalities of the height and duration of the P waves have been described by most authors. Thus in the group of 5 patients reported by Martins de Oliveira and Zimmerman (1959), the duration of the P wave was increased to 0.11 seconds in 2, the amplitude varied from 1.9 to 4.5 mm, and peaking was present in all 5 cases. In the group of 48 patients reported by Noonan *et al.* (1960), abnormal P waves were present in 30 and tended to become more abnormal with increasing age. Elliott *et al.* (1963a) divided their cases into those with a small communication (27 cases), and those with a large communication

TABLE 13.1

ELECTRICAL AXIS AND P WAVE [a]

Number of tracings and age	Electrical axis							P wave [b]			
	0°–90°	90°–150°	150°–180°	180°–220°	220°–270°	270°–360°	Indeterminate	N	R	L	C
35 1st Day	5	22	8	0	0	0	0	26	8	1	0
30 2nd Day	1	22	7	0	0	0	0	25	5	0	0
17 3rd Day	0	14	2	1	0	0	0	14	3	0	0
6 4th Day	0	3	3	0	0	0	0	3	3	0	0
7 5th Day	0	5	2	0	0	0	0	5	2	0	0
12 6th Day	2	6	2	2	0	0	0	8	4	0	0
3 7th Day	1	2	0	0	0	0	0	2	1	0	0
29 1–2 Weeks	0	23	4	2	0	0	0	20	9	0	0
50 3 Weeks–3 months	1	25	15	7	1	0	1	25	24	1	0
18 4–6 Months	1	9	3	1	4	0	0	6	10	0	2
16 6 Months–1 year	0	5	5	3	3	0	0	8	7	0	1
19 1–3 Years	1	8	5	2	3	0	0	7	11	1	0
15 3–10 Years	0	4	3	3	4	1	0	5	9	0	1
2 Above 10 years	0	0	2	0	0	0	0	0	2	0	0
Total	12	148	61	21	15	1	1	154	98	3	4

[a] Group I–162 patients, 259 tracings.
[b] N, normal; R, right; L, left; C, combined.

TABLE 13.2

ELECTRICAL AXIS AND P WAVE [a]

Number of tracings and age		Electrical axis							P wave [b]			
		0°–90°	90°–150°	150°–180°	180°–220°	220°–270°	270°–360°	Indeterminate	N	R	L	C
0	1st Day	0	0	0	0	0	0	0	0	0	0	0
0	2nd Day	0	0	0	0	0	0	0	0	0	0	0
3	3rd Day	0	3	0	0	0	0	0	1	2	0	0
1	4th Day	0	1	0	0	0	0	0	0	1	0	0
0	5th Day	0	0	0	0	0	0	0	0	0	0	0
0	6th Day	0	0	0	0	0	0	0	0	0	0	0
0	7th Day	0	0	0	0	0	0	0	0	0	0	0
5	1–2 Weeks	0	3	1	1	0	0	0	3	2	0	0
4	3 Weeks–3 months	0	3	1	0	0	0	0	3	1	0	0
2	4–6 Months	0	2	0	0	0	0	0	0	2	0	0
2	6 Months–1 year	0	1	1	0	0	0	0	1	1	0	0
5	1–3 Years	0	4	1	0	0	0	0	4	1	0	0
4	3–10 Years	0	4	0	0	0	0	0	0	3	0	1
1	Above 10 years	0	0	0	0	0	1	0	1	0	0	0
	Total	0	21	4	1	0	1	0	13	13	0	1

[a] Group II–14 patients, 27 tracings.
[b] Abbreviations as in Table 13.1.

TABLE 13.3
ELECTRICAL AXIS AND P WAVES [a]

Number of tracings and age	Electrical axis							P wave [b]			
	0°–90°	90°–150°	150°–180°	180°–220°	220°–270°	270°–360°	Indeterminate	N	R	L	C
7 1st Day	2	4	0	1	0	0	0	6	1	0	0
5 2nd Day	0	4	0	1	0	0	0	4	1	0	0
6 3rd Day	0	4	1	0	0	1	0	2	4	0	0
4 4th Day	1	3	0	0	0	0	0	4	0	0	0
3 5th Day	2	1	0	0	0	0	0	3	0	0	0
4 6th Day	2	2	0	0	0	0	0	2	2	0	0
5 7th Day	3	1	0	0	0	1	0	3	2	0	0
18 1–2 Weeks	6	10	0	0	0	2	0	9	9	0	0
54 3 Weeks–3 months	20	25	5	0	0	3	1	29	25	0	0
25 4–6 Months	8	9	1	0	2	3	2	11	14	0	0
17 6 Months–1 year	1	8	0	3	2	1	2	5	11	0	1
25 1–3 Years	1	11	3	3	0	3	4	9	13	2	1
21 3–10 Years	0	6	3	5	4	1	2	5	9	1	6
9 Above 10 years	0	2	4	2	1	0	0	0	5	0	4
Total	46	90	17	15	9	15	11	92	96	3	12

[a] Group III–113 patients, 203 tracings.
[b] Abbreviations same as in Table 13.1.

TABLE 13.4

ELECTRICAL AXIS AND P WAVE [a]

Number of tracings and age	Electrical axis							P wave [b]			
	0°–90°	90°–150°	150°–180°	180°–220°	220°–270°	270°–360°	Indeterminate	N	R	L	C
2 1st Day	0	1	0	1	0	0	0	1	1	0	0
0 2nd Day	0	0	0	0	0	0	0	0	0	0	0
3 3rd Day	1	1	0	0	0	1	0	0	3	0	0
0 4th Day	0	0	0	0	0	0	0	0	0	0	0
2 5th Day	1	0	0	0	0	1	0	1	1	0	0
1 6th Day	1	0	0	0	0	0	0	1	0	0	0
0 7th Day	0	0	0	0	0	0	0	0	0	0	0
7 1-2 Weeks	4	0	2	0	1	0	0	5	2	0	0
12 3 Weeks-3 months	4	3	0	1	1	2	1	6	6	0	0
11 4-6 Months	3	5	0	2	0	0	1	3	7	0	1
16 6 Months-1 year	2	7	0	3	1	1	2	6	9	0	1
15 1-3 Years	1	9	1	0	3	1	0	1	14	0	0
19 3-10 Years	0	8	4	0	4	3	0	5	13	0	1
4 Above 10 years	0	3	0	1	0	0	0	0	2	0	2
Total	17	37	7	8	10	9	4	29	58	0	5

[a] Group IV—43 patients, 92 tracings.
[b] Abbreviations same as in Table 13.1.

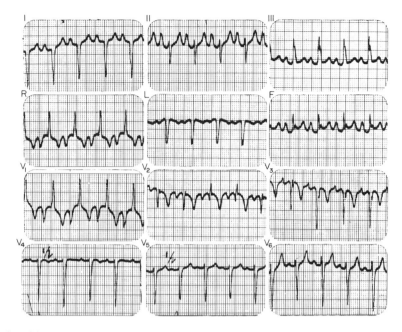

Fig. 13.7. Tall and pointed P waves in lead II, signifying right atrial hypertrophy in the electrocardiogram of 11-year-old patient with transposition and ventricular septal defect.

(21 cases). In their first group the P waves were abnormal in 12 of the 27, while in their second group they were normal in 14 patients.

Khoury *et al.* (1966) attributed the P wave changes after surgical creation of an atrial septal defect to an actual increase in atrial work secondary to a step-up in bidirectional shunting or to the traumatic affect of surgical excision of the atrial septum. El-Said *et al.* (1972) studied the P waves in the electrocardiograms of 60 patients who survived the Mustard procedure. In 54 patients, atrial depolarization waves having the scaler configuration of sinus P waves were seen at one time or another postoperatively. Comparison of these P waves with the preoperative sinus P waves revealed a highly significant decrease in the maximal P wave amplitude without significant change in the maximal width. The mean frontal plane axis of these P waves remained the same as preoperatively. The authors pointed out that some of the P waves seen postoperatively which appeared to be sinus in configuration may actually be of ectopic origin because of (1) the abnormally small amplitude and (2) persistence of the shape of these sinus-like P waves during subsequent attacks of supraventricular tachycardias, and the occurrence of sinus-like P waves in patients whose S-A node was later found to be degenerated histologically.

THE ELECTRICAL AXIS

Table 13.5 shows the distribution of the electrical axis in the whole series while Tables 13.1 to 13.4 show the distribution of the electrical axis in the four groups. Regardless of the anatomy of the ventricular septum, and the presence or absence of pulmonary stenosis, in 385 of the 581 tracings studied, the electrical axis was between 90° and 180°. Left or indeterminate axis deviation was observed mostly in Groups III and IV. Thus, of the 26 tracings which showed left axis deviation (270°–360°), 15 were in Group III and 9 in Group IV, and of the 16 with indeterminate axis 11 were in Group III, and 4 in Group IV.

THE P–R INTERVAL

A prolonged P–R interval was observed in 101 tracings; 45 in Group I, 5 in Group II, 31 in Group III, and 20 in Group IV (Tables 13.6–13.9).

No definite conclusion could be drawn from these findings. However, longer P–R intervals tended to occur in older patients.

VENTRICULAR HYPERTROPHY PATTERN

Of the 259 tracings in Group I a normal pattern was present in 28, right ventricular hypertrophy in 208, left ventricular hypertrophy in 1, and combined ventricular hypertrophy in 22 (Table 13.6) (Figs. 13.8 and 13.9).

Of the 27 tracings in Group II, a normal pattern was present in 1, right ventricular hypertrophy in 24, and combined hypertrophy in 2 (Table 13.7) (Fig. 13.10).

Of the 203 tracings in Group III, a normal pattern was seen in 24, right ventricular hypertrophy in 102, left ventricular hypertrophy in 5, and combined hypertrophy in 72 (Table 13.8) (Figs. 13.11 and 13.12).

Of the 92 tracings in Group IV, a normal pattern was seen in 7, right ventricular hypertrophy in 56, left ventricular hypertrophy in 4, and combined hypertrophy in 25 (Table 13.9) (Figs. 13.13 and 13.14).

In the whole group of 581 tracings, a normal pattern was seen in 57, right ventricular hypertrophy in 393, left ventricular hypertrophy in 10, and combined ventricular hypertrophy in 121.

TABLE 13.5

THE ELECTRICAL AXIS

Group	0°–90°	90°–150°	150°–180°	180°–220°	220°–270°	270°–360°	Indeterminate
Intact septum Group I, 259 tracings	12	148	61	21	15	1	1
Intact septum and pulmonary stenosis Group II, 27 tracings	0	21	4	1	0	1	0
Ventricular septal defect Group III, 203 tracings	46	90	17	15	9	15	11
Ventricular septal defect and pulmonary stenosis Group IV, 92 tracings	17	37	7	8	10	9	4
Total	75	296	89	45	34	26	16

TABLE 13.6
P–R Interval, Ventricular Hypertrophy, and Q Waves [a]

Age	P–R Interval		Ventricular hypertrophy pattern [b]				Slurring RV$_1$	Q Waves [c]	
	Normal	Prolonged	N	R	L	C		V$_1$	V$_6$
1st Day	34	1	15	19	1	0	9	0	5
2nd Day	28	2	5	24	0	1	11	0	4 (1)
3rd Day	16	1	3	13	0	1	1	0	3 (1)
4th Day	4	2	0	6	0	0	2	0	2
5th Day	7	0	1	6	0	0	5	0	1
6th Day	11	1	1	11	0	0	3	0	3
7th Day	2	1	0	3	0	0	1	0	0
1–2 Weeks	24	5	2	24	0	3	8	0	13 (3)
3 Weeks–3 months	46	4	1	40	0	9	10	1	20 (8)
4–6 Months	13	5	0	17	0	1	3	2 (1)	4 (1)
6 Months–1 year	12	4	0	13	0	3	4	2	4 (2)
1–3 Years	14	5	0	16	0	3	4	5 (3)	6 (2)
3–10 Years	4	11	0	14	0	1	5	7 (2)	1 (1)
Above 10 years	0	2	0	2	0	0	0	2 (2)	0
Total	215	44	28	208	1	22	66	19	66

[a] Group I—162 patients, 259 tracings.
[b] Abbreviations same as in Table 13.1.
[c] In parentheses if 2mm or more.

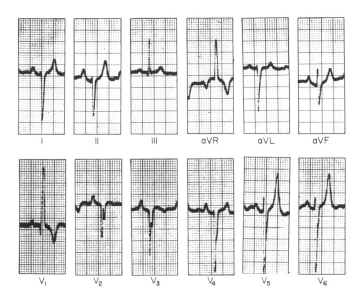

Fig. 13.8. The electrocardiogram of a 10-year-old patient with transposition and intact ventricular septum showing right axis deviation, right ventricular hypertrophy, and qR pattern in lead VI.

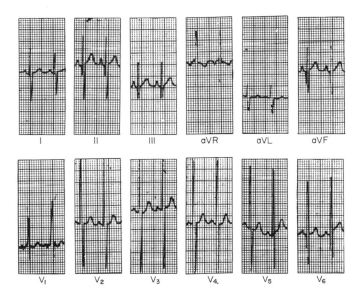

Fig. 13.9. Combined ventricular hypertrophy in a 3-month-old infant with transposition, intact ventricular septum, and a large patent ductus.

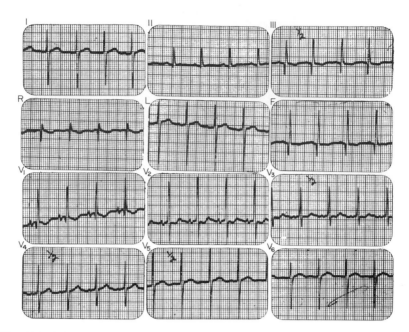

Fig. 13.10. The electrocardiogram of a 2-year-old child with transposition, intact ventricular septum, and left ventricular outflow tract obstruction showing right axis deviation and right ventricular hypertrophy.

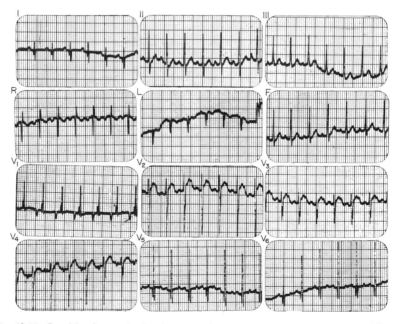

Fig. 13.11. Combined ventricular hypertrophy in a 10-month-old infant with transposition and ventricular septal defect.

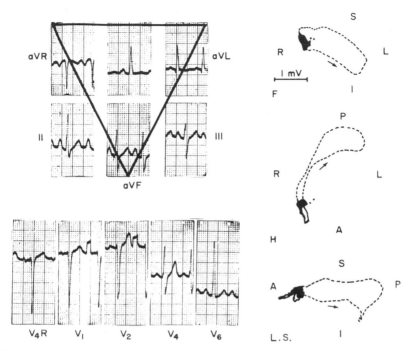

Fig. 13.12. The electrocardiogram and vectorcardiogram of a 2-year-old child with transposition, and complete interruption of the aortic arch showing left ventricular hypertrophy. A, anterior; I, inferior; L, left; S, superior; F, frontal; H, horizontal; L.S., left sagittal; P, posterior; R, right.

In the whole group, slurring of the R wave in lead V_1 or a pattern of rsR' in this lead was observed in 199 tracings; 66 in Group I, 5 in Group II, 94 in Group III, and 34 in Group IV (Tables 13.6 to 13.9).

Q waves in lead V_1 (qR pattern) were seen in 48 tracings; 19 in Group I, 5 in group II, 14 in Group III, and 10 in Group IV. Q waves in lead V_6 were observed in 210 tracings; 66 in Group I, 4 in Group II, 100 in Group III, and 40 in Group IV (Tables 13.6 to 13.9).

Among the different precordial patterns only two could correlate to the pathology of the ventricular septum. Thus, while a pattern of combined ventricular hypertrophy was observed in 8.4% of tracings of patients with an intact ventricular septum (Groups I and II), it occurred in 32.8% of tracings of patients with a ventricular septal defect (Groups III and IV). Similarly a pattern of left ventricular hypertrophy was seen mainly in the presence of a ventricular septal defect, since of the 10 trac-

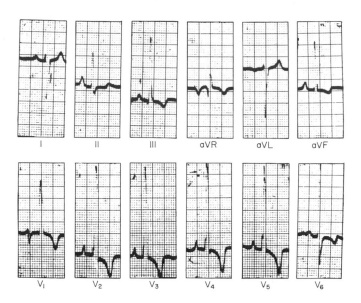

Fig. 13.13. The electrocardiogram of 29-year-old patient with transposition, ventricular septal defect, and pulmonary stenosis showing right axis deviation, and combined atrial and ventricular hypertrophy. Note inversion of the T waves in leads III, VF, and V_{1-6}.

ings with this pattern, 9 were in Groups III or IV. These two patterns, however, should be regarded as only being suggestive of a ventricular septal defect, for the case of transposition with an intact ventricular septum reported by Pung *et al.* (1955) showed "left heart preponderance." Keith *et al.* (1958) pointed out that hypertrophy of both ventricles, or of the left ventricle alone, was the rule in patients with a ventricular septal defect and large pulmonary blood flow. Combined ventricular hypertrophy was not observed in cases with an intact ventricular septum reported by Noonan *et al.* (1960), but among their 37 patients with a ventricular septal defect, 10 showed this electrocardiographic pattern. In the series of Elliott *et al.* (1963a), cases with a ventricular septal defect were associated with biventricular hypertrophy at least twice as frequently as were cases with an intact ventricular septum.

Keith *et al.* (1958) observed a qR pattern in V_1 in 3 of their cases; 2 with a single ventricle and 1 with an intact ventricular septum. Elliott *et al.* (1963a) pointed out that in their series a Q wave was seen in V_1 only in patients with a small communication. In this series Q waves in V_1 were observed in 48 tracings with an incidence of about 7% in each of Groups I, III, and IV. The incidence of Q waves in V_1 was 18% in Group II.

Watson and Keith (1962) found Q waves of 2 mm or more in lead V_6 in 15% of their patients with complete transposition of the great arteries, while Elliott *et al.* (1963a) observed it in 15% of their patients with a small communication, and in 85% of their patients with a large communication. In this series a Q wave in V_6 of 2 mm or more was observed in 67 tracings; 19 in Group I, 1 in Group II, 39 in Group III, and 8 in Group IV.

No definite pattern could be correlated to the presence or absence of pulmonary stenosis, since the incidence of right, left, or combined ventricular hypertrophy was nearly identical in Groups III and IV.

Keith *et al.* (1958) pointed out that whereas at birth the electrocardiogram is usually within normal limits in uncomplicated cases of transposition, complex forms always have pathological changes. When death occurs early the electrocardiogram may remain normal or only slightly changed. They stressed that signs of right ventricular hypertrophy in the newborn infant may only be represented by the presence of upright T waves in the precordial leads. They thought that the statement of Campbell and Suzman (1951), and Astley and Parsons (1952) that the electrocardiogram in transposition is indistinguishable from that in Fallot's

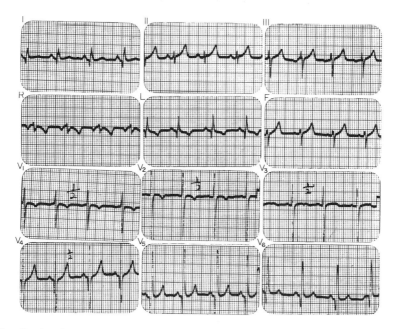

Fig. 13.14. The electrocardiogram of a 10-year-old patient with transposition, ventricular septal defect, and pulmonary stenosis showing left axis deviation and left ventricular hypertrophy.

TABLE 13.7
P–R Interval, Ventricular Hypertrophy, and Q Waves [a]

Age	P–R Interval		Ventricular hypertrophy pattern [b]				Slurring RV$_1$	Q Waves [c]	
	Normal	Prolonged	N	R	L	C		V$_1$	V$_6$
1st Day	0	0	0	0	0	0	0	0	0
2nd Day	0	0	0	0	0	0	0	0	0
3rd Day	3	0	1	2	0	0	0	0	1
4th Day	0	1	0	1	0	0	1	0	1
5th Day	0	0	0	0	0	0	0	0	0
6th Day	0	0	0	0	0	0	0	0	0
7th Day	0	0	0	0	0	0	0	0	0
1–2 Weeks	5	0	0	5	0	0	1	0	0
3 Weeks–3 months	4	0	0	3	0	1	0	0	1
4–6 Months	2	0	0	2	0	0	1	0	0
6 Months–1 year	1	1	0	2	0	0	0	2	0
1–3 Years	4	1	0	4	0	1	0	2 (2)	0
3–10 Years	2	2	0	4	0	0	1	1	1 (1)
Above 10 years	1	0	0	1	0	0	1	0	0
Total	22	5	1	24	0	2	5	5	4

[a] Group II—14 patients, 27 tracings.
[b] Abbreviations same as in Table 13.1.
[c] In parentheses if 2mm or more.

TABLE 13.8
P-R Interval, Ventricular Hypertrophy, and Q Waves [a]

Age	P-R Interval		Ventricular hypertrophy pattern [b]				Slurring RV₁	Q Waves [c]	
	Normal	Prolonged	N	R	L	C		V₁	V₆
1st Day	7	0	3	4	0	0	3	0	2
2nd Day	4	1	3	2	0	0	3	0	2
3rd Day	6	0	4	1	1	0	3	0	1
4th Day	4	0	3	1	0	0	0	0	2
5th Day	3	0	1	1	0	1	1	1	0
6th Day	3	1	0	3	1	0	3	0	0
7th Day	5	0	1	2	0	2	2	1	4 (1)
1–2 Weeks	16	2	3	9	0	6	7	0	8 (2)
3 Weeks–3 months	52	2	3	25	0	26	19	1	32 (17)
4–6 Months	25	0	0	9	2	14	8	1	16 (4)
6 Months–1 year	15	2	1	11	0	5	11	3 (1)	6 (3)
1–3 Years	19	6	0	14	1	10	16	2 (2)	12 (5)
3–10 Years	13	8	1	15	0	5	13	3 (3)	11 (4)
Above 10 years	1	8	1	5	0	3	5	2	4 (3)
Total	173	30	24	102	5	72	94	14	100

[a] Group III—113 patients, 203 tracings.
[b] Abbreviations same as in Table 13.1.
[c] In parentheses if 2mm or more.

TABLE 13.9
P-R Interval, Ventricular Hypertrophy, and Q Waves [a]

Age	P-R Interval		Ventricular hypertrophy pattern [b]				Slurring RV$_1$	Q Waves [c]	
	Normal	Prolonged	N	R	L	C		V$_1$	V$_6$
1st Day	2	0	1	1	0	0	0	1	0
2nd Day	0	0	0	0	0	0	0	0	0
3rd Day	3	0	1	1	1	0	0	0	0
4th Day	0	0	0	0	0	0	0	0	0
5th Day	2	0	1	1	0	0	0	0	2
6th Day	1	0	1	0	0	0	0	0	0
7th Day	0	0	0	0	0	0	0	0	0
1–2 Weeks	7	0	0	3	0	4	1	0	2 (1)
3 Weeks–3 months	10	2	0	7	0	5	1	1	6 (1)
4–6 Months	10	1	1	6	0	4	2	2	6 (1)
6 Months–1 year	14	2	0	11	0	5	8	2 (1)	7 (1)
1–3 Years	11	4	0	13	0	2	8	4 (1)	7
3–10 Years	10	9	2	9	3	5	11	0	10 (4)
Above 10 years	2	2	0	4	0	0	3	0	0
Total	72	20	7	56	4	25	34	10	40

[a] Group IV—43 patients, 92 tracings.
[b] Abbreviations same as in Table 13.1.
[c] In parentheses if 2mm or more.

tetralogy, is valid only in older children and adolescents with transposition. The findings in this series support this opinion, since the majority of patients with a normal ventricular precordial pattern were under the age of 2 weeks. Similar findings have been reported by Calleja *et al.* (1965) .

In the present series a pattern of right ventricular hypertrophy was seen in 67.6% of the patients, left ventricular hypertrophy in 18%, combined ventricular hypertrophy in 20.7%, and normal pattern in 9.9%. Among the 53 patients with complete transposition reported by Calleja and Hosier (1960) , right ventricular hypertrophy was present in 60%, left ventricular hypertrophy in 15% and combined ventricular hypertrophy in 9%. They considered the electrocardiogram normal in 13%. Of the 48 patients reported by Noonan *et al.* (1960) , right ventricular hypertrophy occurred in 60%, combined ventricular hypertrophy in 21%, left ventricular hypertrophy in 13%, and a normal pattern in 6%. On the other hand, in the group of 54 patients reported by Elliott *et al.* (1963a) , right ventricular hypertrophy was present in 52%, combined ventricular hypertrophy in 45%, left ventricular hypertrophy in 1.5%, and Wolff-Parkinson-White syndrome in 1.5%.

In 1955, Anderson and Adams pointed out that cases with a ventricular septal defect frequently show the amplitude of the R waves in lead V_1 to be less than 75% of the total RS amplitude. When the R waves in lead V_1 approach 100% of the total RS amplitude, absence of such defect is indicated. Vliers (1966) pointed out that if the R/S ratio in V_6 exceeds 1 the probability of the presence of a ventricular septal defect or a patent ductus is high. On the other hand, if this ratio is less than 1, a ventricular septal defect is unlikely. In this series no attempt has been made to study the height of the R waves in relation to the total RS amplitude in lead V_1, because 39 tracings in Group 3 had no S wave in this lead.

THE PRECORDIAL T WAVES AND THE S-T SEGMENT

Tables 13.10 to 13.13 show the direction of the T wave in leads V_1 and V_6 in the four groups. The most common pattern was positivity of the T waves in leads V_1 and V_6 in the younger age groups, and negativity in lead V_1 and positivity in lead V_6 of these waves in the older ones.

Notching of the T wave in leads V_4, V_5, or V_6 was noticed in 26 tracings; 11 in Group I, 1 in Group II, 13 in Group III, and 1 in Group IV. Marked abnormality of the S-T segment, unrelated to heart surgery was observed in 1 patient in this series (Fig. 13.15) .

The present series suggests that the most common precordial T wave abnormality in complete transposition of the great arteries is negativity of

TABLE 13.10

PRECORDIAL T WAVES [a]

Age	$+V_1 +V_6$	$+V_1 -V_6$	$-V_1 +V_6$	$-V_1 -V_6$
1st Day	16	9	9	1
2nd Day	11	7	10	2
3rd Day	9	5	2	1
4th Day	2	2	0	2
5th Day	2	4	1	0
6th Day	3	6	2	1
7th Day	1	0	2	0
1–2 Weeks	13	12	2	2
2 Weeks–3 months	27	13	8	2
3–6 Months	9	2	7	0
6 Months–1 year	8	1	7	0
1–3 Years	2	4	13	0
3–10 Years	1	0	11	3
Above 10 years	0	0	2	0
Total	104	65	76	14

[a] Group I, 259 tracings.

this wave in the right precordial leads in adults, and positivity of this wave in these leads in infants and children. Zuckermann *et al.* (1951) suggested that negative T waves in the left precordial leads and positive T waves in the right precordial leads occur in transposition. Among the 48 patients of Noonan *et al.* (1960) 40% had a normally inverted T wave in lead V_4R, but 60% had a normal upright T wave in lead V_6. A flat-

TABLE 13.11

PRECORDIAL T WAVES [a]

Age	$+V_1 +V_6$	$+V_1 -V_6$	$-V_1 +V_6$	$-V_1 -V_6$
1st Day	0	0	0	0
2nd Day	0	0	0	0
3rd Day	1	0	1	1
4th Day	0	0	1	0
5th Day	0	0	0	0
6th Day	0	0	0	0
7th Day	0	0	0	0
1–2 Weeks	5	0	0	0
2 Weeks–3 months	0	2	2	0
3–6 Months	1	0	1	0
6 Months–1 year	0	0	2	0
1–3 Years	1	0	4	0
3–10 Years	1	0	4	0
Above 10 years	0	0	0	0
Total	9	2	15	1

[a] Group II, 27 tracings.

TABLE 13.12
PRECORDIAL T WAVES [a]

Age	$+V_1 +V_6$	$+V_1 -V_6$	$-V_1 +V_6$	$-V_1 -V_6$
1st Day	3	1	2	1
2nd Day	4	0	1	0
3rd Day	3	0	2	1
4th Day	1	1	2	0
5th Day	1	2	0	0
6th Day	3	0	0	1
7th Day	3	1	0	1
1–2 Weeks	10	7	1	0
2 Weeks–3 months	31	14	7	2
3–6 Months	11	7	5	2
6 Months–1 year	5	2	10	0
1–3 Years	8	1	15	1
3–10 Years	3	0	14	4
Above 10 years	1	0	8	0
Total	87	36	67	13

[a] Group III, 203 tracings.

tened, biphasic, or inverted T wave in lead V_6 occurred in 8 of their 12 cases with a ventricular septal defect and large pulmonary blood flow. Sodi-Pallares (1958a,b) suggested other T wave changes in transposition: (1) higher positive T waves in the right than in the left precordial leads, (2) normal positive T waves in V_1 and V_2 and flat T waves in V_5 and V_6, and (3) notched T waves in the left precordial leads. In the

TABLE 13.13
PRECORDIAL T WAVES [a]

Age	$+V_1 +V_6$	$+V_1 -V_6$	$-V_1 +V_6$	$-V_1 -V_6$
1st Day	1	0	0	1
2nd Day	0	0	0	0
3rd Day	2	1	0	0
4th Day	0	0	0	0
5th Day	1	1	0	0
6th Day	1	0	0	0
7th Day	0	0	0	0
1–2 Weeks	1	4	1	1
2 Weeks–3 months	4	6	2	0
3–6 Months	7	1	3	0
6 Months–1 year	12	0	4	0
1–3 Years	3	0	11	1
3–10 Years	4	0	15	0
Above 10 years	0	0	3	1
Total	36	13	39	4

[a] Group IV, 92 tracings.

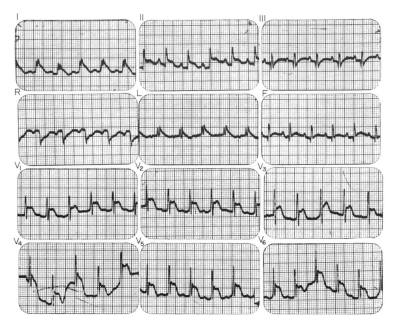

Fig. 13.15. The electrocradiogram of a 10-day-old infant with transposition and a ventricular septal defect showing marked S-T segment elevation in the precordial and standard limb leads. The tracing was obtained before surgical creation of an atrial septal defect.

group of 54 patients of Elliott *et al.* (1963a) notched T waves in lead V_6 were seen in 2, and positive T waves higher in the right precordial leads than in the left precordial leads in 9. Casellas Bernat *et al.* (1968) suggested that flattening of the T wave, its initial negativity, or its notching may suggest the diagnosis in a large number of cases. In the present series, T wave changes, other than flattening or inversion, occurred in a small proportion of patients and were considered insignificant in the diagnosis of transposition.

THE EVOLUTION OF THE ELECTROCARDIOGRAM

During the first week of life the majority of the tracings in Group I showed an electrical axis between 90° and 180°. Between the third week and the third month 17% (8/50) had developed extreme right axis deviation (180°–270°). After the age of 6 months, about 60% showed an axis between 90° and 180°, and 40% between 180° and 270°. During the first day of life 47% showed a normal ventricular hypertrophy pattern. This incidence drops to 7.5% by the age of 1 week and to 2.5% by the age of 3 months. Isolated right ventricular hypertrophy occurred in 78% of all tracings. It was observed in about 50% of the tracings at the age of 1 day and in 100% above the age of 10 years. During the first 2 weeks, the incidence of isolated right ventricular hypertrophy increases steeply because of the equally rapid disappearance of tracings with a normal ventricular hypertrophy pattern. The incidence of right ventricular hypertrophy in the age group 3 weeks to 3 years was 80%. During the first 3 months, about 37% of the tracings showed a flat, biphasic, or inverted TV_6, 44% positive V_1 and V_6, and 19% negative TV_1 and positive $T V_6$. From 3 months to 1 year, 50% showed positive V_1 and V_6 and 40% negative V_1 and positive V_6. After the age of 1 year, 72% showed negative $T V_1$ and positive $T V_6$, and 8% positive $T V_1$ and $T V_6$.

The number of tracings in Group II was too small to allow valid conclusions to be made on the evolution of the electrocardiogram in this group. Regardless of the age, most tracings showed an electrical axis between 90° and 150°, and right ventricular hypertrophy. About 50% of all tracings showed negative $T V_1$ and positive $T V_6$.

During the first week of life 33% of the tracings in Group III showed an axis between 0° and 90°, and 50% between 90° and 150°. Near equal distribution of tracings in these two groups of axis deviation persisted until the age of 6 months. After this age there was a shift to the right and all but 2 showed an electrical axis more than 90°. In addition, in the age group 6 months to 1 year 35% of the tracings showed extreme right axis deviation (180° to 270°). From the age of 1 to 10 years the incidence of axis deviation remained essentially constant and about 60% showed an axis between 90° and 180°, 35% had extreme right axis deviation, and 15% showed left or indeterminate axis deviation. During the first week of life 42% of the tracings showed normal ventricular hypertrophy, 42% right ventricular hypertrophy, and 16% left or combined hypertrophy. From the age of 1 week to 6 months, 50% of the tracings showed combined hypertrophy, 42% right ventricular hypertrophy, and 18% normal pattern. After the age of 6 months, 59% of the tracings showed right ventricular hypertrophy and 33% combined ventricular hypertrophy. During the first 6 months, about 30% of the tracings showed flat, negative or biphasic $T V_6$, 54% positive $T V_1$ and $T V_6$, and 16% negative $T V_1$ and positive $T V_6$. After the age of 6 months, about 23.5% showed positive $T V_1$ and $T V_6$, and 65% showed negative $T V_1$ and positive $T V_6$.

During the first week, the electrical axis of Group IV was mainly distributed to the two ranges 0°–90° and 90°–150°. From the first week to 6 months, 37.5% of the tracings showed an axis between 0° and 90°, 27.5% between 90° and 150°, and 35% between 180° and 360°. Between 6 months and 1 year, 44% of the tracings were between 90° and 150° and 25% between 180° and 270°. After the age of 1 year all but one had an electrical axis more than 90°, and 66% were in the range 90°–180°, 21% between 180° and 270°, and 10.5% between 270° and 360°. During the first week, a normal ventricular hypertrophy pattern occurred in 50% of the tracings and right ventricular hypertrophy pattern in 37.5%. From the first week to 6 months, 53% showed right ventricular hypertrophy and 43% combined ventricular hypertrophy. From 6 months to 1 year, 68% showed right ventricular hypertrophy and 31% combined ventricular hypertrophy. Above the age of 1 year, 68% showed right ventricular hypertrophy, 18% combined ventricular hypertrophy, 8% left ventricular hypertrophy, and 6% normal pattern. During the first 6 months, 43% of the tracings showed flat, negative, or biphasic T V_6. From 6 months to 1 year, 75% showed positive T V_1 and T V_6, and 25% negative T V_1 and positive T V_6. After this age, 18.5% had positive T V_1 and T V_6, whereas 75% had negative T V_1 and positive T V_6.

The findings in this series suggest that initially more patients with a ventricular septal defect will have combined ventricular hypertrophy and leftward axis than patients with an intact ventricular septum. As pulmonary vascular obstruction or left ventricular outflow tract obstruction increases in severity, older patients in all groups will show more rightward axis and right ventricular hypertrophy. Initially a significant number of patients showed flat, inverted, or biphasic T V_6. This finding was not so commonly observed in older age groups. Three factors, singly or in combination, could explain it: (1) early palliation and improvement in the arterial oxygen saturation, (2) development of pulmonary vascular obstruction or pulmonary stenosis thus diminishing diastolic overloading of the left ventricle, and (3) early death of cases with small communications.

Wimmer and Latschewa (1969) pointed out that at birth the electrocardiogram is normal. At the end of 1 month, patients with an intact ventricular septum develop right ventricular hypertrophy. Those with a large ductus or a ventricular septal defect develop combined ventricular hypertrophy. Patients with a ventricular septal defect and pulmonary stenosis have right ventricular hypertrophy from the first day of life.

Hemodynamics and Electrocardiogram

Cabrera and Monroy (1952) and Cabrera and Gaxiola (1959) studied the relation between the electrocardiogram and the hemodynamics in heart diseases in general, and described patterns for the electrocardiographic recognition of systolic and diastolic overloading of the right and left ventricles. In systolic overloading of the heart, stronger contractions occur because of increased resistance to ejection of blood. Diastolic overloading indicated an increase of the volume of blood filling the ventricle during diastole. The electrocardiographic pattern of systolic overloading of the left ventricle is characterized by delayed repolarization of that ventricle, producing a negativity of the T waves and/or S-T segment in the left ventricular leads. Diastolic overloading of the left ventricle is recognized by the high delayed R wave in V_5 and V_6 with deep S waves in V_2 and V_3, and a high positive T wave in V_5 and V_6. Systolic overloading of the right ventricle increases the voltage of the R wave in V_1, and the QRS in this lead may present a RS, Rs, or qR pattern with or without slurring or notching of the R wave. Diastolic overloading of the right ventricle is recognized by the presence of RSR' or a multiphase QRS pattern in V_1. Agustsson et al. (1957) pointed out that diastolic overloading of the left ventricle may be represented by deep Q waves and tall R waves and tall peaked upright T waves in leads II, III, VF, and V_6. Systolic overloading of the left ventricle may be presented by an initial Q wave followed by tall R waves with intrinsicoid deflection greater than 0.04 seconds and associated with flattened or inverted T waves in these leads. Luna and Crow (1961) correlated the degree of pulmonary hypertension to the morphology of the QRS in lead V_1. When the right ventricular pressure was greater than the left ventricular pressure, 75% of their cases had a qR pattern. With balanced ventricular pressure, 77% of their cases had an initial slurring of the upstroke of the R wave. When the pressure in the left ventricle exceeded that in the right ventricle, 75% of their tracings had a clean R wave. Watson and Keith (1962) confirmed the concept that a deep Q wave in the left precordial leads is one of the features of left ventricular diastolic overloading and stressed that a Q V_6 is the most frequent single indication of left ventricular diastolic overloading, and a change in its depth is a most useful indication of a change in the left ventricular diastolic overloading. They pointed out that this sign is more characteristic of left ventricular diastolic overloading than the tall peaked T wave, the latter being frequently absent even in the presence of clear evidence of left ventricular diastolic overload. In their view, the amplitude of the R in V_6 increases in both left ventricular systolic and diastolic overloading, whereas Q V_6 is either normal or diminished in left ventricular systolic overloading.

If the electrocardiogram in complete transposition of the great arteries is to be viewed from a hemodynamic point, three facts must be stressed.

1. In all cases with a large ventricular septal defect (or a large duc-

tus), with or without pulmonary stenosis or pulmonary vascular obstruction, the pressure in the two ventricles is equal and is at the systemic level.

2. In all cases with an intact ventricular septum, the pressure in the right ventricle is at a systemic level.

3. In most cases with an intact ventricular septum the left ventricular pressure is lower than that in the right ventricle. Only when severe pulmonary stenosis, or severe pulmonary vascular obstruction is associated may the pressure in the left ventricle be higher than that in the right.

Accordingly, all cases of transposition have systolic overloading of the right ventricle. By definition, systolic overloading of the left ventricle means the development of a systolic pressure higher than normal in the cavity of this ventricle. Except in the case already mentioned, systolic overloading of the left ventricle is uncommon in complete transposition. Electrocardiographically, therefore, the basic pattern of complete transposition is that of systolic overloading of the right ventricle.

It has been shown elsewhere (Shaher, 1964) that a large pulmonary or systemic blood flow, which is not a function of blood shunt, may occur in transposition. Accordingly, electrocardiographic evidence of diastolic overloading of either ventricles may be superimposed on the basic right ventricular systolic overload pattern. With diastolic overloading of the left ventricle deep Q waves and tall R waves make their appearance in V_6. With diastolic overloading of the right ventricle, multiphasic QRS patterns in V_1 may occur. Thus, whereas cases with large pulmonary blood flow tend to show evidence of diastolic overloading of the left ventricle, cases with severe pulmonary stenosis or severe pulmonary vascular obstruction do not usually show this pattern. Since, as pointed out earlier, systolic overloading of the right ventricle is present in all cases of transposition, the occurrence of tracings which do not show systolic overloading of the right ventricle, suggest hypoplasia of this ventricle (Riemenschneider et al., 1968).

THE SIZE OF ASSOCIATED DEFECTS AND THE ELECTROCARDIOGRAM

Elliott et al. (1963a) studied the electrocardiogram in complete transposition, in relation to the size of the associated defects. They divided their patients into those with a "small communication," and those with a "large communication." It seemed important to them "to work from a functional rather than from a primary anatomic point of view, and to consider the influence of absence of flow through the ductus arteriosus, as well as through the ventricular septum." It has been shown elsewhere

(Shaher, 1964) that the pulmonary and the systemic blood flows are not a function of blood shunting in complete transposition. Moreover, whereas the pulmonary and the systemic blood flows vary within a wide range, the shunt (effective pulmonary blood flow) in each case was small and limited and varied within a narrow range. With these points in mind, it is difficult to see how variations in the size of the communication would produce variable electrocardiographic patterns. Moreover, the interpretation of anatomy in terms of flow is difficult to accept, since a large ductus arteriosus or a large ventricular septal defect with transposition of the great arteries does not necessarily mean a large amount of blood flowing through it. Since the amount of blood exchanged between the two circuits (effective pulmonary blood flow) in transposition is always small, a specific electrocardiogram pattern of a large communication (ventricular septal defect or patent ductus) is not related to the amount of blood passing through it, but is related to the equalization of pressure in the two ventricles which occurs under such circumstances. Similarly, a specific electrocardiographic pattern of the group with a small communication (intact ventricular septum, small ventricular septal defect or small ductus) is related to the higher pressure in the right ventricle than that in the left ventricle, which occurs in most patients in this group. These two electrocardiographic patterns may or may not be modified by diastolic overloading patterns of either or both ventricles.

References

Abbott, M. E. (1936). "Atlas of Congenital Cardiac Disease." American Heart Association, New York.

Aberdeen, E. (1971). Correction of uncomplicated cases of transposition of the great arteries. *Brit. Heart J. Suppl.* 33, 66–68.

Aberdeen, E., Waterston, D. J., Carr, I., Graham, G., Bonham-Carter, R. E., and Subramarian, S. (1965). Successful 'correction' of transposed great arteries by Mustard's operation. *Lancet.* i, 1233.

Agustsson, M. G., DuShane, J. W., and Swan, H. J. C. (1957). Ventricular septal defect in infancy and childhood. Clinical and physiologic study of 19 cases. *Pediatrics* 20, 848.

Aitchison, J. D., Duthie, R. J., and Young, J. S. (1955). Palpable venous pulsations in a case of transposition of both arterial trunks and complete heart block. *Brit. Heart J.* 17, 63.

Anderson, R. C., and Adams, P., Jr. (1955). Differentiation of associated cardiac defects in transposition of the great vessels. *Lancet* 75, 60.

Anderson, R. C., Lillehei, C. W., and Lester, R. G. (1957). Corrected transposition of the great vessels of the heart. *Pediatrics* 20, 626.

Astley, R., and Parsons, S. (1952). Complete transposition of the great vessels. *Brit. Heart J.* 14, 13.

Cabrera, E., and Gaxiola, A. (1959). A critical re-evaluation of systolic and diastolic overloading patterns. *Progr. Cardiovasc. Dis.* **2,** 219.

Cabrera, E., and Monroy, J. R. (1951). Systolic and diastolic loading of the heart. *Amer. Heart J.* **43,** 661.

Calleja, H. B., and Hosier, D. M. (1960). Complete transposition of the great vessels: An electrocardiographic and anatomic correlation. *Circulation* **22,** 730.

Calleja, H. B., Hosier, D. M., and Grajo, M. Z. (1965). The electrocardiogram in complete transposition of the great vessels. *Amer. Heart J.* **69,** 31.

Campbell, M., and Suzman, S. (1951). Transposition of the aorta and pulmonary artery. *Circulation* **4,** 329.

Casellas Bernat, A., Sanchis Aldas, J., and Roca Leop, J. (1968). El electrocardiograma en la transposition aislada de los grandes vasos. *Arch. Inst. Cardiol. Mex.* **38,** 551.

Corvacho, A. (1968). Transposition of the great vessels. *Amer. J. Cardiol.* **21,** 797.

Dack, S. (1960). The electrocardiogram and vectorcardiogram in ventricular septal defect. *Amer. J. Cardiol.* **5,** 199.

Daicoff, G. R., Schiebler, G. L., Elliott, L. P., Van Mierop, L. H. S., Bartley, T. D, Gessner, I. H., and Wheat, M. W. (1969). Surgical repair of complete transposition of the great arteries with pulmonary stenosis. *Ann. Thorac. Surg.* **7,** 529.

Dickson, R. W., and Jones, J. P. (1948). Congenital heart block in an infant with associated multiple congenital cardiac malformations. *Amer. J. Dis. Child.* **75,** 81.

Elliott, L. P., Anderson, R. C., Tuna, N., Adams, P., Jr., and Neufeld, H. N. (1963a). Complete transposition of the great vessels. II. An electrocardiographic analysis. *Circulation* **27,** 1118.

Elliott, L. P., Taylor, W. J., and Schiebler, G. L. (1963b). Combined ventricular hypertrophy in infancy: vectorcardiographic observations with special reference to the Katz-Wachtel phenomenon. *Amer. J. Cardiol.* **11,** 164.

El-Said, G., Rosenberg, H. S., Mullins, C. E., Hallman, G. L., Cooley, D. A., and Mc-Namara, D. G. (1972). Dysrhythmias after Mustard's operation for transportation of the great arteries. *Amer. J. Cardiol.* **30,** 526.

Gerbode, F., Selzer, A., Hill, J. D., and Ålberg, T. (1967). Transposition of the great arteries: surgical repair of a complicated case in a 36-year-old woman. *Ann. Surg.* **166,** 1016–1020.

Hamilton, S. D., Bartley, T. D., Miller, R. H., Schiebler, G. L., and Marriott, H. J. L. (1968). Disturbances in atrial rhythm and conduction following the surgical creation of an atrial septal defect by the Blalock-Hanlon technique. *Circulation* **38,** 73–81.

Ingham, D. W., and Willius, F. A. (1938). Congenital transposition of the great arterial trunks. *Amer. Heart J.* **15,** 482.

Isaacson, R., Titus, J. L., Merideth, J., Feldt, R. H., and McGoon, D. C. (1972). Apparent interruption of atrial conduction pathways after surgical repair of transposition of the great arteries. *Amer. J. Cardiol.* **30,** 533.

Katz, L. N., and Wachtel, H. (1937). The diphasic QRS type of electrocardiogram in congenital heart disease. *Amer. Heart J.* **13,** 202.

Katz, L. N., Langendorf, R., and Pick, A. (1952). "Introduction to the Interpretation of the Electrocardiogram," p. 59. The University of Chicago Press, Chicago, Illinois.

Keith, J. D., Rowe, R. D., and Vlad, P. (1958). "Heart Disease in Infancy and Childhood," 1st Ed. MacMillan, New York.

Khoury, G. H., Shaher, R. M., Fowler, R. S., and Keith, J. D. (1966). Preoperative and postoperative electrocardiogram in complete transposition of the great vessels. *Amer. Heart J.* **72,** 199.

Kossmann, C. E., and Johnston, F. D. (1935). The precordial electrocardiogram. I. The potential variations of the precordium and of the extremities in normal subjects. *Amer. Heart J.* **10**, 925.

Luna, R. L., and Crow, E. W. (1961). Correlation of degree of pulmonary hypertension with morphology of the QRS in lead V1 in cases with evidence of systolic overloading of the right ventricle. *Amer. Heart J.* **62**, 481.

Martins de Oliveira, J., and Zimmerman, A. (1959). Auricular overloadings. Electrocardiographic analysis of 193 cases. *Amer. J. Cardiol.* **3**, 453.

Noonan, A., Nadas, A. S., Rudolph, A. M., and Harris, G. B. C. (1960). Transposition of the great arteries. A correlation of clinical, physiologic and autopsy data. *N. Engl. J. Med.* **263**, 592.

Paul, O., Myers, G. S., and Campbell, J. A. (1951). The electrocardiogram in congenital heart disease. *Circulation* **3**, 564.

Pung, S., Gottstein, W. K., and Hirsch, E. F. (1955). Complete transposition of the great vessels in a male aged 18 years. *Amer. J. Med.* **18**, 155.

Riemenschneider, T. A., Vincent, W. R., Ruttenberg, H. D., and Desilets, D. T. (1968). Transposition of the great vessels with hypoplasia of the right ventricle. *Circulation* **38**, 386–402.

Schiebler, G. L., Edwards, J. E., Burchell, H. B., DuShane, J. W., Ongley, P. A., and Wood, E. H. (1961). Congenital corrected transposition of the great vessels: A study of 33 cases. *Pediatrics Suppl.* **27**, 851.

Scott, O., and Franklin, D. (1963). The electrocardiogram in the normal infant. *Brit. Heart J.* **25**, 44.

Shaher, R. M. (1964). The haemodynamics of complete transposition of the great vessels. *Brit. Heart J.* **26**, 343.

Shaher, R. M., and Deuchar, D. C. (1966). The electrocardiogram in complete transposition of the great vessels. *Brit. Heart J.* **28**, 265.

Sodi-Pallares, D., and Calder, R. M. (1956). "New Bases of Electrocardiography," p. 225. Mosby St. Louis, Missouri.

Sodi-Pallares, D., Pileggi, F., Cisneros, F., Ginefra, P., Portillo, B., Medrano, G., and Bisteni, A. (1958a). The mean manifest electrical axis of the ventricular activation process (AQRS) in congenital heart disease. *Amer. Heart J.* **55**, 681.

Sodi-Pallares, D., Portillo, B., Cisneros, F., de la Cruz, M. V., and Acosta, A. R. (1958b). Electrocardiography in infants and children. *Pediat. Clin. N. Amer.* **5**, 871.

Vince, D. J., and Keith, J. D. (1961). The electrocardiogram in ventricular septal defect. *Circulation* **23**, 225.

Vliers, A. C. (1966). Quelques remarques sur l'electrocardiogramme dans la transposition des gros vaisseaux. *Arch. Mal. Coeur Vaiss.* **59**, 1089–1098.

Watson, D. G., and Keith, J. D. (1962). The Q wave in lead V6 in heart disease of infancy and childhood, with special reference to diastolic loading. *Amer. Heart J.* **63**, 629.

Wimmer, M., and Latschewa, W. T. (1969). Das EKG bei kompletter transposition der grossen gefasse. *Z. Kreislaufforsch*, **58**, 1177–1193.

Wood, P. (1956). "Diseases of the Heart and Circulation," 2nd Ed. Eyre and Spottiswoode, London.

Ziegler, R. F. (1951). "Electrocardiographic Studies in Normal Infants and Children." Thomas, Springfield, Illinois.

Zuberbuhler, J. R., and Bauersfeld, S. R. (1967). Unusual arrhythmia after corrective surgery for transposition of the great vessels. *Amer. Heart J.* **73**, 752–755.

Zuckermann, R., Cisneros, F., and Novelo, S. (1951). El electrocardiograma en algunas cardiopatias congenitas. *Arch. Inst. Cardiol. Mex.* **21**, 61. (Cited by Elliott *et al.*, 1963.)

Chapter 14

THE VECTORCARDIOGRAM

The Frank vectorcardiograms of 58 patients in this series were available; 16 in Group I, 4 in Group II, 24 in Group III, and 14 in Group IV. Of these 58 vectorcardiograms, 50 have already been reported (Khoury *et al.*, 1967).

The vectorcardiograms were analyzed in the frontal, horizontal, and left sagittal plane projections in all cases (Fig. 14.1). Measurements were made of the angular direction and magnitude of the instantaneous time vectors at 10-millisecond intervals, and of the maximum and half-area QRS-T angle in all planes. The spatial QRS-T angle was calculated from Helm and Fowler's (1953) trigonometric tables. Detailed measurements of these parameters in 50 tracings will be found in the tables of Khoury *et al.* (1967). The ages of the patients ranged from 4 days to 13 years as tabulated as follows:

Age of patient	Number of patients
Under 2 months	7
2–6 Months	7
6 Months–1 year	2
1–2 Years	15
2–5 Years	17
6–9 Years	6
9–13 Years	4
	58

Vectorcardiographic Criteria

The diagnostic criteria for ventricular hypertrophy described by Donoso *et al.* (1955), Berengovich *et al.* (1960), Dack (1960), Hugenholtz *et al.* (1962), Elliott *et al.* (1963), Castellanos *et al.* (1964), and Khoury *et al.* (1967) have been used and are summarized below.

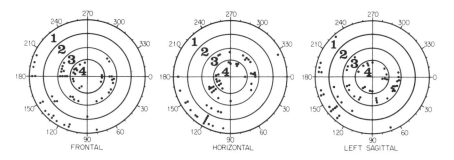

Fig. 14.1. Scattergram of the angular direction of the frontal, horizontal, and left sagittal planes as seen in the four groups. (1) Intact ventricular septum, 16 patients; (2) intact ventricular septum and pulmonary stenosis, 4 patients; (3) ventricular septal defect, 24 patients; (4) ventricular septal defect and pulmonary stenosis, 14 patients.

RIGHT VENTRICULAR HYPERTROPHY

1. Spatial orientation of the half-area and maximum QRS vector to the right, anteriorly or posteriorly, either inferiorly or superiorly.

2. Clockwise inscription of the QRS loop in the horizontal plane after the age of 3 months.

3. Anterior orientation of the maximum T vector in the horizontal plane after the age of 1 week.

4. A wide spatial QRS-T angle above the limits of normal for age.

5. Increased magnitude of the maximum rightward vector above the normal limits.

LEFT VENTRICULAR HYPERTROPHY

1. Spatial orientation of the half-area and maximum QRS vector to the left posteriorly, either inferiorly or superiorly, plus increased magnitude of the maximum QRS vector above the normal limits.

2. Significant posterior deflection of the 0.02 and 0.03 QRS vector in the horizontal plane.

3. Anterior and rightward orientation of the maximum T vector in the horizontal plane.

4. A wide spatial QRS-T angle above the normal limits for age.

COMBINED VENTRICULAR HYPERTROPHY

1. A large, anterior counterclockwise QRS loop in the horizontal plane, with the half-area QRS vector directed to 90°.

2. A large wide open leftward oriented anterior and posterior counterclockwise QRS loop in the horizontal plane.

3. Accentuation of the initial forces (prominent Q loop) in the presence of a clockwise inscription of the QRS loop in the horizontal plane.

4. Figure of eight QRS loop in the horizontal plane, with the terminal appendage directed rightward and posteriorly and inscribed clockwise.

Findings

GROUP I (16 PATIENTS)

Frontal Plane

In all cases, the inscription of the QRS loop was clockwise. The initial forces were directed to the left and inferiorly. The half-area QRS vector was oriented to the right and inferiorly in 11 cases, and superiorly in 5. In 1 patient with a large patent ductus arteriosus, the half-area vector was directed to the left and inferiorly.

Horizontal Plane

The initial 0.01 second QRS vectors were directed leftward and anteriorly. The half-area QRS vector was oriented to the right and anteriorly in 15 patients, with clockwise inscription of the QRS loop. In one case of a large patent ductus arteriosus, the QRS loop trajectory was counterclockwise, and the half-area was directed to the left and posteriorly. The terminal QRS vectors were oriented to the right either anteriorly or posteriorly.

Left Sagittal Plane

The inscription of the QRS loop was counterclockwise in 8 cases, clockwise in 4, and had a figure of eight configuration in 4. The half-area QRS vector was directed mainly anteriorly, and either inferiorly or superiorly.

T Vector

The spatial maximum T vector was oriented leftward, inferiorly, mainly anteriorly or superiorly.

Ventricular Hypertrophy Patterns

Isolated right ventricular hypertrophy was the predominant pattern (Fig. 14.2). It was evident in 12 out of the 16 patients. Combined ventricular hypertrophy was present in 2 patients. One of these 2 patients had a large patent ductus arteriosus. Two neonates had vectorcardiograms which were considered normal for the age.

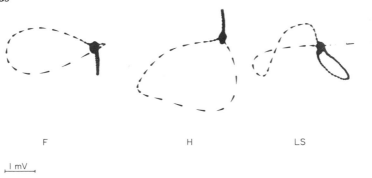

F   H   LS

| 1 mV

Fig. 14.2 The vectorcardiogram of a 5-year-old patient with transposition and intact ventricular septum. The maximum QRS vector is directed superiorly, anteriorly, and rightward. It is consistent with marked right ventricular hypertrophy. The direction of the loop is represented by the pointed ends of the dashes. F, frontal plane; H, horizontal plane; LS, left sagittal plane.

GROUP II (4 PATIENTS)

Frontal Plane

The inscription of the QRS loop was clockwise. The half-area QRS vector was oriented to the right and inferiorly.

Horizontal Plane

The QRS loop was clockwise in 3 patients and had a figure of eight in 1, in whom the initial forces were increased in magnitude and inscribed counterclockwise. The half-area QRS vector was directed to the right and anteriorly. The mean magnitude of the maximum QRS vector was directed mainly anteriorly and inferiorly.

Left Sagittal Plane

The inscription of the QRS loop was clockwise in 2 patients and counterclockwise in the other 2. The half-area QRS vector was directed mainly anteriorly and inferiorly.

T Vector

The maximum T vector was directed inferiorly and anteriorly in 3, and posteriorly in 1.

Ventricular Hypertrophy Patterns

Isolated right ventricular hypertrophy was present in 3 patients, and combined ventricular hypertrophy in 1.

GROUP III (24 PATIENTS)

Frontal Plane

The inscription of the QRS loop was clockwise in 14 patients, counterclockwise in 10. The initial forces were directed inferiorly either to the right or left. The half-area QRS vector showed a wide scatter. It was oriented to the left and superiorly in 5 patients; to the left and inferiorly in 6; to the right and inferiorly in 4; and to the right and superiorly (marked right axis deviation) in 9 patients.

Horizontal Plane

The inscription of the QRS loop was counterclockwise in 14, clockwise in 7, and had figure of eight in 3, with initial counterclockwise inscription of the loop. The initial 0.01 second QRS vectors were directed anteriorly and either to the right or left.

The half-area vector was widely distributed (Fig. 14.1). In 15 of 24 patients it was directed to the left and posteriorly.

Left Sagittal Plane

The inscription of the QRS loop was counterclockwise in 18 patients, clockwise in 4, and had a figure of eight in 2. The half-area vector was directed mainly posteriorly, either superiorly or inferiorly.

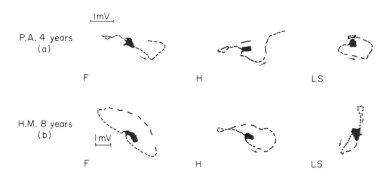

Fig. 14.3. The vectorcardiograms of two patients with transposition and ventricular septal defect. (a) The maximum QRS vector is directed leftward, posteriorly, and inferiorly with counterclockwise inscription of the QRS loop in all planes. (b) The maximum QRS vector is directed leftward, posteriorly and superiorly (left axis deviation). The terminal rightward vectors are increased in magnitude. The tracings are consistent with combined ventricular hypertrophy. F, frontal plane; H, horizontal plane; LS, sagittal plane. From Khoury *et al.* (1967), by permission of American Heart Association, Inc.

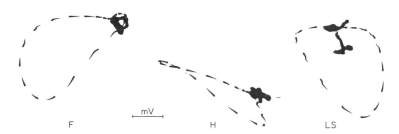

Fig. 14.4. The vectorcardiogram of 2-year-old child with transposition and ventricular septal defect. The maximum QRS vector is directed rightward, inferiorly and anteriorly. The tracing is consistent with marked right ventricular hypertrophy. The direction of the loop is represented by the pointed end of the dashes. Abbreviations same as used previously in Fig. 14.3.

T Vector

The spatial orientation of the maximum T vector was to the left, inferiorly, and either anteriorly or posteriorly.

Ventricular Hypertrophy Patterns

The vectorcardiogram was consistent with combined ventricular hypertrophy patterns in 16 patients (Fig. 14.3), right ventricular hypertrophy in 4 (Fig. 14.4), left ventricular hypertrophy in 3 (Fig. 14.5), and within normal limits for the age of 5 days in 1 (Fig. 14.6). The striking feature in this group was the variability in the spatial orientation of the QRS loop. Six main vectorcardiographic patterns were encountered:

1. The QRS loop was projected to the left and posteriorly, either superiorly or inferiorly, with increased magnitude of the rightward vectorial

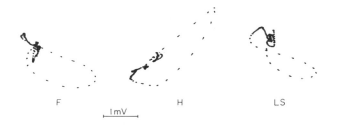

Fig. 14.5. The vectorcardiogram of an 11-year-old patient with transposition and ventricular septal defect. The maximum QRS vector is directed leftward, inferiorly and posteriorly. The inscription is clockwise in the horizontal plane. The tracing is consistent with left ventricular hypertrophy. The direction of the loop is represented by the pointed end of the dashes. Abbreviations same as previously used.

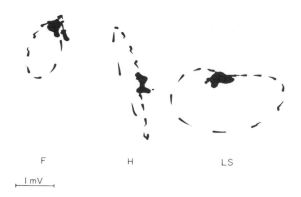

F   H   LS

⊢ I mV ⊣

Fig. 14.6. The vectorcardiogram of a 5-day-old infant with transposition and ventricular septal defect. The tracing is within normal limits for the age. The direction of the loop is represented by the pointed end of the dashes. Abbreviations same as previously used.

forces. This pattern indicating combined ventricular hypertrophy was noticed in 8 patients.

2. In 3 patients the QRS loop was oriented mainly to the right, posteriorly and superiorly, with counterclockwise inscription in the horizontal plane.

3. The QRS loop was oriented leftward and inferiorly with equal anterior and posterior projection, and counterclockwise inscription in the horizontal plane. This pattern was seen in 3 patients.

4. In the horizontal plane the QRS loop had a figure of eight configuration with the initial part being counterclockwise and terminal forces clockwise and directed to the right and posteriorly. The electrocardiographic counterpart of these last two patterns is a large diphasic complex in the midprecordial leads referred to as the Katz-Wachtel sign. This pattern was seen in 2 patients.

5. In 4 patients the QRS loop was oriented to the right and anteriorly with clockwise inscription in the frontal plane, indicating right ventricular hypertrophy.

6. In 3 patients, the QRS loop was spatially oriented to the left, posteriorly, either superiorly or inferiorly. The voltage of the maximum QRS vector was increased above normal, indicating left ventricular hypertrophy.

GROUP IV (14 PATIENTS)

Frontal Plane

The inscription of the QRS loop was counterclockwise in 6 cases, clockwise in 6, and had a figure of eight configuration in 2. The half-area

QRS vector was widely scattered, but oriented mainly to the right either superiorly or inferiorly. In 1 case it was directed to the left and superiorly (left axis deviation).

Horizontal Plane

The QRS loop was counterclockwise in 7 patients, clockwise in 6, and a figure of eight in 1. The half-area QRS vector was widely scattered. It was oriented to the right and anteriorly in 6 cases, to the left and posteriorly in 5, and to the right and posteriorly in 3.

Left Sagittal Plane

The QRS loop was counterclockwise in 7, clockwise in 4, and had a figure of eight configuration in 2. The half-area vector was directed anteriorly or posteriorly, either superiorly or inferiorly.

T Vector

The spatial maximum T vector was directed leftward, inferiorly, either anteriorly or posteriorly.

Ventricular Hypertrophy Patterns

Combined ventricular hypertrophy was present in 7 patients (Fig. 14.7). In 2 out of the 7, the inscription of the QRS loop in the horizontal plane was clockwise, but the initial forces (Q loop) were increased in magnitude and directed to the right and anteriorly. Vectorcardiographic patterns of isolated right ventricular hypertrophy were present in 5 patients. Pure left ventricular hypertrophy was found in 2 patients. In one

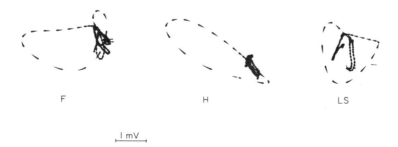

F   H   LS

| 1 mV |

Fig. 14.7. The vectorcardiogram of a 1½-year-old child with transposition, ventricular septal defect, and pulmonary stenosis. The maximum QRS vector is directed rightward, inferiorly and posteriorly. The inscription is clockwise in the frontal and horizontal planes. The tracing is consistent with marked right ventricular hypertrophy. The direction of the loop is represented by the pointed end of the dashes. Abbreviations as in Fig. 14.3.

case, the initial vectors were directed to the right and anteriorly but with clockwise inscription, which is the reverse of normal; they then continued in a counterclockwise fashion.

Discussion

In Groups I and II the vectorcardiogram showed clockwise inscription of the QRS loop in the horizontal plane and was consistent with isolated right ventricular hypertrophy. The findings were not different from the electrocardiographic findings in the same groups. On the other hand, in Group III the vectorcardiogram portrayed a higher incidence of combined ventricular hypertrophy when correlated to the scalar electrocardiogram. Since most patients with transposition and a ventricular septal defect have systemic pressure in the left ventricle, and increased pulmonary blood flow, the vectorcardiogram appears to be superior to the scalar electrocardiogram in expressing the presence of concomitant left ventricular hypertrophy. Moreover, in the horizontal plane the vectorcardiogram exhibited certain diagnostic features characteristic of a relatively large interventricular communication. These were counterclockwise inscriptions of the QRS loop and increased magnitude of the initial vectorial forces which were directed to the right and anteriorly producing a prominent Q wave in the left precordial leads. The significance of such a finding has been well demonstrated by several authors in volume load lesion of the left ventricle (Toscano-Barbosa and DuShane, 1959; Cabrera and Gaxiola, 1959; Elliott *et al.*, 1963a). Also in the frontal plane, the half-area QRS vector tended to be directed to the left either superiorly or inferiorly with high incidence of counterclockwise inscription of the loop. In Group IV the vectorcardiogram was not specific except for a significantly wide spatial QRS-T angle.

Of the whole group of 58 patients pure left ventricular hypertrophy patterns with left axis deviation were noted in 4 patients; 2 in Group III, and 2 in Group IV. This pattern could be explained on the basis of hypoplasia of the right ventricle (Riemenschneider *et al.*, 1968) or the presence of atrioventricularis communis type of ventricular septal defect (Shaher *et al.*, 1967).

Each of 11 patients with intact ventricular septum and relatively low peak systolic pressure in the left ventricle reported by Mair *et al.* (1970a,b) showed isolated right ventricular hypertrophy manifested by a large open clockwise horizontal plane QRS vector loops directed predominately to the right and anteriorly. The frontal plane QRS loops were inscribed in a clockwise manner. Of their 17 patients with systemic pressure in the left ventricle (16 with ventricular septal defect and 1 with intact ventricular septum and pulmonary stenosis), the horizontal plane QRS loops of 14 were counterclockwise or of a figure of eight configuration. Two of the remaining 3 patients had large initial counterclockwise deflections to the left, with the maximal vector directed to the left and anteriorly. Eight of the 16 patients with ventricular septal defects had counterclockwise frontal plane QRS loops. The authors pointed out that the vectorcardiograms were not helpful in separating patients with large pulmonary blood flows from those with pulmonary stenosis, pulmonary artery bands, or severe pulmonary vascular disease. From this point of view, they suggested that serial vectorcardiograms are not reliable as a means of detecting progression of pulmonary vascular disease in transposition.

Restieaux *et al.* (1970) used the maximal spatial vectors to the left and right to quantitate the degree of left and right ventricular hypertrophy in patients with transposition. Of their 44 patients with an intact ventricular septum, 38 had left ventricular pressure one-half or less of the right ventricular pressure. The left maximal spatial vector was 0.9 mV and the right 1.94 mV. Rotation in the horizontal plane was clockwise in all and the frontal plane was predominantly clockwise. The remaining 6 had pulmonary vascular obstruction and the ventricular pressures were equal. The left maximal spatial vector was 1.8 mV and the horizontal plane rotation was counterclockwise. In their 50 patients with a ventricular septal defect, the ventricular pressures were equal. The left maximal spatial vector was 1.56 mV and the right 1.96 mV. Rotation in the horizontal plane was counterclockwise in 40, and clockwise in 10. Rotation in the frontal plane was predominantly clockwise. The authors pointed out that the combination of a moderately low left maximal spatial vector with clockwise rotation in the horizontal plane has proved to be a reliable indicator that the left ventricular pressure is lower than the right. The detection of an increasing left maximal spatial vector or change in the horizontal plane rotation toward counterclockwise would suggest increasing left ventricular pressure. A further report on this group of patients was made by Restieaux *et al.* (1972). The authors added that provided the hematocrit was not excessively elevated, a counterclockwise loop in the horizontal plane was associated with a high left ventricular pressure (greater than 70% of the right ventricular pressure), whereas a clockwise horizontal loop indicated a left ventricular pressure less than 70% of the right ventricular pressure.

References

Berengovich, J., Bleifer, S., Donoso, E., and Grishman, A. (1960). The vectorcardiogram and electrocardiogram in ventricular septal defect with special reference to the diagnosis of combined ventricular hypertrophy. *Brit. Heart J.* **22**, 205.

Cabrera, E., and Gaxiola, A. (1959). A critical re-evaluation of systolic and diastolic overloading patterns. *Progr. Cardiovasc. Dis.* **2**, 219.

Castellanos, A., Lemberg, L., Gosslin, A., and Castellanos, A., Jr. (1964). Combined ventricular enlargement during the first months of life: Vectorcardiographic study of the T loop. *Amer. J. Cardiol.* **12**, 767.

Dack, S. (1960). The electrocardiogram and vectorcardiogram in ventricular septal defect. *Amer. J. Cardiol.* **5**, 199.

Donoso, E., Sapin, S. O., Braunwald, E., and Grishman, A. (1955). Study of the electrocardiogram and vectorcardiogram in congenital heart disease: II. Vectorcardiographic criteria for ventricular hypertrophy. *Amer. Heart J.* **50**, 674.

Elliott, L. P., Anderson, R. C., Tuna, N., Adams, P., Jr., and Neufeld, H. N. (1963a). Complete transposition of the great vessels: II. Electrocardiographic analysis. *Circulation* **27**, 118.

Elliott, L. P., Taylor, W. J., and Schiebler, G. L. (1963b). Combined ventricular hypertrophy in infancy: Vectorcardiographic observations with special reference to the Katz-Wachtel phenomenon. *Amer. J. Cardiol.* **11**, 164.

Helm, R. A., and Fowler, N. O., Jr. (1953). Simplified method for determining the angle between two spatial vectors. *Amer. Heart J.* **45**, 835.

Hugenholtz, P. G., Lees, M. M., and Nadas, A. S. (1962). The scalar electrocardiogram, vectorcardiogram in assessment of congenital aortic stenosis. *Circulation* **26**, 79.

Khoury, G. H., Shaher, R. M., and Fowler, R. S. (1967). The vectorcardiogram in complete transposition of the great vessels. Analysis of fifty cases. *Circulation* **35**, 178–194.

Mair, D. D., Macastney, F. J., Weidman, W. H., Ritter, D. G., Ongley, P. A., and Smith, R. E. (1970a). The vectorcardiogram in complete transposition of the great arteries: correlation with anatomic and hemodynamic findings and calculated left ventricular mass. *Proc. 11th Intern. Vectrocardiography Symp.*, pp. 610–623. North Holland, Amsterdam.

Mair, D. D., Macartney, F. J., Weidman, W. H., Ritter, D. G., Ongley, P. A., and Smith, R. E. (1970b). The vectorcardiogram in complete transposition of the great arteries: correlation with anatomic and hemodynamic findings and calculated left ventricular mass. *J. Electrocardiol.* **3**, 217–229.

Restieaux, N., Ellison, R., and Nadas, A. S. (1970). Assessment of left ventricular pressure in transposition of the great arteries by the Frank electrocardiogram. *Amer. J. Cardiol.* **25**, 124.

Restieaux, N., Ellison, R. C., Albers, W. H., and Nadas, A. S. (1972). The Frank electrocardiogram in complete transposition of the great arteries. Its use in assessment of left ventricular pressure. *Amer. Heart J.* **83**, 219.

Riemenschneider, T. A., Vincent, W. R., Ruttenberg, H. D., and Desilets, D. T. (1968). Transposition of the great vessels with hypoplasia of the right ventricle. *Circulation* **38**, 386.

Shaher, R. M., Puddu, G. C., Khoury, G., Moes, C. A. F., and Mustard, W. T. (1967). Complete transposition of the great vessels with anatomic obstruction of the outflow tract of the left ventricle. Surgical implication of anatomic findings. *Amer. J. Cardiol.* **19**, 658.

Toscano-Barbosa, E., and DuShane, J. W. (1959). Ventricular septal defect: correlation of electrocardiographic and hemodynamic findings in 60 proved cases. *Amer. J. Cardiol.* 3, 721.

Chapter 15

CHEST ROENTGENOGRAM

In 1932, Fanconi recognized the importance of a narrow vascular pedicle in the radiological diagnosis of complete transposition of the great arteries. He pointed out that this appearance was due to the aorta being in front of and parallel to the pulmonary artery. He also noted the progressive enlargement of the heart which occurs over a period of months. Taussig (1938, 1960) pointed out that in transposition the pulmonary artery lies behind the aorta and the outstanding diagnostic radiological feature is the narrow vascular pedicle in the frontal projection. When the child is rotated into the left anterior oblique position, the pulmonary artery lies parallel to the aorta and thereby the shadow cast by these vessels is increased in depth. In infancy the contour of the heart frequently resembles an egg. The aorta seldom arises as far to the left as does the normal pulmonary artery, hence the slight concavity of the upper border of the cardiac silhouette to the left of the sternum. Both ventricles are usually enlarged and dilatation of the superior vena cava is common. Taussig described rhythmic changes in the size of the right atrium, independent of the heart rate, which may be observed due to the piling up of blood on one side of the heart. In addition, she pointed out that the vascular markings in infancy are normal or slightly increased and extend from the hilar region to nearly the periphery of the lungs. Many small discrete circular shadows due to the blood vessels viewed end-on, may be observed. In the presence of pulmonary stenosis the pulmonary artery is a fair-sized vessel and the vascular markings are heavier than those in Fallot. When the aorta is so rotated that it occupies the position of the normal pulmonary artery, there is marked fullness of the pulmonary conus. With enormous dilatation of the pulmonary artery, the heart is slightly enlarged, and huge blotchy shadows extend far out into the lung fields. Under such circumstances it is the excessive vascularity of the lung fields combined with absence of fullness of the pulmonary conus which indicates that the pulmonary artery is transposed. Hilar dance may be present. Rarely, however, the main pulmonary artery is so dilated that it gives the appearance of fullness of the pulmonary conus. In 1949, Eek pointed out that the radiological diagnosis of transposition of the great arteries is simple since the narrow vascular pedicle and the enlarged egg-shaped heart appear as early as the first few months of life. On the other hand, Castellanos *et al.* (1950) thought that the cardiac outline has no value whatsoever in the diagnosis of this condition. Similarly, Kerley (1951) thought that since the great vessels in infants cannot normally be identified by chest radiography, there is little prospect of diagnosing their anomalies without angiocardiography. Campbell and Suzman (1951) found that the heart in transposition is nearly always enlarged, and the deep pulmonary bay of Fallot's tetralogy was almost always absent. Two-thirds of their cases showed some concavity and one-third showed moderate or great convexity in the pulmonary region. The prominence on the left cardiac border which occurred in the majority of their patients, indicated enlargement of the infundibulum of the right ventricle. Dilatation of the pulmonary arteries and general mottling of the lung fields were other features present in most of their cases. In 1951, Campbell pointed out that marked pulsation of the pulmonary arteries may be visible out to the periphery of the lungs, and 4 of his 7 cases had an obvious hilar dance. Abrams *et al.* (1951) reviewed the literature and summarized the important diagnostic features of transposition: (1) a large heart with right and left ventricular enlargement, (2) a cephalolateral bulge in the left midcardiac border, (3) a narrow mediastinal shadow in the frontal projection which widens in the left anterior oblique projection, and (4) prominence of the pulmonary arterial branches. They emphasized, however, that these findings are applicable only within the first few years of life and that these criteria may not be sufficient to establish the diagnosis in older age groups. Astley and Parsons (1952) found three important features the presence of any one of which strongly suggests transposition: (1) a narrow vascular pedicle, (2) a long bulge of a special type caused by the transposed aorta in the left middle segment, and (3) a concave middle segment associated with pulmonary plethora. They thought that normal or oligemic lungs suggest a patent foramen ovale and a patent ductus arteriosus, or pulmonary stenosis. "Congested" lungs indicate a ventricular septal defect. Keith *et al.* (1953) emphasized that at birth the heart in transposition is close to normal in size and shape. After 3 to 4 weeks of life the heart becomes enlarged to a considerable degree to both the right and left with the left cardiac surface assuming a convex border. In their view, the left cardiac border can readily be shown at postmortem as composed of the left ven-

TABLE 15.1
INTACT SEPTUM [a]

	Cardiothoracic ratio (%)					Shape of heart			Vascular pedicle			Vascularity		
	40–50	51–55	56–60	61–65	65 or more	Egg	Nonspecific	Hump	Narrow	Normal	Broad	Diminished	Normal	Increased
1st Day	6	8	17	9	0	12	28	6	22	15	3	12	25	3
2–7 Days	3	9	8	5	0	11	14	8	15	6	4	12	7	6
1 Week–1 month	2	7	14	8	0	24	7	10	23	5	3	11	8	12
1–6 Months	3	2	5	13	6	14	15	6	17	3	9	6	5	18
6 Months–1 year	1	1	4	1	1	2	6	2	2	3	3	1	0	7
1–3 Years	2	0	9	4	3	5	13	4	9	6	3	3	1	14
3–10 Years	1	0	0	2	0	1	2	2	1	2	0	1	0	2
Above 10 years	0	0	0	1	0	0	1	0	1	0	0	0	0	1
Total	18	27	57	43	10	69	86	38	90	40	25	46	46	63

[a] 155 roentgenograms.

tricle. When this ventricle hypertrophies after birth, it often enlarges upward to the point of obscuring the pulmonary artery in either the anteroposterior or lateral view. The narrow great vessel area is then due to the tip of the arch of the aorta with the vertebral column above it. The pulmonary artery is buried in the cardiac shadow below the aorta and below the point where the left cardiac border meets the great vessel or supracardiac shadow. Cooley and Sloan (1956) thought that in young children and infants, cardiac enlargement may not be a prominent feature and a number of variations or additional defects may alter the cardiac contour: (1) double superior vena cava, partial anomalous pulmonary venous drainage, or anomalous drainage of the superior or inferior vena cava into the left atrium, (2) pulmonary stenosis which diminishes the pulmonary vascularity, and (3) rotational or torsional dextrocardia with a resultant variation in the heart contour. According to Keith *et al.* (1958), when the infundibulum of the right ventricle lies at the extreme

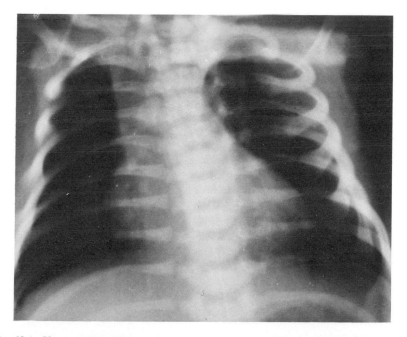

Fig. 15.1. Chest roentgenogram of a 1-day-old infant with transposition and intact ventricular septum showing nonspecific cardiac enlargement and diminished pulmonary vascularity.

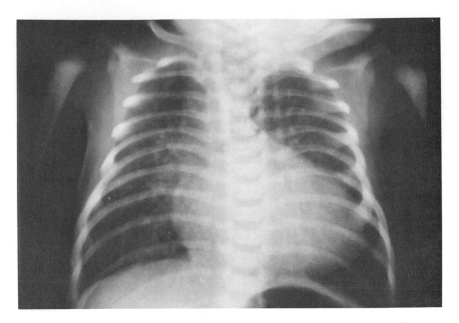

Fig. 15.2. Chest roentgenogram of a 3-week-old infant with intact ventricular septum showing an egg-shaped heart, narrow vascular pedicle, and increased pulmonary vascularity.

left and the ascending aorta protrudes forming the left border of a wide vascular pedicle, transposition with either pulmonary stenosis or single ventricle may be found. Little or no cardiac enlargement was observed in their patients who survived the first 18 months and the aortic arch was most frequently on the left. Among 50 patients with complete transposition of the great arteries, Noonan *et al.* (1960) observed passive pulmonary congestion in 10. She stressed that none of the radiological criteria are specific for complete transposition because small infants with normally related great vessels but with severe pulmonary stenosis may have a narrow vascular pedicle; the bulge of the left border of the heart is also a characteristic finding in corrected transposition, and a dilated pulmonary infundibular chamber may give a similar picture. Moreover, pulmonary plethora in the presence of a concave pulmonary artery segment may occur in persistent truncus arteriosus. According to Kerley (1951), the aortic arch in transposition cannot be outlined because it runs in a wide curve close to the midline in the sagittal plane. In addition, atresia of the left branch of the pulmonary artery occurs in many cases so that there is plethora in the right lung and ischemia in the left. If there is severe pul-

TABLE 15.2

INTACT SEPTUM AND PULMONARY STENOSIS [a]

	Cardiothoracic ratio (%)					Shape of heart			Vascular pedicle			Vascularity		
	40–50	51–55	56–60	61–65	65 or more	Egg	Nonspecific	Hump	Narrow	Normal	Broad	Diminished	Normal	Increased
1st Day	0	0	0	0	0	0	0	0	0	0	0	0	0	0
2–7 Days	1	1	1	0	0	1	2	0	3	0	0	1	1	1
1 Week–1 month	0	0	1	0	0	0	1	0	1	0	0	0	1	0
1–6 Months	0	0	0	0	0	0	0	0	0	0	0	0	0	0
6 Months–1 year	0	0	0	0	0	0	0	0	0	0	0	0	0	0
1–3 Years	0	1	0	2	0	0	0	3	3	0	0	0	2	1
3–10 Years	0	0	3	0	0	1	0	2	3	0	0	0	0	3
Above 10 years	0	0	0	0	0	0	0	0	0	0	0	1	0	0
Total	1	2	5	2	0	5	5	5	10	0	0	1	4	5

[a] 10 Roentgenograms.

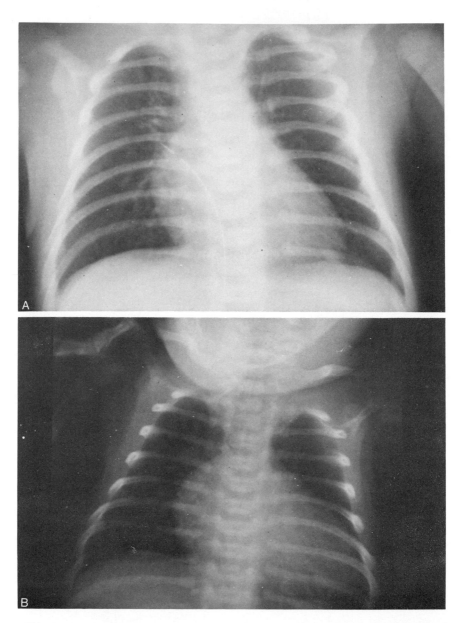

Fig. 153. Serial chest radiographs of an infant with transposition and intact ventricular septum demonstrating progressive cardiac enlargement. (A) 1 day; (B) 3 weeks; (C) 6 weeks; (D) 4 months. Pericardial effusion was found at surgical creation of atrial septal defect at 4 months.

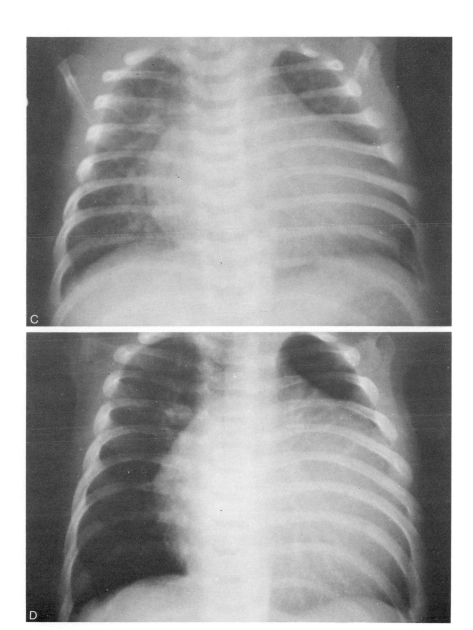

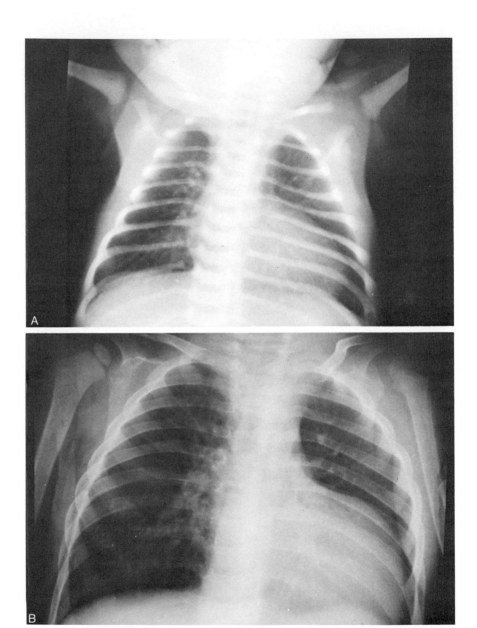

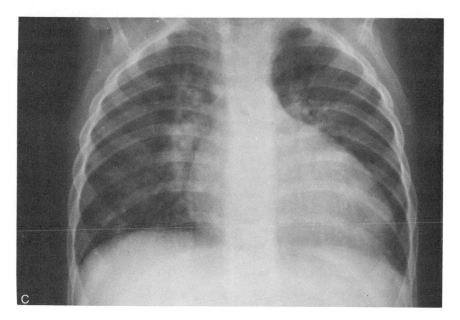

Fig. 15.4. Chest roentgenogram of transposition, intact ventricular septum and pulmonary stenosis. (A) 3-day-old infant. Egg-shaped heart and normal pulmonary vascularity. (B) Same patient at 1 year. A hump at the left cardiac border was seen; there was normal pulmonary vascularity. (C) Another 1-year-old child. Nonspecific configuration, cardiac enlargement, and increased pulmonary vascularity.

monary stenosis or pulmonary atresia there may be no plethora, while if pulmonary hypertension develops the plethora partially disappears. Perloff (1970) pointed out that when severe pulmonary stenosis is present, the cardiac size is relatively unimpressive. The lung fields are clear since pulmonary blood flow is normal or reduced and pulmonary venous congestion absent. The vascular pedicle remains narrow since poststenotic dilation of the pulmonary artery is not seen on the film even if present. A right aortic arch has a tendency to occur with pulmonic stenosis and ventricular septal defect but not with other forms of complete transposition.

In this series, 366 chest X-rays were available; 155 in Group I, 10 in Group II, 136 in Group III, and 65 in Group IV. According to the age of the patient each group was further subdivided into eight subgroups as follows: the first day, 2–7 days, 1 week to 1 month, 1–6 months, 6–12 months, 1–3 years, 3–10 years, and above 10 years. The following parameters were studied in each roentgenogram: the cardiothoracic ratio, the shape of the heart, the vascular pedicle, the pulmonary vascularity,

TABLE 15.3
VENTRICULAR SEPTAL DEFECT [a]

	Cardiothoracic ratio (%)					Shape of heart			Vascular pedicle			Vascularity		
	40-50	51-55	56-60	61-65	65 or more	Egg	Nonspecific	Hump	Narrow	Normal	Broad	Diminished	Normal	Increased
1st Day	0	2	3	2	0	1	6	0	4	1	2	3	3	1
2-7 Days	0	5	6	3	1	2	13	1	8	4	3	3	5	7
1 Week-1 month	2	1	5	6	2	7	9	2	10	5	1	1	1	14
1-6 Months	0	1	17	13	10	26	15	15	32	6	3	3	1	37
6 Months-1 year	0	1	2	4	3	4	6	4	6	1	3	0	0	10
1-3 Years	0	3	9	4	5	4	17	1	9	4	8	1	0	20
3-10 Years	0	4	7	4	3	3	15	3	8	7	3	0	0	18
Above 10 years	2	0	4	1	1	0	8	1	3	1	4	0	0	8
Total	4	17	53	37	25	47	89	27	80	29	27	11	10	115

[a] 136 roentgenograms.

and the thymic shadow. The findings in the four groups have been summarized in Tables 15.1 to 15.4. Excluded from this study were X-rays
taken after the Blalock-Taussig or Pott's anastomosis, banding of the pulmonary artery, or the Mustard procedure.

Findings

GROUP I (TABLE 15.1)

During the first day of life 71% of the patients in Group I had a cardiothoracic ratio of 60% or less and a nonspecific cardiac configuration
(Fig. 15.1). An egg-shaped heart was seen in 29%, and a narrow vascu-

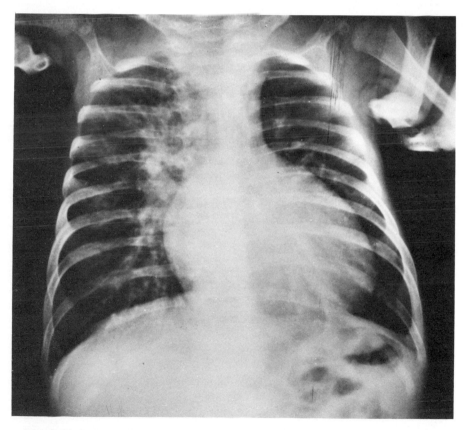

Fig. 15.5. Chest radiography of a 3-month-old infant with transposition and ventricular septal defect showing cardiac enlargement, egg-shaped heart, narrow vascular
pedicle, and increased pulmonary vascularity.

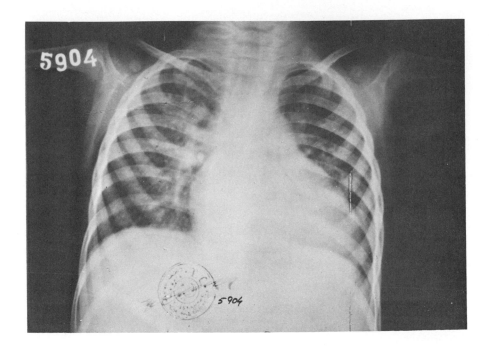

Fig. 15.6. Chest roentgenogram of a 4-year-old child with transposition and ventricular septal defect. Note nonspecific cardiac configuration, normal pulmonary vascular pedicle, and increased pulmonary vascularity.

lar pedicle in 48%. The pulmonary vascularity was essentially normal in 66% and diminished in 34%. From the first week to the first month an egg-shaped heart with a narrow vascular pedicle was seen in the majority of the chest X-rays (Fig. 15.2). Between the ages of 1 and 6 months, the majority showed significant cardiac enlargement (more than 60%) and increased pulmonary vascularity (Fig. 15.3). Although 62% of the patients in this age group had a narrow vascular pedicle, only 50% showed an egg-shaped cardiac configuration. After the age of 6 months, significant cardiac enlargement, a narrow vascular pedicle, and an egg-shaped heart were seen in 30 to 50% of the patients. However, excessive pulmonary vascularity was observed in the majority. A hump at the left cardiac border was seen in 25.5% of the cases in this group. A thymic shadow was observed in 15 cases, and dilatation of the pulmonary artery and increased pulmonary vascularity on the right as compared to the left in 1. A prominent main pulmonary arterial segment was seen in 2 cases. Cardiac configuration suggestive of pericardial effusion was observed in 1 (Fig. 15.3D).

TABLE 15.4

VENTRICULAR SEPTAL DEFECT AND PULMONARY STENOSIS [a]

	Cardiothoracic ratio (%)					Shape of heart			Vascular pedicle			Vascularity		
	40–50	51–55	56–60	61–65	65 or more	Egg	Nonspecific	Hump	Narrow	Normal	Broad	Diminished	Normal	Increased
1st Day	2	0	0	0	1	1	2	1	2	1	0	2	0	1
2–7 Days	1	0	3	0	0	2	2	0	3	1	0	3	1	0
1 Week–1 month	1	1	1	1	0	1	3	0	2	2	0	2	0	2
1–6 Months	1	4	4	5	0	5	9	2	8	4	2	3	1	10
6 Months–1 year	0	2	1	4	3	4	6	1	5	4	1	3	1	6
1–3 Years	2	1	6	4	3	7	9	4	6	8	2	4	1	11
3–10 Years	2	5	0	3	1	5	6	1	7	4	0	0	1	10
Above 10 years	2	0	0	0	1	0	3	0	3	0	0	1	0	2
Total	11	13	15	17	9	25	40	9	36	24	5	18	5	42

[a] 65 Roentgenograms.

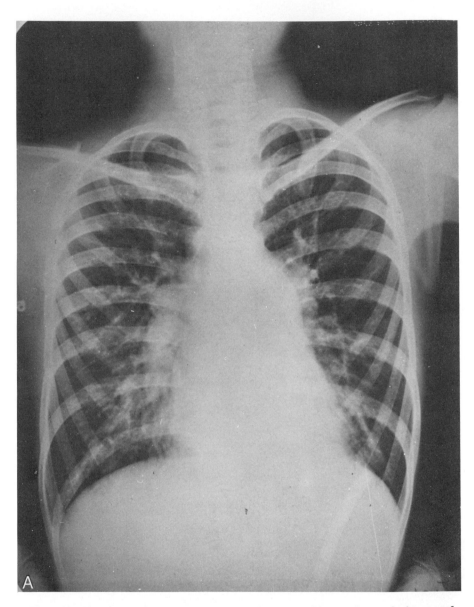

Fig. 15.7. Chest radiograph of a patient with transposition and ventricular septal defect. (A) At 14 years of age showing no cardiac enlargement, prominent pulmonary artery segment, and increased pulmonary vascularity. (B) At the age of 26 years showing nonspecific cardiac enlargement, prominent pulmonary artery segment, and increased vascularity.

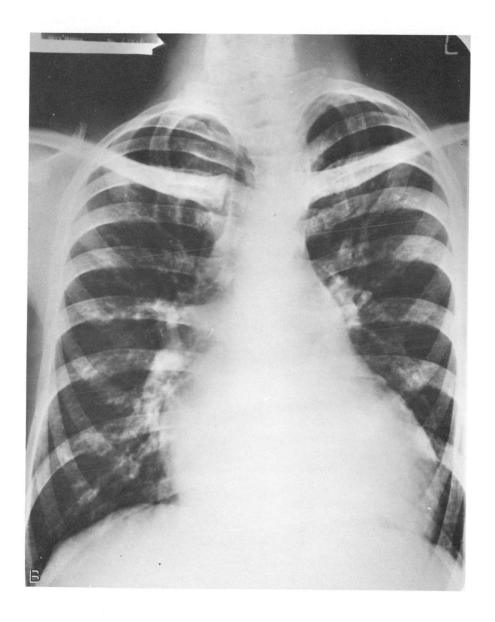

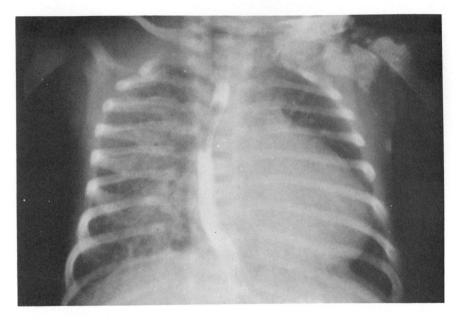

Fig. 15.8. Chest radiograph of a 1-month-old infant with transposition and ventricular septal defect. Note increased vascularity on the right as compared to the left.

GROUP II (TABLE 15.2)

Only 10 chest roentgenograms were available in this group (Fig. 15.4). An egg-shaped heart was seen in 5, a narrow vascular pedicle in all, a normal or diminished pulmonary vascularity in 5, and increased vascularity in 5. A hump at the left cardiac border was seen in 33% of the cases. A thymic shadow was not observed in any case in this group.

GROUP III (TABLE 15.3)

During the first day of life all patients in this group had a nonspecific cardiac configuration and the pulmonary vascularity was normal in 43%, diminished in 43%, and increased in 14%. A narrow vascular pedicle occurred in 50% and significant cardiac enlargement in 28%. After the first day the incidence of an egg-shaped heart, narrow vascular pedicle, and prominent vascularity increased so that in the age group 1–6 months a cardiothoracic ratio of more than 60% occurred in 65%, an egg-shaped heart in 67%, a narrow vascular pedicle in 78%, and increased pulmonary vascularity in 89% (Fig. 15.5). In the age group 1–10 years the majority had a cardiothoracic ratio of less than 60%, nonspecific cardiac configuration, a normal or broad vascular pedicle, and an increased pulmonary vascularity (Fig. 15.6). Above the age of 10 years a cardiothoracic ratio of less than 50% occurred in 28%, a narrow vascular pedicle in 43%, and nonspecific cardiac configuration and increased pulmonary vascularity in all (Fig. 15.7). A hump at the left cardiac border was seen

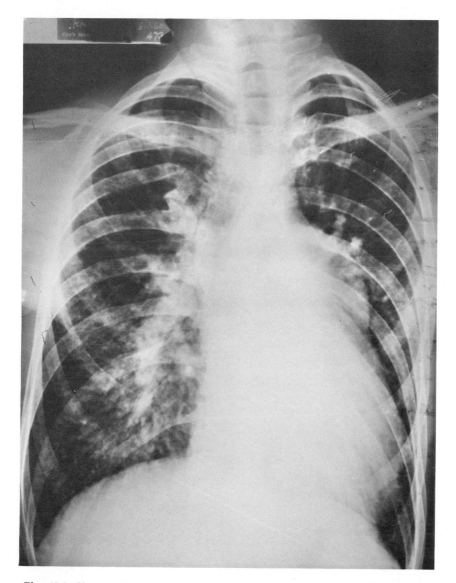

Fig. 15.9. Chest radiograph of a 24-year-old patient with transposition and ventricular septal defect showing marked prominence of the pulmonary arterial segment.

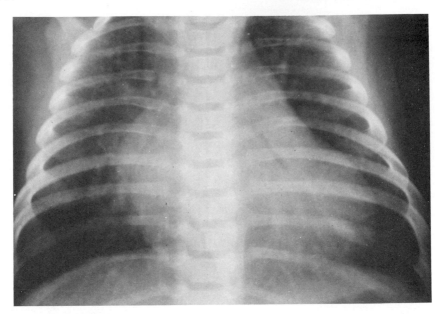

Fig. 15.10. Chest radiograph of a 2-month-old infant with transposition, ventricular septal defect, and pulmonary stenosis showing cardiac enlargement, prominent pulmonary artery segment, and increased vascularity.

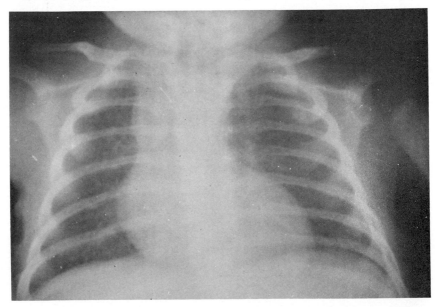

Fig. 15.11. Chest radiograph of a 2-month-old infant with transposition, ventricular septal defect, and pulmonary stenosis showing slight cardiac enlargement and diminished pulmonary vascularity.

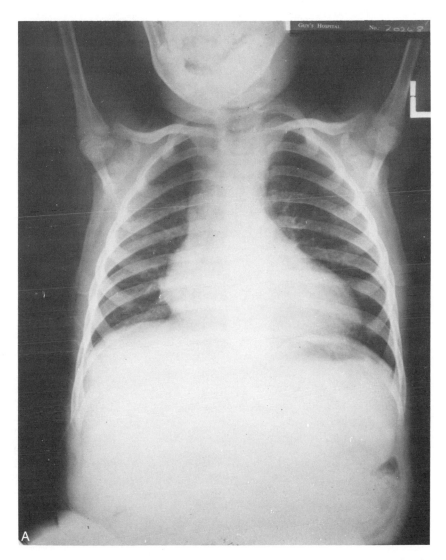

Fig. 15.12. Transposition, ventricular septal defect and pulmonary stenosis above the age of 1 year. (A) Chest radiograph of a 4-year-old patient showing slight cardiac enlargement and diminished pulmonary vascularity. (B) Chest radiograph of a 15-year-old patient showing no cardiac enlargement, and normal pulmonary vascularity. (C) Chest radiograph of a 29-year-old patient showing marked cardiac enlargement and diminished pulmonary vascularity.

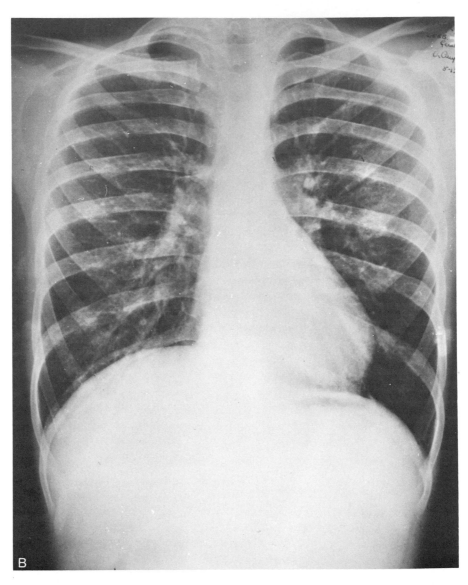

B

in 20.5% of the cases. A thymic shadow was observed in 1, and dilatation of the right pulmonary artery and increased pulmonary vascularity on the right as compared to the left in 1 (Fig. 15.8). A prominent main pulmonary arterial segment was seen in 5 cases (Fig. 15.9). Cardiac configuration suggestive of pericardial effusion was observed in 1 case (Fig. 15.10).

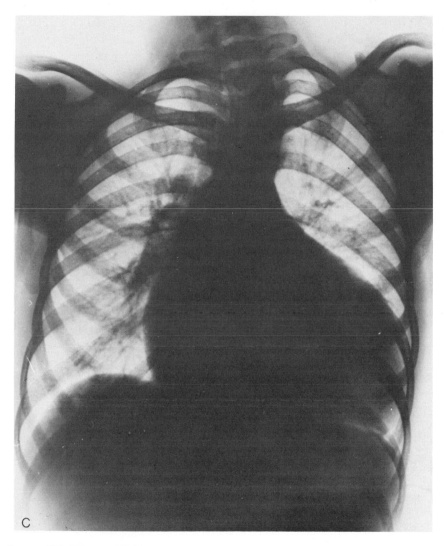

C

Group IV (Table 15.4)

The main radiological features of Group IV in the first day of life were a small heart, nonspecific cardiac configuration, a narrow vascular pedicle, and diminished pulmonary vascularity. However, in the age group 1–6 months a cardiothoracic ratio of more than 60% occurred in 33%, an egg-shaped heart in 33%, a narrow vascular pedicle in 57%, and increased pulmonary vascularity in 71% (Fig. 15.11). Only 21% in this age group had diminished pulmonary vascularity (Fig. 15.12). After the

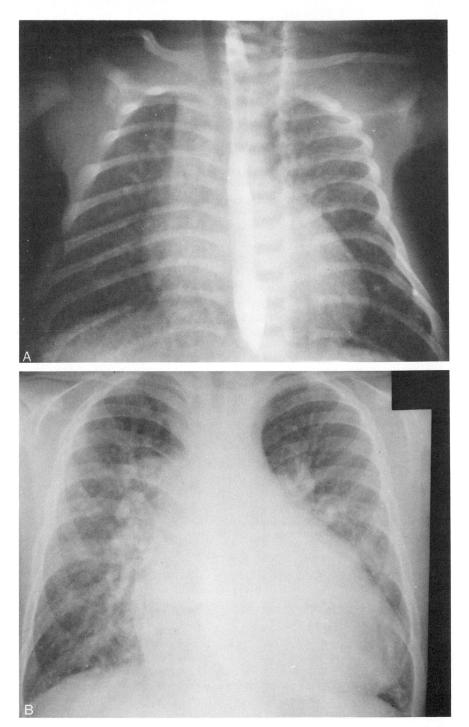

Fig. 15.13. Serial chest radiographs of a patient with transposition and ventricular septal defect demonstrating the development of pericardial effusion. (A) 2 weeks;

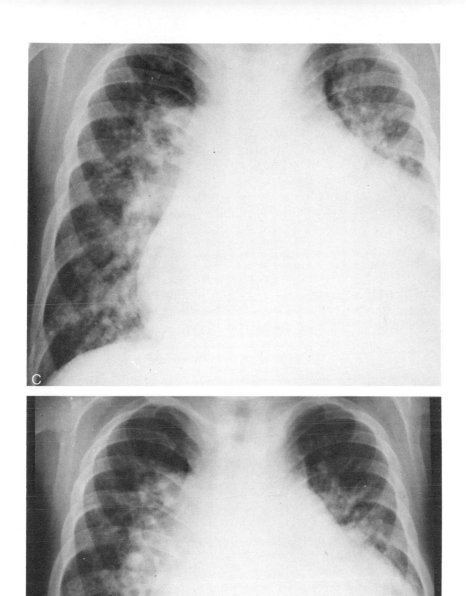

(B) 7 years; (C) at 11 years; (D) at 11½ years after drainage of the pericardial effusion.

age of 1 year, between 56 and 66% had a cardiothoracic ratio of less than 60% and a nonspecific cardiac configuration. The vascular pedicle was narrow and the pulmonary vascularity diminished in the majority (Fig. 15.13). A hump at the left cardiac border was seen in 14%. A thymic shadow was observed in 2, and dilatation of the right pulmonary artery and increased pulmonary vascularity on the right as compared to the left in 5. A long bulge at the left cardiac border similar to that seen with congenitally corrected transposition was seen in 1 case.

Discussion

The present findings confirm the conclusions of Keith *et al.* (1953), Gyllensworth and Lodin (1954), Carey and Elliott (1964), and Elliott and Schiebler (1968) that the heart may appear normal or nearly so for a very short time after birth. As pointed out by Gallaher, *et al.* (1966), cardiomegaly in patients with an intact ventricular septum was unusual during the first week of life. However, the present findings do not support their conclusion that the configuration of the heart was of little diagnostic significance in the age group 1–6 weeks since most patients in this age group in this study had an egg-shaped heart with a narrow vascular pedicle. Between the age of 1 and 6 months, cardiac enlargement, an egg-shaped heart, a narrow vascular pedicle, and increased pulmonary vascularity were seen in the majority of patients in Groups I and III. After this age the majority had nonspecific cardiac configuration and normal or broad vascular pedicle, but the pulmonary vascularity remained excessive in all patients in Group III and in most patients in Group I. Astley (1971) reviewed the plain film findings at the earliest examination in a series of infants in whom transposition was subsequently confirmed. The findings were typical in 39%, suggestive in 37%, and atypical of transposition in 24%. The proportion of atypical findings was very much dependent on the age; under one-fifth have typical findings in the first 2 days of life, but the proportion increased subsequently. Whereas Toole *et al.* (1960) reported that the pulmonary vascularity was increased in most cases with an intact ventricular septum Noonan *et al.* (1960) thought that these cases tend to have the vascular pattern either slightly diminished or top normal. The pulmonary vasculature was moderately to markedly increased in their cases with a ventricular septal defect and either pulmonary vascular obstruction or large pulmonary blood flow. According to Carey and Elliott (1964), patients less than 1 month of age with an intact ventricular septum and a narrow or closed ductus arteriosus showed no obvious increase in the pulmonary vasculature. Cases with an intact septum and a wide open ductus arteriosus usually showed an increase in pulmonary vascularity. After the age of 1 month the pulmonary vascularity was increased in all their patients regardless of the presence or absence of a patent ductus. Increased pulmonary vascularity was observed in 15 of their 17 patients with a ventricular septal defect. Significant cardiac enlargement and increased pulmonary vascularity occurred in a substantial number of patients in Group IV in this series. Similar findings in patients with pulmonary stenosis have been reported by Mehrizi *et al.* (1966). A long bulge at the left cardiac border similar to that seen with congenitally corrected transposition was seen in one patient in this series. This finding was described in 4 of the 14 cases reported by Astley and Parsons (1952) and in 9 of the 50 patients of Noonan *et al.* (1960).

References

Abrams, H. L., Kaplan, H. S., and Purdy, A. (1951). Diagnosis of complete transposition of the great vessels. *Radiology* **57**, 500.

Astley, R. (1971). The early plain film diagnosis of transposition of the great arteries. *Ann. Radiol.* **14**, 183.

Astley, R., and Parsons, S. (1952). Complete transposition of the great vessels. *Brit. Heart J.* **14**, 13.

Campbell, M. (1951). Visible pulsation in relation to blood flow and pressure in the pulmonary artery. *Brit. Heart J.* **13**, 438.

Campbell, M., and Suzman, S. (1951). Transposition of the aorta and pulmonary artery. *Circulation* **4**, 329.

Carey, L. S., and Elliott, L. P. (1964). Complete transposition of the great vessels. Roentgenographic findings. *Amer. J. Roentgenol.* **91**, 529.

Castellanos, A., Pereiras, P., and Garcia, O. (1950). Angiography: Anatomoroentgenological forms of the transposition of the great vessels. *Amer. J. Roentgenol.* **64**, 255.

Cooley, R. N., and Sloan, R. D. (1956). "Radiology of the Heart and Great Vessels." Williams & Wilkins, Baltimore, Maryland.

Eek, S. (1949). Roentgenological examination of morbus coeruleus. *In* "Morbus Coeruleus." (S. Mannheimer, ed.) . P. 58. Karger, Basel.

Elliott, L. P., and Schiebler, G. L. (1968). A roentgenolic-electrocardiographic approach to cyanotic forms of heart disease. *Pediat. Clin. N. Amer.* **18**, 1133.

Fanconi, G. (1932). Die Transposition der Grossen Gefässe. (Das charakteristische Rontgenbild). *Arch. Kinderheilk.* **95**, 202.

Gallaher, M. E., Fyler, D. C., and Lindesmith, G. G. (1966). Transposition with intact ventricular septum. Its diagnosis and management in the small infant. *Amer. J. Dis. Child.* **111**, 248.

Gyllensward, A., and Lodin, H. (1954). The value of selective angiocardiography in the diagnosis of complete transposition of the great vessels. *Acta Radiol.* **42**, 189.

Keith, J. D., Neill, C. A., Vlad, P., Rowe, R. D., and Chute, A. L. (1953). Transposition of the great vessels. *Circulation* **7**, 830.

Keith, J. D., Rowe, R. D., and Vlad, P. (1958). "Heart Disease in Infancy and Childhood," 1st Ed. MacMillan, New York.

Kerley, P. (1951). Cardio-vascular system. *In* "A Text Book of X-Ray Diagnosis" (S. C. Shanks and P. Kerley, ed.), 2nd Ed. P. 121.

Mehrizi, A., Rowe, R. D., Hutchins, G. M., and Folger, G. M., Jr. (1966). Transposition of the great vessels with pulmonary stenosis and ventricular septal defect. *Bull. Johns Hopkins. Hosp.* **119**, 200.

Noonan, A., Nadas, A. S., Rudolph, A. M., and Harris, G. B. C. (1960). Transposition of the great arteries. A correlation of clinical, physiologic and autopsy data. *N. Engl. J. Med.* **263**, 592.

Perloff, J. (1970). "Clinical Recognition of Congenital Heart Disease" P. 540. Saunders, Philadelphia, Pennsylvania.

Taussig, H. B. (1938). Complete transposition of the great vessels. Clinical and pathologic features. *Amer. Heart J.* **16**, 728.

Taussig, H. (1960). "Congenital Malformation of the Heart," 2nd Ed. The Commonwealth Fund, New York.

Toole, A. L., Glenn, W. W. L., Fisher, W. H., Whittemore, R., Ordway, N. K., and Vidone, R. A. (1960). Operative approach to transposition of the great vessels. *Surgery* **48**, 43.

Chapter 16

THE HEMODYNAMICS OF TRANSPOSITION

The hemodynamic findings in 215 cardiac catheterizations form the basis of this chapter. Excluded from this study are 10 cardiac catheterizations performed after the Mustard procedure. There were 91 studies in Group I, 14 in Group II, 73 in Group III, and 37 in Group IV (Table 16.1).

A ventricular septal defect was accepted as being present if this defect was demonstrated by angiocardiography or autopsy, or if the pulmonary artery was intubated from the right ventricle during cardiac catheterization. Pulmonary stenosis was diagnosed if there was a gradient of 40 mm Hg or more across the pulmonary valve or infundibulum of the left ventricle, or if left ventricular angiography demonstrated narrowing of the outflow tract of the left ventricle or pulmonary valve.

A left-to-right shunt was considered to be present if there was an increase of 5% or more in oxygen saturation at any level. A right-to-left shunt was considered to be demonstrated when the sample of blood from the left side of the heart or a systemic artery had an oxygen saturation of 5% or more, less than the pulmonary venous sample or less than 90% if the pulmonary venous sample was not obtained.

In calculating the pulmonary blood flow in previous publications, the author (Shaher, 1964; Shaher and Kidd, 1966) used the left ventricular blood sample instead of the pulmonary arterial blood sample in cases in which the pulmonary artery had not been entered. In the present series no attempt has been made to calculate the actual pulmonary, systemic, and effective pulmonary blood flows. There are a number of reasons for this: (1) the pulmonary artery has not been entered in a significant number of patients; (2) the oxygen consumption was not measured in any patient and it was elected not to assume one (Rudolph and Cayler, 1958) to avoid conclusions based on an assumed oxygen uptake; (3) as has been recently emphasized by Burchell (1966), calculation of the pulmonary

TABLE 16.1
DISTRIBUTION OF 215 CARDIAC CATHETERIZATIONS

Group	Studies not preceded by heart surgery	Follow-up studies on unoperated patients	Initial studies on operated patients	Follow-up studies after palliative surgery
Group I (91 Studies)	66	0	13	12
Group II (14 Studies)	8	1	0	5
Group III (73 Studies)	53	5	7	8
Group IV (37 Studies)	30	1	1	5
Total	157	7	21	30

blood flow in transposition could, on occasion, be difficult to estimate when the left ventricular and pulmonary artery saturations are extremely high and there is an unknown and almost indeterminable amount of admixture from the desaturated systemic circulation via the bronchial arteries; and (4) the different hemoglobin values obtained in patients with transposition renders interpretation of the blood flows difficult.

Mild sedation (Smith *et al.,* 1958) before cardiac catheterization was given to all patients except those in the first 2 months of life. Depending on the age of the patient at the time of cardiac catheterization each group was divided into 3 subgroups as follows: 0–2 weeks, 2 weeks to 1 year, and above 1 year.

The Pulmonary, Systemic, and Effective Pulmonary Blood Flows (Fig. 16.1)

In complete transposition of the great arteries the aorta arises from the right ventricle and the pulmonary artery arises from the left ventricle. Two blood circuits exist: the pulmonary and systemic. In the systemic circuit, mixed venous blood returns to the right atrium and ventricle, and through the aorta most of it is redistributed to the body. In the pulmonary circuit pulmonary venous blood returns to the left atrium and ventricle, and through the pulmonary artery, most of it is recirculated to the lungs. Communications between the pulmonary and systemic circuits occur in all patients and take the form of a patent foramen ovale, atrial septal defect, ventricular septal defect, or patent ductus arteriosus. Through

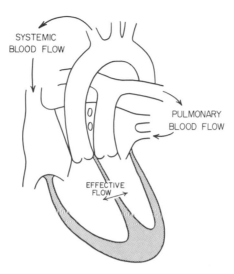

Fig. 16.1. Diagrammatic illustration of the pulmonary, systemic, and effective blood flows in transposition.

these communications oxygenated blood from the lungs reaches the systemic circuit and deoxygenated blood from the body reaches the lungs. In transposition of the great arteries the systemic blood is derived from two sources. The major portion of the systemic blood flow is composed of mixed venous blood that has been recirculated to the aorta. A limited amount of blood reaching the aorta is highly saturated pulmonary venous blood that has been shunted from the lungs through the associated defect. Similarly the pulmonary blood flow is derived from two sources. The major portion of this blood flow is composed of pulmonary venous return that has been recirculated to the lungs through the pulmonary artery. A limited amount of blood reaching the pulmonary artery is systemic venous blood that has been shunted from the systemic circuit through the associated defects. Because of the separate nature of these two circuits, any shunt which occurs between them has to be bidirectional and equal in both directions (Shaher, 1964). Oxygenation of the blood in the systemic circuit is achieved by exchanging a small part of blood in this circuit with an equal volume of pulmonary venous blood from the pulmonary circuit through the associated defects. This shunt is the effective pulmonary blood flow since it is the volume of mixed venous blood which, after returning to the right atrium, eventually reaches the pulmonary capillaries (Campbell *et al.*, 1949). On the other hand, the actual pulmonary and systemic blood flows, are the volume of blood flowing through the pulmonary artery and aorta per minute, respectively. The following equations, which utilize Fick's principle, could be used for calculation of the pulmonary, systemic, and effective blood flows.

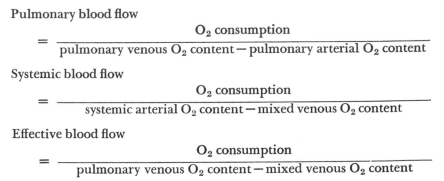

Pulmonary blood flow
$$= \frac{O_2 \text{ consumption}}{\text{pulmonary venous } O_2 \text{ content} - \text{pulmonary arterial } O_2 \text{ content}}$$

Systemic blood flow
$$= \frac{O_2 \text{ consumption}}{\text{systemic arterial } O_2 \text{ content} - \text{mixed venous } O_2 \text{ content}}$$

Effective blood flow
$$= \frac{O_2 \text{ consumption}}{\text{pulmonary venous } O_2 \text{ content} - \text{mixed venous } O_2 \text{ content}}$$

Since the only way oxygenated blood from the lung reaches the systemic circuit is through the associated defects, the systemic arterial oxygen content is directly proportional to the effective pulmonary blood flow (Shaher, 1964). On the other hand, actual measurement of the pulmonary, systemic, and effective blood flows will be inversely proportional to the hemoglobin content of the blood. In a recent publication, Mair et al. (1971) measured the effective pulmonary blood flow and the arterial oxygen saturation in polycythemic and anemic patients with transposition. In the group with anemia the arterial oxygen saturation was lower and effective pulmonary blood flow higher than in the group with polycythemia. Based on this finding the authors challenged the concept that the systemic arterial oxygen saturation is directly proportional to the effective pulmonary blood flow. Needless to say, their conclusion is unjustified since they have only demonstrated that the effective pulmonary blood flow of a group of hypoxic and anemic patients with transposition is higher than the effective pulmonary blood flow of another group of patients with transposition with less hypoxia but with a higher hemoglobin content. Since measurement of the blood flow by the Fick's principle utilizes the hemoglobin content and oxygen capacity and since the blood flow is inversely proportional to the hemoglobin content the conclusions of Mair and associates seem to be unnecessarily artefactual.

Catheterization of the Pulmonary Artery;
The Pulmonary and Bronchial Blood Flows

Until fairly recently it was believed that cardiac catheterization contributes little to the diagnosis of complete transposition of the great arteries (Campbell et al., 1949; Blalock and Hanlon, 1950; Abrams et al.,

1951; Lillehei and Varco, 1953; Keith *et al.*, 1958; Helwig, 1966). With the advent of successful surgical correction of transposition, it has become increasingly obvious that more information is needed to understand its hemodynamics and the hemodynamic effects of the associated lesions. Thus measurement of pulmonary arterial pressure will allow assessment of the severity of pulmonary stenosis if the left ventricular pressure is also known. Morever, since 1966 when Ferencz emphasized the high incidence of pulmonary vascular disease in transposition of the great arteries, assessment of the pulmonary and systemic blood flows and resistances has become the most important single factor in the selection of patients without left ventricular outflow obstruction for complete surgical correction. The intubation of the aorta from the right ventricle is fairly easy to do in transposition. However, since the pulmonary artery arises from the left ventricle, this vessel is less likely to be intubated, particularly in patients with an intact ventricular septum. Stimulated by the need to accurately measure the pulmonary blood flow, Carr and Wells (1966) used a flow-guided cardiac catheter to intubate the pulmonary artery. They used this technique successfully on twenty occasions in 20 children with transposition. Rahimtoola *et al.* (1966) reported 23 patients in whom pulmonary arterial pressure and oxygen saturation were obtained by the percutaneous suprasternal puncture technique. Complications included systemic hypertension in 1, and widening of the mediastinum in 3 patients. However, this method requires a general anesthetic, the use of which may not be desirable particularly if measurement of blood flows and resistances is the main object of the study. With the use of a "floppy wire" and "J wire," Celermajer *et al.* (1970) were able to catheterize the pulmonary artery in 7 of their 9 patients with transposition. The authors emphasized the safety of the method and that it can be used during the first year of life. A similar technique to catheterize the pulmonary artery utilizing the Lehman catheter, Formocath, and a guide wire was used by Pickering *et al.* (1972). Kelly *et al.* (1971), Black (1972), and Stanger *et al.* (1972) used a double-lumen floatation catheter (Swan *et al.* 1970) to enter the pulmonary artery in patients with transposition. The balloon catheter was guided into the left atrium and ventricle through an atrial septal defect. It required minor manipulation in the left ventricle before the pulmonary artery could be entered. In cases with transposition and ventricular septal defect in whom prograde venous catheterization of the pulmonary artery is unsuccessful, Mullins *et al.* (1972) recommend retrograde femoral arterial catheterization by the precutaneous sheath technique as a safe and effective method of entering this vessel. Parsons *et al.* (1971) indicated that until they obtained a Muller ASIC catheter, the pulmonary artery was seldom entered.

When a blood sample is obtained from the pulmonary artery and vein,

TABLE 16.2

SUMMARY OF HEMODYNAMIC FINDINGS IN 157 UNOPERATED PATIENTS [a]

Age	LV/RV pressure ratio				Mean atrial pressure relationship			Atrial shunt		Ventricular shunt	
	Less than 50%	50-75%	75-100%	More than 100%	Higher RA	Higher LA	Equal	RA to LA	LA to RA	RV to LV	LV to RV
Group I (66 Patients)											
0-2 w (41 Patients)	7/22	9/22	6/22	—	—	13/26	13/26	6/15	36/38	—	—
2 w-1 y (18 Patients)	1/8	5/8	2/8	—	1/12	6/12	5/12	2/8	12/13	—	—
Above 1 y (7 Patients)	6/7	1/7	—	—	—	1/7	6/7	4/5	5/5	—	—
Group II (8 Patients)											
0-2 w (3 Patients)	—	—	1/1	—	—	—	1/1	1/2	2/2	—	—
2 w-1 y (2 Patients)	—	—	—	2/2	—	—	1/1	2/2	—	—	—
Above 1 y (3 Patients)	2/3	1/3	—	—	—	—	2/2	2/2	1/2	—	—
Group III (53 Patients)											
0-2 w (12 Patients)	2/7	1/7	2/7	2/7	—	2/6	4/6	1/5	8/11	2/4	9/12
2 w-1 y (32 Patients)	1/26	—	24/26	1/26	—	11/16	5/16	1/17	15/31	2/14	22/30
Above 1 y (9 Patients)	1/6	—	3/6	2/6	—	—	4/4	3/3	1/8	2/3	8/8
Group IV (30 Patients)											
0-2 w (2 Patients)	—	—	—	—	—	—	—	2/2	—	—	1/2
2 w-1 y (13 Patients)	—	—	10/10	—	1/7	2/7	4/7	1/8	3/11	3/7	10/13
Above 1 y (15 Patients)	—	—	12/12	—	—	—	11/11	9/11	4/12	3/10	7/13

[a] LV, left ventricle; RV, right ventricle; RA, right atrium; LA, left atrium; w, weeks; y, year.

the pulmonary blood flow could be calculated using the Fick's principle. However, as pointed out earlier, calculation of the pulmonary blood flow in transposition could, on occasion, be difficult to estimate when the left ventricular and pulmonary artery saturations are extremely high and there is an unknown and almost indeterminable amount of admixture from the desaturated systemic circulation via the bronchial arteries. It is likely that in the future the use of ventricular volume measurements (Graham *et al.*, 1971), thermodilution (Tynan 1972a) and radioactive isotopes (Hurley *et al.*, 1970) will shed more light on the problem of measurement of the pulmonary blood flow in transposition.

Pressures, Shunts, and Flows

The following observations on the hemodynamics are based on the results of cardiac catheterization of 157 patients. None has had heart surgery or balloon atrial septostomy before cardiac catherization. There were 66 patients in Group I, 8 in Group II, 53 in Group III, and 30 in Group IV. Table 16.2 summarizes the hemodynamic data in the four groups. Since complete hemodynamic details were not available in several studies, percentages refer to the number of patients in whom particular information was available.

GROUP I (66 PATIENTS; TABLES 16.2 AND 16.3)

The pulmonary artery was not entered in any patient in Group I. There were 41 patients in the age group 0–2 weeks. During the first 2 weeks of life 68% (15/22) had a left ventricular pressure 50% or more of right ventricular pressure. One-half of the patients had a higher mean left than right atrial pressure (13/26) while the remaining one-half had equal mean atrial pressures (13/26). Representative samples from the cavae and atria were obtained in 38. Of these 38 patients, no blood shunting at the atrial level was observed in 2 while the remaining 36 showed a left-to-right shunt at the atrial level. Of these 36, a left ventricular sample was available in 15. Of these 15, 6 had an additional right-to-left interatrial shunt.

There were 18 patients in the age group 2 weeks to 1 year. Of the 8 patients in whom the pressures in the two ventricles were obtained, the pressure in the left ventricle was at systemic levels in 2, between 50 and 70% of right ventricular pressure in 5, and less than 50% of right ventricular pressure in 1. Of the 12 patients, in whom both atrial pressures were obtained, 6 had higher mean left than right, 1 higher mean right

TABLE 16.3

HEMODYNAMIC DATA ON UNOPERATED PATIENTS [a,b]

Patient no.	Age [a]	Hb	O₂ cap.	Blood O₂ saturation %								Pressures						PVD Grades 1-4 and age [c]
				SVC	RA	RV	Ao	PV	LA	LV	PA	RA	LA	RV	Ao	LV	PA	
1	1 d	18.5	24.8	20	20	36	22	97	96	97	—	8	12	65/10	60/45	50/15	—	—
2	1 d	15.6	21.2	21	40	37	—	98	98	—	—	7	12	40/10	40/25	—	—	—
3	1 d	—	—	34	26	52	44	99	96	—	—	2	8	60/10	60/40	40/0	—	—
4	1 d	15.5	20.7	18	39	32	30	95	92	92	—	6	6	70/0	80/55	40/0	—	—
5	2 d	14.6	18.7	15 IVC	34	39	—	—	79	—	—	8	8	60/0	—	—	—	1 (4 d)
6	2 d	—	—	12	16	26	20	100	100	93	—	4	10	56/10	52/35	32/2	—	1 (4 d)
7	2 d	12.6	16.6	40	42	31	34	96	—	94	—	6	8	47/10	50/36	35/8	—	—
8	2 d	20	26.8	37	42	43	48	99	99	99	—	0	3	60/0	63/40	52/0	—	—
9	2 d	17.4	23.5	26	29	44	45	98	—	—	—	5	—	64/8	68/53	—	—	N (6 d)
10	2 d	17.8	23.8	24	47	43	42	95	89	83	—	6	8	67/0	65/35	45/0	—	—
11	2 d	16.0	21.7	23	33	37	37	—	96	97	—	0	0	64/5	65/44	65/5	—	—
12	2 d	11.1	14.9	20	43	40	59	95	94	—	—	12	14	82/13	93/40	—	—	—
13	3 d	17.9	24.0	33	42	52	53	92	—	—	—	0	2	65/0	67/47	33/2	—	—
14	3 d	16.8	22.5	22	27	23	37	98	—	90	—	1	—	75/2	75/45	40/5	—	—
15	3 d	18.6	25	30	38	20	34	98	98	—	—	0	8	47/5	47/30	—	—	—
16	3 d	16.7	22.3	10	21	27	21	100	—	—	—	5	8	71/6	71/55	29/0	—	—
17	3 d	15.6	20.9	15	45	32	20	—	—	—	—	0	—	94/5	85/50	—	—	—
18	3 d	18.5	25	20	20	29	33	99	100	97	—	2	—	80/0	78/53	37/0	—	1 (3 d)
19	4 d	18.6	25	28	40	46	40	—	97	96	—	10	15	60/20	60/40	40/12	—	—
20	4 d	—	—	37	—	40	42	—	86	91	—	4	4	65/4	65/35	55/2	—	1 (2 w)
21	5 d	—	—	—	—	64	—	—	—	—	—	—	—	70/10	—	45/10	—	1 (6 d)
22	5 d	—	—	53	41	—	—	100	100	—	—	—	—	70/5	—	—	—	1 (9 d)
23	5 d	13.0	17.6	26 IVC	41	33	33	100	85	91	—	4	—	74/10	75/43	—	—	—
24	5 d	22.2	30.0	24 IVC	34	56	54	99	—	93	—	5	8	80/5	85/60	25/4	—	—
25	6 d	15.3	20.6	27	33	31	34	—	100	—	—	3	3	65/0	67/50	22/0	—	1 (8 d)
26	6 d	—	—	60	70	74	64	—	98	—	—	3	6	50/6	48/30	—	—	1 (2 w)
27	1 w	18.2	24.4	39	40	60	54	—	81	83	—	5	6	95/3	95/68	74/5	—	—

No.	Age																	
28	1 w	—	—	—	—	52	—	—	90	—	—	—	—	65/0	65/40	35/0	—	1 (3 w)
29	1 w	16.8	21.8	17 IVC	31	22	30	—	—	—	—	6	—	99/7	—	45/74	—	—
30	8 d	21	28	20	27	30	25	100	92	96	—	6	—	96/5	93/67	40/3	—	—
31	8 d	—	—	13	38	20	21	98	—	—	—	0	2	90/7	90/60	—	—	—
32	8 d	—	—	20	27	30	25	100	97	—	—	6	—	96/5	93/57	20/0	—	—
33	9 d	—	—	25	25	37	34	98	—	—	—	9	20 PV	92/9	86/15	—	—	N (17 d)
34	10 d	21.7	29.6	34	54	62	68	—	—	—	—	2	—	52/5	50/4	—	—	—
35	10 d	16.0	21.2	35	41	54	52	—	100	—	—	5	—	100/0	90/55	—	—	1 (2 y)
36	10 d	14.3	19.3	24	31	30	34	98	—	—	—	4	5	77/9	78/43	—	—	1 (12 d)
37	10 d	—	—	31	35	33	39	100	100	—	—	2	12	82/5	80/60	—	—	—
38	11 d	—	—	48 IVC	71	70	75	—	—	—	—	5	4	67/9	66/34	40/10	—	1 (2 m)
39	11 d	—	—	60 IVC	68	57	50	—	—	97	—	4	4	75/0	68/38	—	—	—
40	12 d	—	—	—	51	51	—	98	97	—	—	3	—	50/10	—	40/20	—	1 (24 d)
41	12 d	—	—	31	45	47	—	—	—	—	—	2	—	85/5	—	—	—	1 (14 d)
42	16 d	—	—	—	44	35	—	—	100	—	—	7	7	62/10	—	—	—	2 (24 d)
43	3 w	12.4	16.7	30	56	62	56	98	97	—	—	3½	8	—	75/41	—	—	1 (25 d)
44	3 w	—	—	46	70	67	—	—	—	—	—	10	—	100/6	—	50/15	—	—
45	3 w	19.5	26.2	28 IVC	38	36	51	—	100	98	—	10	10	85/10	75/35	—	—	2 (1 m)
46	3 w	—	—	41 IVC	47	42	39	96	88	95	—	—	30	75/8	60/40	—	—	—
47	1 m	—	33.6	39	39	39	39	—	—	—	—	—	—	60/0	—	—	—	1 (1 m)
48	1 m	25	—	31	56	48	46	100	—	—	—	—	—	—	—	90/0	—	—
49	5 w	—	—	—	12	57	34	—	93	—	—	5	10	110/0	85/60	—	—	1 (2½ m)
50	5 w	15	20.2	15	30	24	—	100	—	—	—	—	—	90/0	—	—	—	—
51	6 w	18.8	25.3	10	—	43	46	—	100	—	—	5	—	72/0	—	35/5	—	—
52	6 w	—	—	—	—	—	—	—	—	—	—	5	11	55/5	—	70/0	—	—
53	2 m	12.5	16.8	42	65	62	61	—	—	—	—	4	4	75/0	75/40	—	—	—
54	3 m	—	—	47	60	59	59	—	—	84	—	0	9	70/0	—	45/12	—	—
55	4 m	—	—	—	—	55	—	84	—	—	—	6	—	85/15	80/50	55/0	—	4 (6½ m)
56	4 m	—	—	—	—	44	—	97	—	97	—	4	6	75/0	—	50/5	—	1 (17 m)
57	4½ m	17.6	23.7	32	51	50	50	99	97	99	—	6	3	70/10	65/40	40/6	—	—
58	5 m	12.1	16.4	50	51	51	65	89	88	88	—	8	8	100/10	100/70	—	—	—

TABLE 16.3 (continued)

Patient No.	Age[a]	Hb	O₂ Cap.	Blood O₂ saturation %								Pressures						PVD Grades 1–4 and age[a]
				SVC	RA	RV	Ao	PV	LA	LV	PA	RA	LA	RV	Ao	LV	PA	
59	5 m	19.5	26.4	27	32	58	60	100	100	—	—	3	5	97/0	97/63	—	—	—
60	13 m	14.0	18.9	57	77	79	79	100	95	98	—	3	4	80/7	95/53	35/6	—	—
61	13 m	15.5	20.7	45	55	56	58	98	85	85	—	4	4	80/5	80/60	35/6	—	(2 y, 4 m)
62	4 y 4 m	—	—	—	34	48	48	—	—	94	—	6	4	80/0	80/50	35/0	—	—
63	4 y 6 m	13.9	18.8	13	23	29	25	98	100	—	—	3	3	95/7	91/53	—	—	3 (4½ y)
64	4 y 9 m	—	—	43	64	71	—	—	93	87	—	3	2	80/0	—	28/0	—	—
65	9 y	—	—	51	65	68	73	—	—	86	—	2	5	95/0	—	35/0	—	—
66	16 y	—	—	56	72	70	70	—	94	81	—	2	2	82/2	80/52	50/1	—	—

[a] Group I, 66 patients.

[b] Ao, aorta; Cap., capacity; Hb, hemoglobin; IVC, inferior vena cava; LA, left atrium; LV, left ventricle; PA, pulmonary artery; PV, pulmonary vein; PVD, pulmonary vascular disease; RA, right atrium; RV, right ventricle; SVC, superior vena cava.

[c] d, days; m, months; w, weeks; y, years.

than left, and 5 had equal mean atrial pressures. A left-to-right atrial shunt was detected in 12 of 13 cases, and a right-to-left atrial shunt in 2 of 8 cases in whom these informations were available. There was no definite relationship between the direction of the blood shunt and atrial pressures.

There were 7 patients above the age of 1 year. All but 1 case had a left ventricular pressure less than 50% of right ventricular pressure. Equal or near equal mean atrial pressures with a bidirectional shunt at the atrial level was observed in 4 of the 5 in whom this measurement was available. In the remaining patient, only left-to-right shunt was discovered.

A study of blood samples obtained from the cavae, aorta, left ventricle, and pulmonary veins suggests that in the majority of these patients the pulmonary blood flow is higher than the systemic blood flow. Flow gradients across the outflow tract of the left ventricle in some patients with an intact ventricular septum have been described by Aberdeen and Carr (1968), Black (1972), and Tynan (1972a). The low mixed venous blood oxygen saturation found in almost all patients in this group, suggests that the effective pulmonary blood flow is markedly diminished. Some patients with a small effective pulmonary blood flow have excessive blood flows in the pulmonary and systemic circuits. Graham *et al.* (1971) studied left heart volumes and systolic output in transposition. The majority of patients who had an intact ventricular septum and were less than 6 months of age showed normal end-diastolic volumes and systolic output while patients more than 6 months of age had elevated volumes and outputs. The authors pointed out that this finding may be partially accounted for by a progressive decrease in pulmonary vascular resistance. In addition, alterations in total blood volume and dynamics of atrial shunting also may play roles in this increase in volume and output during the first year.

GROUP II (8 PATIENTS; TABLES 16.2 AND 16.4)

The number of patients in this group was too small to allow any definite conclusions to be made. The pulmonary artery was not entered in any case. Of the 6 patients in whom the left ventricle was catheterized, the ratio between left and right ventricular pressures was less than 50% in 2, 50–70% in 1, 75–100% in 1, and more than 100% in 2. The mean atrial pressures were equal or near equal in 4 patients in whom this information was available. Three had a left-to-right shunt and 5 had right-to-left atrial shunting. The systemic, pulmonary, and effective pulmonary arteriovenous oxygen differences in this group were not materially different from those in Group I.

TABLE 16.4
HEMODYNAMIC DATA ON UNOPERATED PATIENTS [a,b]

Patient no.	Age	Hb	O₂ cap.	Blood O₂ saturation %								Pressures						PVD Grades 1–4 and age
				SVC	RA	RV	Ao	PV	LA	LV	PA	RA	LA	RV	Ao	LV	PA	
67	9 d	22.4	30	30	42	42	42	—	89	—	—	8	6	60/5	70/40	—	—	—
68	10 d	14.7	20	27	50	60	69	96	94	96	—	—	—	63/10	52/48	52/12	S. 25/9	—
69	2 w	13.4	18	7	9	13	13	—	—	—	—	10	—	75/0	75/42	—	—	N (14 m)
70	5 w	—	—	40 IVC	42	—	40	100	87	87	—	—	4	91/0	—	97/0	—	—
71	2 m	—	—	16	20	18	18	—	86	79	—	9	9	110/10	105/65	120/10	—	3 (3 y)
72	1 y	12.9	17.4	32	30	58	34	97	96	92	—	4	4	105/5	105/68	48/5	—	—
73	1 y 2 m	—	—	—	—	—	—	—	—	—	—	—	—	—	83/55	51/4	—	N (3 y 4 m)
74	1 y 6 m	15.2	22	30 IVC	42	54	52	—	78	88	—	3	3	64/0	84/42	26/0	—	—

[a] Group II, 8 patients.
[b] All abbreviations same as indicated in Table 16.3. N, normal; S, surgery.

TABLE 16.5
Hemodynamic Data on Unoperated Patients [a,b]

Patient no.	Age	Hb	O_2 cap.	Blood O_2 saturation %								Pressures						PVD Grades 1–4 and age	Size of VSD at autopsy
				SVC	RA	RV	Ao	PV	LA	LV	PA	RA	LA	RV	Ao	LV	PA		
75	2 d	20.1	27	20	37	30	46	98	—	77	—	4	8	60/6	60/45	28/4	—	1 (8 d)	2 x 2 mm
76	4 d	20.1	27	37	41	66	58	—	99	98	—	2	1	70/0	70/50	50/0	—	—	Cl. Spon.
77	5 d	17.3	23	54	63	75	68	90	89	85	—	4	6	55/15	55/35	50/15	—	—	2 x 2 mm
78	5 d	14.6	19.6	24	37	60	71	—	—	—	—	15	—	75/15	70/40	—	—	—	—
79	7 d	19.3	26.1	25	34	58	66	—	—	—	—	3	—	79/1	70/49	—	—	—	—
80	8 d	—	—	52	80	80	—	—	—	—	87	—	—	70/10	—	75/10	40/20	3 (3½ m)	—
81	7 d	19.3	26.1	25	34	58	66	—	—	—	—	3	—	79/1	70/49	—	—	—	—
82	9 d	14.7	19.8	0	0	13	26	—	96.5	—	—	—	6	86/9	93/60	39/2	—	—	Cl. Spon.
83	10 d	—	—	12	20	20	20	—	—	—	—	9	—	70/0	69/38	—	—	N (2 w)	2 x 2 mm
84	12 d	16.2	21.8	40	42	76	85	100	96	91	—	3	8	88/5	90/70	85/4	—	2 (10 m)	15 x 10 mm; 6 x 3 mm
85	13 d	—	—	—	41	46	43	—	—	—	—	5	—	64/7	65/44	—	—	—	—
86	14 d	19.5	26.4	37	72	82	82	99	85	93	—	10	10	74/5	74/54	80/7	—	—	—
87	15 d	—	—	57	60	17	—	90	—	—	85	12	—	65/10	—	—	52/30	2 (2 m)	—
88	17 d	—	—	24	27	77	26	84	—	82	—	1	4	85/5	80/45	85/10	—	—	—
89	17 d	12.5	16.7	41	55	68	73	—	87	80	82	6	—	63/3	60/40	48/5	—	—	—
90	18 d	—	—	35	38	56	71	—	—	—	89	0	20	87/0	110/73	—	106/60	1 (8 m)	20 x 25 mm
91	3 w	—	—	40	28	74	50	94	99	99	—	4	6	70/0	60/40	60/20	60/40	—	—
92	22 d	12	16.1	56	68	47	76	—	93	94	82	3	—	85/3	85/60	85/5	—	N (1 m)	3 x 4 mm
93	23 d	—	—	31	37	—	49	—	—	—	89	—	—	78/0	80/45	—	—	N (1 m)	4 x 2 mm
94	24 d	10.5	14.2	39	45	77	72	—	93	95	—	7	7	—	—	—	—	—	—
95	1 m	13.6	18.4	33	63	68	72	—	97	96	89	6	12	100/6	108/55	100/6	99/42	1 (1 m)	10 x 5 mm
96	1 m	20.2	27.5	58	67	66	74	—	97	97	95	5	16	45/10	50/35	45/10	45/35	—	—
97	1 m	18.6	25.0	20	26	46	54	—	97	97	97	3	7	80/10	80/40	40/5	—	—	—
98	1 m 2 d	—	—	46 IVC	52	—	—	—	97	99	—	—	—	50/0	—	50/0	—	1 (5 m)	2 x 2 mm

TABLE 16.5 (continued)

Patient no.	Age	Hb	O_2 cap.	SVC	RA	RV	Ao	PV	LA	LV	PA	RA	LA	RV	Ao	LV	PA	PVD Grades 1–4 and age	Size of VSD at autopsy
				Blood O_2 saturation %								Pressures							
99	2 m	10.7	14.4	40	43	47	59	96	96	—	—	2	4	72/6	80/34	—	—	—	—
100	1 m 3 w	—	—	30	40	42	—	—	92	83	—	2	—	70/0	—	70/0	52/28	2 (2 m)	—
101	2 m	15.3	20.6	42	65	58	79	—	90	91	—	12	14	80/10	66/55	80/10	—	—	—
102	2 m 2 w	12.1	16.1	27	30	52	55	—	—	—	72	7	—	80/4	75/60	80/4	65/30	—	—
103	2 m	—	—	58 IVC	69	82	81	—	—	—	—	6	—	65/0	65/25	—	—	—	8 x 8 mm
104	2 m	13.1	17.6	46	70	69	66	—	—	91	—	—	—	80/10	—	—	—	3 (2 y 1 m)	10 x 5 mm
105	2 m	13.1	17.6	34	64	68	57	—	—	87	—	4	—	75/5	75/40	75/5	—	—	2 x 2 mm
106	2½ m	—	—	30	40	65	77	—	98	96	—	1	6.5	80/0	75/35	76/5	—	4 (2 y)	—
107	2½ m	12.5	16.8	54	47	75	76	96	—	94	—	3	—	95/9	95/60	95/9	—	—	—
108	3 m	10.1	13.5	45	73	70	67	—	—	—	83	6	8	85/0	75/50	—	75/40	3 (4 y 3 m)	10 x 10 mm
109	4 m	—	—	48	49	70	60	—	97	96	—	2	—	69/0	72/46	71/0	—	3 (2 y)	6 x 7 mm
110	4 m	—	—	—	41	55	60	—	—	88	—	6	—	90/6	85/53	95/0	—	1 (4½ m)	6 x 6 mm
111	5 m	—	—	41	41	54	72	—	—	80/4	—	6	8	80/6	—	80/4	—	1 (5 m)	10 x 5 mm
112	5½ m	—	—	41	69	77	50	95	91	93	86	5	7	95/5	105/55	90/0	85/42	—	—
113	6 m	20.9	28.4	34	33	45	72	—	93	90	—	4	10	80/0	80/50	80/0	—	—	—
114	6 m	15.8	21.2	52	52	76	—	—	—	—	90	2	—	80/5	76/47	—	63/31	—	—
115	6 m	—	—	50	50	—	A. 73 / D. 86	—	98	—	88	5	8.5	86/5	99/40	—	84/42	—	—
116	6 m	—	—	20	18	55	73	—	—	90	79	3	—	70/5	—	—	70/35	2 (7 m)	6 x 10 mm
117	7 m	11.7	15.8	47	46	60	66	—	92	—	91	3	8	85/0	100/53	100/0	78/44	B. 3 (2½ y)	—
118	9 m	—	—	48	43	42	74	—	—	—	—	6	—	90/10	85/60	—	—	—	—
119	1 y 3 m	—	—	45	47	70	69	—	—	—	—	—	—	70/5	70/50	—	—	—	—
120	2 y 5 m	—	—	60	61	72	62	98	—	90	—	6	—	63/2	60/39	—	—	—	—
121	3 y 1 m	17.8	26.8	45	47	64	73	—	94	90	92	3	5	95/0	95/65	95/0	—	—	—
122	4 y	24.5	33	60	66	76	73	—	—	92	—	2	—	100/5	98/80	82/0	15/5	—	—
123	4 y 7 m	17.5	23.7	28	29	47	44	—	—	92	—	1	—	106/0	106/66	—	—	B. 3 (5 y)	—

124	4 y 9 m	—	—	—	62	—	—	—	—	—	7	—	130/17	134/68	107/9	108/66	B. 3 (5 y)	—
125[d]	4 y 10 m	—	58	72	A.72 and D.78	—	—	95	92	92	9	11	90/7	90/65	110/5	—	—	—
126	7 y 3 m	19.3	25.9	45	47	77	—	—	92	82	10	8	110/10	—	105/14	—	—	—
127	11 y	—	—	59	54	51	62	—	92	79	6	8	110/0	110/60	120/0	—	3 (11 y)	15 x 15 mm

[a] Group III, 53 patients.
[b] VSD, ventricular septal defect; Cl. Spon., closed spontaneously. All other abbreviations as in Table 16.3.
[c] Patient 115 has complete interruption of aortic arch.
[d] A, ascending; D, descending; B, biopsy.

GROUP III (53 PATIENTS; TABLES 16.2 AND 16.5)

The pulmonary artery was catheterized in 16 patients in this group. There were 12 patients in the age group 0–2 weeks. Of the 7 in whom the ratio between right and left ventricular pressures was obtained, this ratio was 75% or more in 4 (Table 16.2). The size of the ventricular septal defect is seen in Table 16.5. Of the 6 in whom right and left atrial pressures were obtained, 4 had equal mean pressures and 2 had higher left than right. A left-to-right shunt at atrial and ventricular levels were observed in the majority. Right-to-left shunt occurred at the atrial level in 20% and at ventricular level in 50%.

There were 32 patients in the age group 2 weeks to 1 year. Of the 26 in whom the two ventricular pressures were recorded, all but 1 had a systemic pressure in the left ventricle. The size of the ventricular septal defect is shown in Table 16.5. It is note worthy that in 2 cases with systemic pressure in left ventricle this defect measured 2×2 mm². The majority had a higher left than right atrial pressure. A left-to-right atrial shunting was observed in 15 of the 31 in whom this information could be obtained. A step-up in the oxygen saturation at right ventricular level with or without a left-to-right shunt at the atrial level, was noted in 22 patients. Of the 14 patients in whom blood samples were obtained from both ventricles, a right-to-left ventricular shunt was demonstrated in 2.

There were 9 patients above the age of 1 year. Of the 6 in whom the pressure in both ventricles was obtained, the left ventricular pressure was equal or higher than systemic levels in 5. In the remaining patient, the left ventricular angiogram showed a small ventricular septal defect, and the left ventricular–right ventricular pressure ratio was less than 50%. The mean atrial pressures were essentially equal. A right-to-left atrial shunt was detected in 3 cases in whom sufficient data was available. A left-to-right shunt was detected at the atrial level in 1, and at ventricular level in 8. Of the 3 in whom left atrial and ventricular blood samples were obtained, 2 showed a right-to-left ventricular shunting.

A study of the arteriovenous oxygen saturation difference in the two circuits suggests that during the first 2 or 3 years of life the pulmonary blood flow exceeds the systemic blood flow in the majority. After this age, some patients had diminished pulmonary and increased systemic blood flows. Mixed venous blood samples suggest that the effective pulmonary blood flow in this group is slightly larger than the effective pulmonary blood flow in the group with an intact ventricular septum. A flow gradient of 15 to 35 mm Hg between the left ventricle and pulmonary artery was recorded in 6 of the 10 patients in whom these pressures were obtained. Graham *et al.* (1971) pointed out that their patients with transposition and ventricular septal defect without pulmonary stenosis had increased left ventricular volumes and systolic outputs with the average values significantly greater than for the group with an intact ventricular septum.

GROUP IV (30 PATIENTS; TABLES 16.2 AND 16.6)

The pulmonary artery was catheterized in 8 patients. There were 2 patients in the age group 0–2 weeks. Both had a left-to-right atrial shunting.

Thirteen patients were in the age group 2 weeks–1 year. Systemic pressure in the left ventricle was noted in all. Of the 7 in whom right and left atrial pressures were obtained, 4 had equal pressures, 2 had higher left than right, and 1 had higher right than left. Of the 11 patients in whom sufficient data were available, 3 had a left-to-right atrial shunt. Of the 8 in whom a left atrial blood sample was obtained, a right-to-left atrial shunt was present in 1. Additional right-to-left ventricular shunting was observed in 3, and left-to-right ventricular shunting in 10.

Fifteen patients were above the age of 1 year. The pressure in the left ventricle was at systemic levels where this information was available. The mean atrial pressures were equal in all. Nine of 11 cases had a right-to-left, and 4 of 12 had a left-to-right atrial shunting. A left-to-right ventricular shunt was observed in 7 of 13 cases and a right-to-left shunt at the same level in 3 of 10.

A gradient of 48 mm Hg or more between the pulmonary artery and left ventricle was noted in 8 patients in whom the pulmonary artery was entered at cardiac catheterization. Blood samples from this vessel suggest that the pulmonary blood flow in this group is lower than the pulmonary blood flow of the group with a ventricular septal defect without pulmonary stenosis. Mixed venous blood samples also suggest that the effective pulmonary blood is lower in this group than Group III. Left heart volumes and systolic output performed by Graham *et al.* (1971) suggest that these measurements have normal values in patients with a ventricular septal defect and pulmonary stenosis.

Relationship between Patency of the Ductus Arteriosus and Left Ventricular Pressure

The relationship between patency of the ductus arteriosus and left ventricular pressure was studied in 56 cases with an intact ventricular sep-

TABLE 16.6

Hemodynamic Data on Unoperated Patients [a,b]

Patient no.	Age	Hb	O₂ cap.	Blood O₂ saturation %								Pressures						PVD Grades 1–4 and age	Size of VSD at autopsy
				SVC	RA	RV	Ao	PV	LA	LV	PA	RA	LA	RV	Ao	LV	PA		
128	6 d	—	—	46	62	61	—	—	93	—	82	4	4	80/3	—	—	40/10	—	—
129	11 d	16.6	22.3	16 IVC	21	27	25	—	—	—	—	5	5	98/8	98/54	—	—	N (1 m)	5 x 5 mm
130	5 w	12.8	17.1	56	73	73	77	—	—	—	—	5	—	79/0	79/49	—	—	—	—
131	2 m	15.4	20.6	20	22	—	59	100	100	—	—	3	6	72/2	76/45	72/2	—	—	—
132	2 m	15.3	20.6	51	56	49	60	96	95	87	90	6	10	60/10	60/40	60/10	12/10	—	—
133	2 m	14	18.6	15	22	39	48	—	100	97	—	4	6	70/8	65/40	70/8	—	—	—
134	2 m	15	20.2	—	32	35	33	—	—	—	—	—	—	73/2	—	79/5	—	—	—
135	4 m	12.4	16.7	38	44	51	—	96	97	86	—	6	3	52/2	—	54/4	—	1 (2 y)	9 x 7 mm
136	4½ m	11.9	15.5	46	42	65	64	—	—	85	—	3	—	80/0	70/45	80/0	—	—	—
137	5 m	—	—	36	37	—	44	—	98	97	87	7	—	88/9	107/63	90/12	25/15	—	—
138	6 m	—	—	42	45	50	59	—	94	90	63	3	4	80/0	75/45	75/15	8/3	—	—
139	8 m	12.4	16.5	31	31	53	42	97	85	88	78	4	4	80/0	75/45	80/8	30/12	—	—
140	1 y 2 m	13.9	18.8	47	47	47	68	98	98	93	—	5	7	100/0	100/60	100/0	—	—	—
141	1 y 4 m	—	—	—	26	37	42	—	—	—	—	8	—	100/0	100/65	—	—	—	—
142	1 y 11 m	18.1	24.2	39 IVC	35	49	45	—	—	—	—	—	—	—	45/60	—	—	4 (4 y)	12 x 3 mm
143	2 y	—	—	56	60	65	68	98	90	86	—	9	—	93/0	95/55	98/5	—	—	—
144	2 y	16.8	22.5	57 IVC	52	70	64	97	98	—	—	7	5	99/5	99/58	98/5	—	—	—
145	2 y 4 m	13.4	18.0	37	36	43	40	97	98	—	—	—	8	90/8	93/50	—	—	—	—
146	3 y 1 m	—	—	—	30	35	39	—	—	—	—	3	3	90/5	90/6	80/0	—	Thrombi	16 x 10 mm
147	3 y 2 m	19.3	26	49	49	49	61	—	68	72	—	8	8	90/0	95/55	90/0	—	—	—
148	3 y 9 m	9.9	13.3	35	35	42	38	97	88	65	—	13	13	95/10	95/70	95/10	—	2 (3 y 10 m)	15 x 4 mm
149	3 y 9 m	21.3	28.7	51	51	59	64	99	77	85	—	7	7	92/2	95/70	100/0	—	Thrombi	10 x 10 mm
150	5 y 2 m	19.0	25.4	50 IVC	45	54	54	98	87	84	—	3	3	97/5	88/52	102/8	—	—	—

151	6 y 1 m	15.9	22	50	65	62	65	95	92	86	—	4	6	90/0	90/56	90/0	—	—	—
152	6 y 11 m	—	—	57	65	66	81	97	90	91	—	5	5	85/5	95/55	85/5	—	—	—
153	7 y 3 m	14.2	19.0	59	68	77	78	94	89	89	84	4	2	118/2	102/65	120/0	10/1	—	—
154	8 y	—	—	70	85	83	85	99	99	98	90	5	5	110/0	105/70	110/0	18/10	—	—
155	9 y 9 m	—	—	—	—	44	40	—	—	—	—	3	—	105/0	—	105/75	—	—	3 (11 y)
156	9 y 7 m	19.4	26.2	44	45	57	66	95	70	77	77	4	4	85/5	85/55	85/5	12/5	—	—
157 [c]	11 y 4 m	—	87.5	90	84	84	—	—	—	—	—	—	105/10	110/70	—	—	—	2 (11 y)

[a] Group IV, 30 patients.

[b] All abbreviations same as in Table 16.3 and Table 16.5

[c] Patient 157 with total anomalous pulmonary drainage into left superior vena cava.

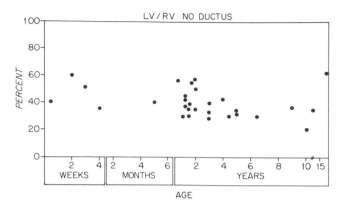

Fig. 16.2. Ratio between left and right ventricular pressures in 29 patients with intact ventricular septum and no ductus arteriosus.

tum. All cases in which there was evidence of obstruction to left ventricular outflow by angiography or postmortem examination were eliminated. In each case, the state of the ductus arteriosus was determined by angiocardiography or autopsy examination. Of the 56 cases, the ductus was patent in 27 and closed in 29. The relationship between right and left ventricular pressures in these two groups is illustrated in Fig. 16.2 and 16.3.

TWENTY-SEVEN CASES WITH A PATENT DUCTUS

In 7 of these cases (26%) left ventricular pressures were 80% or more of the systemic pressure, in 8 (29.5%) they were between 60 and 80%, in 10 (37%) between 40 and 60%, and in 2 (7.5%) less than 40% of the systemic pressure. None of these children was more than 5 months of age.

TWENTY-NINE CASES WITH A CLOSED DUCTUS

No patient in this group had systemic pressures in the left ventricle, 2 (7%) had left ventricular pressure between 60 and 70% of right ventricular pressure, 12 (41%) between 40 and 60%, and 15 (52%) between 20 and 40% systemic pressures. The ages in this group varied from 3 days to 16 years, the majority being above 1 year of age.

The present findings suggest two possibilities. First, the presence of a patent ductus arteriosus very largely determines the presence of pulmonary hypertension in the group with an intact ventricular septum (Shaher and Kidd, 1968). This was demonstrated in the first group with a patent

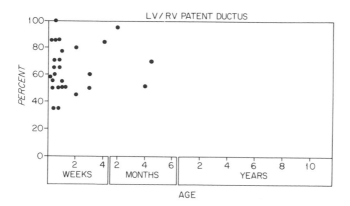

Fig. 163. Ratio between left and right ventricular pressures in 27 patients with intact ventricular septum and patent ductus arteriosus.

ductus since 55.5% of the cases had left ventricular pressures of 60% or more of systemic pressures. On the other hand, in the second group with a closed ductus, 93% of the cases had left ventricular pressures less than 60% of systemic pressures. Second, patients with a patent ductus were investigated at the stage when both fetal pulmonary hypertension and patent ductus were present, and patients with a closed ductus were investigated after the ductus had spontaneously closed and the pulmonary vascular resistance had regressed with evolution of the pulmonary vascular bed. This possibility is suggested by the fact that most patients with a patent ductus were less than 2 weeks of age, whereas most patients with a closed ductus were more than 1 year of age. It seems reasonable, however, to conclude that in the majority of patients with an intact septum the ductus is small and is closed by the age of 1 year. In a few cases a large ductus is responsible for the production of pulmonary hypertension at systemic levels during the first year of life. After this age, the ductus probably has no role in the production of pulmonary hypertension in the group with an intact septum.

The Mechanism of Blood Exchange

Several views have been expressed about the mechanism of blood exchange in transposition of the great arteries. Becker and Brill (1948) and Ebel and Lynxwiller (1951) pointed out that when both the foramen ovale and ductus arteriosus are patent, the blood flows from the right to the left atrium, and from the pulmonary artery to the aorta. With an associated atrial septal defect there is a bidirectional atrial shunting; with a ventricular septal defect the shunt is from left-to-right during systole, and from right-to-left during ventricular diastole. Astley and Parsons (1952) stated that the shunt through the ventricular septal defect is from right-to-left, and through the bronchial veins from left-to-right. Wood (1956) pointed out that if the pulmonary vascular resistance is more or less normal, a ventricular septal defect allows venous blood from the right ventricle to enter the left ventricle and pulmonary artery, where it mixes with oxygenated blood from the left atrium. If there is no atrial septal defect the pulmonary circulation is flooded, the only escape being through the bronchial anastomotic veins. With an atrial septal defect the pulmonary circulation is still excessive, but less so, oxygenated blood escaping into the right atrium and then to the right ventricle and aorta. If the pulmonary vascular resistance is raised, or if there is associated pulmonary stenosis, the right-to-left interventricular shunt is limited or reversed according to the degree of obstruction to pulmonary flow; the interatrial shunt is adjusted accordingly, being proportionately limited or reversed, respectively. When the defects are large, bidirectional shunts may occur at the atrial or ventricular level. Kjellberg *et al.* (1959) pointed out that with a large ventricular septal defect the pressure in the two ventricles is equalized. The volume and direction of the shunt are determined by the total resistance in the two vascular systems. The relationship between the pulmonary and systemic resistances probably varies considerably with respiration. In a patient with an intact ventricular septum the authors demonstrated a right-to-left interatrial shunt during ventricular diastole, and a left-to-right shunt during ventricular systole. They explained this phenomenon on the basis of the low resistance to filling of the left ventricle which will result in unusually rapid fall in the left atrial pressure at the opening of the mitral valve. This permits a right-to-left interatrial shunt. Since the left atrium is less distensible than the right, pressure is higher in the former during ventricular systole, and a left-to-right interatrial shunt occurs. The greater respiratory variations in left atrial pressure also permits a periodic change in the direction of the shunt. A similar view on the mechanism of blood shunting in transposition was expressed by Gotsman (1965). This author investigated a patient with transposition, intact ventricular septum, and surgical atrial septal defect. Venous angiography, which demonstrated intermittent opacification of the right atrium, suggested that there was a left-to-right shunt during part of the cardiac cycle with a right-to-left shunt during the remainder of the cycle. According to Taussig (1960), if there are no intracardiac abnormalities, the foramen ovale and the ductus arteriosus, which are normally patent at birth, are the only possible pathways for the crossing of the two circulations. Blood will flow from the aorta to the pulmonary artery. Since the valve which covers the foramen ovale closes from left-to-right, all the blood from the left atrium will flow into the left ventricle and from there it is again pumped to the lungs. Since all the blood which goes to the lungs is returned to the left side of the heart, the pressure in the left ventricle and in the pulmonary artery will eventually rise. When the pressure in the pulmonary artery exceeds that in the aorta, the direction of the flow of blood through the ductus arteriosus will be reversed and blood will flow from the pulmonary artery to the systemic circulation. The blood so shunted is returned to the right atrium. The pressure on the right side of the heart will rise, while that on the left will fall. As soon as the pressure in the right atrium exceeds that in the left atrium, the valve covering the foramen ovale will be forced open and blood will flow from the right atrium to the left, thus raising the pressure in the left atrium and the left ventricle and the pulmonary artery. Afterward blood will continue to flow from the pulmonary artery through the ductus arteriosus to the descending aorta and from the right atrium through the foramen ovale to the left atrium. She pointed out that in transposition the blood tends to pile up on one side of the circulation. Thus, while the pressure on one side steadily rises, that on the other side must fall. Whenever the pressure on one side exceeds that on the other, the direction of the shunt will be reversed. In addition, she as well as Edwards (1960) believed that in complete transposition of the great arteries the resistance in the pulmonary vascular bed probably regulates the amount of blood which is directed to the two circulations. Taussig emphasized that pulmonary hypertension is the rule except when there is also pulmonary stenosis. Abbott (1936) and Astley and Parsons (1952) expressed similar views and pointed out that the direction of the shunt is from the right atrium to the left atrium, and from the ductus arteriosus to the aorta. On the other hand, McElroy *et al.* (1947) thought that there was much evidence to discredit this assumption. Fowler and Ordway (1952) and Keith *et al.* (1958) found that these patients usually have a left-to-right shunt at the atrial level, and the former authors said that they had never seen the clinical picture of differential cyanosis in patients with transposition of the great arteries and an intact ventricular septum.

Several authors (Lenkei *et al.* 1959; Keith *et al.*, 1958; Kjellberg *et al.*, 1959) have found that in cases of complete transposition of the great arteries, the two atrial pressures are often different. Noonan *et al.* (1960) further noticed that in a group of patients with complete transposition associated with severe pulmonary stenosis and the systemic blood flow exceeding the pulmonary blood flow, the mean right atrial pressure was often higher than the mean left atrial pressure. In another group of patients with low pulmonary vascular resistance and pulmonary blood flow exceeding the systemic blood flow, they noticed that the mean left atrial pressure was often higher than the mean right atrial pressure.

In 1964, Shaher found that the effective pulmonary blood flow in transposition was extremely limited, but the actual flows in the pulmonary and the systemic circuits varied within a large range. This finding excluded the possibility that the shunt, i.e., the effective flow is responsible for the high flows in the pulmonary and the systemic circuits, and it did not support the suggestion of Astley and Parsons (1952), Wood (1956), Kjellberg *et al.* (1959), Taussig (1960), Ferencz (1966), and others that the volume and the direction of the shunt in transposition of the great arteries is determined by the total resistances in the two circuits. Had this been so, the shunt (effective flow) and, consequently, the pulmonary blood flow would increase in exactly the same proportions as the pulmonary vascular resistance drops, which is not the case. Shaher (1964) also demonstrated that in patients with a large ventricular septal defect, a relationship existed between the actual pulmonary blood flow and the effective pulmonary blood flow. Patients with pulmonary blood flow more than the systemic blood flow had larger effective blood flows than those with pulmonary blood flow less than systemic blood flow. It was also shown that there was an inverse relationship between pulmonary and systemic blood flows in patients with a large ventricular septal defect. Patients with a high pulmonary blood flow (low pulmonary vascular resistance or mild pulmonary stenosis) had a low systemic blood flow, and patients with low pulmonary blood flow (severe pulmonary vascular obstruction or severe pulmonary stenosis) had a high systemic blood flow. Shaher (1964) advanced the theory that when the pulmonary vascular resistance is not elevated a left-to-right shunt will occur at atrial level and a further left-to-right shunt at ventricular level may occur during diastole. An equivalent right-to-left shunt returns to the pulmonary circuit during right ventricular systole. If only a ventricular septal defect is present, the shunt is probably from left ventricle to right ventricle during ventricular diastole, and from the right ventricle to the pulmonary circuit during systole. In patients with high pulmonary vascular resistance or severe left ventricular outflow obstruction, the effective flow is diminished and a hyperkinetic systemic circulation develops secondary to tissue anoxia. This would result in a rise in the mean right atrial pressure above that in the left atrium and probably also an increase in the right ventricular diastolic pressure above that in the left ventricle. Consequently, a right-to-left shunt occurs at atrial level and probably a further right-to-left shunt at ventricular level during diastole. A left-to-right shunt from the left ventricle to the systemic circuit occurs during systole. If only a ventricular septal defect is present, a right-to-left shunt probably occurs at ventricular level during diastole and an equal left-to-right shunt from the left ventricle to the systemic circuit probably occurs during systole. It was also pointed out that when the ventricular septum is intact an aorta to pulmonary artery shunt occurs through the ductus and an equivalent left-to-right atrial shunt occurs through a foramen ovale. Bidirectional shunt occurs at the atrial level in patients with a large atrial septal defect. It was emphasized that patients with a hyperkinetic systemic circulation (Campbell and Suzman, 1951; Cleland *et al.*, 1957; Noonan *et al.*, 1960; Deuchar, 1962) either have small associated defects, or a large ventricular septal defect with severe pulmonary vascular obstruction or severe pulmonary stenosis. The mechanism of production of a hyperkinetic systemic circulation in these cases was thought to be related to severe tissue anoxia, and peripheral vasodilation secondary to a small bidirectional shunt (effective flow).

In 1971, Carr confirmed the views of Kjellberg *et al.* (1959) and Gotsman (1965) on the mechanism of atrial shunting in 10 children with transposition, intact ventricular septa, and atrial septal defects. He demonstrated a higher pressure in the left atrium than the right atrium during ventricular systole and a higher pressure in the right atrium than the left atrium during ventricular diastole. He concluded that the shunt at the atrial level in these cases was left-to-right in ventricular systole, and right-to-left in ventricular diastole. In patients with isolated ventricular septal defects, Jarmakani *et al.* (1968) have shown that the direction of shunting across the septal defect is determined by the instantaneous pressure difference between them. Rashkind (1971) used angiocardiography in 12 patients with complete transposition of the great arteries and a ventricular septal defect to study the mechanism of blood exchange in these cases. He concluded that instantaneous pressure difference between the two ventricles, produced by early activation of the left ventricle, will give rise to an early systolic shunt from the left ventricle to the right ventricle and to a late systolic shunt from the right ventricle to the left ventricle. However, as pointed out by Brown *et al.* (1965) injection of contrast media in the circulation will bring about significant changes in the circulatory dynamics in man. Moreover, injection of such media under high pressure into the right or left ventricles in transposition might temporarily alter the direction of the shunt between the two ventricles. Such an event is likely to occur especially if the ventricular pressures are equal or near equal. As pointed out earlier, about 90% of patients with a ventricular septal defect in this series had systemic or near systemic pressure in the left ventricle. Moreover, the theory that early activation of the left ventricle is the method by which blood is exchanged in transposition with a ventricular septal defect, does not explain the fact that some patients with a ventricular septal defect have a left-to-right, right-to-left, or bidirectional atrial shunt. Indeed, in some patients with a large ventricular septal defect the only step-up in oxygen saturation is found at right atrial level.

At the time of this writing, it would seem that most neonates with an intact ventricular septum have an aorta to pulmonary artery shunt through a patent ductus arteriosus and a left-to-right atrial shunt through a patent foramen ovale. The presence, in some patients, of higher left than right mean atrial pressure could be attributed to the presence of a small foramen ovale since after surgical creation of an atrial septal defect the atrial pressures equalizes (Shaher and Kidd, 1966). In slightly older infants, and in all children above the age of 1 year, a bidirectional shunt occurs at the atrial level. The mechanism of production of this shunt is probably as suggested by Kjellberg *et al.* (1959), Gotsman (1965), and Carr (1971). In most patients, the ductus has no role in the blood exchange between the two circuits after the age of 1 year. The method of blood exchange in patients with a ventricular septal defect is probably more compound. As observed by various workers (Wood, 1956; Noonan *et al.*, 1960; Shaher, 1964) an associated atrial shunt tends to be from left-to-right when the pulmonary vascular resistance is low, or bidirectional or from right-to-left when there is severe pulmonary stenosis or severe pulmonary vascular obstruction. This finding, probably related to increased resistance of the left or right ventricles to filling, respectively, could be an important factor in the mechanism of the blood shunting in these cases. The role of the bronchial arterial collateral circulation in the mechanism of blood exchange is not completely understood. Needless to say that while the net shunt in transposition has to be bidirectional and equal, in the presence of bronchial collateral circulation or a patent ductus the intracardiac shunt is likely to be predominant in one direction.

The factors that might influence the intercirculatory mixing (effective pulmonary blood flow) in patients with complete transposition were investigated by Mair and Ritter (1972). These authors studied the hemodynamic data from 100 patients all 1 year old or older. They confirmed the views of Shaher (1964) on the relationship between total pulmonary blood flow and effective pulmonary blood flow, and on the mechanism of production of hyperkinetic systemic circulation. They pointed out that in the group of patients they studied, intercirculatory mixing in those with only one anatomic communication between the two circuits was generally equally good whether the communication was an atrial or ventricular septal defect. The average mixing in patients with two communications was only slightly greater than that in patients with one communication. Their figures revealed that for the 25 patients with an atrial septal defect only, there was a significant direct relation between total pulmonary flow and effective pulmonary flow. There was also a significant relation between these indexes for the 35 patients with communications at two or more levels. The only group in which there was no statistically significant relation between these two indexes was that of 33 patients with a ventricular septal defect as their only potential mixing site. The authors thought that the reason for the lack of relation in this group may be variations in the position of the septal defect. Their figures also showed that of those patients with a total pulmonary flow index of less than 6.5, only 35% achieved an effective flow index of 1.5 or greater and only 3% achieved an effective index of 2.0 or greater. In patients with a total pulmonary flow index greater than 6.5, the corresponding figures were 73% and 32%. The effective flow was larger in the group of patients with a communication at only one site and increased total pulmonary blood flow than in the group of patients with two sites of communication but with relatively decreased total pulmonary blood flow. The authors pointed out that other contributing factors that might affect intercirculatory mixing include the actual size of the septal defects, location of the defects on the atrial and ventricular septa, blood viscosity, and perhaps the relative compliances of the two ventricles. Unusually good mixing is often achieved by patients who have a ventricular septal defect that extends posteriorly to a position beneath the pulmonary artery. They postulated that if a patient with a large defect has poor mixing despite increased total pulmonary blood flow, the defect may be in a disadvantageous position for mixing, probably anterior in the muscular septum. However, Shaher *et al.* (1973) reported the case of an 11¼-year-old patient with transposition. Autopsy examination showed a large supracristal ventricular septal defect immediately beneath the aortic valve. The authors concluded that the long survival of this patient was partly related to the position of the ventricular septal defect, for a significant amount of left ventricular output must have entered directly the ascending aorta.

Follow-up Hemodynamic Studies on Unoperated Patients

Follow-up cardiac catheterization was carried out on 7 patients who had had no form of heart surgery; 1 in Group II, 5 in Group III, and 1 in

TABLE 16.7

FOLLOW-UP HEMODYNAMIC STUDIES ON 7 UNOPERATED PATIENTS [a]

Group	Patient no.	Age	Hb	O₂ cap.	Blood O₂ saturation %								Pressures						Other data
					SVC	RA	RV	Ao	PV	LA	LV	PA	RA	LA	RV	Ao	LV	PA	
II	73	1 y 2 m	—	—	—	—	—	—	—	—	—	—	—	—	—	83/55	51/4	—	
		3 y 3 m	14.4	19.4	25	35	39	61	99	94	86	—	6	6	100/0	105/65	65/10	—	
III	87	15 d	—	—	57	60	—	—	90	—	—	85	12	—	65/10	—	—	52/30	
		2½ m	—	—	40	49	61	—	—	—	—	81	2	—	68/0	—	—	68/26	
		5 y 6 m	20.3	27.3	58	62	78	75	—	—	—	84	0	—	77/0	84/70	108/0	79/57	
	108	3 m	10.1	13.5	45	73	70	76	—	—	—	83	6	—	85/0	75/50	—	75/40	
		7 m	15.2	20.5	52	65	71	73	—	—	—	84	8	—	80/0	80/60	—	80/40	Grade 3 PVD at 4 y and 3 m VSD 10 x 10 mm
		4 y	—	—	58	62	72	71	—	—	—	—	5	—	85/0	85/50	—	—	
	115	6 m	—	—	50	50	—	A. 73 D. 86	—	98	—	88	5	8.5	86/5	99/40	—	84/42	Interrupted aortic arch
		4 y	17.1	23.1	55	56	65	A. 68 D. 73	—	—	81	74	5	—	100/0	100/50 100/60	100/0	100/60	
	120	2 y 5 m	—	—	60	61	72	69	—	—	—	—	6	—	63/2	60/39	—	—	
		5 y 6 m	24.2	32.8	56	56	60	66	—	—	—	—	2	—	90/0	96/68	—	—	
	122	4 y	24.6	33	60	66	76	73	98	—	92	92	2	—	100/5	98/80	32/0	15/5	
		9½ y	—	—	48	56	66	64	—	89	92	92	5	6	94/9	100/56	50/0	50/30	
		13 y	18.5	24.8	33	44	48	55	—	—	—	—	5	—	80/0	80/50	—	—	
IV	132	2 m	—	—	51	56	49	60	96	95	87	90	6	10	60/10	60/40	60/10	12/10	Left ventricular infundibulum
		2 y 1 m	16.1	21.6	35	42	35	44	93	93	86	87	4	12	90/0	70/40	90/0	20/10	60/0

[a] All abbreviations same as given in Tables 16.3 and 16.5.

Group IV (Table 16.7). Follow-up cardiac studies were performed twice on each of 3 patients in Group III, and once on each of the remaining 4 patients. The age of the patients at the initial studies varied between 15 days and 5 years, and at the final studies between 3 and 13 years.

Follow-up cardiac catheterization performed 2 years after the initial studies on the patient in Group II demonstrated no significant change in the severity of left ventricular outflow tract obstruction (Table 16.7). Of the 5 patients in Group III, the systemic arterial oxygen saturation in the follow-up studies diminished in 4 patients in whom this information was available (Table 16.7). The systemic arteriovenous oxygen saturation difference diminished in 3 and increased in 1 patient. In 4 patients the pulmonary artery was entered in both initial and follow-up studies. The blood oxygen saturation in this vessel had remained unchanged in 3, and had diminished in 1. In 3 the pulmonary arterial pressure was at systemic levels in both studies and in 1 of these 3 patients a pressure gradient of 29 mm Hg between the pulmonary artery and the left ventricle was detected in the follow-up studies. In the fourth patient a 17 mm Hg gradient across the pulmonary valve was detected in the initial studies. The follow-up studies on this patient demonstrated moderate pulmonary hypertension and equal systolic pressures in the pulmonary artery and left ventricle. Follow-up studies performed 2 years after the initial studies on the patient in Group IV showed no essential change in the systemic or pulmonary arteriovenous oxygen saturation difference (Table 16.7). Similarly the ratio between pulmonary arterial and left ventricular systolic pressures had remained unchanged. In the follow-up studies, however, the effective pulmonary arteriovenous oxygen saturation difference had increased and a pulmonary subvalvular gradient of 30 mm Hg had developed.

No attempt has been made to include hemodynamic studies performed after balloon septostomy or palliative heart surgery in this section for the following reasons. Surgical creation of an atrial septal defect, by improving blood mixing between the two circuits, will diminish the calculated pulmonary blood flow and give a false impression of an elevated pulmonary vascular resistance. Banding of the pulmonary artery will diminish the pulmonary blood flow and pressure, and a systemic artery–pulmonary artery shunt will increase pulmonary artery blood flow and pressure. Plauth *et al.* (1970) reported the follow-up cardiac catheterization on 65 patients with complete transposition of the great arteries. Of these 64 patients, 51 have had palliative operations. The authors defined pulmonary stenosis as a peak systolic pressure gradient of 20 mm Hg or more between the main pulmonary artery and the left ventricle and pulmonary arterial hypertension as pulmonary arterial systolic pressure 50% or more of systemic arterial pressure or left ventricular systolic pressure greater than 75% of systemic pressure in the absence of pulmonary stenosis. The authors found left ventricular outflow tract obstruction in 28% of their patients with an intact ventricular septum and 50% of those with a ventricular septal defect. Pulmonary arterial hypertension or pulmonary vascular obstruction or both were present in about half of the patients with an intact ventricular septum and all the patients with a large ventricular septal defect without pulmonary artery banding or pulmonary stenosis. In this series the incidence of pulmonary arterial hypertension in the group with an intact ventricular septum was low. Of the 28 patients above the age of 1 year (Table 16.3; see also Tables 16.8, 16.15, and 16.16), only 2 had a left ventricular pressure more than 50 mm Hg and none had a left ventricular pressure greater than 75% of systemic pressure. Some pressure gradients described by Plauth and associates could possibly be regarded as flow gradients. This mechanism could explain the disappearance or diminution of gradients in the final studies of 3 of their patients with a ventricular septal defect. Tynan (1972) reported the hemodynamic findings, modified only by balloon atrial septostomy, in 42 cardiac catheterizations performed on 19 patients with complete transposition and an intact ventricular septum. All patients were under 3 months of age at the initial investigation. The pulmonary artery was entered in all cases. The pulmonary artery systolic pressure and pulmonary-to-systemic vascular resistance ratios were significantly higher under 9 weeks than over this age. The major fall in pulmonary vascular resistance appeared to occur in the first four weeks of life. On the other hand, changes in the ratio between pulmonary and systemic blood flows showed no clear cut pattern. In 11 cases there was an overall rise, in 4 an overall fall, and 4 showed no overall change. A systolic pressure gradient of 5 mm Hg or more between the left ventricle and the pulmonary artery was found in 35 of the investigations. The 7 investigations in which a pressure difference of less than 5 mm Hg was found were all performed during the first 2 weeks of life. After the age of 14 days, the range of pressure gradient was from 8 to 35 mm Hg with a median of 13 mm Hg. The author emphasized that (1) maturation of the pulmonary circulation after birth in simple transposition is similar to that demonstrated in the normal human infant, (2) a systolic pressure gradient from the ventricle to the pulmonary artery is a usual finding in uncomplicated transposition, (3) no systematic distribution of pulmonary-to-systemic flow ratios or age related changes in these ratios could be demonstrated. However, as has been pointed out earlier, surgical creation of an atrial septal defect, by improving the

TABLE 16.8

HEMODYNAMIC DATA BEFORE AND AFTER SURGICAL CREATION OF AN ATRIAL SEPTAL DEFECT IN 9 PATIENTS WITH AN INTACT VENTRICULAR SEPTUM [a]

Patient no.	Age	Hb	O₂ cap.	Blood O₂ saturation %								Pressures					
				SVC	RA	RV	Ao	PV	LA	LV	PA	RA	LA	RV	Ao	LV	PA
23	5 d	13	17.6	26 IVC	41	33	33	100	85	—	—	4	—	74/10	75/43	—	—
	1 y 5 m	14.8	20	50	74	75	76	96	83	84	—	5	4	80/5	80/45	30/5	—
35	10 d	21.7	29.6	35	41	54	52	—	—	—	—	5	—	100/0	90/55	—	—
	2 y	12.8	17.1	70 IVC	73	67	68	98	89	88	—				—	—	—
37	10 d	14.3	19.3	31	35	33	39	98	100	—	—	2	5	82/5	80/60	—	—
	1 y 2 m	15.1	20.2	43	79	72	70	95	95	80	—	4	4	80/0	80/45	25/0	—
48	1 m	25	33.6	31	56	48	46	—	—	—	—				—	—	—
50	1½ y	15.6	21	41	30	56	55	—	89	91	—	1	3	99/6	90/49	31/2	—
	1 m 1 w	15	20.2	15	12	24	34	100	100	—	—	5	10	90/0	85/60	—	—
51	23 m	10.9	14.6	48	40	62	62	99	92	88	—	6	6	122/0	140/4	65/4	—
	6 w	18.8	25.3	10	30	43	—	—	—	—	—	—		72/0	—	—	—
58	2 y 2 m	14.8	19.8	50	63	66	67	98	91	92	—	3	3	76/3	90/52	44/0	—
	5 m	12.1	16.4	50	51	51	65	89	88	88	—	8	8	100/10	100/70	40/6	—
59	4 y 7 m	15.2	20.4	55	65	76	76	96	96	87	—	5	5	90/6	125/90	25/6	—
	5 m	19.5	26.4	27	32	58	60	100	100	—	—	3	5	97/0	97/63	—	—
60	1 y 4 m	14.8	19.8	53	67	73	75	94	87	88	—	5	7	80/7	80/50	33/9	—
	13 m	14.0	18.9	57	77	79	79	100	95	98	—	3	4	80/7	95/53	35/6	—
	2 y 2 m	13.6	18.4	49	73	74	73	100	93	91	—	2	3	96/5	103/55	48/3	—

[a] All abbreviations same as in Tables 16.3 and 16.5.

TABLE 16.9

HEMODYNAMIC DATA BEFORE AND AFTER SURGICAL CREATION OF AN ATRIAL SEPTAL DEFECT IN 5 PATIENTS WITH INTACT VENTRICULAR SEPTUM AND LEFT VENTRICULAR OUTFLOW TRACT OBSTRUCTION [a]

Patient no.	Age	Hb	O₂ cap.	Blood O₂ saturation %								Pressures					
				SVC	RA	RV	Ao	PV	LA	LV	PA	RA	LA	RV	Ao	LV	PA
67	9 d	22.4	30	30	42	42	42	—	89	—	—	8	6	60/5	70/40	—	—
	1 y 11 m	16.7	22.5	45	54	62	58	—	83	85	—	6	6	83/10	83/51	64/11	—
69	2 w	13.4	18	7	9	13	13	—	—	—	—	10	—	75/0	75/42	—	—
	8 m	15	20.1	48	65	66	67	99	88	87	—	3	2	100/6	94/53	40/5	—
70	5 w	—	—	40 IVC	42	—	40	100	87	87	—	—	4	91/0	—	97/0	—
	3 y 3 m	19.1	23.8	41	54	54	61	98	83	85	—	5	5	85/0	95/50	105/0	—
72	1 y	12.9	17.4	32	30	58	34	97	96	92	—	4	4	105/5	105/68	48/5	—
	2½ y	18.6	25.2	57	80	79	82	98	91	88	—	5	5	90/10	100/60	60/5	—
74	1½ y	15.2	22	30 IVC	42	54	52	—	78	88	—	3	3	64/0	84/42	26/0	—
	2 y 10 m	17.2	23.1	31	42	46	42	98	77	85	85	6	7	90/3	98/54	56/3	11/7

[a] Abbreviations same as in Tables 16.3 and 16.5.

blood mixing between the two circuits, will diminish the calculated pulmonary blood flow. Since the follow-up studies of Tynan (1972) were performed after balloon atrial septostomy, his conclusions on the pulmonary and systemic blood flows seem unjustified.

Spontaneous Closure of Ventricular Septal Defect

Spontaneous closure of a ventricular septal defect occurred in 3 patients in this series, after surgical creation of an atrial septal defect in 2, and after surgical creation of an atrial septal defect and banding of the pulmonary artery in 1 (see Tables 16.10 and 16.14). Initially both patients with a surgical atrial septal defect had low systolic left ventricular pressure. Follow-up studies demonstrated that the left ventricular–right ventricular systolic pressure ratio had diminished in 1 and had remained unchanged in the other. In the third patient preoperative hemodynamic data were not obtained before surgical creation of an atrial septal defect and banding of the pulmonary artery but preoperative angiocardiography demonstrated a ventricular septal defect. Postoperative studies demonstrated spontaneous closure of the defect and a left ventricular pressure 175% of systemic pressure.

Spontaneous closure of a ventricular septal defect associated with transposition of the great arteries was first reported by Shaher et al. (1965). Li et al. (1969) reported 7 patients with transposition in whom autopsy or clinical data suggested spontaneous closure of the defect. They pointed out that spontaneous closure of ventricular septal defects in transposition is likely to increase as survival in this condition is helped by modern medical and surgical therapy. Of the 10 patients reported by Dobell et al. (1969), spontaneous closure of a small ventricular septal defect occurred in 1. Of the 43 patients with a ventricular septal defect reported by Plauth et al. (1970), spontaneous closure of the defect was documented in 7, and in 2 others the defect had clearly become much smaller. The earliest documented closure in their material occurred between 2 days and 8 months and the latest between 4 and 9 years of age. The authors pointed out that as a predictor of ventricular septal defect narrowing or closure, the level of left ventricular pressure was not particularly helpful. In their view, angiocardiographic demonstration of a small defect or a low initial systemic saturation, is the best indicator of small or closing defects. Parsons et al. (1971) reported that of their 19 cases with transposition and ventricular septal defect spontaneous closure of this defect occurred in 5. Of the 60 infants of Paul (1971) spontaneous closure of the defect was observed in 5.

TABLE 16.10

HEMODYNAMIC DATA BEFORE AND AFTER SURGICAL CREATION OF AN ATRIAL SEPTAL DEFECT IN 6 PATIENTS WITH A VENTRICULAR SEPTAL DEFECT[a]

Patient No.	Age	Hb	O₂ Cap.	Blood O₂ saturation %								Pressures						Size of VSD	PVD Grades 1–4 and Age
				SVC	RA	RV	Ao	PV	LA	LV	PA	RA	LA	RV	Ao	LV	PA		
76	4 d	20.1	27	37	41	66	58	—	99	98	—	2	1	70/0	70/50	50/0	—		
	6 m	15.1	20.1	34	50	55	53	96	86	85	—	8	8	85/0	80/43	40/0	—	Cl. spont	
81	7 d	19.3	26.1	25	34	58	66	93	—	—	77	3	—	79/1	70/49	—	—		Biopsy
	4 y 6 m	17.9	24	47	56	70	69	—	95	—	—	6	6	90/0	90/60	—	90/45		Grade 3 (5 y)
82	9 d	14.7	19.8	0	0	13	26	—	96.5	—	—	—	6	86/9	93/60	39/2	—		
	13 m	13.6	18.4	53	76	75	78	98	95	90	—	5	5	80/8	95/50	37/9	—	Cl. spont	
104	2 m	13.1	17.6	46	70	69	—	—	98	91	—	—	—	80/10	—	—	—		Grade 3
	2 y	16.7	22.4	41	63	69	66	98	—	88	—	5	5	80/0	80/55	87/0	—	10 x 5 mm	(2 y 1 m)
114	6 m	15.8	21.4	52	52	76	72	—	—	—	90	2	—	80/5	76/47	—	63/31		
	2 y 10 m	14.7	19.7	59	71	73	72	—	94	91	80	4	4	—	87/51	84/0	71/49		
123	4 y 7 m	17.5	23.7	28	29	47	44	—	—	—	—	1	—	106/0	106/66	—	—		Biopsy
	5 y 9 m	20.1	27	44	56	65	70	95	85	84	80	2	2	90/0	95/7	93/0	70/50		Grade 3 (5 y)

[a] Abbreviations same as in Tables 16.3 and 16.5.

TABLE 16.11

Hemodynamic Data Before and After Surgical Creation of an Atrial Septal Defect in 4 Patients with Ventricular Septal Defect and Pulmonary Stenosis [a]

Patient No.	Age	Hb	O₂ Cap.	Blood O₂ saturation %								Pressures						Size of VSD	PVD Grades 1-4 and Age
				SVC	RA	RV	Ao	PV	LA	LV	PA	RA	LA	RV	Ao	LV	PA		
133	2 m	14	18.6	15	22	39	48	—	100	97	—	4	6	70/8	65/40	70/8	—		
	1 y 2 m	14.6	19.6	44	59	64	70	99	88	83	—	6	6	70/6	93/56	73/6	—		
134	2 m	15.1	20.2	—	32	35	33	—	—	—	83	—	—	73/2	—	79/5	—		
	2 y 3 m	14.2	19	45	79	76	77	96	—	81	83	5	5	110/8	112/65	111/8	20/7		
135	4 m	12.4	16.7	38	44	51	—	96	97	86	—	6	3	52/2	—	54/4	—		
	2 y 3 m	10	13.4	33	33	36	47	98	94	81	—	—	—	—	—	—	—	9 x 7 mm	Grade 1 (2 y 3 m)
142 [b]	1 y 11 m	18.1	24.2	39 IVC	35	49	45	—	—	—	—	—	—	—	45/60	—	—	12 x 3 mm	Grade 4 (4 y)
	4 y 5 m	21.3	28.5	52	71	69	69	100	99	87	72	10	10	127/23	100/80	114/20	93/27		

[a] Abbreviations same as in Tables 16.3 and 16.5.
[b] Patient 142 with a subvalvular diaphragm.

Hemodynamic Effects of Palliative Cardiac Surgery

SURGICAL CREATION OF AN ATRIAL SEPTAL DEFECT

Thirty-five patients were investigated by cardiac catheterization 6 months to 4 years after surgical creation of an atrial septal defect. Of these 35 patients, cardiac catheterizations before surgery were carried out on 24. The postoperative hemodynamic findings in the group without preoperative hemodynamic data will be presented separately.

Of the 24 patients with preoperative hemodynamic data, 14 had an intact ventricular septum (5 with left ventricular outflow tract obstruction) and were classified as Group I, and 10 had a ventricular septal defect (4 with left ventricular outflow tract obstruction) and were classified as Group II (Tables 16.8–16.11). Preoperative and postoperative systemic arterial oxygen saturation, atrial pressures, and systemic, pulmonary, and effective arteriovenous difference were compared only when available. Since none of the postoperative cardiac catheterizations were carried out within weeks after surgical creations of an atrial septal defect, some of the postoperative findings could be attributed to the changing hemodynamics of transposition brought about by aging. Closing or closure of a

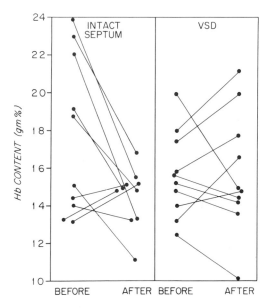

Fig. 16.4 Hemoglobin (Hb) content before and after surgical creation of an atrial septal defect in 10 patients with intact ventricular septum, and 10 patients with a ventricular septal defect. (VSD).

patent ductus, diminution or closure of a ventricular septal defect, development or increase in the severity of pulmonary vascular obstruction, and development or increase in the severity of left ventricular outflow tract obstruction, may, singly or in combination, affect the postoperative hemodynamics. In addition, since most preoperative cardiac catheterizations were carried out on older patients with transposition, neither the pre- nor postoperative findings could be compared to studies performed during the neonatal period or to studies performed after balloon atrial septostomy. To eliminate the factor of changing hemoglobin content and blood oxygen capacity on flows, only the pre-and postoperative pulmonary, systemic, and effective arteriovenous oxygen saturation differences have been studied.

Hemoglobin (Fig 16.4)

In Group I, the hemoglobin diminished in 7 and increased in 3, while in Group II it diminished in 5 and increased in 5 cases.

Systemic Arterial Oxygen Saturation (Fig. 16.5)

In Group I the systemic arterial oxygen saturation increased in 12 and diminished in 2, while in Group II it diminished in 3 and increased in 5 cases.

Left Atrial Pressure (Fig. 16.6)

In Group I the mean left atrial pressure diminished in 4, increased in 4, and remained unchanged in 1 case. In Group II it diminished in 2, increased in 1, and remained unchanged in 1.

Right Atrial Pressure (Fig. 16.7)

In Group I the mean right atrial pressure diminished in 4 and increased in 6 cases. In Group II it increased in 4 in whom this measurement was available.

Left Atrium–Right Atrium Pressure Gradient (Fig. 16.8)

Essentially equal pressures were noted postoperatively in all patients in whom these measurements were available. Preoperative pressure gradients of 3 mm Hg or more were abolished by the operation.

The Effective Arteriovenous Oxygen Saturation Difference (Fig. 16.9)

In Group I, the effective arteriovenous oxygen saturation difference diminished in 11, and was unchanged in 2, while in Group II it diminished in 6 and was unchanged or slightly increased in 2 cases.

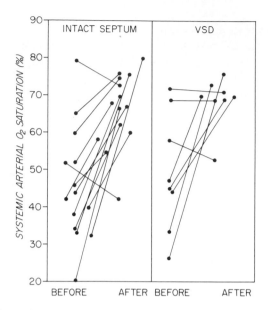

Fig. 16.5. Systemic arterial oxygen saturation before and after surgical creation of an atrial septal defect in 14 patients with intact ventricular septum and 8 patients with a ventricular septal defect. (VSD).

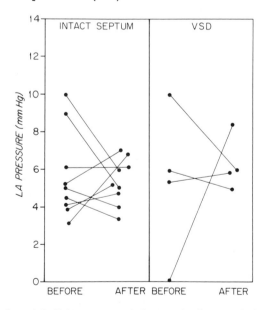

Fig. 16.6. Left atrial (LA) pressure before and after surgical creation of an atrial septal defect in 9 patients with intact ventricular septum, and 4 patients with ventricular septal defect. (VSD).

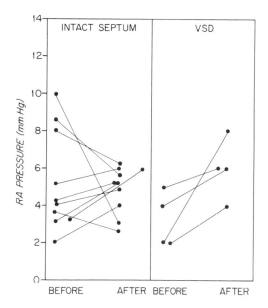

Fig. 16.7. Right atrial (RA) pressures before and after surgical creation of an atrial septal defect in 10 patients with intact ventricular septum and 4 patients with ventricular septal defect.

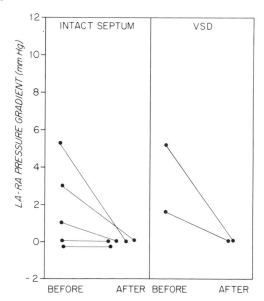

Fig. 16.8. Pressure gradient between mean left and right atrial pressures before and after surgical creation of atrial septal defect in 5 patients with intact septum and 2 patients with ventricular septal defect (VSD).

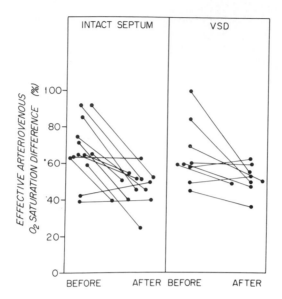

Fig. 16.9. Effective arteriovenous oxygen saturation difference before and after surgical creation of atrial septal defect in 13 patients with intact septum and 9 patients with ventricular septal defect (VSD).

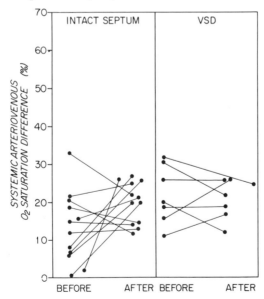

Fig. 16.10. Systemic arteriovenous oxygen saturation difference before and after surgical creation of atrial septal defect in 12 patients with intact ventricular septum and 7 patients with ventricular septal defect (VSD).

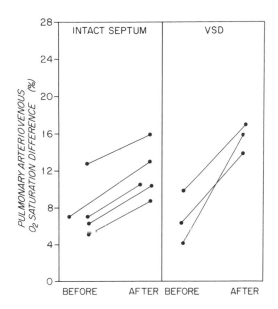

Fig. 16.11. Pulmonary arteriovenous oxygen saturation difference before and after surgical creation of atrial septal defect in 5 patients with intact ventricular septum and 3 patients with ventricular septal defect (VSD).

The Systemic Arteriovenous Oxygen Saturation Difference (Fig. 16.10)

In Group I the systemic arteriovenous oxygen saturation difference increased in 7, diminished in 3, and was unchanged in 2 cases. In Group II it increased in 2, diminished in 3, and was unchanged in 2.

The Pulmonary Arteriovenous Oxygen Saturation Difference (Fig. 16.11)

This measurement increased in all patients in whom it was available.

Ventricular Pressures

Pre- and postoperative right and left ventricular pressures were available on 10 patients, 5 in Group I and 5 in Group II. Of the 5 in Group I, left ventricular pressure remained less than 50% of right ventricular pressure in 2 and had risen in 3 with left ventricular outflow tract obstruction. In 3 cases, with a ventricular septal defect, left ventricular pressure, at or near systemic level in the preoperative studies, was unchanged in the postoperative studies. In the remaining 2 it had fallen from 72 to 47% of right ventricular pressure in 1, and remained less than 50% of the right ventricular pressure in 1.

The postoperative hemodynamic data on 11 patients who had not had preoperative cardiac catheterizations are shown in Table 16.12. Of the 9

TABLE 16.12

INITIAL HEMODYNAMIC DATA OBTAINED AFTER SURGICAL CREATION OF AN ATRIAL SEPTAL DEFECT [a]

Patient no.	Age	Hb	O₂ Cap.	Blood O₂ saturation %								Pressures						PVD Grades 1-4 and Age
				SVC	RA	RV	Ao	PV	LA	LV	PA	RA	LA	RV	Ao	LV	PA	
A. 9 patients with an intact ventricular septum (no pulmonary stenosis)																		
158	10 m	10.1	13.7	38	40	57	48	93	92	80	—	5	5	78/0	87/50	45/0	—	N (1½ y)
159	1 y 9 m	12.1	16.3	52	65	73	70	97	96	86	—	7	8	85/4	90/52	46/2	—	—
160	2 y	16	21.6	48	67	74	75	97	91	85	—	8	8	90/10	770/50	32/10	—	—
161	3 y	20.2	28.2	59	74	77	70	97	91	93	—	5	5	90/10	90/55	30/10	—	—
162	3 y 2 m	—	—	48	50	63	—	97	83	83	—	1	2	87/0	—	36/5	—	—
163	3 y 5 m	17	23	69	79	77	75	100	95	92	—	4	4	81/6	81/58	25/6	—	—
164	5 y	20.1	26.7	62	71	72	71	99	92	90	—	4	6	98/6	98/62	33/5	—	—
165	6 y 6 m	24.6	33.5	60	81	69	70	94	92	90	—	7	7	100/5	80/40	30/10	—	—
166	10 y 1 m	17.5	23.4	59	63	73	76	97	93	86	—	4	3	107/0	90/50	22/0	—	—
B. 2 patients with a ventricular septal defect (no pulmonary stenosis)																		
167 [b]	1 y 2 m	14.3	19.3	50	65	62	64	97	85	84	—	5	5	95/0	95/10	102/0	—	3 (15 m)
168	3 y 9 m	17.1	23	53	60	66	69	96	95	91	—	7	7	105/0	105/54	100/0	—	B 3 (4 y)

[a] B, biopsy; Eff., effective; N, normal; Pul, pulmonary; Syst., systemic. All other abbreviations same as in Tables 16.3 and 16.5.

[b] Size of VSD at autopsy: 3 x 3 mm.

with an intact ventricular septum (Group I), equal or near equal mean right and left atrial pressures were observed in all. Of the 8 patients in whom the systemic arterial oxygen saturation was available, this measurement was 70% or more in 7, and 48% in 1. The ratio between left ventricular systolic pressure and systemic arterial pressure was less than 50% in 8, and 58% in 1. Of the 2 with a ventricular septal defect, equal mean right and left atrial pressures were present in both. The systemic arterial oxygen saturation was 64% in one, and 69% in the other. Left ventricular pressures were at systemic arterial levels in both.

It would seem that surgical creations of an atrial septal defect brings about considerable changes in the hemodynamics of both the pulmonary and the systemic circulations. The most obvious of these are an increase in the bidirectional blood shunting, improvement in the systemic arterial oxygen saturation, and diminution of the calculated pulmonary blood flow. Other changes also involve the left atrial pressure, the systemic blood flow, and the hemoglobin content.

The most significant of the hemodynamic changes (since most other changes were secondary to it) was the increase in the bidirectional shunting as evidenced by a diminution of the effective arteriovenous oxygen saturation difference. This means that more oxygenated blood from the lungs reached the systemic circuit and more reduced blood reached the lungs for oxygenation. Theoretically, if the pulmonary venous blood saturation remains unchanged, the increase in the bidirectional blood shunt will increase the arteriovenous oxygen difference across the lungs and the calculated pulmonary blood flow should diminish. The present findings show that this was the case in the 7 cases in whom this measurement was available. However, at the time of this writing there is no evidence that this apparent diminution in the calculated pulmonary blood is associated with an elevation of the pulmonary vascular resistance. In all probability the change in the calculated flow simply is the result of admixture of a larger amount of systemic venous blood with the pulmonary venous blood in the left side of the heart.

Significant improvement in the arterial oxygen saturation occurred in the majority of patients in the two groups. Of the 5 patients in whom no postoperative improvement in the systemic arterial oxygen saturation occurred, the long interval between the heart operation and the re-study or unsatisfactory surgical result could be the underlying mechanism producing this phenomenon in 4. In the fifth patient a ventricular septal defect had spontaneously closed between the two studies. Whatever the anatomy of the atrial and ventricular septa, no improvement was observed in the arterial oxygen saturation when this was 70% or more preoperatively.

The systemic arteriovenous oxygen saturation difference and consequently the systemic blood flow showed no uniform response to the surgically created defect. In the majority in whom improvement in the systemic arterial saturation occurred postoperatively, the oxygen saturation of the mixed venous blood either increased to the same extent or exceeded the increase of the systemic arterial oxygen saturation. Accordingly, the arteriovenous oxygen saturation difference in the systemic circuit in these cases either remained the same or diminished. There were 7 patients who were extremely hypoxic and improved after operation. Preoperatively they had a small systemic arteriovenous oxygen saturation difference and large systemic blood flow. Improvement of systemic arterial saturation in these cases was accompanied by an increase in the arteriovenous oxygen saturation difference and lowering of the systemic blood flow. In 5 patients in whom the systemic arterial oxygen saturation did not improve or deteriorate after operation, the systemic arteriovenous oxygen saturation difference diminished in 3, slightly increased in 1, and did not change in 1.

Changes in atrial pressures were not remarkable. Thus although atrial pressures were equalized as a result of the surgical procedure, lowering of the mean left atrial pressure more than 3 mm Hg occurred in only 3 patients. No significant change in the left atrial pressure occurred in 60% of patients in whom this measurement was available pre- and postoperatively.

The hemodynamic effects of balloon atrial septostomy are essentially identical to those resulting from surgical creation of an atrial septal defect. Rashkind and Miller (1968) measured the left atrial to right atrial pressure gradients before and after septostomy in 11 patients. A decrease in the "a" wave gradient was recorded in 9 and a reduction in mean pressure gradient was demonstrated in 10. In 20 patients the mean increase in the arterial oxygen saturation after the procedure was 23%. In 15 patients with an intact ventricular septum, mean saturations of 41% increased to 64% after the procedure. In 5 patients with "large" ventricular septal defects, mean saturations of 53% increased to 74%. Of the 9 patients who underwent balloon atrial septostomy by Dobell *et al.* (1969), pre- and postseptostomy atrial pressures were available in 6. Of these 6 patients a left atrial–right atrial pressure gradient was present in 4 before and in 1 after septostomy. Significant increase in the systemic arterial oxygen saturation was observed in all patients in whom this measurement was performed before and after the procedure. Tynan *et al.* (1969) measured the systemic arterial oxygen saturation before and immediately after balloon atrial septostomy in 38 patients with transposition. The mean saturation before septostomy was 48% and the mean saturation after it was 67%; the mean rise was 13%. The mean systemic arterial oxygen saturation before septostomy was 61% in those with a ventricular septal defect and 46% in those with an intact ventricular septum. The mean saturation after septostomy was 71% in cases with a ventricular septal defect, and 63% in cases with an intact ventricular septum. The authors pointed out that the presence of subvalvular pulmonary obstruction did not appear to alter the initial response to septostomy in 5 patients in whom it was diagnosed at a subsequent investigation. Of the 31 patients with adequate data reported by Baker *et al.* (1971), 19 showed a rise of 10% or greater, 9 had a step-up of 5 to 9%, and 3 increased less than 5%. Mean and "a" wave pressure gradients were measured from left atrium to right atrium in 33 patients. Eleven (33%) showed a decrease of 4 mm Hg or more. The authors pointed out that a large atrial septal defect was less critical in the group with a ventricular septal defect than in the group with an intact ventricular septum. Of their 7 patients with a ventricular septal defect, the size of the atrial defect was less than 12 mm and none had required surgical septectomy. On the other hand, of the group with an intact septum 7 had atrial defect less than 12 mm in diameter and all eventually required surgical septectomy because of hypoxic spells and/or failure to thrive.

THE EDWARDS PROCEDURE

Four patients in Group I underwent repositioning of the right pulmonary veins as suggested by Edwards *et al.* (1964) (Table 16.13). Preoperative hemodynamic studies were carried out on 2. All patients were 4 weeks of age or less at the second cardiac catheterization. Equalization of the atrial pressures were noted in 3. In the fourth patient no preoperative hemodynamic studies were obtained, but postoperatively a 5 mm Hg gradient was present between the right and left atria. The 2 patients with preoperative data showed a moderate improvement in the systemic arterial saturation. On the other hand, the 2 without preoperative studies had a postoperative systemic arterial oxygen saturation of 26 and 31%, respectively. Compared to patients studied after surgical creation of an atrial septal defect, the 4 patients in this group showed a large pulmonary arteriovenous oxygen saturation difference suggesting a markedly reduced pulmonary blood flow.

It would seem that repositioning of the pulmonary veins coupled with closure of the atrial septum will deplete the pulmonary circuit of a significant amount of the circulating blood. This appeared to be the underlying mechanism of the production of severe systemic arterial desaturation and

TABLE 16.13
Edwards Procedure [a,b]

Patient no.	Age	Hb	O₂ cap.	Blood O₂ saturation %								Pressures					
				SVC	RA	RV	Ao	PV	LA	LV	PA	RA	LA	RV	Ao	LV	PA
A. Hemodynamic data before and after procedure																	
14	3 d	16.8	22.5	22	27	23	37	98	—	90	—	1	—	75/2	75/45	40/5	—
	3 w	11.4	15.4	41	47	48	62	97	80	81	—	5	5	90/5	80/45	42/0	—
24	5 d	22.2	30	24 IVC	34	56	54	99	—	91	—	5	8	80/5	85/60	25/4	—
	24 d	13.9	18.6	31	41	64	65	94	76	78	—	3	1	82/4	82/48	28/3	—
B. Initial hemodynamic data after procedure																	
169	16 d	14.6	19.5	18	26	28	26	99	67	73	—	5	5	92/7	90/62	40/6	—
170	18 d	13.7	18.4	13	21	38	31	92	52	72	—	8	3	92/6	92/53	48/10	—

[a] All patients with an intact ventricular septum.
[b] All abbreviations same as in Tables 16.3 and 16.5.

a large pulmonary arteriovenous oxygen saturation difference. The presence of postoperative high right atrial pressure in 1 is a supportive evidence of this hypothesis. The 2 who showed moderate improvement in the systemic arterial saturation probably had a large patent foramen ovale.

BANDING OF THE PULMONARY ARTERY AND CREATION OF AN ATRIAL SEPTAL DEFECT

Cardiac catheterizations were carried out on 5 patients in Group III with a surgical atrial septal defect and pulmonary artery banding (Table 16.14). Preoperative hemodynamic studies were available on 2. The pulmonary artery was entered in 1 patient in the preoperative studies and in none in the postoperative studies. Postoperatively, the 2 patients with preoperative studies had lost the gradient between the left and right atria, and all patients had equal mean atrial pressures postoperatively. The ventricular pressure remained equal in 2 patients with preoperative studies. Of the remaining 3 patients, ventricular pressures were equal in 2. In the third patient, postoperative studies demonstrated spontaneous closure of a ventricular septal defect, previously documented by angiography, and a left ventricular pressure 175% of right ventricular pressure. In the 2 with preoperative studies, the systemic arterial oxygen saturation diminished in 1 and improved in the other.

Of the 8 restudied patients with a surgical pulmonary artery band reported by Plauth *et al.* (1970), the pressure distal to the band was normal in 6 and slightly elevated in 2. The pulmonary vascular resistance was normal in all. The authors pointed out that banding of the pulmonary artery had protected the pulmonary vasculature of their patients. Persisting left atrial hypertension in 1 of 2 patients with pulmonary artery banding alone, suggested that atrial septal defect creation could have been beneficial at the time of the original banding. Stark *et al.* (1970) reported the results of banding of the pulmonary artery in 33 children with transposition and ventricular septal defect. At the time of surgery it was possible to lower the pulmonary arterial pressure to below 45 mm Hg in all 15 infants. Ten infants recatheterized after the operation had no evidence of progressive pulmonary vascular disease. In 6 of 18 children older than 1 year the pulmonary arterial pressure at surgery remained higher than 45 mm Hg distal to the band. In 6 recatheterized children, the pulmonary blood flow had decreased from preoperative levels and the ratio between pulmonary and systemic resistances had not changed significantly. The arterial oxygen saturation was decreased after banding of the pulmonary artery in 16 of 20 patients in whom it was measured. The au-

TABLE 16.14
DATA FROM BANDING OF THE PULMONARY ARTERY AND SURGICAL CREATION OF AN ATRIAL SEPTAL DEFECT [a]

Patient no.	Age	Hb	O₂ cap.	Blood O₂ saturation %								Pressures					
				SVC	RA	RV	Ao	PV	LA	LV	PA	RA	LA	RV	Ao	LV	PA
A. Hemodynamic data before and after procedure [b]																	
96	1 m	20.2	27.5	58	67	68	74	—	97	97	95	6	12	45/10	50/35	45/10	45/35
	1½ y	19.2	25.7	46	49	58	58	95	94	81	—	2	2	80/5	80/50	80/5	—
113	6 m	20.9	28.4	34	33	45	50	95	93	90	—	4	10	80/10	80/50	80/0	—
	7 m	13.4	18.1	50	64	67	69	91	92	81	—	3	2	80/0	80/5	75/0	—
B. Initial hemodynamic data obtained after procedure [c]																	
171	2 y	16.9	22.6	65	73	76	76	100	91	92	—	9	9	117/4	120/80	115/3	—
172	3½ y	16.6	22.5	56	60	55	65	97	70	84	—	5	5	110/0	110/60	110/0	—
173 [d]	6½ y	22.4	30.2	38	61	41	48	92	89	87	—	7	7	77/6	75/45	135/0	—

[a] Abbreviations same as in Tables 16.3 and 16.5.
[b] Two patients with ventricular septal defect.
[c] Three patients with ventricular septal defect.
[d] Patient 173: spontaneous closure of ventricular septal defect.

thors pointed out that pulmonary artery banding can prevent the development of pulmonary vascular disease in infants. In children older than 1 year, pulmonary vascular disease can be arrested at the stage it had reached at the time of banding of the pulmonary artery.

BAFFE'S PROCEDURE

Cardiac catheterization was carried out on 5 patients after the venous switching operation described by Baffe (1956) (Table 16.15). Two patients were in Group I, 2 in Group III, and 1 in Group IV. Preoperative studies were available on 1 patient in Group I and 1 patient in Group IV. More or less complete mixing of the systemic and pulmonary venous blood was evident in these patients. In 2 patients the aortic blood samples were more saturated with oxygen than pulmonary artery blood samples. The postoperative ratio between left and right ventricular systolic pressures in each of the 2 patients with an intact ventricular septum was less than 40%. Ventricular pressures were equal or near equal in the 3 patients in Groups III and IV. Postoperative cardiac catheterization on the patient in Group IV demonstrated an increase in the severity of left ventricular outflow tract obstruction.

Comparable hemodynamic findings on 17 children with partially corrected transposition were reported by Hastreiter *et al.* (1966). Almost complete mixing of the two blood streams occurred in all and in 4 the blood oxygen saturation in the aorta was actually higher than that in the pulmonary artery. The authors pointed out that when adequate surgical relief of cyanosis is accomplished, the future hemodynamic course appears to be determined by the type and size of the associated anatomic lesions. Children with an intact ventricular septum or a small ventricular septal defect did not develop pulmonary hypertension. Of their patients with larger ventricular septal defects, a considerable number had significant left ventricular outflow tract obstruction, which, in some, appeared to develop over the years. Seven of 14 cases with ventricular septal defect and no pulmonary stenosis developed a variable degree of pulmonary hypertension and 5 had a significant increase of pulmonary vascular resistance.

THE BLALOCK–TAUSSIG OR POTT'S ANASTOMOSIS

Cardiac catheterization after the Blalock-Taussig anastomosis was carried out on 1 patient in Group I, and after Pott's anastomosis on 1 patient in Group IV (Table 16.16). Preoperative hemodynamic studies were not obtained in both. At the time of surgery, which was performed

TABLE 16.15
BAFFE'S PROCEDURE [a]

Patient no.	Age	Hb	O₂ cap.	Blood O₂ saturation %								Pressures					
				SVC	RA	RV	Ao	PV	LA	LV	PA	RA	LA	RV	Ao	LV	PA
A. Hemodynamic data before and after procedure																	
62 [b]	4 y 4 m	—	—	—	34	48	48	—	—	94	—	6	4	80/0	80/50	35/0	—
	10 y	17.5	23.5	52	83	77	77	99	76	77	—	4	3	85/0	90/70	35/0	—
137 [c]	5 m	—	—	36	37	—	44	—	98	97	87	7	—	88/9	107/63	90/12	25/15
	6 y 5 m	18.7	25.2	53	64	71	71	98	—	—	66	7	—	100/0	100/70	100/0	12/7
B. Initial hemodynamic data after procedure																	
174 [b]	13 y 1 m	17.1	23	56	77	76	76	95	—	82	—	—	4	80/0	80/55	30/0	—
175 [d]	6 y 7 m	12.2	16.6	68	91	88	88	96	89	87	89	—	9	95/9	95/65	75/10	70/30
176 [d]	11 y 3 m	13.2	17.7	47	84	87	87	96	—	85	83	3	—	85/10	85/65	70/5	70/40

[a] Abbreviations same as in Tables 16.3 and 16.5.
[b] Patients with intact ventricular septum.
[c] Patient with ventricular septal defect and pulmonary stenosis.
[d] Patients with ventricular septal defect.

TABLE 16.16

Initial Hemodynamic Data after Blalock–Taussig, and Pott's Anastomosis [a]

Patient no.	Age	Hb	O₂ cap.	Blood O₂ saturation %								Pressures					
				SVC	RA	RV	Ao	PV	LA	LV	PA	RA	LA	RV	Ao	LV	PA
177 [b]	9 y 2 m	21.6	29	41	48	59	57	99	94	89	—	2	2	90/0	90/60	60/0	—
178 [c]	5 y 2 m	19.1	25.7	55	55	66	70	—	—	—	—	4	—	100/0	100/60	—	—

[a] Abbreviations same as in Tables 16.3 and 16.5.

[b] Blalock-Taussig. Intact septum. Biopsy; grade 3 PVD at 9 years 5 months.

[c] Pott's anastomosis; ventricular septal defect and pulmonary stenosis. Pulmonary artery pressure 90 mm Hg at thoracotomy at 5 years 3 months.

TABLE 16.17

Blood pH, P_{O_2} and P_{CO_2} of 8 Patients with an Intact Ventricular Septum [a]

Patient	Age	pH				P_{O_2} (mm Hg)				P_{CO_2} (mm Hg)			
		SVC	PV	Ao	LV-PA	SVC	PV	Ao	LV-PA	SVC	PV	Ao	LV-PA
1	1 d	—	7.37	7.26	—	—	—	20	—	—	21	35	—
2	5 d	—	7.44	7.36	—	—	108	18	—	—	26	33	—
3	1 y 11 m	—	7.39	7.37	—	—	100	51	—	—	35	38	—
4	1 y 2 m	7.35	7.39	7.38	7.37	28	96	40	53	40	31	36	34
5	1 y 4 m	7.37	7.44	7.41	—	30	114	38	—	46	30	43	—
6	1 y 9 m	7.40	7.41	7.37	7.38	32	94	41	54	46	37	42	39
7	8 y 10 m	—	7.39	7.36	—	—	109	27	—	—	29	31	—
8	13 y 1 m	7.368	7.395	7.385	7.375	37	93	44	51	37	32	34	35
Mean		7.37	7.40	7.35	7.375	32	102	35	53	42	30	36.5	36

[a] ASD, atrial septal defect; all other abbreviations same as in Tables 16.3 and 16.5.

Comments (Table 16.17):
- Patient 4: ASD created at 1 month
- Patient 5: ASD created at 2 weeks
- Patient 6: ASD created at 1 week
- Patient 8: Blalock-Taussig, at 4 years; Baffe's operation at 6 years

TABLE 16.18

BLOOD pH, P_{O_2} AND P_{CO_2} OF 7 PATIENTS WITH A VENTRICULAR SEPTAL DEFECT [a]

Patient	Age	pH				P_{O_2} (mm Hg)				P_{CO_2} (mm Hg)				Comments
		SVC	Ao	PV	LV-PA	SVC	Ao	PV	LV-PA	SVC	Ao	PV	LV-PA	
9	6 m	—	7.32	7.42	7.40	—	37	99	58	—	43	29	37	ASD created at 3 weeks
10	11 m	—	7.40	7.42	7.43	—	41	100	57	—	33	26	30	ASD created at 2 months
11	1 y 2 m	7.30	7.29	7.35	7.30	35	40	79	54	47	45	37	42	ASD created at 3 months
12	1 y 3 m	7.42	7.45	7.48	7.44	33	42	96	64	41	38	31	30	
13	2 y	—	7.38	7.41	—	—	38	91	—	—	47	34	—	ASD created at 4 months
14	2 y 11 m	7.31	7.30	7.44	—	31	34	82	—	36	38	28	—	
15	5 y 10 m	7.20	7.39	7.40	7.38	35	36	93	61	36	37	31	34	ASD created at 4½ years
Mean		7.307	7.36	7.41	7.39	33.5	38	91	59	40	40	31	34	

[a] ASD, atrial septal defect. All other abbreviations as in Tables 16.3 and 16.5.

TABLE 16.19

BLOOD pH, P_{O_2}, AND P_{CO_2} OF 4 PATIENTS WITH VENTRICULAR SEPTAL DEFECT AND PULMONARY STENOSIS [a]

Patient	Age	pH				P_{O_2} (mm Hg)				P_{CO_2} (mm Hg)				Comments
		SVC	Ao	PV	LV-PA	SVC	Ao	PV	LV-PA	SVC	Ao	PV	LV-PA	
16	8 m	—	7.365	7.415	7.395	—	14	70	43	—	28.5	17	24.5	ASD [b] created at 6 months
17	1 y 2 m	—	7.40	7.50	—	—	40	102	—	—	37	26	—	
18	3 y 9 m	—	7.38	7.46	—	—	24	93	—	—	45	30	—	
19	3 y 9 m	0	7.35	7.38	7.37	—	41	84	56	—	40	34.3	35.5	
Mean			7.37	7.44	7.38	—	30	87	49.5	—	37.5	27	30	

[a] Abbreviations same as in Tables 16.3 and 16.5.
[b] ASD, atrial septal defect.

at the age of 4 years, the ratio between left and right ventricular systolic pressures in the patient in Group I was 22%. This ratio had increased to 65% at cardiac catheterization performed at the age of 9 years and 2 months. Subsequently, a lung biopsy demonstrated grade 3 pulmonary vascular changes. The postoperative hemodynamic data on the patient in Group IV were incomplete but the systemic arterial oxygen saturation suggested fairly good mixing of the blood streams between the two circuits.

The Acid—Base Balance

The acid—base balance was studied in 19 patients in this series; 8 in Group 1, 7 in Group III, and 4 in Group IV. The results of this study were reported earlier by Shaher and Kidd (1967). Their age at cardiac catheterization ranged from 1 day to 13 years. An atrial septal defect had been surgically created earlier in life in 10, a Blalock—Taussig anastomosis performed in one, and a Baffe's operation in one. Blood samples were taken from the aorta and a pulmonary vein in each case, and, in addition, from the superior vena cava and left ventricle or pulmonary artery in 10. Samples were taken anaerobically in rapid succession into heparinized syringes and were analyzed within 5 minutes for pH, P_{O_2}, and P_{CO_2}. pH was measured using a microglass electrode, P_{O_2} using a Clark-type electrode, and P_{CO_2} using a modified Severinghaus electrode (Instrumentation Laboratories, Inc.). In addition, blood lactate and pyruvate levels were measured in systemic arterial blood in 10 of these 19 patients, using the enzymatic methods described by Scholz et al. (1959) and by Hess (1955). The normal ranges for this method in our laboratory are for pyruvate, 0.2 to 0.7 mg% (0.02–0.08 mEq/liter) and for lactate, 3–11 mg% (0.33–1.22 mEq/liter).

The results of the acid-base balance are given in Tables 16.17 to 16.19. In all three groups the pH of the systemic blood varied on the acid side of normal, while that from the pulmonary circuit was more alkaline. In all three groups the P_{CO_2} of the systemic blood was considerably higher than that in the pulmonary circulation. The mean pH in the 3 groups was: Superior vena cava (SVC), 7.34 ± 0.22; Aorta (Ao), 7.36 ± 014; pulmonary vein (PV), 7.42 ± 0.025; pulmonary artery—left ventricle (PA-LV), 7.39 ± 0.012. Mean P_{CO_2} was: SVC, 41.1 ± 4.3; Ao, 38.4 ± 4.7; PV, 29.7 ± 5.0; PA-LV, 34.2 ± 4.7. The mean P_{O_2} was: SVC, 32.6 ± 2.8; Ao, 35.1 ± 9.6; PV, 94.6 ± 10.7; PA-LV, 55.1 ± 5.4.

The results of lactate and pyruvate measurements are given in Table

TABLE 16.20
BLOOD LACTATES AND PYRUVATES [a]

Patient	Lactate (mg %)	Pyruvate (mg %)	Ratio	P_{O_2}
1	38.25	1.858	20.61	20
2	92.022	3.371	27.3	18
3	6.00	0.410	14.6	51
5	5.051	0.537	9.4	38
6	6.063	0.476	12.9	41
8	6.563	0.330	19.9	44
9	8.313	0.641	12.7	37
11	3.250	0.378	8.4	40
15	6.313	0.376	16.7	36
19	8.813	0.732	12.0	41

[a] Samples from systemic artery.

16.20. The results were within normal limits except in patients 1 and 2. They were the youngest patients and were clinically the most severely ill.

The systemic arterial oxygen saturation and the mean left atrial pressure are given in Table 16.21. In Group I, the systemic arterial oxygen saturation varied from 21 to 76%, with an average of 62%. In Group III, the systemic arterial saturation varied from 53 to 73%, with an aver-

TABLE 16.21
LEFT ATRIAL PRESSURE AND SYSTEMIC ARTERIAL OXYGEN SATURATION

Patient	Left atrial pressure	Systemic arterial saturation
1	8	21
2	5	33
3	5	79
4	4	70
5	2	67
6	8	70
7	2	57
8	4	76
9	8.5	53
10	9	73
11	5	64
12	7.5	65
13	5	66
14	5	62
15	2	70
16	4	40
17	6	70
18	13	38
19	7	63

age of 65%. In Group IV, the systemic arterial saturation varied from 38 to 70%, with an average of 53%. Apart from patient 18, the mean left atrial pressure in all remaining 18 patients was normal.

Sunico et al. (1960) measured the acid–base balance in the systemic circuit of 14 patients with complete transposition of the great arteries securing, however, a sample from the pulmonary vein in only 1 of them. Gootman et al. (1963) reported a study in 4 patients with cyanotic congenital heart disease, 1 of whom had transposition of the great arteries. All had in common a markedly reduced effective pulmonary blood flow and pulmonary venous blood samples were obtained in each case.

Regardless of the anatomy of the associated defects in each patient in this series, the systemic arterial sample had a lower pH and a higher P_{CO_2} than that obtained from the pulmonary veins. From the point of view of the pulmonary venous blood, therefore, hyperventilation is implied. Since the systemic arterial P_{CO_2} and pH in complete transposition result from the admixture of a large amount of systemic venous blood with a low pH and P_{O_2} and high P_{CO2} with a small amount of pulmonary venous blood (effective flow) with a high pH and P_{O_2} and low P_{CO_2} which has crossed through the associated defects, the hyperventilation helps to maintain a normal systemic arterial acid-base status or only slightly toward the acid side. The hyperventilation may thus be considered as a barely effective respiratory compensation for systemic acidosis. It is similarly obvious that the pulmonary arterial P_{CO_2} and pH result from the admixture of a large amount of pulmonary venous blood with a small amount of systemic venous blood which has crossed through the associated defects.

Huckabee (1958) has shown that anaerobic tissue metabolism begins to assume significance at systemic arterial P_{O_2} levels below 35 mm Hg. At these levels the lactic acid–pyruvic acid relationship is disturbed, resulting in a greater proportion of lactic acid. This is supported by the present series in that patients 1 and 2 with the lowest arterial P_{CO_2} had the highest lactates and lactate/pyruvate ratios.

Talner and his co-workers (1965) studied the acid–base balance in the systemic circuit of 20 patients with congenital heart disease who were in heart failure. Three of these patients had transposition of the great arteries. They concluded that the occurrence of systemic acidosis in these cases must be respiratory in origin since all the patients they studied shared the features of large pulmonary blood flow and pulmonary congestion. They suggested that pulmonary congestion, giving rise to diminished lung compliance and airway obstruction, produced respiratory acidosis.

The data from the present series shows that the pulmonary venous P_{CO_2} was low in all cases, suggesting that there was no abnormality in the gaseous exchange mechanisms at the alveolar-capillary level. In addition, pulmonary venous congestion, as evidenced by mean left atrial pressure, was absent in 18 patients. Patient 18, with mildly elevated left atrial pressure, had pulmonary stenosis. Heart failure and pulmonary venous congestion, however, might be expected to increase the abnormalities in the systemic circuit in patients with complete transposition of the great arteries through the mechanism described.

The patients in this series are not truly representative of the entire spectrum of cases with transposition of the great arteries, a large number of whom present early in life with a much more severe disturbance than is demonstrated here. These data present the picture in those children who, because of associated defects—either surgical or congenital—and presumably larger effective pulmonary blood flow, have survived infancy. The disturbance in the severely ill group is likely to be of the same nature but more grave (i.e., with more acidosis in the systemic and more alkalosis in the pulmonary circulation) because of lack of sufficient communication between the two circulations, and complicated by a lactic acidosis due to hypoxia, and congestive heart failure.

The Hemodynamics and Pulmonary Vascular Disease in Transposition

Various authors have commented on the high incidence of pulmonary hypertension in patients with transposition and ventricular septal defect (Shaher and Kidd, 1968; Watson, 1969; Plauth *et al.*, 1970). In this series 90% of Group III patients had pulmonary hypertension at or near systemic levels. The size of the defect alone or the common ejectile force, suggested by Ferencz (1966), cannot be the only factor, since among autopsied cases in this series with pulmonary hypertension at systemic levels a small defect that measured 3 mm or less was found in 4 (Tables 16.5 and 16.12). Such high incidence of pulmonary hypertension has not been reported in isolated ventricular septal defects. According to Keith *et al.* (1967), only 27.5% of patients with an isolated ventricular septal defect develop this complication. Mild-to-moderate pulmonary hypertension is also a feature of patients with an intact ventricular septum during the first few months of life. After this age mild elevation of left ventricular pressure persists in the majority. Indeed, it was the exception rather than the rule to find left ventricular pressures as low as the normal right ventricular pressure in any age group.

From the nature of the two separate blood circuits in transposition, communications between them, like ventricular septal defect or a patent ductus arteriosus, unless very small, will allow the blood to pile up in the pulmonary circuit until the pressures are equalized. This mechanism, suggested by Taussig (1960), probably accounts for the occurrence of pulmonary hypertension at or near systemic levels in the majority of patients with a ventricular septal defect. Patients with an intact ventricular septum and a patent ductus arteriosus behave similarly; a large ductus will give rise to pulmonary hypertension at systemic levels. A smaller ductus, which may not alter the pulmonary arterial pressure in the normal circulation, might elevate the pulmonary arterial pressure in transposition.

Review of the lung sections studied in this series shows that the highest incidence of severe pulmonary vascular obstruction occurred among patients with a ventricular septal defect. Almost all patients above the age of 1 year in this group had severe pulmonary vascular disease. Patients with intact ventricular septa also developed pulmonary vascular disease but less frequently than those with a ventricular septal defect. Pulmonary vascular disease was least common in patients with a ventricular septal defect and pulmonary stenosis, although one of the patients in this series with pulmonary subvalvular diaphragm developed pulmonary hypertension and grade 4 pulmonary vascular changes (Table 16.11) Newfeld *et al.* (1972) correlated the pulmonary vasculature with the hemodynamic findings in patients with transposition. Patients with normal pulmonary artery pressures had either normal vessels, Grade 1 or at most Grade 2 changes. With an intact ventricular septum, only 8 patients showed pulmonary vessel changes greater than Grade 2; 2 Grade 3, and 6 Grade 4. In contrast, with a large ventricular septal defect, Grade 3 and 4 changes were found as early as 6 months of age and were the rule over 1 year. However, of 36 infants under 6 months of age with a large ventricular septal defect, only 1 had Grade 4 and 5 had Grade 3 changes. These findings suggest that the major determinants of pulmonary obstructive disease in transposition are pulmonary arterial hypertension and increased pulmonary blood flow. As pointed out by Ferencz (1966) the impact upon the pulmonary vascular bed of the increased blood flow or a high pressure does not explain fully the gravity of pulmonary arterial disease noted in patients with transposition. Both of these effects can be present in patients with other malformations in whom the pulmonary arterial changes remain more benign. She suggested that in transposition the impact of these influences is aggravated by pulmonary vasoconstriction secondary to anoxia and an elevated pulmonary venous pressure. She pointed out that the work of Enson *et al.* (1964) suggests that the vasomotor response is affected by an increase in hydrogen ion concentration and that the sensitivity of the pulmonary arterial pressure to systemic arterial unsaturation is enhanced at low pH levels. The occurrence of metabolic acidosis in cyanotic infants has been demonstrated by Gootman *et al.* (1963), and in infants with transposition by Shaher and Kidd (1967). Significant elevation of the left atrial pressure is present in some neonates with transposition. After this period, because of palliative surgery, or the presence of a large foramen ovale, most patients have no significant elevation of the left atrial pressure. In this series, the left atrial pressure was normal in all patients who had severe pulmonary vascular obstruction. As pointed out by Ferencz (1966) the normal appearance of the pulmonary veins of these patients suggests that pulmonary venous obstruction is not a major factor in the genesis of the elevated arterial resistance.

The variability of pulmonary vascular disease was examined by Ferencz *et al.* (1971) in patients with atrial septal defect, total anomalous pulmonary venous drainage, ventricular septal defect, and transposition of the great arteries. A progression of "malignancy" pattern was apparent in the diagnostic sequence. Arterial injury was rare in atrial septal defect and occurred occasionally in anomalous venous return and significantly more frequently in ventricular septal defect. In transposition, arterial injury appeared earlier and was more severe than in the other groups. When a ventricular septal defect was associated with transposition, there was a greater incidence of advanced lesions. The severity of pulmonary vascular disease was not clearly related to the levels of pulmonary vascular resistance as judged by clinical or physiologic means. The authors pointed out that anoxia, a cardial feature of transposition, is also present in patients with anomalous pulmonary venous return. Yet the vascular changes are severe in one and benign in the other. From this point of view anoxia is unlikely to be a factor of major significance. They added that the effect of pulmonary venous obstruction appears to be protective with regard to intimal fibrosis except in mitral regurgitation. Since hemodynamic variables provided no explanation for the difference in vulnerability to injury of the arterial bed, knowledge to the vasoconstrictive effect of acidosis suggests that the total internal environment must be considered in the search for a constellation of pathogenetic factors which affect the nature of vascular response to mechanical derangement. Fascinating as this theory may be, it is worthy of note that most of their patients with total anomalous drainage were older than 6 months of age. From this point of view, it seems unlikely that pulmonary hypertension, severe anoxia, pulmonary venous obstruction, and acidosis were a feature of most of these patients. In contrast, most or all of these features occur in transposition. Moreover, their observation that there was a high incidence of pulmonary vascular damage in ventricular septal defect as compared to atrial septal defect emphasizes the role of pulmonary hypertension in the production of pulmonary arteriolar injury.

References

Abbott, M. E. (1936). "Atlas of Congenital Cardiac Disease." American Heart Association, New York.

Aberdeen, E., and Carr, I. (1968). Transposition of the great arteries. In "Modern Trends in Cardiac Surgery." (E. Aberdeen, and G. H. Wooler, eds.). Vol. 2, p. 182. Butterworth, London.

Abrams, H. L., Kaplan, H. S., and Purdy, A. (1951). Diagnosis of complete transposition of the great vessels. Radiology 57, 500.

Astley, R., and Parsons, S. (1952). Complete transposition of the great vessels. Brit. Heart J. 14, 13.

Baffe, T. G. (1956). A new method for surgical correction of transposition of the aorta and pulmonary artery. Surg. Gynecol. Obstet. 102, 227.

Baker, F., Baker, L., Zoltun, R., and Zuberbuhler, J. R. (1971). Effectiveness of the Rashkind procedure in transposition of the great arteries in infants. Circulation 43 (Suppl. 1), 1.

Becker, M. C., and Brill, R. M. (1948). Complete transposition of the great vessels. Arch. Pediat. 65, 249.

Black, I. F. S. (1972). Floating a catheter into the pulmonary artery in transposition. Amer. Heart J. 84, 761.

Blalock, A., and Hanlon, C. R. (1950). The surgical treatment of complete transposition of the aorta and the pulmonary artery. Surg. Gynecol. Obstet. 90, 1.

Brown, R., Rahimtoola, S. H., Davis, G. D., and Swan, H. J. C. (1965). The effect of angiocardiographic contrast medium on circulatory dynamics in man; cardiac output during angiocardiography. Circulation 31, 234.

Burchell, H. B. (1966). Some hemodynamic problems in transposition of the great vessels. Circulation 33, 181.

Campbell, J. A., Bing, R. J., Handelsman, J. C., Griswold, H. E., and Hammond, M. (1949). Physiologic studies in congenital heart disease. Physiologic findings in two patients with complete transposition of the great vessels. Bull. Johns Hopkins Hosp. 84, 269.

Campbell, M., and Suzman, S. (1951). Transposition of the aorta and pulmonary artery. Circulation 4, 329.

Carr, I. (1971). Timing of bidirectional atrial shunts in transposition of the great arteries and atrial septal defect. Circulation 44 (Suppl. 2), 70.

Carr, I., and Wells, B. (1966). Coaxial flow-guided catheterization of the pulmonary artery in transposition of the great vessels. Lancet ii, 318.

Celermajer, J. M., Venables, A. W., and Bowdler, J. D. (1970). Catheterization of the pulmonary artery in transposition of the great vessels. Circulation 41, 1053.

Cleland, W. P., Goodwin, J. F., Steiner, R. E., and Zoob, M. (1957). Transposition of the aorta and pulmonary artery with pulmonary stenosis. Amer. Heart J. 54, 10.

Deuchar, D. C. (1962). Personal communications.

Dobell, A. R. C., Gibbons, J. E., and Busse, E. F. G. (1969). Hemodynamic correction of transposition of the great vessels in infants. *J. Thorac. Cardiovasc. Surg.* 57, 108–114.

Ebel, E. H., and Lynxwiller, C. P. (1951). Complete transposition of the great vessels with patent ductus arteriosus and patent foramen ovale. *Arch. Pediat.* 68, 51.

Edwards, J. E. (1960). Cited by Taussig (1960).

Edwards, W. S., Bargeron, L. M., Jr., and Lyons, C. (1964). Reposition of right pulmonary veins in transposition of great vessels. *J. Amer. Med. Ass.* 188, 522.

Enson, Y., Giuntini, C., Lewis, M. L., Morris, T. Q., Ferrer, M. I., and Harvey, R. H. (1964). The influence of hydrogen ion concentration and hypoxia on the pulmonary circulation. *J. Clin. Invest.* 43, 1146.

Ferencz, C. (1966). Transposition of the great vessels. Pathophysiologic considerations based upon a study of the lungs. *Circulation* 33, 232.

Ferencz, C., Greco, J. M., and Libi-SyLora, M. (1971). Variability of pulmonary vascular disease in certain malformations of the heart. *In* "The Natural History and Progress in Treatment of Congenital Heart Defects." (B. S. L. Kidd and J. D. Keith, eds.), p. 300. Charles C. Thomas, Springfield, Illinois.

Fowler, R. E. L., and Ordway, N. K. (1952). Circulatory dynamics in complete transposition of the great vessels. Physiologic considerations with report of 4 cases. *Amer. J. Dis. Child.* 83, 414.

Gootman, N. L., Scarpelli, E. M., and Rudolph, A. M. (1963). Metabolic acidosis—cyanotic heart disease. *Pediatrics* 31, 251.

Gotsman, M. S. (1965). Creation of an atrial septal defect in transposition of the great vessels. *Thorax* 20, 574–578.

Graham, T. P., Jarmakani, J. M., Canent, R. V., Jr., and Jewett, P. H. (1971). Quantitation of left heart volume and systolic output in transposition of the great arteries. *Circulation* 44, 899–909.

Hastreiter, A. R., Serratto, M., Arevalo, F., and Miller, R. A. (1966). Long-term hemodynamic studies in postoperative patients with transposition of the great vessels. Results of the venous switching operation. *Circulation* 33, 34.

Helwig, J., Jr. (1966). Transposition of the great vessels. *In* "Intravascular Catheterization" (H. A. Zimmerman, Ed.) 2nd Ed., p. 773. Thomas, Springfield, Illinois.

Hess, B. (1955). Bemerkungen zur bestimmung der Brenztraubensaure in menschlichen serum. *Klin. Wochenscho.* 33, 450.

Huckabee, W. E. (1958). Relationship of pyruvate and lactate in hypoxia. III. Effects of breathing low oxygen gases. *J. Clin. Invest.* 37, 264.

Hurley, P. J., Strauss, H. W., and Wagner, H. N., Jr. (1970). Radionuclide angiocardiography in cyanotic congenital heart disease. *Johns Hopkins Med. J.* 127, 46.

Jarmakani, M. M., Edwards, S. B., Spach, M. S., Cannent, R. V., Jr., Capp, M. P., Hagan, M. J., Barr, R. C., and Jain, V. (1968). Left ventricular pressure volume characteristics in congenital heart disease. *Circulation* 37, 879.

Keith, J. D., Rowe, R. D., and Vlad, P. (1958). "Heart Disease in Infancy and Childhood," 1st Ed. MacMillan, New York.

Keith, J. D., Rowe, R. D., and Vlad, P. (1967). "Heart Disease in Infancy and Childhood," 2nd Ed. MacMillan, New York.

Kelly, D. T., Krovetz, L. J., and Rowe, R. D. (1971). Double-lumen flotation catheter for use in complex congenital cardiac anomalies. *Circulation* 44, 910.

Kjellberg, S. R., Mannheimer, E., and Rudhe, U. (1959). "Diagnosis of Congenital Heart Disease," 2nd Ed. Year Book Publ., Chicago, Illinois.

Lenkei, S. C., Swan, H. J. C., and DuShane, J. W. (1959). Transposition of the great vessels with atrial septal defect. A haemodynamic study of two cases. *Circulation* 20, 842.

Li, M. D., Collins, G., Disenhouse, R., and Keith, J. D. (1969). Spontaneous closure of ventricular septal defect. *Can. Med. Ass. J.* 100, 737.

Lillehei, C. W., and Varco, R. L. (1953). Certain physiologic, pathologic and surgical features of complete transposition of the great vessels. *Surgery* 34, 376.

McElroy, J. W., Davis, J. P., and Michelson, R. P. (1947). Complete transposition of the arterial trunks with closed interventricular septum. *Ann. Intern. Med.* 27, 308.

Mair, D. D., and Ritter, D. G. (1972). Factors influencing intercirculatory mixing in patients with complete transposition of the great arteries. *Amer. J. Cardiol.* 30, 653.

Mair, D. D., Ritter, D. G., Ongley, P. A., and Helmholz, H. F. (1971). Hemodynamics and evaluation for surgery of patients with complete transposition of the great arteries and ventricular septal defect. *Amer. J. Cardiol.* 28, 632–640.

Mullins, C. E., Neches, W. H., Reitman, M. J., El-Said, G., and Riopel, D. A (1972). Retrograde technique for catheterization of the pulmonary artery in transposition of the great arteries with ventricular septal defect. *Amer. J. Cardiol.* 30, 385.

Newfeld, E. A., Muster, A. J., and Paul, M. (1972). The pulmonary vascular bed in complete transposition. Hemodynamic–pathologic correlations. *Circulation* 46, Suppl. 2, 97.

Noonan, A., Nadas, A. S., Rudolph, A. M., and Harris, G. B. C. (1960). Transposition of the great arteries. A correlation of clinical, physiologic and autopsy data. *N. Engl. J. Med.* 263, 592.

Parsons, C. G., Astley, R., Burrows, R. G. O., and Singh, S. P. (1971). Transposition of the great arteries. A study of 65 infants followed for 1 to 4 years after balloon septostomy. *Brit. Heart J.* 33, 725.

Paul, M. H. (1971). Transposition of the great arteries: physiologic data. *In* "The Natural History and Progress in Treatment of Congenital Heart Defects." (B. S. L. Kidd and J. D. Keith, eds.), p. 144. Charles C. Thomas, Springfield, Illinois.

Pickering, D., McDonald, P., and Kidd, B. S. L. (1972). Catheterization of the pulmonary artery in transposition of the great arteries: A new technique. *Pediatrics* 47, 1068.

Plauth, W. H., Jr., Nadas, A. S., Bernhard, W. F., and Fyler, D. C. (1970). Changing hemodynamics in patients with transposition of the great arteries. *Circulation* 42, 131.

Rahimtoola, S. H., Ongley, P. A., and Swan, H. J. C. (1966). Percutaneous suprasternal puncture (Radner technique) of the pulmonary artery in transposition of the great vessels. *Circulation* 33, 242.

Rashkind, W. (1971). Shunting at the ventricular level in transposition of the great vessels. *Circulation* 44 (Suppl. 2), 71.

Rashkind, W. J., and Miller, W. W. (1968). Transposition of the great arteries. Results of palliation by balloon atrioseptostomy in thirty-two infants. *Circulation* 38, 453.

Rudolph, A. M., and Cayler, G. G. (1958). Cardiac catheterization in infants and children. *Pediat. Clin. N. Amer.* 5, 907.

Scholz, R., Schmitz, H., Bucher, T., and Lampen, J. D. (1959). Über die Wirkung von Nystatin auf Bacherhafe. *Biochem. Z.* 31, 71.

Shaher, R. M. (1964). The haemodynamics of complete transposition of the great vessels. *Brit. Heart J.* 26, 343.

Shaher, R. M., and Kidd, L. (1966). Hemodynamics of complete transposition of the great vessels before and after the creation of an atrial septal defect. *Circulation* **33**, 3–12.

Shaher, R. M., and Kidd, L. (1967). Acid-base balance in complete transposition of the great vessels. *Brit. Heart J.* **29**, 207.

Shaher, R. M., and Kidd, L. (1968). Effect of ventricular septal defect and patent ductus arteriosus on left ventricular pressure in complete transposition of the great vessels. *Circulation* **37**, 232.

Shaher, R. M., Fowler, R. S., Kidd, B. S. L., Moes, C. A. F., and Keith, J. D. (1965). Spontaneous closure of a ventricular septal defect in a case of complete transposition of the great vessels. *Can. Med. Ass. J.* **93**, 1037.

Shaher, R. M., Farina, M. A., and Bishop, M. (1973) . Long survival in a patient with complete transposition of the great vessels. *N. Y. State J. Med.* In press.

Smith, C., Rowe, R. D., and Vlad, P. (1958). Sedation of children for cardiac catheterization with an ataractic mixture. *Can. Anaesth. Soc. J.* **3**, 35.

Stanger, P., Heymann, M. A., Hoffman, J. I. E., and Rudolph, A. M. (1972). Use of the Swan-Ganz catheter in cardiac catheterization of infants and children. *Amer. Heart J.* **83**, 749.

Stark, J., Tynan, M., Tatooles, C. J., Aberdeen, E., and Waterston, D. J. (1970). Banding of the pulmonary artery for transposition of the great arteries and ventricular septal defect. *Circulation* **41** (Suppl. 2), 116.

Sunico, R. M., Harned, H., Jr., and Ordway, N. K. (1960). Respiratory acidosis in transposition of the great vessels. *Amer. J. Dis. Child.* **100**, 531.

Swan, H. J. C., Ganz, W., Forrester, J., Marcus, H., Diamond, G., and Chonette, D. (1970) . Catheterization of the heart in man with use of a flow-directed balloon-tipped catheter. *New Engl. J. Med.* **283**, 447.

Talner, N. S., Sanyal, S. K., Halloran, K. H., Gardner, T. H., and Ordway, N. K. (1965). Congestive heart failure in infancy. I. Abnormalities in blood gases and acid-base equilibrium. *Pediatrics* **35**, 20.

Taussig, H. (1960). "Congenital Malformation of the Heart," 2nd Ed. The Commonwealth Fund, New York.

Tynan, M. (1972). Transposition of the great arteries. Changes in circulation after birth. *Circulation* **46**, 809.

Tynan, M., Carr, I., Graham, G., and Carter, R. E. B. (1969). Subvalvular pulmonary obstruction complicating the postoperative course of balloon atrial septostomy in transposition of the great arteries. *Circulation* **39**, 223.

Watson, H. (1969). Palliative procedures for transposition of the great arteries. *Brit. Heart J.* **31**, 407.

Wood, P. (1956). "Diseases of the Heart and Circulation," 2nd Ed. Eyre & Spottiswoode, London.

Chapter 17

ANGIOCARDIOGRAPHY

Castellanos *et al.* (1938) were the first to use angiocardiography in the diagnosis of congenital heart disease and were able to diagnose complete transposition of the great arteries during life in a 13-day-old baby. A postmortem angiocardiographic study was done under fluoroscopy with injection of the contrast medium into the left ventricle. This resulted in opacification of the pulmonary artery, the left atrium, and the pulmonary veins. Injection of a larger quantity of the contrast medium resulted in its passage through the ventricular septal defect with opacification of the right ventricle, right atrium, and aorta. In 1947, Castellanos *et al.* correlated angiocardiographic appearances with postmortem examinations and concluded that the diagnosis of complete transposition is absolutely impossible without the former technique. In 1953, Rushmer *et al.* used cineangiocardiography to establish the diagnosis of transposition of the great arteries. It is generally agreed that immediate and massive filling of the anteriorly situated aorta takes place from the right ventricle (Castellanos *et al.*, 1938; Goodwin *et al.*, 1949; Kreutzer *et al.*, 1950; Campbell and Hills, 1950; Abramson, 1950; Keith and Munn, 1950; Dotter and Steinberg, 1951; Abrams *et al.*, 1951; Cooley and Sloan, 1952; Astley and Parsons, 1952; Gasul *et al.*, 1953; Keith *et al.*, 1958). In addition, there is no diminution in the density of the contrast medium in the aorta when compared to that in the right ventricle (Dotter and Steinberg, 1951). According to these authors, the aortic arch, as seen in the lateral view, is wider than normal. In this projection, the right ventricular origin of the aorta is best demonstrated (Cooley and Sloan, 1952; Keith, 1954). In the anteroposterior view, the ascending aorta may be situated at the right cardiac border (Castellanos *et al.*, 1950; Keith *et al.*, 1958), may have a median position (Astley and Parsons, 1952; Abrams and Kaplan, 1956), or may be situated at the left cardiac border in the position normally occupied by the main pulmonary artery (Goodwin *et al.*, 1949; Campbell and Hills, 1950; Castellanos *et al.*, 1950; Campbell and Suzman, 1951; Astley and Parsons, 1952; Goodwin et al., 1953; Gyllensward and Lodin, 1954; Keith, et al., 1958; Shaher et al., 1967a). Keith et al. (1958) pointed out that whereas normally the aortic valve is situated at the level of the 7th thoracic vertebra, in transposition it is usually situated at the level of the 4th thoracic vertebra. According to De Groot (1951) and Abrams and Kaplan (1956) there is poor opacification of the pulmonary artery at the time of visualization of the aorta especially in the presence of pulmonary stenosis, and Goodwin et al. (1953) stressed the posterior situation of this vessel. Cooley and Sloan (1952) pointed out that pulmonary stenosis is usually difficult to demonstrate in transposition. By injecting contrast media in the left atrium, Gyllenward and Lodin (1954) demonstrated the left ventricular origin of the pulmonary artery, and these workers as well as Keith et al. (1958), stressed that injection of such media in the left side of the heart is the method of choice for demonstrating this vessel. According to Cooley and Sloan (1952, 1956) a feature of transposition without pulmonary stenosis is the presence of large pulsating pulmonary vessels which fill with small amounts of dye. The right atrium and the right ventricle are invariably grossly enlarged, and thickening of the right ventricular wall may be evident (Abrams and Kaplan, 1956). According to Abrams and Kaplan (1956) and Gasul et al. (1957) left ventricular enlargement can be assessed by considering the size of the unopacified area posterior to the right ventricle. Cooley and Sloan (1952, 1956), Gasul et al. (1953), and Ingomar and Tersley (1962) pointed out that it is usually difficult on angiocardiography to detect the site of the shunt and to estimate its size; interatrial communications are usually difficult to demonstrate unless exceptionally large. Cooley and Sloan (1952, 1956) and Keith (1954) pointed out that in the presence of a ventricular septal defect direct opacification of the left ventricle from the right ventricle, or a stream of dye passing toward the pulmonary artery from the right ventricle may be observed. According to Keith et al. (1958) all cases with a demonstrable ductus have a shunt from the aorta to the pulmonary artery even in the presence of preductal coarctation. In 1966, Elliott et al. studied the angiocardiographic coronary arterial patterns in transposition complexes and concluded that angiocardiography may be a valuable aid in differentiating one form of transposition from the other. Shaher et al. (1967a) studied the angiograms of patients with complete transposition and left ventricular outflow tract obstruction and recognized three types of subvalvular pulmonary stenosis. Recently, Hallermann et al. (1970) and Deutsch et al. (1970) demonstrated that continuity between the pulmonary and mitral valves could be demonstrated by means of angiocardiography and pointed out that this sign was particularly helpful in differentiating between transposition of the great arteries and other anomalies of the heart. Wesselhoeft *et al.* (1972) used nuclear angiocardiography with a gamma camera, a pinhole collimator, and 99mTc pertechnetate to diagnose transposition of the great arteries. The superior vena cava, right atrium, and right ventricle outline normally, but no pulmonary artery is seen in its normal position. Instead, the clear space which normally exists between the superior vena cava and the pulmonary artery fills immediately after the right ventricle, representing the aorta. In the lateral view the great vessel arising from the anterior ventricle passes down into the abdomen. The left atrium and ventricle outline before the lung phase via the right to left intracardiac shunt. The pulmonary artery is faintly outlined after left ventricular filling and a faint activity is observed in the lungs after pulmonary arterial filling.

Material

The angiocardiograms of 184 patients in this series were available for study; 88 in Group I, 6 in Group II, 65 in Group III, and 25 in Group IV. Angiograms in the anteroposterior and lateral projections were available for all. Selective angiography with injection of the contrast medium into the cardiac chambers was performed in 146 cases. Of these 146, additional angiograms of the ascending aorta were obtained in 22. In the remaining 38 cases, a venous angiogram was obtained and the contrast medium was injected into the superior or inferior vena cava. In 1 patient in this series there was dextrocardia with solitus atria (Fig. 17.1). The findings in 184 angiocardiograms were evaluated as follows.

1. Size of the ventricle
2. Position of the ventricles
3. Position of the aorta to the pulmonary artery
4. Size of the aorta and pulmonary artery
5. Height of the aortic to the pulmonary valves
6. Position of the aortic arch
7. Associated findings
   a. Ventricular septal defect
   b. Atrial septal defect
   c. Patent ductus arteriosus
   d. Left ventricular outflow tract obstruction
   e. Coarctation of the aorta and complete interruption of the aortic arch
   f. The bronchial circulation

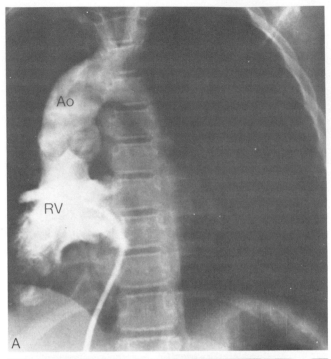

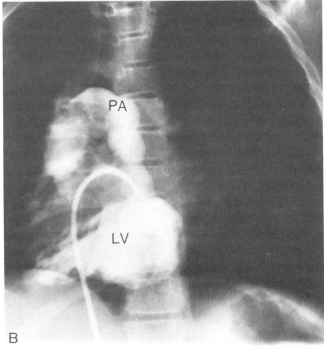

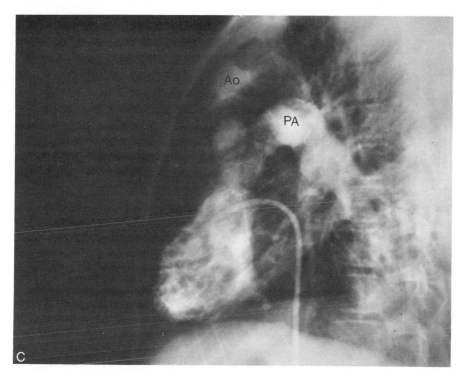

Fig. 17.1. Complete transposition of the great arteries, ventricular septal defect, and pulmonary stenosis in dextrocardia with solitus atria. (A) Aorta arises from right ventricle. (B) Pulmonary artery smaller than aorta arises from the left ventricle. Note poststenotic dilatation of the right pulmonary artery. (C) Left ventricular angiogram in the lateral position demonstrating anterior aorta and posterior pulmonary artery. Ao, aorta; PA, pulmonary artery; RV, right ventricle; LV, left ventricle.

General Findings

Following opacification of the inferior or superior vena cava there was usually opacification of an enlarged right atrium and right ventricle. In all patients with the exception of 2 in this series, the right ventricle lay anterior or anterior and to the right of the left ventricle. In 2 patients, a side to side relationship existed between the ventricles (Fig. 17.2). In most patients the right ventricle appeared smaller than the left ventricle but in

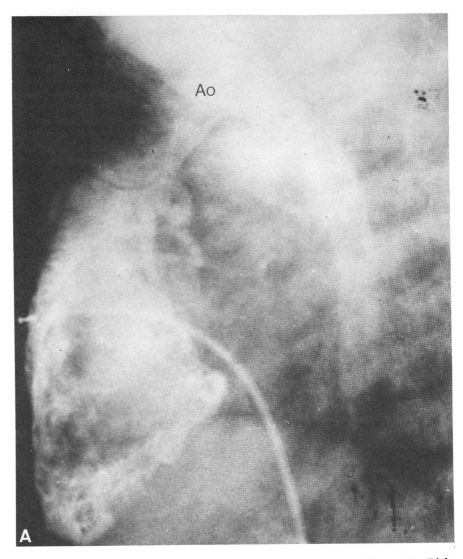

Fig. 17.2. Side by side relationship of the ventricles in transposition. (A) **Right** ventricular angiogram in the lateral position opacifies aorta (Ao). (B) Left ventricular angiogram in the lateral position opacifies pulmonary artery (PA).

some the two ventricles appeared equal in size or the right larger than the left. In a few patients there was hypoplasia of the right ventricle. The aorta arises from the right ventricle and is anteriorly situated (Fig. 17.3). In some patients it coursed upward to the right of the thoracic spine and

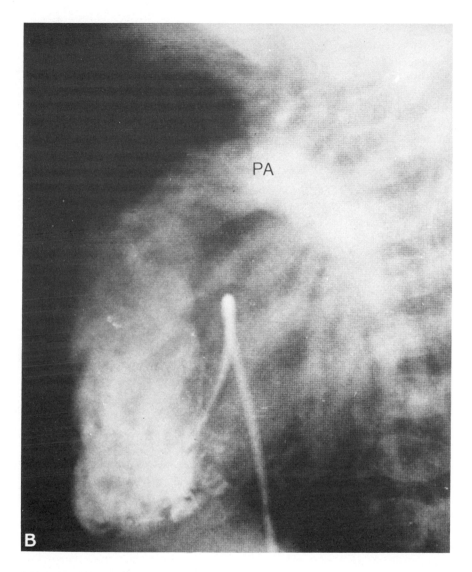

then arched downward to become continuous with the descending thoracic aorta. In other patients, the ascending aorta coursed vertically upward directly in front of the thoracic spine and then arched downward and continued as the descending thoracic aorta. In a few patients, especially those with left ventricular outflow tract obstruction, the origin of the aorta lay to the left of the thoracic spine (Fig. 17.4). The aortic arch is almost always on the left side. Only 4 patients in this series had a right

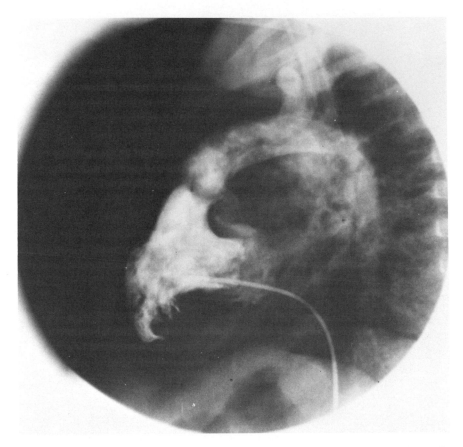

Fig. 17.3. Right ventricular angiogram in the lateral position demonstrating anterior origin of the aorta.

aortic arch. Because the amount of contrast medium that reaches the pulmonary artery through the associated defects is small, the levogram is usually of a poor quality. For good visualization of the left side of the heart and the pulmonary artery, injection of the contrast medium into the left atrium or ventricle is mandatory (Fig. 17.5). The left atrium appears enlarged in most patients. The left ventricle is also enlarged and in this series it was situated posterior and to the left of the right ventricle in all cases but two. It is usually possible to demonstrate by angiocardiography the continuity between the mitral and pulmonary valves. The pulmonary artery arises from the left ventricle and is always posterior to the aorta. Unless left ventricular outflow tract obstruction is associated, the aorta

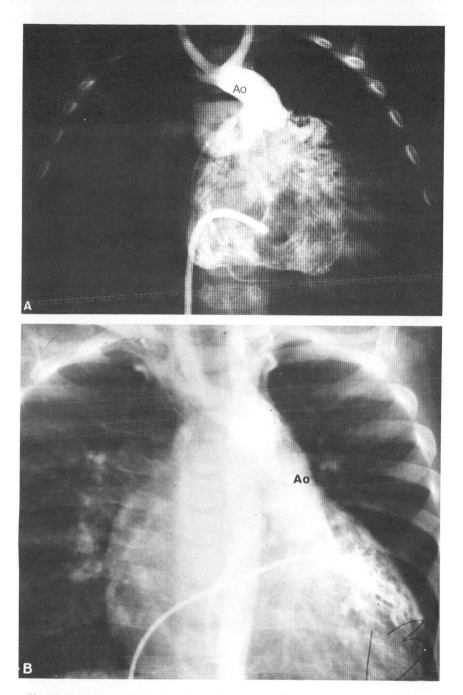

Fig. 17.4. Aorta (Ao) forming the left upper cardiac border in transposition. (A) Intact ventricular septum and patent ductus. (B) Intact ventricular septum and left ventricular outflow tract obstruction. (C) Ventricular septal defect. (D) Ventricular septal defect and left ventricular outflow tract obstruction.

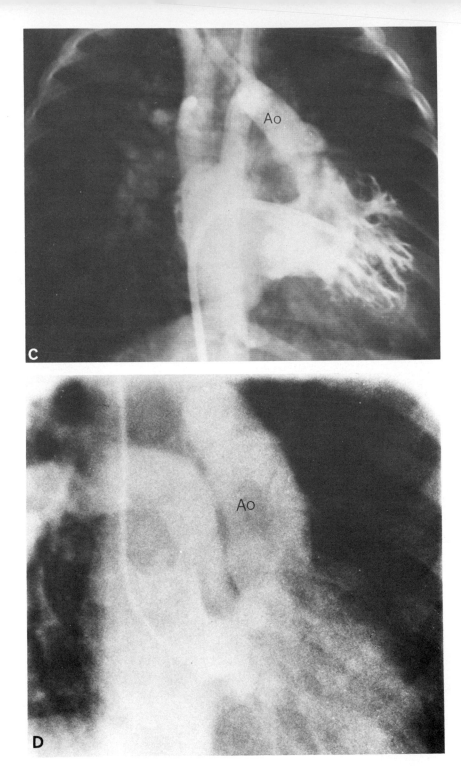

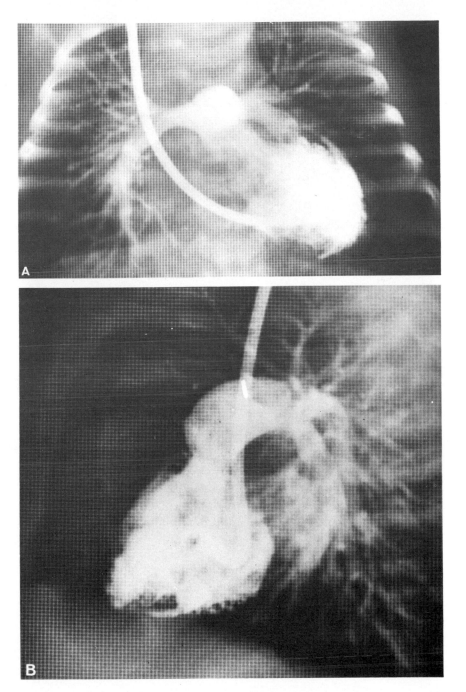

Fig. 175. Origin of the pulmonary artery from the left ventricle in transposition. Left ventricular angiogram in the anteroposterior (A) and lateral (B) positions.

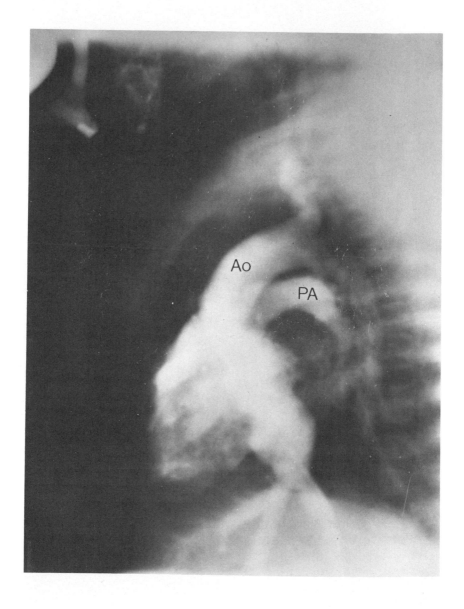

Fig. 17.6. Transposition with ventricular septal defect and pulmonary stenosis. Note the small size of pulmonary artery (PA) compared to aorta (Ao).

usually appears smaller than the pulmonary artery in cases with a ventricular septal defect and the two vessels appear of equal size in cases with an intact septum. When left ventricular outflow tract obstruction is present, the pulmonary artery usually appears smaller than the aorta (Fig. 17.6). The most common relationship between the aorta and the pulmonary artery is that in which the aorta is situated directly anterior or anterior and to the right of the pulmonary artery. Uncommonly the aorta is anterior and to the left of the pulmonary artery.

Selective injection of contrast media into the cardiac chambers and great arteries will allow recognition of the type of associated defects in almost all cases. Atrial septal defects are best visualized in the left oblique or lateral positions with the contrast medium injected into the cavae or the right or left atria (Fig. 17.7). Similarly, ventricular septal defects are

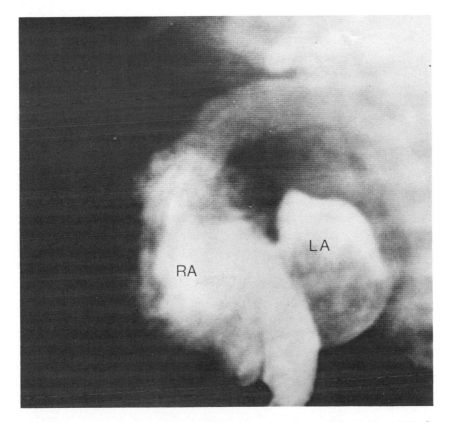

Fig. 17.7. Venous angiogram demonstrating opacification of left atrium (LA) from right atrium (RA) in a case of transportation with intact ventricular septum.

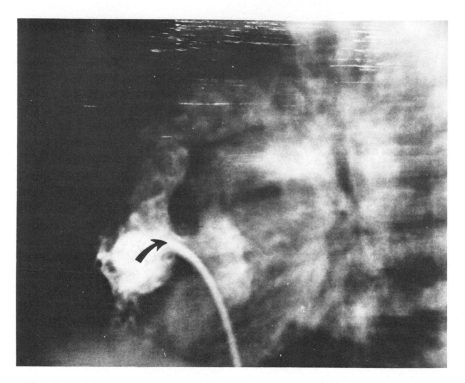

Fig. 17.8. Right ventricular angiogram in the lateral position demonstrating a ventricular septal defect. Arrow points to defect.

best demonstrated in the lateral position and the contrast medium injected into the right or left ventricles (Fig. 17.8) . If the dye is injected into the right ventricle, direct opacification of the left ventricle may occur or a stream of dye passing toward the pulmonary artery from the right ventricle may be observed. Using this technique it should be possible to estimate the size of the defect in the majority of cases. In addition, the type of the defect and its relationship to the semilunar valves could be studied. Patent ductus arteriosus and coarctation of the aorta are shown best by aortography or right ventricular angiography in the left oblique or lateral positions. In these views, the ascending and descending aortae are not superimposed and the state and the size of the ductus arteriosus and the type and severity of coarctation of the aorta could be determined (Fig. 17.9) . In the majority of cases, the flow of blood through the ductus arteriosus is from the aorta to the pulmonary artery (Fig. 17.10) . Obstruction of the outflow tract of the right ventricle, rarely seen in pathological material, has not been described in angiocardiographic studies. Left ventricular outflow tract obstruction is best demonstrated by left ventricular angiography. Obstruction at the pulmonary valve level often reveals a small valve ring and fusion with lack of movement of the valve cusps. The size of the lumen of the valve could also be estimated by the size of the stream of contrast agent passing through the valve. Three types of subvalvular obstruction could be demonstrated by left ventricular angiography: a fibromuscular tunnel producing a relatively long area of fixed narrowing (Fig. 17.11), a subvalvular diaphragm producing a ringlike filling defect beneath the valve (Fig. 17.12A and B), and muscular narrowing of the outflow tract produced by bulging of the ventricular septum (Fig. 17.13A and B). Bulging of the ventricular septum is best studied in the lateral projection. Peripheral stenosis of the pulmonary arteries could be demonstrated by pulmonary arterial or left ventricular angiography.

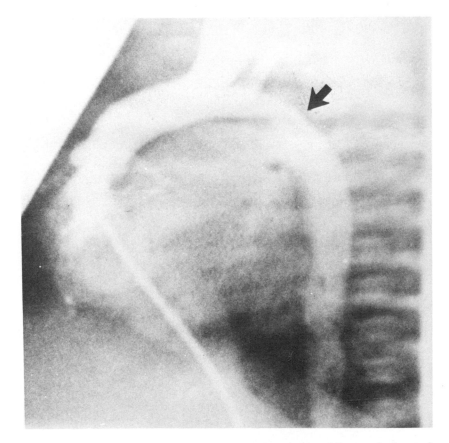

Fig. 17.9 Preductal coarctation of the aorta demonstrated by right ventricular angiography in a patient with transposition, ventricular septal defect, and patent ductus arteriosus. Arrow points to coarctation.

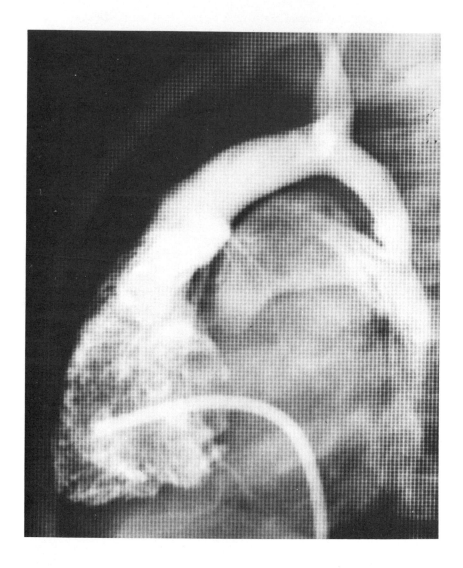

Fig. 17.10. Right ventricular angiogram in the lateral position demonstrating a large patent ductus arteriosus.

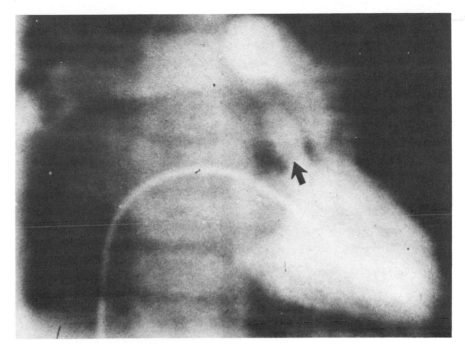

Fig. 17.11. Left ventricular angiogram in the anteroposterior position of a patient with transposition, ventricular septal defect, and left ventricular outflow tract obstruction of the tunnel type. Arrow points to subvalvular obstruction.

GROUP I (TABLE 17.1)

In most patients in this group the left ventricle appeared larger than the right ventricle. In 3 patients the right ventricle appeared hypoplastic. A right ventricle larger than the left ventricle was seen in 2 cases in this group. In all patients the right ventricle was situated anterior and to the right of the left ventricle. Of the 77 patients in whom the external relationship between the aorta and the pulmonary artery could be determined, the aorta lay anterior and to the right of the pulmonary artery in 48, directly anterior in 23, and anterior and to the left in 5 cases. Of the 53 patients in whom the size of the aorta and the pulmonary artery could be assessed, the two vessels were of equal size in 33, the aorta larger than the pulmonary artery in 6, and the pulmonary artery larger than the aorta in 14. A right aortic arch was present in 1 patient and coarctation of the aorta in another. A patent ductus arteriousus was observed on 39 occasions, and in 5 of these it was considered moderate or large. Venous or selective atrial angiography will demonstrate an interatrial communica-

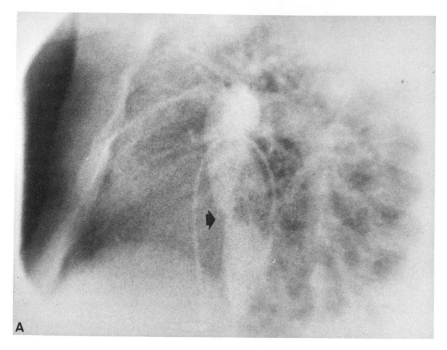

Fig. 17.12. Left ventricular outflow tract obstruction produced by a subvalvular diaphragm (A) with intact ventricular septum; (B) with ventricular septal defect. Arrow points to site of diaphragm.

tion in all. A high aortic valve, at the level of the 4th thoracic vertebral was observed in all patients in this group.

GROUP II (TABLE 17.1)

Of the 5 angiocardiograms in which the size of the ventricles could be assessed, the right ventricle appeared larger than the left ventricle in 4 and the two ventricles were of equal size in 1. The aorta was anterior and to the right of the pulmonary artery in 2, directly anterior in 2, and anterior and to the left in 2. The aorta appeared larger than the pulmonary artery in 2, the pulmonary artery larger than the aorta in 2, and the two vessels were of equal size in 1. A left aortic arch was present in all and a patent ductus in 1. The aortic valve was higher than the pulmonary valve in all. Left ventricular angiography demonstrated narrowing of the outflow tract of this ventricle produced by septal bulging in 4, by pulmonary subvalvular diaphragm in 1, and combined septal bulging and subvalvular diaphragm in 1.

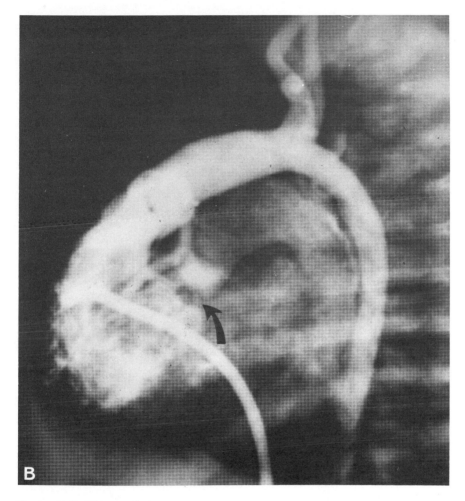

B

GROUP III (TABLE 17.1)

Of the 48 patients in this group in whom the size of the two ventricles could be assessed, the left ventricle was larger than the right in 28, the right larger than the left in 5, and the 2 ventricles of equal size in 15. In 55 of the 57 in whom the relationship of the ventricles could be determined, the right ventricle lay anterior and to the right of the left ventricle. In the remaining 2 the ventricles lay side by side. In the whole group of 65, the aorta was anterior and to the right of the pulmonary artery in 33, directly anterior in 23, and anterior and to the left in 9. When the relative size of the aorta and the pulmonary artery could be determined the

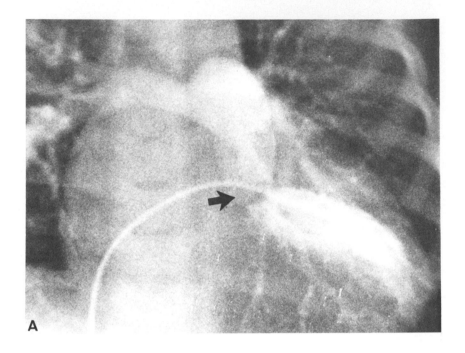

Fig. 17.13. Left ventricular angiogram in the anteroposterior (A) and lateral (B) positions demonstrating outflow tract obstruction of the left ventricle produced by a bulging septum. Arrow points to site of obstruction.

pulmonary artery was larger than the aorta in 46, the two vessels of equal size in 8, and the aorta larger than the pulmonary artery in 2. A right aortic arch was observed in 2 cases. Preductal coarctation of the aorta was observed in 6 and complete interruption of the aortic arch in 2 (Fig. 17.14A and B). Of the two patients with complete interruption of the aortic arch, the interruption occurred distal to the left subclavian artery in 1, and between the left subclavian and left common carotid arteries in 1. A patent ductus arteriosus was observed in 18 cases.

GROUP IV (TABLE 17.1)

Of the 17 cases in whom the size of the ventricles could be determined, the left ventricle was larger than the right in 12, the two ventricles were

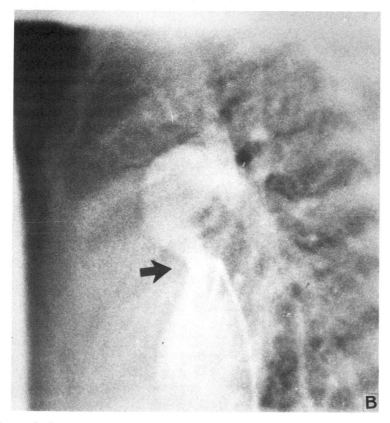

of equal size in 4, and the right ventricle appeared larger than the left ventricle in 1. An anteroposterior relationship of the ventricles was found in all with the ventricles partially overlapping one another. In every instance the aorta lay anterior to the pulmonary artery in the lateral projection. The anteroposterior view showed the aorta to be situated to the right of the pulmonary artery in 11, to the left in 9, and in 4 they lay directly anteroposterior to one another. The aorta was larger than the pulmonary artery in 22 cases, the great vessels were of equal size in 2, while the pulmonary artery was the larger vessel in 1. The aortic valve on both the anteroposterior and lateral projections lay at a slightly higher level than the pulmonary valve in 9 cases, while in 7 it was lower (Fig. 17.15), and in 8 the two valves were at the same level. A right aortic arch was observed in 1 case. Of the 25 angiograms in this series, pulmonary valvular stenosis of moderate to severe degree was shown in 23 and suspected in 1. Definite subvalvular pulmonary stenosis was observed in 15 and suspected in 1; a subvalvular fibromuscular tunnel in 11 and sus-

TABLE 17.1

ANGIOCARDIOGRAPHIC FINDINGS IN 184 STUDIES [a]

	Size of ventricles			Position of ventricle		Relationship of Ao to PA			Size of Ao and PA			Right Ao arch	PDA	Coarct.
	RV larger	LV larger	Equal	A-P	S-S	AR	A	AL	Ao larger	PA larger	Equal			
Group I (88 Patients)	2/31	22/31	7/31	65/65	0/65	48/77	23/77	5/77	6/53	14/53	33/53	1/85	39/78	1
Group II (6 Patients)	4/5	0	1/5	5/5	0	2/6	2/6	2/6	2/5	2/5	1/5	0/5	1/6	0
Group III (65 Patients)	5/48	28/48	15/48	55/57	2/57	33/65	23/65	9/65	2/57	46/57	8/57	2/63	18/58	8
Group IV (25 Patients)	1/17	12/17	4/17	23/23	0	11/25	5/25	9/25	22/25	1/25	2/25	1/25	4/17	0

[a] A, anterior; AL, anterior to left; Ao, aorta; Ao. Arch, aortic arch; A-P, anteroposterior; AR, anterior to right; Coarct, coarctation; LV, left ventricle; PA, pulmonary artery; PDA, patent ductus arteriosus; RV, right ventricle; S-S, side by side.

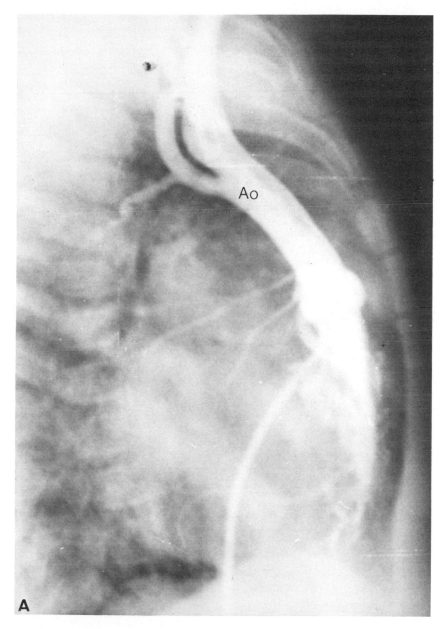

Fig. 17.14. Complete interruption of the aortic arch in each of 2 patients with transposition and ventricular septal defect documented by right ventricular (A) and venous (B) angiography in the lateral position. Ao, aorta.

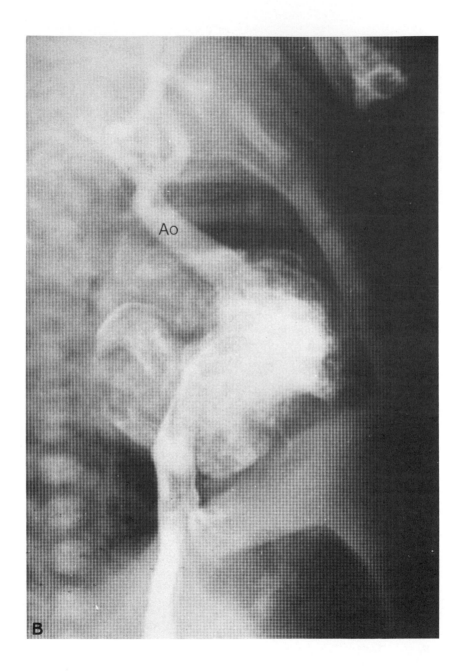

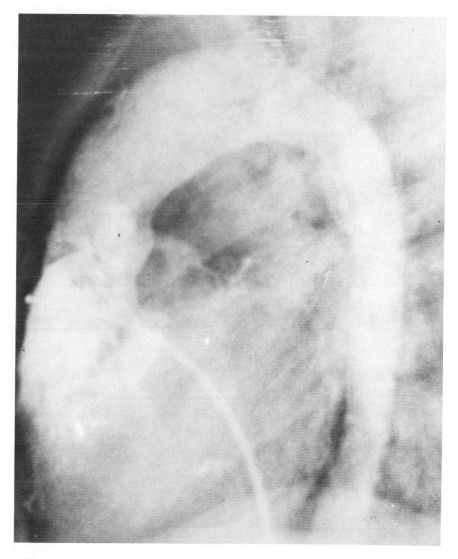

Fig. 17.15. Right ventricular angiogram in the lateral position of a patient with ventricular septal defect and pulmonary stenosis demonstrating low position of the aortic valve.

pected in 1; a subvalvular diaphragm in 1 and suspected in 1; and subvalvular bulging of the septum in 2. The distance between the ventricular septal defect and pulmonary valve could be estimated in 22 patients. It was moderate in 11 with subvalvular fibromuscular stenosis, in 2 with a subvalvular fibrous ring, and in 3 with isolated valvular stenosis. The ventricular septal defect was in close approximation to the valve in 6 patients with isolated pulmonary valve stenosis. A small ductus arteriosus was observed in 4 patients, while significant bronchial circulation to the lungs was not demonstrated in any case. Coarctation of the aorta was not observed in any patient in this study. Poststenotic dilatation involving the pulmonary artery was noted in 17 cases. The right pulmonary artery alone was involved in 14, the main pulmonary artery and right branch in 1, and the main pulmonary artery in 2. Peripheral stenosis of the pulmonary arteries was not observed in this series.

Discussion

Regardless of the presence or absence of a ventricular septal defect or left ventricular outflow tract obstruction, the majority of patients in this series had a larger left than right ventricle. A pattern in which the two ventricles were of equal size was less common. The least common pattern was that in which the right ventricle appeared larger than the left. In only 2 patients in this series the ventricles were situated side by side. In all others an anteroposterior relationship existed with the right ventricle slightly to the right of the left ventricle. A similar relationship between the ventricles has been reported by Carey and Elliott (1964), and Barcia *et al.* (1967).

In most patients in this series the aorta lay anterior and to the right of the pulmonary artery. Less frequently the aorta was directly anterior to the pulmonary artery and the two vessels superimposed in the anteroposterior projection. An aorta ascending along the left upper cardiac border is described as typical of congenitally corrected transposition of the great vessels (Anderson *et al.*, 1957). In the present series this phenomenon was observed in 25 cases of which 11 had left ventricular outflow tract obstruction. Slight rotation of the patient to the left, as suggested by Carey and Elliott (1964) has been excluded in these patients. Most authors agree that when a heart specimen with complete transposition of the great arteries is examined, the aorta always lies to the right of the pulmonary artery (Lev *et al.*, 1961; Elliott *et al.*, 1963). The discrepancy between the autopsy findings and the angiocardiographic findings deserves special consideration. When a heart specimen with transposition is examined with ventricles lying side by side, i.e., right ventricle on the right and left ventricle on the left, the aorta is always to the right of the pulmonary artery. The two vessels may lie side by side or the aorta may be slightly anterior to the pulmonary artery. During life, however, the right ventricle is anterior, though slight overlap of the ventricles may occur, and thus, during life, the aorta is always anterior to the pulmonary artery. Moreover, the aorta may lie to the right, directly in front, or to the left of the pulmonary artery. Only 2 patients in the present series had side to side relationship of the ventricles but in each the aorta was to the right and slightly anterior to the pulmonary artery. An aorta posterior to the pulmonary artery (Van Praagh *et al.*, 1971) was not observed in this series.

Whereas in most patients with an intact ventricular septum the pulmonary artery and aorta were of equal size, in most patients with a ventricular septal defect the pulmonary artery was larger than the aorta. On the other hand, in the majority of patients with a ventricular septal defect and pulmonary valvular or subvalvular fibromuscular stenosis, the aorta was larger than the main pulmonary artery. The author believes that a pulmonary artery smaller than the aorta is diagnostic of left ventricular outflow tract obstruction. The reverse however, i.e., a pulmonary artery larger than the aorta, does not necessarily exclude this diagnosis.

Keith *et al.* (1958) noted that the aortic valve usually lies at a higher level than the pulmonary valve. This finding has been confirmed in patients without left ventricular obstruction in the present series. In patients with a ventricular septal defect and left ventricular outflow tract obstruction the aortic valve was higher than the pulmonary valve in 9, both valves were at the same level in 8, while in 7 the aortic valve was lower than the pulmonary valve. The author does not have a reasonable explanation for this observation.

The incidence of right aortic arch in transposition is low. It was approximately 4–5% in two series (Keith *et al.*, 1958; Elliott *et al.*, 1963). According to Carey and Elliott (1964) the occurrence of a right aortic arch appears to be higher in patients with transposition of the great arteries, ventricular septal defect, and left ventricular outflow tract obstruction. Of the 14 patients with a ventricular septal defect and pulmonary stenosis reported by Mehrizi *et al.* (1966), a right aortic arch was present in 2. Hastreiter *et al.* (1966) pointed out that all their cases with transposition and a right aortic arch had a ventricular septal defect and pulmonary stenosis. Of the 184 angiograms in this series a right aortic arch was observed in 4; 1 in Group I, 2 in Group III, and 1 in Group IV.

The presence of a ventricular septal defect in transposition can be demonstrated by either a right or left ventricular angiogram. Both demonstrate the size and the site of the defect reasonably well. Imamura *et al.* (1971) pointed out that their studies of 14 angiograms of patients with

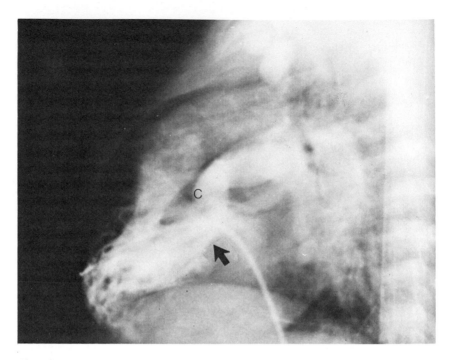

Fig. 17.16. Infracristal ventricular septal defect in transposition and pulmonary stenosis demonstrated by right ventricular angiography in the lateral position. C, crista. Arrow points to ventricular septal defect.

transposition demonstrated two major patterns regarding the position of a ventricular septal defect: either the absence or the presence of a crista supraventricularis. The crista supraventricularis usually appears in the lateral projection as a translucent area just beneath the conjoint region of the aortic and pulmonary cusps. The crista supraventricularis is usually absent when the defect is located above it. On the other hand, when the crista is evident the defect is usually situated between the crista above and the ventricular septum below (Fig. 17.16). Muscular defects are usually seen close to the apex of the ventricles or in a middle portion of the ventricular septum. Injection of the contrast medium in the left ventricle has the advantage of demonstrating the distance of the defect from the pulmonary valve. This information is of particular importance in patients with left ventricular outflow tract obstruction, since those with a ventricular septal defect distant from the pulmonary valve tend to have a fibromuscular tunnel beneath the valve (Shaher *et al.,* 1967a).

A patent foramen ovale or an atrial septal defect is present in the majority of patients with transposition. In the presence of shunt reversal, an interatrial communication can be demonstrated by injecting the contrast medium into the right atrium or the inferior vena cava in the lateral or left oblique position. If the catheter intubates the left atrium, an angiogram in this chamber will also demonstrate the defect. As pointed out by Carey and Elliott (1964) it is often very difficult to distinguish the nature of the communication between the atria in terms of whether the flow was through an atrial septal defect or a patent foramen ovale. However, when the communication is a foramen ovale rather than a surgical atrial septal defect, it is often possible to identify it in the lateral view, as a high but small communication on the atrial septum. Surgical atrial septal defect is often large and its location on the atrial septum appears lower than that of the foramen ovale.

Of the 159 angiocardiograms in which the state of the ductus could be determined, this structure was patent in 62 instances. The highest incidence of a patent ductus was found in Group I (50%), and the lowest in Group IV (23.5%). This finding is probably related to the fact that most Group I patients die at a stage when the ductus is still patent but Group IV patients survive long enough for the ductus to close spontaneously. The ductus appeared small in the majority of the angiograms, and as pointed out by Keith *et al.* (1958) the flow of blood through the ductus was from the aorta to the pulmonary artery. In the 2 patients with complete interruption of the aortic arch the flow of the blood through the ductus was from the pulmonary artery to the descending aorta.

The diagnosis of left ventricular outflow tract obstruction in patients with complete transposition of the great arteries depends upon either the demonstration of a pressure gradient across the pulmonary valve or the subvalvular area or upon the presence of angiocardiographic evidence of narrowing of the pulmonary valve and/or the outflow tract of the left ventricle. Left ventricular angiography, aside from showing the origin of the pulmonary artery from the left ventricle, provides four important points of information: (a) the type of left ventricular outflow tract obstruction; (b) the size of the pulmonary artery and its main branches; (c) the presence or absence and the type of a ventricular septal defect and its distance from the pulmonary valve; (d) the presence or absence of abnormalities of the mitral valve. Right ventricular angiography is also often successful in visualizing the outflow tract of the left ventricle when a ventricular septal defect is present. In the 6 patients with an intact ventricular septum, the obstruction was caused by bulging of the septum alone in 4, by a subvalvular ring in 1, and by combined septal bulging and a subvalvular ring in 1. Neither valve stenosis nor a subvalvular fibromuscular tunnel was observed in this group. Twenty-three of the 25 patients in Group IV had definite narrowing of the pulmonary valve, 1 had probable pulmonary valve stenosis, while the pulmonary valve in the remaining case appeared normal. In addition to valvular stenosis in these 23, in 9 a subvalvular tunnel was also definite, in 1 a tunnel was probable, and in 2 a tunnel plus septal bulging was apparent. The patient with probable valvular stenosis also had a subvalvular diaphragm both of which were confirmed at necropsy, while the patient without valve stenosis had a diaphragm angiocardiographically and at postmortem. These findings confirm the conclusion of Shaher *et al.* (1967b) that when pulmonary stenosis is present in a case of complete transposition with a ventricular septal defect, the pulmonary valve is almost invariably involved. Bulging of the septum, while prevalent in the autopsied series, was not commonly seen angiocardiographically when a ventricular septal defect was present, possibly because of some overlap of the ventricles obscuring this phenomenon.

Poststenotic dilatation of the right pulmonary artery occurred in a sufficient number of patients to be of diagnostic importance in those with a ventricular septal defect. While dilatation involves the main pulmonary artery and the left branch in patients with pulmonary valvular stenosis and normally related great arteries, the right branch tended to be involved in the cases under discussion. As pointed out by Shaher *et al.* (1967a) this phenomenon is due to the fact that when the pulmonary artery arises from the left ventricle, the right branch is aligned with the main pulmonary artery and streaming or jetting of blood is, therefore, directed mainly toward the right branch. Dilatation of the main pulmonary artery was not a common finding, however, and was noted alone in 2 cases and associated with dilatation of the right branch in 1 case. Peripheral stenosis of the pulmonary arteries was not seen in this series but the angiocardiogram of one of the patients reported by Mehrizi *et al.* (1966) revealed severe peripheral stenosis of both pulmonary arteries.

Redundant tricuspid valvular tissue protruded through a ventricular septal defect into the left ventricular outflow tract, and produced severe obstruction to the outflow of blood from the left ventricle in 2 patients reported by Riemenschneider *et al.* (1969). In each of the 2 patients described by the authors, a large asymmetrical filling defect was demonstrated at the anterior border of the left ventricular outflow tract below the pulmonary valve.

Preductal coarctation of the aorta was observed in 7 patients in this series; 1 in Group I and 6 in Group III. The coarctation was in the form of a long segment in 6 and a mild ring of constriction in 1. In 1 patient the left subclavian artery arose from the coarctation area of the aorta. While coarctation of the aorta was observed in only 1 patient in the necropsied series in Group IV it was not seen in the angiocardiographic study of the same group. This suggests that the combination of pulmonary stenosis and coarctation of the aorta rarely occurs in complete transposition of the great arteries. It is of interest to note that of the 6 patients in Group III with preductal coarctation of the aorta a hypoplastic right ventricle was observed in 4.

Complete interruption of the aortic arch occurred in 2 patients in Group III. In 1 patient the interruption occurred distal to the left subclavian artery. A small anastomotic vessel appeared to connect the left subclavian artery to the pulmonary artery. In the second patient the left subclavian artery arose from the descending aorta below the interrupted segment. The right ventricle appeared hypoplastic in both. Of the reported cases of transposition of the great arteries with an interrupted arch, the diagnosis has been confirmed by angiocardiography in the patients reported by Castellanos et al. (1959), Buckley et al. (1965), Bowers et al. (1965), Waldhausen et al. (1969), and Norton et al. (1970).

Prominent bronchial arterial circulation to the lungs in transposition has been demonstrated at autopsy (Cockle, 1863; Cleland et al., 1957) and by injection techniques by several authors (Cudkowicz and Armstrong, 1952; Robertson, 1965). Recently, Ferencz (1966) suggested that the bronchial circulation may be of etiological significance in the development of pulmonary vascular disease in these patients. Such, however, was not observed in any patient in this series. This suggests that aortic root angiography may be necessary to define this circulation (this was done in only 22 patients in this series), that it is microscopic rather than macroscopic, or that it does not have much functional significance in transposition.

References

Abrams, H. L., and Kaplan, H. S. (1956). "Angiocardiographic Interpretation in Congenital Heart Disease," p. 118. Thomas, Springfield, Illnois.

Abrams, H. L., Kaplan, H. S., and Purdy, A. (1951). Diagnosis of complete transposition of the great vessels. *Radiology* 57, 500.

Abramson, H. (1950). Transposition of the great vessels. *Amer. J. Dis. Child.* 79, 1063.

Anderson, R. C., Lillehei, C. W., and Lester, R. G. (1957). Corrected transposition of the great vessels of the heart. *Pediatrics* 20, 626.

Astley, R., and Parsons, S. (1952). Complete transposition of the great vessels. *Brit. Heart J.* 14, 13.

Barcia, A., Kincaid, O. W., Davis, G. D., Kirklin, J. W., and Ongley, P. A. (1967). Transposition of the great arteries. An angiocardiographic study. *Amer. J. Roentgenol.* 100, 249.

Bowers, D. E., Schiebler, G. L., and Krovetz, L. J. (1965). Interruption of the aortic arch with complete transposition of the great vessels. Hemodynamic and angiocardiographic data of a case diagnosed during life. *Amer. J. Cardiol.* **16**, 442.

Buckley, M. J., Mason, D. T., Ross, J., Jr., and Braunwald, E. (1965). Reversed differential cyanosis with equal desaturation of the upper limbs syndrome of complete transposition of the great vessels with complete interruption of the aortic arch. *Amer. J. Cardiol.* **15**, 111.

Campbell, M., and Hills, T. H. (1950). Angiocardiography in cyanotic congenital heart disease. *Brit. Heart J.* **12**, 65.

Campbell, M., and Suzman, S. (1951). Transposition of the aorta and pulmonary artery. *Circulation* **4**, 329.

Carey, L. S., and Elliott, L. P. (1964). Complete transposition of the great vessels. Roentgenographic findings. *Amer. J. Roentgenol.* **91**, 529.

Castellanos, A., Garcia, O., and Gonzalez, E. (1959). Complete interruption of the aortic arch with transposition of the great vessels. (Report of a case diagnosed *in vivo*). *Cardiologia* **34**, 53.

Castellanos, A., Pereiras, R., and Garcia, A. (1938). L'angiocardiographie chez l'enfant. *Presse Med.* **46**, 1474.

Castellanos, A., Perez de los Reyes, R., and Garcia, L. (1947). Comparison of angiocardiographic examinations and autopsy findings. *Rev. Cubana Cardiol.* **8**, 29.

Castellanos, A., Pereiras, P., and Garcia, O. (1950). Angiography: Anatomoroentgenological forms of the transposition of the great vessels. *Amer. J. Roentgenol.* **64**, 255.

Cleland, W. P., Goodwin, J. F., Steiner, R. E., and Zoob, M. (1957). Transposition of aorta and pulmonary artery with pulmonary stenosis. *Amer. Heart J.* **54**, 10.

Cockle, J. (1863). A case of transposition of the great vessels of the heart. *Med. Chir. Trans.* **46**, 193.

Cooley, R. N., and Sloan, R. D. (1952). Angiocardiography in congenital heart disease of cyanotic type. III. Observations on complete transposition of the great vessels. *Radiology* **58**, 481.

Cooley, R. N., and Sloan, R. D. (1956). "Radiology of the Heart and Great Vessels." Williams & Wilkins, Baltimore, Maryland.

Cudkowicz, L., and Armstrong, J. B. (1952). Injection of the bronchial circulation in a case of transposition. *Brit. Heart J.* **14**, 374.

De Groot, J. W. C. (1951). "Angiocardiography as a Diagnostic Aid in Congenital Heart Disease." Keesing, Amsterdam.

Deutsch, V., Shem, T. A., Yahini, J. H., and Neufeld, H. N. (1970). Cardioangiographic evaluation of the relationship between atrioventricular and semilunar valves: Its diagnostic importance in congenital heart disease. *Amer. J. Roentgenol.* **110**, 474–490.

Dotter, C. T., and Steinberg, I. (1951). Angiocardiography. *Ann. Roentgenol.* **20**, 228.

Elliott, L. P., Neufeld, H. N., Anderson, R. C., Adams, P., Jr., and Edwards, J E., (1963). Complete transposition of the great vessels. I. An anatomic study of sixty cases. *Circulation* **27**, 1105.

Elliott, L. P., Amplatz, K., and Edwards, J. E. (1966). Coronary arterial patterns in transposition complexes. Anatomic and angiocardiographic studies. *Amer. J. Cardiol.* **17**, 362.

Ferencz, C. (1966). Transposition of the great vessels. Pathophysiologic considerations based upon a study of the lungs. *Circulation* **33**, 232.

Gasul, B. M., Hait, G., Dillon, R. F., and Fell, E. H. (1957). "The Salient Points and the Value of Venous Angiocardiography in the Diagnosis of the Cyanotic types of Congenital Malformations of the Heart," p. 16. Thomas, Springfield, Illinois.

Gasul, B. M., Weiss, H., Fell, E. H., Dillon, R. F., Fisher, D. L., and Marienfeld, C. J. (1953). Angiocardiography in congenital heart disease correlated with clinical and autopsy findings. *Amer. J. Dis. Child.* 85, 404.

Goodwin, J. F., Steiner, R., and Wayne, E. J. (1949) . Transposition of the aorta and pulmonary artery demonstrated by angiography. *Brit. Heart J.* 11, 279.

Goodwin, J. F., Steiner, R. F., Mounsey, J. D. P., MacGregor, A. G., and Wayne, E. J. (1953). A critical analysis of the clinical value of angiocardiography in congenital heart disease. *Brit. J. Radiol.* 26, 161.

Gyllensward, A., and Lodin, H. (1954). The value of selective angiocardiography in the diagnosis of complete transposition of the great vessels. *Acta Radiol.* 42, 189.

Hallermann, F. J., Kincaid, O. W., Ritter, D. G., and Titus, J. L. (1970). Mitral semilunar valve relationships in the angiography of cardiac malformations *Radiol ogy* 94, 63 68.

Hastreiter, A. R., D'Cruz, I. A., and Cantez, T. (1966). Right-sided aorta. *Brit. Heart J.* 28, 722.

Imamura, E. S., Morikawa, T., Tatsuno, K., Konno, S., Arai, T., and Sakakibara, S. (1971). Surgical considerations of ventricular septal defects associated with complete transposition of the great arteries and pulmonary stenosis. *Circulation* 44, 914.

Ingomar, C. J., and Tersley, E. (1962). Complete transposition of the great vessels. *Brit. Heart J.* 24, 358.

Keith, J. D. (1954). Angiocardiography in infants and children. *Pediat. Clin. N. Amer.* 1, 73.

Keith, J. D., and Munn, J. D. (1950). Angiocardiography in infants and children. New technique. *Pediatrics* 6, 20.

Keith, J. D., Rowe, R. D., and Vlad, P. (1958). "Heart Disease in Infancy and Childhood," 1st Ed. MacMillan, New York.

Kreutzer, R. O., Caprile, J. A., and Wessels, F. M. (1950). Angiocardiography in heart disease in children. *Brit. Heart J.* 12, 293.

Lev, M., Alcalde, V. M., and Baffes, T. G. (1961). Pathologic anatomy of complete transposition of the arterial trunks. *Pediatrics* 28, 293.

Mehrizi, A., Rowe, R. D., Hutchins, G. M., and Folger, G. M., Jr. (1966). Transposition of the great vessels with pulmonary stenosis and ventricular septal defect. *Bull. Johns Hopkins Hosp.* 119, 200.

Norton, J. B., Ullyot, D. J., Stewart, E. T., Rudolph, A. M., and Edmunds, L. H. (1970). Aortic arch atresia with transposition of the great vessels: Physiologic considerations and surgical management. *Surgery* 67, 1011–1016.

Riemenschneider, T. A., Goldberg, S. J., Ruttenberg, H. D., and Cyepes, M. T. (1969). Subpulmonic obstruction in complete (d) transposition produced by redundant tricuspid tissue. *Circulation* 39, 603–609.

Robertson, B. (1965). Microangiographic studies of the lung in transposition of the great arteries. *Acta Paediat. Scand.* 159, 84.

Rushmer, R. F., Crystal, D. K., Tidwell, R. A., Crose, R. F., and Hendron, J. A. (1953). Complete transposition of the great vessels. *J. Pediat.* 42, 189.

Shaher, R. M., Moes, F., and Khoury, G. (1967a) . Radiologic and angiocardiographic findings in complete transposition of the great vessels, with left ventricular outflow tract obstruction. *Radiology* 88, 1092.

Shaher, R. M., Puddu, G. C., Khoury, G., Moes, C. A. F., and Mustard, W. T. (1967b). Complete transposition of the great vessels with anatomic obstruction of the outflow tract of the left ventricle. Surgical implications of anatomic findings. *Amer. J. Cardiol.* **19**, 658.

Van Praagh, R., Perez-Trevino, C., Lopez-Cuellar, M., Baker, F. W., Zuberbuhler, J. R., Quero, M., Perez, V. M., Moreno, F., and Van Praagh, S. (1971). Transposition of the great arteries with posterior aorta, anterior pulmonary artery, subpulmonary conus and fibrous continuity between aortic and atrioventricular valves. *Amer. J. Cardiol.* **28**, 621.

Waldhausen, J. A., Boruchow, I., Miller, W. W., and Rashkind, W. J. (1969). Transposition of the great arteries with ventricular septal defect. Palliation by atrial septostomy and pulmonary artery banding. *Circulation* **39**, 215.

Wesselhoeft, H., Hurley, P. J., Wagner, H. N., Jr., and Rowe, R. (1972). Nuclear angiocardiography in the diagnosis of congenital heart disease in infants. *Circulation* **45**, 77.

Chapter 18

NATURAL HISTORY, PROGNOSIS, CAUSE OF DEATH, AND LONG SURVIVAL

Transposition of the great arteries is the most common cyanotic heart disease presenting early in infancy and is responsible for the majority of the cyanotic heart deaths in this age group. Its prognosis without palliative surgery is extremely poor. Abbott (1936) found that the mean age at death of 49 necrosied cases of transposition to be 1.4 years. Keith *et al.* (1953) found that the average life-span of 44 patients with transposition was 3 months, 50% did not survive the 4th week, and 85% were dead by the end of 6 months. Of the 29 cases reported by Lillehei and Varco (1953), the age ranged between 3 weeks and 6½ years with an average of about 1 year. The average life duration of the 74 cases reported by Keith *et al.* (1958) was 13 weeks. Noonan *et al.* (1960) reported 50 selected patients with transposition of the great arteries. The ages ranged from 12 days to 12 years with an average of 3 years and 4 months. Lev *et al.* (1961) reported 92 cases of transposition associated with normal ventricular architecture. The average age of these patients was about 14 months. Fontana and Edwards (1962) reported 24 cases of complete transposition. The age at death of these patients ranged from 33 hours to 7 years with a median of 7 weeks. Eight patients were 1 month of age or less at the time of death. Only 2 patients lived more than 1 year. In an analysis of Bauer and Astbury's (1944) bibliography of Abbott's cases, Fontana and Edwards (1962) found that the median age at death of 49 patients with transposition was 2 months and the range of survival was 2 days to 16 years. Calleja *et al.* (1964) reported 40 patients with complete transposition of the great arteries. More than 85% died within the first 6 months of postnatal life. Only 2 patients survived the first year. Paul *et al.* (1968) reported that the probability of survival of an infant with this malformation to 100 days of age without palliative intervention was only 30%. Liebman *et al.* (1969) studied the natural history of 742 cases of complete transposition of the great arteries. Their material included single ventricle, mitral atresia, tricuspid atresia, and cor biloculare. The area of the study was the State of California and included 363 cases from 14 selected hospital centers, and 379 cases from death certificates. They found that the age of death for the whole group was as follows: by 1 week, 28.7%; by 1 month, 51.6%; and by 1 year, 89.3%.

Campbell and Suzman (1951) agreed that the prognosis in transposition is poor, and pointed out that if the septal defects are large enough for adequate mixing of the circulations of both sides of the heart, so that the child survives in infancy, there is no reason why it should not survive much longer. Similarly Cooley and Sloan (1952) said that "whereas formerly it was thought that a life-span greater than 18 months was exceptional, it is now evident that a considerable number of patients may live beyond this period and an age of 8 to 10 years or even more is quite compatible with the presence of this anomaly." Of the 35 selected cases of transposition reported by Shaher (1963), 10 patients exceeded the age of 10 years. Campbell (1972) pointed out that the mean age of death of his 8 necropsied cases was 7 years.

At the conclusion of this study there were 409 patients; 201 unoperated and 208 operated. Since heart surgery modifies the natural history of the disease, these two groups of patients have been separately studied.

Age at Death and Age Distribution (Tables 18.1–18.3)

There were 201 unoperated patients in this series. At the conclusion of the study 164 were dead and 37 alive. Of the group of 164 patients, 45.2% died during the first month of life, 69.5% by the third month, 75.5% by the sixth month, and 80.5% by the end of the first year (Table 18.1). Of the group of 37 patients who were alive at the conclusion of the study, 30.5% were 1 year or less, and 69.5% survived to be 1 year or more. Six patients or 16.8% were 10 years or more (Table 18.2). The age distribution of the 201 unoperated patients is shown in Table 18.3. Of these 201 patients, 22% were more than 1 year of age.

The reported incidence of death for transposition of the great arteries is about 90% by the age of 1 year (Keith et al., 1967; Paul et al., 1968; Plauth et al., 1968; and Liebman et al., 1969). Operative deaths, however, were included in the natural history study of transposition by these authors, on the grounds that in a significant number of patients with transposition the operation is a precipitative cause of death. Operative deaths were not included in this study, hence the reported incidence of death of transposition patients by 1 year was higher than the incidence of death by 1 year in this series.

TABLE 18.1
AGE AT DEATH OF 164 UNOPERATED PATIENTS

Group	Months												Years									Above 10 years[a]	Average age[b]
	0-1	1-2	2-3	3-4	4-5	5-6	6-7	7-8	8-9	9-10	10-11	11-12	1-2	2-3	3-4	4-5	5-6	6-7	7-8	8-9	9-10		
Group I (96)	58	15	7	7	2	1	2	0	0	0	0	0	2	0	0	1	0	0	0	0	0	10 y-6 m	95 Patients 2 m, 6 d
Group II (4)	2	0	1	0	0	0	0	0	1	0	0	0	0	0	0	0	0	0	0	0	0		4 Patients 3 m, 1 w, 4 d
Group III (57)	13	11	6	5	4	5	2	0	1	0	0	0	2	1	0	1	1	1	1	0	0	11 y, 18 y 24 y, 25 y 26 y	52 Patients 4 m, 1 w, 2 d
Group IV (7)	1	0	0	0	0	0	0	0	0	0	1	0	0	1	0	0	0	0	0	0	0	11 y, 11 y 21 y, 29 y	3 Patients 1 y, 3 m, 2 w, 1 d
Total (164)	74	26	14	12	6	6	4	0	2	0	1	0	4	2	0	2	0	1	1	0	0	10	

[a] d, Days; m, months; w, weeks; y, years.
[b] Patients above 10 years were excluded from average age.

TABLE 18.2

37 Unoperated, Alive Patients

Group	Months												Years									Above 10 years [a]	Average age
	0-1	1-2	2-3	3-4	4-5	5-6	6-7	7-8	8-9	9-10	10-11	11-12	1-2	2-3	3-4	4-5	5-6	6-7	7-8	8-9	9-10		
Group I (7)	1	2	0	1	0	0	0	0	0	0	0	0	2	0	0	0	0	0	0	0	0	22 y	3 y, 7 m, 3 w, 2 d
Group II None	0	0	0	0	0	0	0	0	0	0	0	0	0	0	0	0	0	0	0	0	0		
Group III (21)	1	1	1	0	0	0	0	0	0	1	0	0	1	1	3	3	0	2	0	1	1	10 y–6 m 13 y, 13½ y 15 y, 16 y	6 y, 1 m, 1 w, 4 d
Group IV (9)	1	0	0	0	0	1	0	0	0	0	0	1	3	0	0	0	1	0	1	0	1		3 y, 2 m, 3 w, 4 d
Total (37)	3	3	1	1	0	1	0	0	0	1	0	1	6	1	3	3	1	2	1	1	2	6	

[a] Abbreviations same as in Table 18.1.

TABLE 18.3

AGE DISTRIBUTION OF 201 UNOPERATED PATIENTS [a]

Group	Months												Years												
	0–1	1–2	2–3	3–4	4–5	5–6	6–7	7–8	8–9	9–10	10–11	11–12	1–2	2–3	3–4	4–5	5–6	6–7	7–8	8–9	9–10	10–15	15–20	20–25	25–30
Group I (103)	59	17	7	8	2	1	2	0	0	0	0	0	4	0	0	1	0	0	0	0	0	1	0	1	0
Group II (4)	2	0	1	0	0	0	0	0	1	0	0	0	0	0	0	0	0	0	0	0	0	0	0	0	0
Group III (78)	14	12	7	5	4	5	2	0	1	1	0	0	3	2	3	4	0	3	0	1	1	5	2	2	1
Group IV (16)	2	0	0	0	0	1	0	0	0	0	1	1	3	1	0	0	1	0	1	1	0	2	0	1	1
Total (201)	77	29	15	13	6	7	4	0	2	1	1	1	10	3	3	5	1	3	1	2	1	8	2	4	2

[a] 164 patients died; 37 alive.

Prognosis in Relationship to the Associated Defects

Of the 201 unoperated patients in this series, 164 were dead at the conclusion of the study. To maintain a homogeneous age distribution, and to avoid including cases of exceptional longevity, 10 patients who survived 10 years or more were excluded from the 164 dying patients. Of the remaining 154 patients there were 95 in Group I, 4 in Group II, 52 in Group III, and 3 in Group IV. The average age at death of these patients is as follows (Table 18.1) : Group I, 2 months and 6 days; Group II, 3 months, 1 week and 2 days; Group III, 4 months, 1 week and 2 days; Group IV, 1 year, 3 months, 2 weeks and 1 day.

During the same period there were 208 operated patients. Of these 208 patients, 64 were still alive at the conclusion of the study (Table 18.4), and 144 were deceased (Table 18.5). The cause of death was related to heart surgery in 141, while 3 who had had successful palliative surgery had subsequently died of independent causes. Of the 141 operative deaths, 10 had had successful palliative surgery and had later died at a second heart operation. These 10 patients and an additional long survivor, whose death at 12 years of age had complicated heart surgery, have been excluded from the average age at death. Of the remaining 130 patients, 73 were in Group I, 7 in Group II, 35 in Group III, and 15 in Group IV. The average age at death of these patients was as follows (Table 18.5) : Group I, 2 months, 1 week, and 4 days; Group II, 1 year, 7 months, and 3 weeks; Group III, 10 months and 4 weeks; Group IV, 2 years, 11 months, and 1 week.

These findings show that the worst prognosis occurred in patients with an intact ventricular septum. A slightly better prognosis occurred in patients with a ventricular septal defect. The addition of left ventricular outflow tract obstruction to each of Groups I and III improved its prognosis. In the four subgroups, however, the average age of operated dying patients was more than the average age of unoperated dying patients. This finding is related to the fact that some older children, who were doing fairly well, had died as a result of the heart surgery. This conclusion is supported by the fact that of 153 unoperated dying patients, 9 were more than 1 year, whereas of the 130 operated dying patients, 26 were more than 1 year.

The relationship between the associated defects and the prognosis of transposition of the great arteries has been extensively discussed in the literature and various views have been expressed. In 1948, Hanlon and Blalock correlated the age of survival of patients with complete transposition of the great arteries to the associated anatomical defects. Their work was mainly based on 85 cases of transposition collected from the litera-

TABLE 18.4

64 Operated, Alive Patients [a]

Group	Months 0-1	1-2	2-3	3-4	4-5	5-6	6-7	7-8	8-9	9-10	10-11	11-12	Years 1-2	2-3	3-4	4-5	5-6	6-7	7-8	8-9	9-10	Above 10 years [b]	Average age [b]
Group I (27)	0	2	0	1	0	1	3	2	0	0	0	1	2	2	3	1	2	0	0	0	3	10 y-5 m 13 y-7 m 14 y-3 m 16 y	4 y, 7 m, 2 w
Group II (4)	0	0	0	0	0	0	0	0	0	0	0	0	0	0	2	0	1	1	0	0	0		4 y, 10 m, 3 d
Group III (20)	0	2	0	0	0	0	0	1	0	1	0	0	3	2	2	2	1	2	1	0	1	11 y	3 y, 9 m, 5 d
Group IV (13)	0	0	0	0	0	0	0	0	0	0	0	0	2	2	1	0	1	3	1	0	1	13 y, 26 y	7 y, 2 m, 1 w
Total (64)	0	4	0	2	0	1	3	3	0	1	0	1	7	6	8	3	5	6	2	0	5	7	

[a] Included are patients corrected by the Mustard operation.
[b] Abbreviations same as in Table 18.1.

TABLE 18.5
AGE DISTRIBUTION OF 141 OPERATIVE DEATHS [a]

| Group | Months | | | | | | | | | | | | Years | | | | | | | | | Patients died at second operation | Average age [d] |
	0–1	1–2	2–3	3–4	4–5	5–6	6–7	7–8	8–9	9–10	10–11	11–12	1–2	2–3	3–4	4–5	5–6	6–7	7–8	8–9	9–10		
Group I (79)	56	13	7	1	2	1	1	1	0	0	0	0	4	1	0	0	0	0	0	0	0	1 y 6 m; 2 y; 2 y; 2 y 4 m; 3 y 3 m; 4 y 2 m	73 Patients 2 m, 1 w, 4 d
Group II (8)	1	1	0	0	0	0	0	0	1	0	0	0	1	2	1	0	0	0	0	0	0	12 y	7 Patients 1 y, 7 m, 3 w
Group III [b] (38)	10	7	5	0	1	0	0	1	0	1	2	0	5	0	0	1	1	0	1	0	0	1 y 3 m; 2 y; 2 y 1 m	35 Patients 10 m, 4 w
Group IV [c] (16)	3	0	0	0	0	0	0	1	1	0	1	0	2	2	1	1	0	1	1	1	0	2 y	15 Patients 2 y, 11 m, 1 w, 4 d
Total (141)	70	13	7	1	2	1	1	3	2	1	3	0	12	5	2	2	1	1	2	1	0	11	

[a] Abbreviations same as in Table 18.1.
[b] Excluded from Group III are 2 operated patients who died of independent causes at the age of 1½ years and 2 years, respectively.
[c] Excluded from Group IV is 1 patient who died of independent cause at the age of 3 years.
[d] Excluded from average age are patients who died at a second heart operation and/or patients above 10 years of age.

ture by Kato (1930). They added 23 cases of their own and 15 other cases reported since Kato's work by other authors. In the whole group of 123 cases, they found that the average age at death in those with transposition and an atrial septal defect was 1 year and 11 months, while in those with transposition and a ventricular septal defect it was 4 years and 9 months. They concluded that the combination of an interatrial septal defect gives the best prognosis for those having transposition of the great arteries. The authors added, however, that the inclusion of 2 individual cases, aged 19 and 56 years, lends an unduly favorable character to the average survival time for the group with combined defects. Without this long surviving pair the average span of the group would be less than 1 year. Based on this observation, Blalock and Hanlon (1950) suggested the surgical therapy for transposition might be to create an atrial septal defect. Similarly, Lillehei and Varco (1953) suggested that the combination of an atrial septal defect gives the best prognosis in transposition of the great vessels.

In 1963, Shaher analyzed the 85 cases collected from the literature by Kato (1930) and which were included among the 123 patients reported by Hanlon and Blalock (1948). It was pointed out that the patient aged 19 years of Nasse (1821) was described as having a foramen ovale, an open ventricular septum, and a contracted pulmonary artery. The patient aged 56 years of age (Hedinger, 1915) was described by Kato as fol-

TABLE 18.6
15 PATIENTS FROM KATO (1930)

Case No.	Author	Age	Associated lesions
3A	Farre, 1814	5 Months	Single ventricle
18	Thore, 1842	11 Days	Single ventricle
21	Mauran, 1827	7 Months–8 days	Pulmonary atresia
33	Buchanan, 1857	4 Years	Overriding aorta
38	Peacock, 1858	8 Months	Single ventricle
39	Martin, 1839	10 Weeks	Doubtful cor biloculare
41	Otto, 1909	7 Month fetus	Single ventricle
70	Bournier, 1907	24 Days	Pulmonary atresia
77	Bissell, 1913–1915	11 Days	Single ventricle
79	Hedinger, 1915	56 Years	Single ventricle and tricuspid atresia
80	Marchand, 1908	21 Years	Single ventricle
82	Robertson, 1915–1917	7 Months	Double outlet RV
83	Jacobson, 1921	7 Months	Large PFO, virtually single atrium [a]
84	Abbott and Dawson, 1924	—	Aortic atresia
86	Ball, 1926	—	Single ventricle

[a] PFO indicates patent foramen ovale.

lows: "The oldest patient with typical transposition was in a case reported by Hedinger, that of a woman, aged 56, who was apparently in good health, except during pregnancy and just prior to death when she showed signs of cardiac failure. This patient had a cor biatriatum biloculare, which condition is also thought to be a beneficial association with a transposition of the great vessels." Moreover, of 15 patients included in Kato's list (Table 18.6) a single ventricle was present in 9, pulmonary atresia in 2, aortic atresia in 1, overriding aorta in 1, double outlet right ventricle in 1, and single atrium in 1. In addition, the case of Chevers (1846–1848) which was included in Kato's list of transposition had normal relationship of the aorta and pulmonary artery. His Cases 38 and 29 are one and the same. The original author, Peacock, described this case in "Transactions of the Pathological Society" in 1855, and later in his book "On Malformations of the Human Heart" in 1858. Furthermore, Kato's Case 14 which was described as having a closed ventricular septum and a nearly closed foramen ovale, was described by the original author, Coliny (1834), as a case of transposition of the great vessels and a ventricular septal defect. The original reports on 3 additional patients included among Kato's list (Mauran, 1827; Schilling, 1857; Gilliat, 1915), could not be traced by the author, for the correct reference was not cited by Kato. Based on these findings, the author (Shaher, 1963) doubted the validity of using such a group of patients for a study of the prognosis of complete transposition of the great arteries. In a selected group of exceptionally long survivors with transposition, Shaher (1963) found that the best prognosis occurred in the group with a large ventricular septal defect, and that the addition of an atrial septal defect to this group, apparently, shortened its life expectancy. This view, however, was criticized by Trusler *et al.* (1964) on the grounds that it was based on a small number of selected patients.

Similar findings emphasizing the poor prognosis of patients with an intact ventricular septum and a slightly better prognosis of patients with a ventricular septal defect have been reported by Boesen (1963), Calleja *et al.* (1964), and Liebman *et al.* (1969). An unfavorable influence exerted by patency of the ductus arteriosus upon the prognosis of transposition has been suggested by Ingomar and Tersley (1962), Calleja *et al.* (1964), Keith *et al.* (1967), and Liebman *et al.* (1969). No attempt was made in the present study to correlate the patency of the ductus to the anatomy of the associated defects, since at autopsy a patent ductus is found in most neonates and young infants with transposition. Review of the pathological material in this series shows that the ductus was small in the majority of cases (see Table 10.13). It seems likely that because of severe anoxia and acidosis the patients die at a stage when the ductus is still open. A clinical support of this view is the improvement that takes place in the condition of neonates with transposition, in whom the ductus is likely to be open, after balloon atrial septostomy or surgical creation of an atrial septal defect. Moreover, very seldom a ductus had to be surgically ligated to control heart failure in those with an intact ventricular septum. Indeed, as pointed out by Plauth *et al.* (1970) persistance of the ductus may contribute to maintenance of a satisfactory systemic arterial saturation beyond the first few weeks of life and that closure of the ductus may result in a precipitous drop in that saturation.

The favorable influence on prognosis exerted by left ventricular obstruction has been suggested by Taussig (1948) and Becker and Brill (1948). Undoubtedly, this effect is secondary to the protective influence of pulmonary stenosis against excessive pulmonary blood flow and pressure in cases with a ventricular septal defect. Although the figures in this series suggest that patients with an intact ventricular septum and pulmonary stenosis might have a better prognosis than patients with an intact septum but without pulmonary stenosis, the number of the patients in Group II was too small to allow any valid conclusions to be made.

Heart Failure and Prognosis

Heart failure in transposition is a sign of grave omen. In the majority of cases it occurred during the first few weeks of life. In some patients it complicated the postoperative course either as a result of arrhythmia or excessive pulmonary blood flow and pressure secondary to a shunt procedure. In older patients with transposition it occurred as a terminal event. Apart from postoperative heart failure, all unoperated patients who developed this complication died. Infants who survived heart failure were those who underwent successful balloon atrial septostomy or surgical creation of an atrial septal defect with or without banding of the pulmonary artery. In 2 patients in Group I and 4 in Group III, a large patent ductus had to be ligated to control the symptoms and signs of heart failure. In older children with transposition acute bronchitis or pneumonia precipitated heart failure. Heart failure in neonates, unless treated by balloon atrial septostomy or surgical creation of an atrial septal defect, almost always followed a very rapid downhill course and ended in the death of the patient after a few days. In older patients the course of this complication was less acute. The oldest patient in this series, 29 years of age, was noted to develop intermittant ankle edema for 8 years prior to her death.

Keith (1956) analyzed 304 cases of heart failure in the pediatric age group. Of these 304 cases, 71 had complete transposition of the great arteries. The author pointed out that when heart failure occurs during the first week of life, 85% die in the following weeks or months. Transposition of the great arteries is the second leading cause of death in this group. When the onset of failure occurs between the first week and the first month, 66% will die in the near future. Transposition of the great arteries is the second leading cause of death in this group. When the age of onset is 1–2 months, 58% will die shortly thereafter. Transposition of the great arteries is the leading cause of death from heart failure in this group. When the age of onset of failure is 2–6 months, 50% will die shortly. Transposition of the great arteries is the second leading cause of death in this group. Of the 37 patients who developed heart failure described by Noonan *et al.* (1960), 28 were below the age of 18 months and 9 were above the age of 18 months. Twenty-one patients (75%) in their first group died, while 7 (78%) in their second group survived. McCue and Young (1961) reported their experience with 115 patients under the age of 2 years in heart failure. Of these 115 patients, 11 had complete transposition of the great arteries. All 11 patients with this diagnosis died. A high mortality rate among infants with transposition in heart failure has also been reported by Blumenthal and Andersen (1959) and Goldblatt (1962).

Cause of Death

The cause of death of 308 patients in this series is shown in Table 18.7. Heart surgery, heart failure, pneumonia or other lung conditions, and anoxia were the four major causes of death, respectively. Heart surgery was the cause of death in less than one-half of the deaths in Groups I and III, and in more than two-thirds of the deaths in Groups II and IV. Heart failure was the cause of death in 33.5% in Group I, and 27.3% in Group III. On the other hand, anoxia accounted for 16.8% of the deaths in Group I, and 3.2% of the deaths in Group III. Lung problems were the cause of death in 24 patients; pneumonia in 19, and lung atelectasis in 5. Lung conditions were the cause of death in 5.7% in Group I, and 12.6% in Group III. Hemorrhage was the cause of death of 8 patients; intracranial in 3, pulmonary in 3, and gastrointestinal in 2. Eight patients died of infection; infected meningocele in 1, gastroenteritis in 3, brain abscess in 2, lung abscesses in 1, and subacute bacterial endocarditis in 1. In 4 patients, cardiac catheriza-

TABLE 18.7

CAUSE OF DEATH

Group	Surgery	Heart failure	Anoxia	Pneumonia and other lung conditions	Hemorrhage	Infection	Cardiac catheter	Sudden death	Others
Group I (175 Patients)	79	60	19	10	4	1	2	—	—
Group II (12 Patients)	8	2	—	1	—	1	—	—	—
Group III (97 Patients)	38	27	3	12	3	5	1	2	6
Group IV (24 Patients)	16	1	1	1	1	1	1	—	2
Total (308 Patients)	141	90	23	24	8	8	4	2	8

tion was the immediate cause of death. In 1 of these 4 gangrene of the foot complicated the procedure. Sudden death occurred in 2 other patients. Of the other causes that accounted for the death of 8, intestinal obstruction occurred in 2 (duodenal atresia in 1, and mesenteric artery thrombosis in 1), thoracotomy or appendicectomy in 3, stroke or thrombosis of the venous sinuses in 2, and a road accident in 1.

In the group of patients reported by Keith *et al.* (1958), heart failure was responsible for the deaths of 49%, anoxia for 17%, and surgery for 27%. Liebman *et al.* (1969) reported that anoxia was the most common cause of death in patients with an intact septum, while congestive heart failure was the leading cause in those with a ventricular septal defect and increased pulmonary blood flow. On the other hand, operation was the most common cause in the ventricular septal defect groups with pulmonary vascular obstruction and with pulmonary stenosis. Other primary causes of deaths in their series were 11 due to cardiac catheterization, 5 due to cerebrovascular accidents, either thrombosis with infarction or subarachnoid hemorrhage, and 1 each due to spontaneous pneumothorax, massive gastrointestinal bleeding from a stomach ulcer, and a saddle thromboembolism at the bifurcation of the aorta. A rare cause of death in transposition is acute myocardial infarction (Bernreiter, 1958), and acute coronary insufficiency (Messeloff and Weaver, 1951).

Long Survival in Transposition

Survival in transposition is determined by the size of the associated defects, the pulmonary vascular resistance, and the presence or absence of left ventricular outflow tract obstruction. Unoperated cases rarely survive more than 1 year. In the present series 17 patients survived more than 10 years of age without palliative or totally corrective heart surgery (Table 18.8). Unoperated reported cases with survival longer than 10 years is in Table 18.9.

In this group of long survivors complications secondary to relative aging, high hematocrit, and pulmonary hypertension, tended to be obvious. A frequent cause of death has been severe pulmonary or gastrointestinal hemorrhage. In 1 patient the cause of death was severe bleeding after thoracotomy. Cerebrovascular accidents occurred fairly frequently and a brain abscess was the cause of death of one. One patient developed gout. In most patients effort tolerance was markedly diminished, but some remained fairly active, and 1 patient used to take rock-and-roll classes until he died after appendicectomy at the age of 26 years. One patient was doing well until he died in a road accident at the age of 24 years.

TABLE 18.8

17 UNOPERATED PATIENTS WITH MORE THAN 10 YEARS SURVIVAL

Group	Age	SEX	Diagnosis and findings [a]
I	10 Years–6 months	F	Autopsy; ASD
	22 Years, alive	M	Angio.; ASD
II	12 Years	M	Autopsy; common atrium
III	10½ Years	M	Angio; VSD
	11 Years	M	Autopsy; VSD
	13 Years	M	Angio.; VSD
	13½ Years	M	Angio.; VSD
	15 Years	F	Angio.; VSD
	16 Years	F	Angio.; VSD
	18 Years	M	Autopsy; VSD
	24 Years	M	Autopsy; VSD
	25 Years	F	Autopsy; VSD
	26 Years	M	Autopsy; VSD
IV	11 Years	F	Autopsy; VSD, PS
	11 Years	M	Autopsy; VSD, PS
	21 Years	F	Autopsy; VSD, PS
	29 Years	F	Autopsy; VSD, PS

[a] Angio, angiogram; ASD, atrial septal defect; PS, pulmonary stenosis; VSD, ventricular septal defect.

TABLE 18.9

REPORTED UNOPERATED CASES WITH 10 YEARS OR MORE SURVIVAL

Author	Age (years)	SEX	FINDINGS [a]
Dorning (1890)	10	M	PFO
Emanuel (1906)	11	—	PFO
Keith (1912), Case 5	16	—	VSD, PS, PFO
Lewis and Abbott (1915)	21	—	VSD
Alexander and White (1947)	17	—	PFO
Brown (1950)	20	M	VSD
Campbell and Suzman (1951)	24	F	VSD, PS
Messelof and Weaver (1951)	38	—	PAPVD, VSD, PFO
Nichol and Segal (1951)	29	F	VSD, PDA, PS
Vogelsang (1953)	19	M	PFO
Massachusetts Hospital (1953)	16	F	VSD, PDA, PFO, PS, Brain abscess
Heim de Balsac and Eman-Zade (1954)	15	—	—
Pung et al. (1955)	18	M	PFO, PS
Wood (1956)	33	—	—
Best and Heath (1958), Case 5	14	M	PS (no details)
Levine and Harvey (1959)	17	M	PAPVD (no details)
Senning (1959), Case 2	10	M	VSD, PS
Froment et al. (1960)	26	M	PFO
Barnard et al. (1962)	16	F	ASD
Fisher et al. (1962)	20–40	—	—
Nice et al. (1964)	10	F	VSD
Folger et al. (1964)	14	F	—
Ferencz (1966)	21	—	—
Gasul et al. (1966)	47	—	ASD
Hightower et al. (1966)	16	—	ASD
Gerbode et al. (1967)	36	F	PAPVD, ASD, PDA

[a] ASD, atrial septal defect; PAPVD, partial anomalous pulmonary venous drainage; PDA, patent ductus arteriosus; PFO, patent foramen ovale; PS, pulmonary stenosis; VSD, ventricular septal defect.

References

Abbott, M. E. (1936). "Atlas of Congenital Cardiac Disease." American Heart Association, New York.

Abbott, M. E., and Dawson, W. T. (1924). The clinical classification of congenital cardiac disease, with remarks upon its pathological anatomy, diagnosis and treatment. *Int. Clin.* 4, 156.

Alexander, F., and White, P. D. (1947). Four important congenital cardiac conditions causing cyanosis to be differentiated from the tetralogy of Fallot: tricuspid atresia, Eisenmenger's complex, transposition of the great vessels, and a single ventricle. *Ann. Intern. Med.* 27, 64.

Ball, R. P. (1926). *Amer. J. Dis. Child.* **32**, 84. (Cited by K. Kato, 1930.)

Barnard, C. N., Schrire, V., and Beck, W. (1962). Complete transposition of the great vessels. Successful complete correction. *J. Thorac. Cardiovasc. Surg.* **43**, 768.

Bauer, D., and Astbury, E. C. (1944). Congenital cardiac disease: Bibliography of the 1,000 cases analysed in Maude Abbott's Atlas with an index. *Amer. Heart J.* **27**, 688.

Becker, M. C., and Brill, R. M. (1948). Complete transposition of the great vessels. *Arch. Pediat.* **65**, 249.

Bernreiter, M. (1958). Myocardial infarction in an infant with transposition of the great vessels. *J. Amer. Med. Ass.* **167**, 459.

Best, P. V., and Heath, D. (1958). Pulmonary thrombosis in cyanotic heart disease without pulmonary hypertension. *J. Pathol. Bacteriol.* **75**, 281.

Bissell, W. W. (1913–1915). Transposition of the arterial trunks, patent interventricular septum and rudimentary right ventricle. *Trans. Chicago Pathol. Soc.* **9**, 162.

Blalock, A., and Hanlon, C. R. (1950). The surgical treatment of complete transposition of the aorta and the pulmonary artery. *Surg. Gynecol. Obstet.* **90**, 1.

Blumenthal, S., and Andersen, D. H. (1959). Congestive heart failure in children. *J. Chronic Dis.* **9**, 590.

Boesen, I. B. (1963). Complete transposition of the great vessels: Importance of septal defects and patent ductus; analysis of 132 patients dying before age 4. *Circulation* **28**, 885.

Bournier, (1907). *Bull. Mein. Soc. Anat. (Paris).* (Cited by K. Kato, 1930.)

Brown, J. W. (1950). "Congenital Heart Disease," 2nd Ed. Staples Press, London.

Buchanan, G. (1857). Malformation of the heart cyanosis. *Trans. Pathol. Soc. London* **8**, 149.

Calleja, H. B., Hosier, D. M., and Grajo, M. Z. (1964). Anatomical ventricular hypertrophy patterns in complete transposition of the great vessels. *Brit. Heart J.* **26**, 642.

Campbell, M. (1972). Natural history of cyanotic malformations and comparison of all common cardiac malformations. *Brit. Heart J.* **34**, 3–8.

Campbell, M., and Suzman, S. (1951). Transposition of the aorta and pulmonary artery. *Circulation* **4**, 329.

Chevers, N. (1846–1848). Case illustrating the earliest stage of the malformation usually known as distribution of the descending aorta from the pulmonary artery. *Trans. Pathol. Soc. London* **1**, 55.

Coliny, M. (1834). Vice de conformation du coeur. *Arch. Gen. Med.* **5**, 284.

Cooley, R. N., and Sloan, R. D. (1952). Angiocardiography in congenital heart disease of cyanotic type. III. Observations on complete transposition of the great vessels. *Radiology* **58**, 481.

Dorning, J. (1890). A case of transposition of the aorta and pulmonary artery with patent foramen ovale; death at 10 years of age. *Trans. Amer. Pediat. Soc.* **2**, 46.

Emanuel, J. G. (1906). Three specimens of congenital deformity of the heart. *Rep. Soc. Stud. Dis. Child.* **6**, 240.

Farre, J. R. (1814). Pathological Researches, Essay No. 1, Malformations of the Human Heart, p. 29. London.

Ferencz, C. (1966). Transposition of the great vessels. Pathophysiologic considerations based upon a study of the lungs. *Circulation* **33**, 232.

Fisher, J. M., Wilson, W. R., and Theilens, E. O. (1962). Recognition of congenital heart disease in the fifth to eighth decades of life. *Circulation* **25**, 821.

Folger, G. M., Jr., Roberts, W. C., Mehrizi, A., Shah, K. D., Glancy, D. L., Carpenter, C. C. J., and Esterly, J. R. (1964) . Cyanotic malformations of the heart with pheochromocytema. A report of five cases. *Circulation* **29**, 750.

Fontana, R. S., and Edwards, J. E. (1962) . "Congenital Cardiac Disease: A review of 357 Cases Studied Pathologically." Philadelphia and London: Saunders, Philadelphia, Pennsylvania.

Froment, R., Perrin, A., and Brun, F. (1960). Transposition complete des gros vaisseaux de la base chex un adulte avec dolicho-mega-coronaires. *Arch. Mal. Coeur Vaiss.* **53**, 449.

Gasul, B. M., Arcilla, R. A., and Lev, M. (1966). "Heart Disease in Children." Lippincott, Philadelphia, Pennsylvania.

Gerbode, F., Selzer, A., Hill, J. D., and Aberg, T. (1967). Transposition of the great arteries: surgical repair of a complicated case in a 36-year-old woman. *Ann. Surg.* **166**, 1016–1020.

Gilliat, W. (1915). *J. Anat. Physiol.* **50**, 10. (Cited by K. Kato, 1930.)

Goldblatt, E. (1962). Treatment of cardiac failure in infancy: review of 350 cases. *Lancet* **ii**, 212.

Hanlon, R. C., and Blalock, A. (1948). Complete transposition of the aorta and the pulmonary artery. Experimental observations on venous shunts as corrective procedures. *Ann. Surg.* **127**, 385.

Hedinger, E. (1915). *Zentralbl. Allg. Pathol. Pathol. Anat.* **26**, 529. (Cited by K. Kato, 1930.)

Heim de Balsac, R., and Emam-Zade, A. M. (1954). Les transpositions vasculaires. *In* "Traites des Cardiopathies Congenitales." (E. Donzelot and F. D'Allaines, eds.) , pp. 848–889. Masson and Cie, Paris.

Hightower, B. M., Weidman, W. H., and Kirklin, J. W. (1966). Open intracardiac repair for complete transposition of the great arteries. *Circulation* **33**, 19–27.

Ingomar, C. J., and Tersley, E. (1962). Complete transposition of the great vessels. *Brit. Heart J.* **24**, 358.

Jacobson, V. C. (1921). Deviation of the aortic septum: complete transposition of great vessels, with report of two cases in infants. *Amer. J. Dis. Child.* **21**, 176.

Kato, K. (1930). Congenital transposition of cardiac vessels: a clinical and pathologic study. *Amer. J. Dis. Child.* **39**, 363.

Keith, A. (1912). Six specimens of abnormal heart. *J. Anat. Physiol.* **46**, 211.

Keith, J. D. (1956). Congestive Heart Failure. *Pediatrics* **18**, 491.

Keith, J. D., Neill, C. A., Vlad, P., Rowe, R. D., and Chute, A. L. (1953). Transposition of the great vessels. *Circulation* **7**, 830.

Keith, J. D., Rowe, R. D., and Vlad, P. (1958). "Heart Disease in Infancy and Childhood." 1st Ed. MacMillan, New York.

Keith, J. D., Rowe, R. D., and Vlad, P. (1967). "Heart Disease in Infancy and Childhood." 2nd Ed. MacMillan, New York.

Lev, M., Alcalde, V. M., and Baffes, T. O. (1961). Pathologic anatomy of complete transposition of the arterial trunks. *Pediatrics* **28**, 293.

Levine, S. A., and Harvey, W. P. (1959). "Clinical Auscultation of the Heart." Saunders, Philadelphia, Pennsylvania.

Lewis, F. T., and Abbott, M. (1915). Reversed torsion of the human heart. *Anat. Rec.* **9**, 103.

Liebman, J., Cullum, L., and Belloc, N. B. (1969). Natural history of transposition of the great arteries. Anatomy and birth and death characteristics. *Circulation* **40**, 237–262.

Lillehei, C. W., and Varco, R. L. (1953) . Certain physiologic, pathologic and surgical features of complete transposition of the great vessels. *Surgery* **34**, 376.

McCue, C. M., and Young, R. B. (1961). Cardiac failure in infancy. *J. Pediat.* **58**, 330.

Marchand, F. (1908). *Verh. Deut. Ges. Pathol.* **12**, 174. (Cited by E. Hedinger.)

Martin. (1859). Cited by J. Cockle (1863). *Med. Chir. Trans.* **46**, 193.

Massachusetts General Hospital Case Records. Weekly Clinicopathological exercises: Case 39351. (1953). *N. Engl. J. Med.* **249**, 371.

Mauran, J. (1827). *Phil. J. Med. Phys. Sci.* **14**, 253. (Cited by K. Kato, 1930).

Messeloff, C. R., and Weaver, J. C. (1951). A case of transposition of the large vessels in an adult who lived to the age of 38 years. *Amer. Heart J.* **42**, 467.

Nasse, C. F. (1821). *Leichenoffnungen Diag. Pathol. Anat.* (Cited by K. Kato, 1930.)

Nice, C. M., Jr., Daves, M. L., and Wood, G. H. (1964). Changes in bone associated with cyanotic congenital cardiac disease. *Amer. Heart J.* **68**, 25.

Nichol, A. D., and Segal, A. J. (1951). Complete transposition of the main arterial stems. *J. Amer. Med. Ass.* **147**, 645.

Noonan, A., Nadas, A. S., Rudolph, A. M., and Harris, G. B. C. (1960). Transposition of the great arteries. A correlation of clinical, physiologic and autopsy data. *N. Engl. J. Med.* **263**, 592.

Otto, W. (1909). *Virchows Arch. Pathol. Anat. Physiol.* **196**, 127. (Cited by K. Kato, 1930.)

Paul, M. H., Muster, A. J., Cole, R. B., and Baffes, T. G. (1968). Palliative management for transposition of the great arteries: 1957–1967. *Ann. Thorac. Surg.* **6**, 321.

Peacock, T. B. (1855). Case of malformation of the heart. Both auricles opening into the left ventricle, and transposition of the aorta and pulmonary artery. *Trans. Pathol. Soc. London* **6**, 117.

Peacock, T. B. (1858). "On Malformation of the Human Heart," 1st Ed. Churchill, London.

Plauth, W. H., Jr., Nadas, A. S., Bernhard, W. F., and Gross, R. E. (1968). Transposition of the great arteries. Clinical and physiological observations on 74 patients treated by palliative surgery. *Circulation* **37**, 316–330.

Plauth, W. H., Jr., Nadas, A. S., Bernhard, W. F., and Fyler, D. C. (1970). Changing hemodynamics in patients with transposition of the great arteries. *Circulation* **42**, 131–142.

Pung, S., Gottstein, W. K., and Hirsch, E. F. (1955). Complete transposition of the great vessels in a male aged 18 years. *Amer. J. Med.* **18**, 155.

Robertson, J. J. (1915–1917). *Heart* **6**, 99. (Cited by K. Kato, 1930.)

Schilling, E. (1857). Cited by Kato (1930).

Senning, A. (1959). Surgical correction of transposition of the great vessels. *Surgery* **45**, 966.

Shaher, R. M. (1963). Prognosis of transposition of the great vessels with and without atrial septal defect. *Brit. Heart J.* **25**, 211.

Taussig, H. B. (1948). Tetralogy of Fallot, especially care of cyanotic infant and child. *Pediatrics* **1**, 307.

Thore. (1842). *Arch. Gen. Med.* **15**, 316. (Cited by K. Kato, 1930.)

Trusler, G. A., Mustard, W. T., and Fowler, R. S. (1964). The role of surgery in the treatment of transposition of the great vessels. *Can. Med. Ass. J.* **91**, 1096–1100.

Vogelsang, A. (1953). Transposition of the great arteries with patent foramen ovale. *Can. Med. Ass. J.* **69**, 625.

Wood, P. (1956). "Diseases of the Heart and Circulation," 2nd Ed. Eyre and Spottiswoode, London.

Chapter 19

MEDICAL MANAGEMENT AND BALLOON ATRIAL SEPTOSTOMY

Transposition of the great arteries in the neonatal period should be regarded as a medical emergency. Patients with transposition presenting after the first month of life are usually less acutely sick. Most patients with transposition who develop severe cyanosis and congestive heart failure during the first few days of life have an intact ventricular septum or a small ventricular septal defect. The management of these critically sick infants is directed toward control of heart failure, hypoxia, and correction of the acid–base balance and hypothermia. On arrival to the hospital the infant should be put in an isolette incubator with an oxygen concentration maintained as high as possible. An intravenous infusion of 1/3 saline in 5% dextrose should be started at once. If the infant is seen during the first day or two of life the umbilical artery should be catheterized to provide constant information on the acid–base balance and blood gases. Digitalis and diuretics should be given to control heart failure. While getting ready for cardiac catheterization, which should be done as an emergency procedure, acidosis and electrolyte imbalance should be corrected. As pointed out by Benzig *et al.* (1969) the blood sugar should be determined and hypoglycemia corrected since a low blood sugar could be a factor in aggravating heart failure. Because of the low risk involved at atrial septostomy (Rashkind and Miller, 1966), this procedure should be performed as soon as the diagnosis has been established by cardiac catheterization. Unless the systemic arterial saturation is exceptionally high, i.e., 75% or more, this procedure should be done on all infants with transposition. Atrial septostomy will improve acidosis, anoxia, and heart failure. In addition, by reducing left atrial hypertension, it will diminish pulmonary venous congestion and improve tachypnea and cyanosis. Although angiocardiography will demonstrate a small ductus in the majority of neonates with transposition, occasionally this structure is large and might give rise to persistent heart failure after successful atrial septostomy. At cardiac catheterization an aortic angiogram is essential to investigate the size of the ductus and to rule out coarctation of the aorta. Patients with severe hypoxia will show marked improvement after atrial septostomy. On the other hand, heart failure caused by excessive pulmonary blood flow and pressure in patients with a large ventricular septal defect or a large patent ductus arteriosus with or without coarctation of the aorta may not show significant improvement after this procedure. This group of patients with persistent heart failure should be considered for division of the ductus or banding of the pulmonary artery. Coarctation of the aorta, if present, should be corrected at the same time. After atrial septostomy, the infant should be monitored in the intensive care unit and oxygen in relatively high concentration should be continued. The acid-base balance and blood gases should be determined frequently and acidosis should be corrected by intravenous sodium bicarbonate. As the condition of the infant improves, oxygen concentration should be diminished and finally it could be discontinued. The infant should stay in the hospital until heart failure has been satisfactorily controlled. In most of these patients, digitalis has to be continued for 1, 2, or several years.

Patients with transposition of the great arteries and left ventricular outflow tract obstruction do not usually get into trouble in the neonatal period. In this group of patients balloon atrial septostomy should be performed too at the initial cardiac catheterization unless, because of the age of the patient, the procedure is considered unsafe.

All patients with transposition of the great arteries should be followed up at fairly short but regular intervals. Increase in the severity of cyanosis should prompt repeated cardiac catheterization, since development of left ventricular outflow tract obstruction, diminution in the size of atrial or ventricular septal defects, spontaneous closure of ventricular septal defects, development of pulmonary vascular obstruction, or a nonfunctioning surgical shunt could be responsible. If the child remains well cardiac catheterization should be repeated between the ages of 6 months and 1 year and again at the age of 2 years.

During the follow-up period lung infections should be treated promptly and adequately since very often pneumonia or acute bronchitis precede congestive heart failure. Prompt correction of the acid-base balance and dehydration should minimize central nervous system complications. Regular and frequent checkups by the pediatrician is an important aspect of the medical care of these children.

The Rashkind Procedure

An important contribution to the medical management of transposition of the great arteries was made by Rashkind and Miller (1966). The closed technique of rupturing the foramen ovale by repeatedly withdrawing a balloon-tipped catheter from the left atrium to the right atrium gives excellent palliation and carries low mortality rate in infants with transposition. Further comments on the procedure were published by Watson and Rashkind (1967), Rashkind and Miller (1968a), Rashkind (1970a,b; and 1971a,b,c) and Mullins et al. (1972).

According to Rashkind (1971b) the procedure is performed in the following manner. In most instances, surgical exposure of the femoral vein is required. In a newborn infant less than 48 or 72 hours of age, the umbilical vein has been used by Abinader et al. (1970) for both the diagnostic catheterization as well as balloon septostomy. A double-lumen No. 6.5 French catheter is advanced to the right atrium and across the foramen ovale into the left atrium or a pulmonary vein. The location of the catheter in the left atrium is verified by one or more of the following procedures: angiocardiography, determination of a high level of oxygen saturation in blood samples obtained from a chamber with atrial pressure, recognition of the posterior position of the catheter tip at the upper left cardiac border, and entry of the catheter tip into a pulmonary vein. The balloon is inflated with dilute radiopaque iodine solution to a diameter of 1.0 to 1.5 cm and is then rapidly withdrawn across the atrial septum with an abrupt, short tug (Fig. 19.1). During withdrawal, the septum is displaced toward the inferior vena cava. The pullback motion is designed to carry the balloon in a single movement from the left atrium to the right atrial-inferior vena cava junction. It is then pushed cephalad into the right atrial cavity and deflated. Using gradually increasing balloon volumes, the procedure is repeated five to ten times until no resistance is perceived during withdrawal of a balloon inflated to a diameter of 1.5 to 2.0 cm. It is important to repeat this procedure several times until no further resistance is met on pullback, until a satisfactory arterial oxygen saturation is obtained, or until the left atrial to right atrial "a" wave pressure gradient has been abolished.

Mullins et al. (1972) suggested the following useful cardiac catheterization protocol for infants with transposition:

A. Establish diagnosis
B. Perform balloon septostomy
C. Obtain essential information

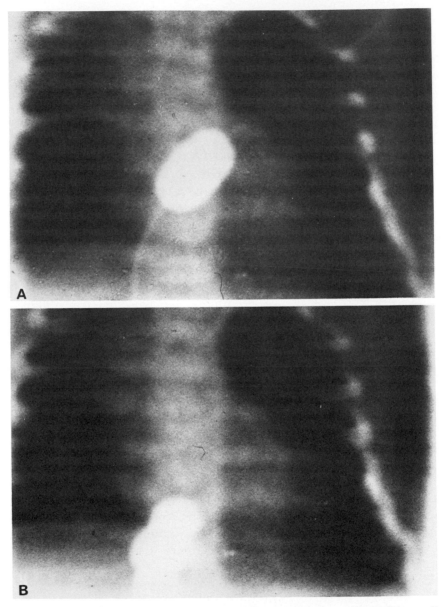

Fig. 19.1. Balloon atrial septostomy. (A) Balloon in left atrium. (B) Balloon pulled through the foramen ovale and wedged into inferior vena cava which produced the lower constriction in the balloon. The upper constriction is produced by the foramen ovale.

     1. Pressure data
       a. Left atrium to right atrium withdrawal pressure both before
         and after septostomy.
       b. Left ventricular verus right ventricular pressure.
     2. Associated Defects
       a. Patent ductus
       b. Ventricular septal defect
       c. Severe pulmonary stenosis
   D. Obtain additional useful information
     1. Pressure and oxygen saturation
       a. All cardiac chambers and great vessels
       b. Before and after septostomy
     2. Pressure gradient in mild to moderate pulmonary stenosis.

COMPLICATIONS OF THE PROCEDURE

Rashkind (1970a,1971b) emphasizes that this procedure carries all the hazards of cardiac catheterization in infants and children. Perforation of atrial wall was reported by Venables (1966), Parsons *et al.* (1971), Rashkind (1971b), Baker *et al.* (1971), and Neches *et al.* (1972). Rashkind points out that this hazard can be minimized by softening the distal half of the catheter in hot water prior to use. Inability to insert the balloon catheter into the femoral vein should be overcome by making the skin incision high enough to obtain a vein of large diameter. Withdrawal of the inflated balloon from either ventricle can produce serious damage to the atrioventricular valves. Balloon rupture of the tricuspid valve occurred in one of the patients of Baker *et al.* (1971). Using a double-lumen catheter, this hazard is prevented by checking the pressures and oxygen saturations. If a single-lumen catheter is necessary, left atrial position is verified by catheterization of a pulmonary vein or by measurement of the pressure wave transmission through the partly inflated balloon to distinguish between atrial and ventricular pressure. Damage to a pulmonary vein from balloon distention is avoided by slow inflation, which results in gentle extrusion of the entire tip into the left atrial cavity. Rashkind points out that rupture of the balloon is a rather common phenomenon and one must be extremely careful to remove all air bubbles from the balloon catheter to prevent air embolization. Vogel (1970) reported an infant with transposition of the great arteries in whom a piece of rubber from the balloon embolized the ostium of the right renal artery completely occluding it. Inability to deflate the catheter balloon after septostomy was reported by Scott (1970), Ellison *et al.* (1970) and Hohn and Webb (1972). This complication was caused by retraction of the balloon due to movement of the proximal tethering during septostomy. Rashkind suggests that this complication could be managed by inserting a sharp stylet wire inside a very fine catheter to the inferior vena cava–right atrial junction. The wire tip then can be advanced just beyond the catheter, and the balloon-tipped catheter pulled against the wire tip until the balloon ruptures. Zamora *et al.* (1970) reported 2 patients in whom thrombosis of the inferior vena cava complicated the procedure. None of these children had a history suggesting acute caval thrombosis. Absence of clinical and pathological evidence of distant embolization suggested to the authors a slowly developing thrombosis. Hawker *et al.* (1971) reported 3 other patients with transposition in whom thrombosis of the inferior vena cava followed balloon septostomy. The authors advocated the use of the saphenous rather than the femoral vein for balloon atrial septostomy, because effort should be made not only to preserve as many veins as possible, but also to minimize the risk of thrombosis of the inferior vena cava. Intraabdominal hemorrhage complicating this procedure was reported by Ehmke *et al.* (1970). The relevance of levo-position of the right atrial appendage to balloon septostomy was discussd by Tyrrell and Moes (1971). These authors emphasized that in this condition the catheter may appear to conform to the criteria of a left atrial position yet still be in the right atrial appendage.

OTHER INSTRUMENTS USED FOR ATRIAL SEPTOSTOMY

The Rashkind catheters are more frequently used for atrial septostomy than any other type of balloon catheters. Singh *et al.* (1969) pointed out that No. 5 or No. 6 Fogarty embolectomy catheters could be used for this procedure. These catheters have acron tips which are sometimes easier to introduce than the Rashkind No. 6½ catheters. They are also cheaper but do have the slight disadvantage that they need filling with contrast medium to make them radiopaque and they do not have a second lumen. Clarkson *et al.* (1972) used a Fogarty embolectomy catheter to perform septostomy in 5 patients. This method was found to be unsatisfactory as 3 of the 5 had an inadequate atrial communication created. Hawker *et al.* (1971) used an Edwards No. 6 double-lumen catheter in all their cases. A catheter, the distal end of which can be pulled into a rigid triangular-shaped instrument was used by Girod (1971) to perform atrial septostomy. In this technique a teflon sheath is percutaneously introduced through the femoral vein to the left atrium. A triangle catheter is advanced through the sheath and a triangle is formed in the left atrium. The catheter is then withdrawn to the right atrium. Of the 7 patients reported by Girod, the oxygen saturation increased in 2. In 2 other patients an atrial defect, freshly made, was observed at subsequent surgery. In 1 patient the catheter could not be passed through the sheath. In 3 patients no resistance was met during catheter withdrawal, and the oxygen saturation did not rise. In 1 patient, during withdrawal, the catheter tubing tore and was removed during atrial septectomy. The author pointed out that the triangle catheter, with and without cutting edges, may be useful in some patients requiring atrial septostomy. The fact, however, that the triangle catheter could be introduced percutaneously, makes it an important contribution worthy of further clinical trials.

RESULTS OF PALLIATION BY BALLOON ATRIAL SEPTOSTOMY

The immediate efficacy of the balloon septostomy in producing adequate palliation of transposition of the great vessels is emphasized in the literature. Muster *et al.* (1967) used this technique on 33 patients with transposition. Of the 15 with an intact ventricular septum, 9 survived with clinical improvement, 3 required additional palliative surgery, and 3 died later. Of the 8 with a ventricular septal defect, 1 survived without additional surgery and 7 required banding of the pulmonary artery; 4 patients survived. Their 5 patients with ventricular septal defect and pulmonary stenosis have had adequate septostomies. Balloon atrial septostomy was used by Gerard *et al.* (1968) on 7 babies between the ages of 2 and 15 days with satisfactory results in 5 cases. Venables (1968) reported the result of 12 completed procedures and pointed out that the main problem was atrial perforation which occurred three times. Despite this complication he thought that the procedure offers the opportunity to increase the salvage of hypoxic infants with transposition. All 31 patients reported by Rashkind and Miller (1968b) survived balloon atrial septostomy without complications; 26 had effective immediate palliation and 22 were long-term survivors. Of the 37 patients palliated at The Hospital For Sick Children, London, and reported by Tynan (1968), there were 9 deaths during the first hospital admission. Singh *et al.* (1969) reported their experience with 38 infants palliated by balloon atrial septostomy. Thirty-four survived the procedure and 4 died on the same day. Disturbances in the rhythm of the heart was the cause of death in these 4. Five patients died between 1 day and 6 weeks after septostomy, of operative mortality as a result of subsequent Blalock-Hanlon operation in 3, and of severe bronchopneumonia in 2. There were 5 late deaths: after Blalock-Hanlon operation in 1, cerebral thrombosis in 2, undetermined cause of death in 2. The results of palliation seemed satisfactory in the 24 patients who were seen in the follow-up. A further report on balloon septostomy from the Hospital For Sick Children, London, was given by Tynan *et al.* (1969). Fourty-one patients had this procedure and the result was considered adequate in 36, inadequate in 2, and equivocal in 3. There were 10 hospital deaths, only one of these occurring in the absence of an additional cardiac lesion. Massive hemorrhage into the thymus appeared to be the cause of death in this case. Five of the 10 deaths occurred in patients who had operations for additional cardiac lesions. Eight patients were reinvestigated because of increasing cyanosis developing after an initial good result from the septostomy. No cardiac cause was found in 1, an inadequate septostomy in 1, raised pulmonary vascular resistance in 1, and left ventricular outflow tract obstruction in 5. Tamer *et al.* (1969) performed balloon septostomy in 8 infants with transposition and intact ventricular septum. Six infants survived from 2 to 10 months with significant clinical improvement. Dobell *et al.* (1969) reported their experience with balloon atrial septostomy on 9 infants with transposition. All patients survived and the procedure was dramatically effective in increasing mixing and in decompressing a high pressure left atrium. Further palliation by surgical creation of an atrial septal defect was performed in 3 patients months after septostomy. Newfeld *et al.* (1970) reported their experience with 10 infants palliated by balloon septostomy. Death occurred following attempted banding of the pulmonary artery in 2 patients with a ventricular septal defect. The remaining 8 patients, all with an intact ventricular septum, were alive and doing well. One of these required a surgical septostomy at 5 months of age after 2 balloon septostomies during the first 2 weeks of life. Porstmann *et al.* (1970) reported on 40 babies suffering from complete transposition of the great arteries. Thirty-one of them were subjected to balloon atrial septostomy. The survival rate after a technically successful septostomy was 81%. Muster *et al.* (1970) encountered significant complications in over 30% of the 57 infants in their series before they reached what had been previously considered an optimum age for corrective surgery (2 or 3 years of age). Some of these complications involved changes in the hemodynamic status of the patient such as spontaneous closure of atrial or ventricular septal defects or the development of left ventricular outflow tract obstruction. Other problems were thromboembolism, chronic hypoxia, or uncontrolled heart failure. Venables (1970) further commented on the results of 26 complete balloon septostomies. Of 7 deaths following this procedure, 3 were clearly or probably related to it or to its failure to produce an adequate septal defect, while 4 were unrelated. Atrial perforations occurred on 4 occasions. The author pointed out that apparently adequate initial defects do not guarantee satisfactory long-term palliation, since 4 of 11 infants followed for more than 6 months after effective initial palliation have required surgical procedures to provide more adequate atrial mixing of blood. He added that despite this, the procedure appears to offer considerable advantage over initial surgical procedures to create atrial defects. Zamora *et al.* (1970) performed balloon atrial septostomy on 9 infants with an intact ventricular septum. A continuously deteriorating clinical course, however, made emergency surgical septectomy necessary within a few hours. Parsons *et al.* (1971) gave additional information on the group of patients studied at Birmingham, England. Of their 65 consecutive cases, a second septostomy was needed on 18 occasions. There were 32 deaths in this group; 5 immediate, 25 intermediate, and 2 late. Of the 5 immediate deaths, 4 resulted from cardiac arrest and 1 from perforated atrium. Of the 25 intermediate deaths, 9 resulted directly from thrombosis mainly of the cerebral vessels, 7 from heart failure, 4 from inadequate relief from septostomy, 2 from surgical septectomy, and in 3 patients the cause of death was unexplained. There were 2 late deaths after Mustard's operation. Baker *et al.* (1971) reported the immediate and long-term efficacy of the balloon atrial septostomy in a series of 43 patients with transposition. There were 7 technical failures. In 3 patients the balloon catheter could not be inserted. In the remaining 4, balloon rupture of the tricuspid valve occurred in 1, perforation of the atrial wall in 1, inability to deflate the balloon in 1, and subarachnoid hemorrhage following multiple balloon ruptures in 1. In 5 patients no improvement was seen following the procedure. Thirty-one patients were considered initial successes. The authors pointed out that in spite of the improved survival rate with balloon septostomy, complications have occurred frequently. Five patients have had cerebrovascular accidents, and 7 others have shown seizure activity. Six infants have had episodes of severe dyspnea and lethargy and 6 others have had pneumonia. Diminution in the size of or spontaneous closure of the atrial septal defect was shown at cardiac catheterization in 2. A total of 13 patients required late surgical septectomy with only 1 death. The authors concluded that balloon atrial septostomy is initially effective and relatively safe, but in those with intact ventricular septum surgical septectomy is often required. In their experience, balloon catheter measurement of the interatrial opening was helpful in predicting the necessity for surgical septectomy. Rashkind (1971b) reported the results of balloon atrial septostomy in 60 patients with transposition seen at The Children's Hospital of Philadelphia. Of these 60 patients, 51 (85%) improved from their first hospital admission and were discharged. Nine patients died in the hospital on the first admission and, in 1 of these, death was considered a procedural failure since it resulted from perforation of the right atrium by the balloon catheter. The remaining 8 patients had adequate atrial septostomies but death was related to other factors. Of the 51 infants who had improved and were discharged 48 had effective long-term palliation. Of these 48 patients, 6 died subsequent to total correction of their heart condition, and 21 have had total corrections. Repeat balloon septostomy was performed on 4 patients. Eight patients developed strokes, with 3 deaths. Half of the strokes occurred in children under 1 year of age. Six were preceded by severe infections. Tynan (1971) analyzed the survival chances of 80 infants with transposition of the great arteries palliated by balloon septostomy. The hospital death rate was considerably less than that of surgically treated patients in the same institution. However, the number of late deaths brought total survival figures from both methods of treatment to similar levels. Of the 60 patients who underwent balloon atrial septostomy by Paul (1971), there were 5 early deaths and 4 late deaths that were not associated with subsequent surgical intervention. Of the 5 early deaths, 4 were due to procedural failure and 1 to excessive respiratory depression from sedation. Of the 4 late deaths, 1 resulted from progressive pulmonary vascular obstruction, and 3 from cerebrovascular accidents. Subsequently, 20 infants required palliative surgery; surgical atrial septal defect in 13, patent ductus ligation in 1, pulmonary artery banding in 3, and systemic to pulmonary artery shunt in 3. Reassessment of the systemic arterial blood oxygen saturation at various intervals demonstrated a mean of 59.7 ± 9.6 percent when the highest values are selected for the group with an intact ventricular septum. The group mean for this value was 50.1 ± 8.7 percent when the lowest values observed for each individual were considered. For the ventricular septal defect group, there was little individual variation and the group follow-up mean arterial blood oxygen saturation was 74.5 ± 11.8 percent. Using a No. 5 Edwards dilatation or Rashkind catheter, Clarkson *et al.* (1972) performed atrial septostomy in 22 patients. One patient died as a result of excessive blood loss during the procedure. Early in the series, 3 patients appeared clinically unsatisfactory and had a surgical creation of an atrial septal defect after the septostomy with 1 death occurring. At the time of the septectomy the atrial defect was large in 1 patient but was inadequate in 2 who had an anatomically small fossa ovalis. There were 2 late deaths among the surviving 20 patients who left the hospital. Two other patients survived 3 episodes of cerebral thrombosis. Information concerning the size of the interratrial communication was obtained at subsequent surgery or autopsy in 20 of the 22 patients. The diameter of defect was 10 mm or more in 9, 7–9 mm in 5, and 6 mm or less in 6. Neches *et al.* (1972) performed balloon septostomy in 45 infants with transposition. Twenty-seven patients had an intact ventricular septum, while 18 had a ventricular septal defect alone or in combination with other lesions. One infant died during attempted septostomy as the result of perforation of the right atrial appendage. Forty-one patients were considered to have had initial improvement, while 3 had an unsatisfactory result. Nine patients required a second septostomy 3 weeks to 11 months after the initial procedure. Six infants, exclusive of those who had a second septostomy, required further palliation. Thirty patients did not have palliative procedures performed subsequent to the initial septostomy. A total of 12 deaths occurred in these 45 patients; one as a complication of the procedure, 3 during the first week following the procedure, 3 after palliative procedures, 2 after total correction, and 3 late deaths. Thirty-three patients were alive from 3 to 46 months following the initial septostomy. Of these 33 patients, 6 under went total correction. Of the remaining 27 patients, 8 had palliative surgery, 2 had repeat septostomy, and 17 had no further palliative procedures. Of the 33 survivors, 2 developed cerebrovascular accidents at 3 and 7 months of age, respectively. The authors considered balloon atrial septostomy a safe and effective means of immediately palliating 91% of infants with transposition. Beuron et al. (1972) performed balloon atrial septostomy in 91 infants. Transposition of the great arteries was present in 86, and total anomalous pulmonary venous drainage in 5. The death rate in these two groups was markedly lowered by the procedure. However, the number of deaths from other complications before the age for total correction had been reached remained high.

The efficacy of balloon septostomy in palliating infant with transposition has also been emphasized by others, such as Jordan and McCarthy (1967) 1 case, Watson and Rashkind (1967), Parenzan et al. (1967), Watson (1968), Rashkind and Miller (1968a), Lemoine (1968), Pernot et al. (1967), 3 cases, Webb and Hohn (1969), and Kidd et al. (1971). DeGuzman and Silver (1970) reported a neonate with transposition and ventricular tachycardia. After atrial septostomy the patient improved clinically and ventricular tachycardia gradually reverted to sinus rhythm within 48 hours.

Tynan (1972) pointed out that increasing cyanosis is a poor guide to atrial septal defect adequacy after balloon atrial septostomy, because the size of the atrial septal defect is not the only determinant of arterial oxygen saturation. He analyzed the relationship between the systemic arterial oxygen saturation and the ratio between pulmonary and systemic blood flows by linear regression in 14 patients before and 27 patients after balloon atrial septostomy. A direct relationship existed only when an atrial septal defect was present. He pointed out that since arterial oxygen saturation and atrial pressures as unreliable in assessing atrial septal defect adequacy the relationship between arterial oxygen saturation and the ratio between pulmonary and systemic blood flows provides a valuable method of making this assessment. If, in the presence of low systemic arterial oxygen saturation the flow is also low, then the atrial septal defect is adequate. But if the flow ratio is high, the atrial septal defect is too small. Needless to say, Tynan's conclusions apply only to cases without left ventricular outflow obstruction for an infant with transposition; severe pulmonary stenosis and a small atrial septal defect might have the combination of low systemic arterial oxygen saturation and low pulmonary-to-systemic flow ratio.

In the present series, atrial septostomy was performed on 11 infants with transposition; 10 in Group I, and 1 in Group III. The procedure was considered a failure in 5; inability to insert the catheter in 2, rupture of the tricuspid valve in 1, and no significant enlargement of the foramen ovale in 2. One patient with an intact ventricular septum died of severe acidosis and autopsy demonstrated a large atrial defect produced by the balloon catheter. Of the 5 survivors, 2 required surgical septectomies 3–6 months after the procedure, 2 required repeat balloon septectomy after 2 months, 1 underwent banding of the pulmonary artery and surgical creation of an atrial septal defect 2 months after septostomy, and 1 is alive and well 1 year after the initial palliation.

As pointed out by various workers balloon atrial septostomy gives excellent initial results in a significant number of infants with transposition. Since the risks involved at this procedure are low, all infants with transposition should have balloon septostomy at the same time of the initial cardiac catheterization. Adequacy of palliation after this procedure is determined by adequacy of rupture of the foramen ovale by the balloon catheter. After the first 6 months of life, surgical creation of an atrial septal defect or total surgical correction should be considered if interatrial shunting is inadequate.

References

Abinader, E., Zeltzer, W., and Riss, E. (1970). Transumbilical atrial septostomy in the newborn. *Amer. J. Dis. Child.* 119, 354.

Baker, F., Baker, L., Zoltun, R., and Zuberbuhler, J. R. (1971). Effectiveness of the Rashkind procedure in transposition of the great arteries in infants. *Circulation* 43 (Suppl. 1), 1.

Benzing, G., III, Schubert, W., Hug, G., and Kaplan, S. (1969). Simultaneous hypoglycemia and acute congestive heart failure, *Circulation* 40, 209.

Beuren, A. J., Keutel, J., Gandjour, A., et al. (1972). Kunstlicher vorhofseptumdefeckt nach Rashkind. Ergebnisse bei 91 patienten. *Deut. Med. Wochschr.* 97, 148.

Clarkson, P. M., Barratt-Boyes, B. G., Neutze, J. M., and Lowe, J. B. (1972). Results over a ten year period of palliation followed by corrective surgery for complete transposition of the great arteries. *Circulation* 45, 1251.

DeGuzman, A., and Silver, W. (1970) . Ventricular tachycardia and transposition of the great arteries. Occurrence in an infant 1 hour of age and favorable response to septostomy. *Amer. J. Dis. Child.* **119**, 278.

Dobell, A. R. C., Gibbons, J. E., and Busse, E. F. G. (1969). Hemodynamic correction of transposition of the great vessels in infants. *J. Thorac. Cardiovasc. Surg.* **57**, 108.

Ehmke, D. A., Durnin, R. E., and Lauer, R. M. (1970). Intra-abdominal hemorrhage complicating a balloon atrial septostomy for transposition of the great arteries. *Pediatrics* **45**, 289.

Ellison, R. C., Plauth, W. H., Jr., Gazzaninga, A. B., and Fyler, D. C. (1970). Inability to deflate catheter balloon: a complication of balloon atrial septostomy. *J. Pediat.* **76**, 604.

Gerard, R., Monties, J. P., Baille, Y., *et al.* (1968). Le traitement Durgence de la transposition des gros vaisseaux par la methode de Rashkind. *Marseille Med.* **105**, 677.

Girod, A. (1971). Use of triangle catheter instrument for atrial septostomy. *Circulation* **44** (Suppl. 2), 70.

Hawker, R. E., Celermajer, J. M., Cartnill, T. B., and Bowdler, J. D. (1971). Thrombosis of the inferior vena cava following balloon septostomy in transposition of the great arteries. *Amer. Heart J.* **82**, 593–595.

Hohn, A. R., and Webb, H. M. (1972). Balloon deflation failure: A hazard of "medical" atrial septostomy. *Amer. Heart J.* **83**, 389.

Jordan, S. C., and McCarthy, C. (1967). Haemodynamic consequences of atrial septostomy without thoracotomy in an infant with transposition of the great arteries. *Lancet* **i**, 310–311.

Kidd, B. S. L., Tyrell, M. J., and Pickering, D. (1971) . Transposition 1969. *In* "The Natural History and Progress in Treatment of Congenital Heart Defects". (B. S. L. Kidd and J. D. Keith, eds.) , P. 127. Charles C. Thomas, Springfield, Illinois.

Lemoine, G. (1968). La Chirurgie des cardiopathies congenitales dans les premieres semaines de la vie. *Sem. Hop.* **44**, 2887–2894.

Mullins, C. E., Neches, W. H., and McNamara, D. G. (1972). The infant with transposition of the great arteries. I. Cardiac catheterization protocol. *Amer. Heart J.* **84**, 597.

Muster, A. J., Cole, R. B., and Paul, M. (1967). Non-surgical creation of atrial septal defect. Clinical, physiologic and pathologic observations in 32 infants with transposition of the great arteries. Presented at the Proc. Pediat. Cardiol. Section Acad. Pediat., October, Washington, D.C.

Muster, A. J., Levin, S. E., Cole, R. B., *et al.* (1970). The modified history of transposition of the great arteries following non-surgical atrial septostomy. *Amer. J. Cardiol.* **25**, 118.

Neches, W. H., Mullins, C. E., and McNamara, D. G. (1972). The infant with transposition of the great arteries. II. Results of balloon atrial septostomy. *Amer. Heart J.* **84**, 603.

Newfeld, E. A., Eisenberg, R. N., and Young, D. (1970). Transposition of the great arteries. The changing prognosis. *Amer. J. Dis. Child.* **120**, 320–323.

Parenzan, L., Bianchetti, L., and Pasolini, G. (1967). La 'settostomia atriale' mediante il catetere con palloncino de Rashkind-Miller. Efficace nuova techica per il trattamento della trasposizione die grossi vasi nel neonato e nel lattante. *Minerva Pediat.* **19**, 1928–1932.

Parsons, C. G., Astley, R., Burrows, F.G.O., and Singh, S. P. (1971). Transposition of the great arteries. A study of 65 infants followed for 1 to 4 years after balloon septostomy. *Brit. Heart J.* **33**, 725.

Paul, M. H. (1971). Transposition of the great arteries: physiologic data. *In* "The Natural History and Progress in Treatment of Congenital Heart Defects." (B. S. L. Kidd and J. D. Keith, eds.), p. 144. Charles C. Thomas, Springfield, Illinois.

Pernot, C., Worms, A. M., Fall, M., and Pierson, M. (1967). L'atrioseptostomie de Rashkind dans le traitement des nouveaux—nes atteints de transposition complete des gros vaissexux. *Ann. Med. Nancy* **6**, 792.

Porstmann, W., Barthel, I., Motsch, K., and Munster, W. (1970). Transatriale septostomie mit ballon-kathetern zur palliativbehandlung der kompletten transposition der grossen gefasse. *Deut. Gesundheitsw.* **25**, 2361.

Rashkind, W. J. (1970a). The complications of balloon atrioseptostomy. *J. Pediat.* **76**, 649.

Rashkind, W. J. (1970b). Transposition of the great arteries. *In* "Current Pediatric Therapy" (S. S. Gellis and B. M. Kagan, Ed.), Vol. 4, p. 223. Saunders, Philadelphia, Pennsylvania.

Rashkind, W. J. (1971a). Palliative procedures for transposition of the great arteries. *Brit. Heart J.* **33**, 69.

Rashkind, W. J. (1971b). Transposition of the great arteries. *Pediat. Clin. N. Amer.* **18**, 1075.

Rashkind, W. J. (1971c). Balloon atrial septostomy for transposition of the great arteries: technique and follow-up. *In* "The Natural History and Progress in Treatment of Congenital Heart Defects." (B. S. L. Kidd and J. D. Keith, eds.), p. 138. Charles C. Thomas, Springfield, Illinois.

Rashkind, W. J., and Miller, W. W. (1966). Creation of an atrial septal defect without thoracotomy. *J. Amer. Med. Ass.* **196**, 991.

Rashkind, W. J., and Miller, W. W. (1968a). Atrial septostomy by balloon catheter in transposition of the great arteries. *Bull. Ass. Cardiol. Pediat. Europ.* **4**, 30.

Rashkind, W. J., and Miller, W. W. (1968b). Transposition of the great arteries. Results of palliation by balloon atrioseptostomy in thirty-one infants. *Circulation* **38**, 453.

Scott, O. (1970). A new complication of Rashkind balloon septostomy: a short report. *Arch. Dis. Child.* **45**, 716.

Singh, S. P., Astley, R., and Burrows, F. G. O. (1969). Balloon septostomy for transposition of the great arteries. *Brit. Heart J.* **31**, 722–726.

Tamer, D. F., Martin, R. A., and Hernandez, F. A. (1969). Balloon atrial septostomy for transposition of the great vessels in infancy. *J. Fl. Med. Ass.* **56**, 258–260.

Tynan, M. J. (1968). Balloon atrial septostomy. *Arch. Dis. Child.* **43**, 744.

Tynan, M. J. (1971). Survival of infants with transposition of great arteries after balloon atrial septostomy. *Lancet* **i**, 621.

Tynan, M. (1972). Assessment of atrial septal defect adequacy in transposition of the great arteries. *Circulation* **45** and **46**, Suppl. 11, 97.

Tynan, M. J., Carr, I., Graham, G., and Carter, R. E. B. (1969). Subvalvular pulmonary obstruction complicating the postoperative course of balloon atrial septostomy in transposition of the great arteries. *Circulation* **39**, 223.

Tyrrell, M. J., and Moes, C. A. F. (1971). Congenital levoposition of the right atrial appendage. Its relevance to balloon septostomy. *Amer. J. Dis. Child.* **121**, 508.

Venables, A. W. (1966). Complete transposition of the great vessels in infancy with reference to palliative surgery. *Brit. Heart J.* **28**, 335.

Venables A. W. (1968). Creation of atrial septal defects by the balloon catheter technique in infants with complete transposition of the great vessels. *Aust. Paediat. J.* **4**, 236.

Venables, A. W. (1970). Balloon atrial septostomy in complete transposition of great arteries in infancy. *Brit. Heart J.* **32**, 61.

Vogel, J. H. K. (1970). Balloon embolisation during atrial septostomy. *Circulation* **42**, 155.

Watson, H. (1968). Atrial septostomy. *Bull. Ass. Cardiol. Pediat. Europ.* **4**, 27.

Watson, H., and Rashkind, W. J. (1967). Creation of atrial septal defects by balloon catheter in babies with transposition of the great arteries. *Lancet* **i**, 403–405.

Webb, H. M., and Hohn, A. R. (1969). Balloon catheter palliation for infants with transposed great arteries. Report of two cases with successful balloon atrial septostomy. *J. S. C. Med. Ass.* **65**, 1–4.

Zamora, R., Moller, J. H., Lucas, R. V., Jr., and Castaneda, A. R. (1970). Complete transposition of the great vessels. Surgical results of emergency Blalock-Hanlon operation in infants. *Surgery* **67**, 706–710.

Chapter 20

THE SURGICAL MANAGEMENT
OF TRANSPOSITION

Various operative procedures have been used or suggested for the surgical management of complete transposition of the great arteries. These procedures are discussed below.

In this series there were 208 operated patients. A total of 271 operations were performed. There were 141 surgical deaths and the overall surgical mortality was 68%. Tables 20.1 and 20.2 show the type and number of heart operations performed.

Methods of Increasing the Pulmonary Blood Flow

ANASTOMOSIS BETWEEN A SYSTEMIC ARTERY
AND THE PULMONARY ARTERY

In 1945, Blalock and Taussig published their pioneer work on the surgical treatment of patients with pulmonary stenosis or atresia. They found that the condition of these patients could be improved by increasing the blood flow to the lungs by end to side anastomosing of the subclavian artery to the pulmonary artery. Potts *et al.* (1946) modified Blalock and Taussig's operation by side to side anastomosis of the aorta to the pulmonary artery, and, in 1948, Potts and Gibson reported the results of this operation on 45 patients. The advantages and disadvantages of the Potts modification have been discussed by Baker *et al.* (1949). Because of certain anatomical peculiarities various modifications have been introduced:

1. End to side subclavian–pulmonary artery anastomosis (Blalock, 1947)

2. Division of a pulmonary artery upper lobe branch with end to end anastomosis of the proximal end to the subclavian artery (Shumacker, 1951)

TABLE 20.1
HEART SURGERY [a]

Group	Blalock–Hanlon	ASD inflow occlusion	Edwards	PDA ligation	PA band	Coarctation resection	Senning	Mustard	SVC to LA
I	60	8	9	3	1	0	2	21	0
II	6	1	0	0	0	0	0	3	0
III	29	3	2	5	18	3	2	7	1
IV	6	0	0	0	0	0	0	3	0
Total	101	12	11	8	19	3	4	34	1

[a] ASD, atrial septal defect; LA, left atrium; PA, pulmonary artery; PDA, patent ductus arteriosus; SVC, superior vena cava.

3. End to side union with the aorta with or without a vascular graft (Potts and Smith, 1949; Gross *et al.*, 1949; Johnson *et al.*, 1949).

4. Ligation and division of the right main pulmonary artery and anastomosing its distal end to the side of the descending aorta (Shumacker and Mandelbaum, 1962).

5. Interposition of a graft between the ascending aorta and either the right or left main pulmonary artery (Shumacker and Mandelbaum, 1962).

6. Anastomosis between the ascending aorta and the right pulmonary artery (Waterston, 1962).

Of these surgical procedures, the Blalock-Taussig and Waterston procedures have been used in transposition more frequently than the other modifications. The major disadvantages of Pott's anastomosis are the difficulties in closing it at the time of total correction (Sirak and Britt, 1962) and the danger that pulmonary vascular disease may develop if the shunt is large (Paul *et al.*, 1961). While the Blalock–Taussig opera-

TABLE 20.2
HEART SURGERY [a]

Group	Pulmonary valvotomy	Glenn	Pott's	Blalock–Taussig	Baffe	Graft	Switch-over	Internal carotid to cor. artery	Thoracotomy	PV to RA
I	1	0	1	3	3	6	6	1	4	1
II	1	2	0	2	0	1	0	0	0	0
III	0	0	0	2	7	1	3	0	1	3
IV	6	6	4	6	2	1	1	0	2	1
Total	8	8	5	13	12	9	10	1	7	5

[a] Cor, coronary; PV, pulmonary vein, RA, right atrium.

tion provides effective palliation for most patients with inadequate pulmonary blood flow over 1 year of age the surgical results in infants have not been satisfactory (Harris *et al.,* 1964; Kaplan *et al.,* 1968; Sommerville *et al.,* 1969; Bernhard *et al.,* 1971). The Waterston anastomosis is carried out intrapericardially since, at this location, the vascular structures are of sufficient size to permit satisfactory anastomosis in the small infant. In addition, the shunt is centrally located in the mediastinum and can be closed with little difficulty at the time of open correction of the cardiac defects (Cooley and Hallman, 1966; Edwards *et al.,* 1966; Bernhard *et al.,* 1971). The disadvantages of Waterston operation are that it may be difficult to control the size of the stoma and that it is easy to kink the right pulmonary artery and selectively perfuse part of, or only the right lung (Sommerville *et al.,* 1969).

In the present series 5 patients underwent a Pott's anastomosis, 1 in Group I, and 4 in Group IV. Four patients died in the immediate postoperative course of heart failure. The only survivor improved after the surgery, but at thoracotomy, 3 years later, she was found to have pulmonary hypertension at systemic levels. A biopsy of the lungs demonstrated grade 3 pulmonary vascular changes. The Blalock–Taussig anastomosis was performed on 12 patients; 3 in Group I, 2 in Group II, 2 in Group III, and 5 in Group IV. An atrial septal defect was created at the same time in 4. Six patients died as a result of the surgical procedure and the overall mortality was 50%. Of the 3 in Group I, 1 died and 2 survived. Subsequent cardiac catheterization in 1 demonstrated moderate elevation of the left ventricular pressure. At total surgical correction in 1, utilizing the Mustard procedure, grade 3 pulmonary vascular changes were found. Of the 2 patients in Group II, 1 died in the immediate postoperative course. The second, a 12-year-old boy, with a common atrium and transposition, developed congestive heart failure after surgery. He died 3 months later after ligation of the anastomosis. Both patients in Group III had had banding of the pulmonary artery and surgical creation of an atrial septal defect 2–4 years before the Blalock–Taussig shunt. Both survived and cyanosis and effort tolerance showed improvement. Of the 2 survivors in Group IV, 1 was doing well 14 years after the shunt procedure and the other died 2 years later of subacute bacterial endocarditis. A continuous murmur of a functioning anastomosis was heard in all survivors. The Waterston anastomosis was not used on any patients in the present series.

Of the reported cases, 1 patient of Astley and Parsons (1952) underwent a Blalock–Taussig's anastomosis with considerable improvement, and the authors wondered whether it might be necessary to create an artificial stenosis of the pulmonary artery in cases with a ventricular septal defect. In a group of 32 patients with transposition of the great arteries reported by Murphy *et al.* (1955), 6 had pulmonary stenosis and were treated with either Blalock's or Pott's operation. Three of these survived and did moderately well. Baffes *et al.* (1957) operated on 6 patients with pulmonary stenosis using either of these two operations; 5 patients survived with improvement. Cleland *et al.* (1957) operated on 8 patients with pulmonary stenosis (1 with single ventricle) using the Blalock operation in 7 and Pott's modification in 1. Five survived with considerable improvement. The authors pointed out that despite the striking changes in the physical capacity, there has been little change in the hemoglobin level and only a slight diminution in cyanosis. They attributed these findings to the fact that the aorta arising from the right ventricle, continues to receive a large proportion of venous blood. Collins *et al.* (1959) reported their results on 17 patients with transposition of the great vessels. In 2 infants with pulmonary stenosis, a Blalock's operation was performed resulting in death in 1 and improvement in the other. Noonan *et al.* (1960) reported 4 patients with transposition and pulmonary stenosis in whom a shunt procedure was accomplished. Two survived with a slight improvement. Hallman and Cooley (1964) anastomosed a systemic artery to the pulmonary artery in 6 patients; 3 patients survived. Sterns *et al.* (1964a) reported a case of transposition with pulmonary stenosis who, at the age of 3 years, was treated by the Blalock-Taussig operation and the creation of an atrial septal defect. The patient improved after the operation and survived 8 years. Of the 16 patients operated upon by Sterns *et al.* (1964b) a subclavian–pulmonary artery shunt was performed in 1 patient with pulmonary stenosis with improvement. Reed (1965) used the Potts operation on 2 patients with transposition and pulmonary stenosis. One died immediately after the operation while the other survived with improvement.

Somerville *et al.* reported (1969) that of the 30 patients with cyanotic heart disease who had Waterston anastomoses, a 6-year-old patient had transposition, multiple ventricular septal defects, and pulmonary stenosis. Improvement was dramatic, but the continuous murmur, documented after operation, disappeared 7 months later, and aortography confirmed that the anastomosis was not patent. The authors pointed out that among their 30 patients there was a tendency for preferential perfusion of the right lung, and unilateral pulmonary edema occurred in some patients. A side to side anastomosis between the ascending aorta and the right pulmonary artery was created in 80 infants and 61 older children with a variety of cyanotic cardiac abnormalities associated with pulmonary stenosis or atresia by Bernhard *et al.* (1971). Of the 15 with transposition and pulmonary stenosis, 10 patients survived the surgical procedure. Of these 15 patients, a side to side anastomosis between the ascending aorta and the main pulmonary artery was performed in 5 neonates with 3 survivors. Severe hypoxemia was the major indication for surgery in the infant group while surgery was undertaken on an elective basis in older children. The authors pointed out that Waterston anastomosis is the procedure of choice in infants under 1 year of age and that it is also of value in older patients if a Blalock–Taussig shunt cannot be performed.

Braunwald *et al.* (1966) suggested a new palliative operation for transposition of the great arteries and ventricular septal defect. A systemic pulmonary artery shunt is created, and the main pulmonary artery ligated. The operation converts transposition to a functional equivalent of truncus arteriosus with normal or nearly normal pulmonary blood flow. This procedure was carried out in a patient with transposition, mild pulmonary stenosis, and ventricular septal defect. Postoperatively the patient showed considerable clinical improvement and significant elevation of arterial oxygen saturation.

ANASTOMOSIS BETWEEN THE SUPERIOR VENA CAVA AND THE RIGHT PULMONARY ARTERY

The possibility of completely bypassing the right side of the heart has intrigued several workers during the past 25 years. Starr *et al.* (1943) and Bakos (1950) charred the right ventricle of dogs using electrocautery without producing a rise in the central venous pressure. Kagan (1952) destroyed the outer wall of the right ventricle of dogs by means of an electrothermocautery and concluded that a normal contractile right ventricular wall is not necessary for the maintenance of a normal circulation. Donald and Essex (1954) ligated the right coronary artery in dogs which deprived 50–75% of the right ventricular myocardium of its coronary arterial blood supply and found that this did not result in extensive changes in the mean pulmonary or systemic arterial blood pressure. They obtained similar results in animals by injecting the right coronary arterial system with vinyl acetate which inactivates 59–95% of the right ventricular myocardium. Rodbard and Wagner (1949) anastomosed the right atrial appendage to the pulmonary artery in dogs and found that in acute experiments if the pulmonary artery is ligated on the cardiac side proximal to the anastomosis, the venous pressure maintained the venous return through the lungs. Jamison *et al.* (1954) placed a pump of 50 ml reservoir capacity in the systemic circuit between the left auricular appendage and the left common carotid artery on each of 10 dogs so that the systemic circulation was maintained by the pump during complete cardiac arrest resulting from experimentally produced ventricular fibrillation. The arterial pressure was maintained and the blood was forced through the right heart and pulmonary circuit. They suggested that the left ventricle may be able to take over the work of the right ventricle.

The physiological basis of these experiments was summarized by Rodbard and Wagner (1949) who pointed out that comparative analysis of the physiology of the pulmonary and systemic pressures of several classes of vertebrates indicates that the pulmonary vascular tree is a circuit of very low resistance. The pulmonary arterial pressure is of the order of 25/10 mm Hg in fish, amphibia, reptiles, birds, and mammals, while the systemic pressure varies according to the class and body temperature. These data suggest that pumping the venous blood through the lungs might be supplied adequately by the venous pressure alone. Furthermore, in the presence of a congenital or acquired stenosis of the tricuspid or pulmonary valves, a right atrium–pulmonary artery shunt by bypassing the right ventricle might provide a means of complete oxygenation of the entire venous return.

On the other hand, the experimental work of Rose et al. (1955a,b) in which they attempted to shunt the entire venous return past the right ventricle directly into the pulmonary artery, demonstrated that the right ventricle is an essential pump for the maintenance of normal flows and pressures in the intact circulation. When they acutely excluded the right ventricle by ligating the pulmonary artery, the resulting elevated venous pressure was not capable of maintaining adequate lung perfusions. Patino et al. (1956) attempted to completely bypass the right ventricle but none of the animals survived the operation. Recently, however, Robicsek et al. (1963) were able to experimentally bypass the right heart by anastomosing the superior vena cava to the right pulmonary artery and transplanting the inferior vena cava into the left atrium. In this way they were able to exclude the right heart from the circulation for a period as long as 7 days without significant changes in the arterial and venous pressures. In experiments by Nuland et al. (1958) to divert the entire inferior vena cava blood to the pulmonary artery, the increased resistance to blood flow caused excessive pooling of the venous blood peripherally which resulted in systemic arterial hypotension and death in some animals. Animals that survived this shunt developed ascites in the postoperative period.

In recent years partial bypass of the right heart by means of anastomosing the superior vena cava to the distal end of the right pulmonary artery has been shown by several workers to be compatible with long sur-

vival in animals. Experiments of this nature have been published by Carlon *et al.* (1951), Glenn and Patino (1954), Patino *et al.* (1956), Robicsek *et al.* (1956), Glenn (1958), Nuland *et al.* (1958), Robicsek *et al.*
(1958), and Sanger *et al.* (1959). Bakulev and Kolesnikov (1959)
pointed out that experimental and clinical anastomosis between the superior vena cava and the right pulmonary artery had been practiced in the
Soviet Union as early as 1951.

Carlon *et al.* (1951) pointed out that the blood flow to the lungs, after
anastomosing the superior vena cava to the distal end of the pulmonary
artery, is held up by a moderate increase of the venous pressure in the
upper half of the body, by thoracic suction, and by expansion and collapse of the lungs. Glenn and Patino (1954) were able to show a prompt
fall in pressure in the occluded superior vena cava after opening the
shunt between it and the right pulmonary artery. Furthermore, experiments by Patino *et al.* (1956), and Nuland *et al.* (1958) showed that the
venous flow through the shunt will not exceed 30–40% of the total systemic venous return. Robicsek *et al.* (1958) investigated some animals
after completion of the anastomosis and found that the average pressure
in the superior vena cava was a few millimeters Hg higher than normal
but was not significant and caused no untoward symptoms. Moreover, the
pulmonary vascular resistance was considerably lower on the side of the
anastomosis than in the contralateral lung. They believed that active dilatation of the pulmonary vessels by a reflex process takes place after this
operation.

Lindskog *et al.* (1962) advocated superior vena cava–distal pulmonary artery shunt for the following conditions:

1. Anomalous drainage of the superior vena cava into the left atrium
2. Obstruction of the venae cavae, congenital or acquired
3. Tricuspid atresia or stenosis
4. Ebstein's anomaly of the tricuspid valve
5. Single ventricle (with pulmonary stenosis congenital or acquired).
6. Bilocular heart
7. Transposition of the great arteries (with pulmonary stenosis congenital or surgical)
8. Fallot's tetralogy (a few specific cases)

The authors, and Redo (1964), stressed that the operation is contraindi-
cated in the presence of pulmonary hypertension or if the pulmonary artery has a diameter which is one-half or less than that of the superior
vena cava.

Robicsek *et al.* (1956), and Bakulev and Kolesnikov (1959) compared and contrasted this anastomosis to the classical Blalock–Taussig operation and pointed out that:

1. Superior vena cava–pulmonary artery anastomosis decreases the work of the right side of the heart whereas Blalock's operation increases the work of the heart.

2. Superior vena cava–pulmonary artery anastomosis delivers venous blood to the lungs, while Blalock's operation delivers mixed arterial blood to the lungs.

3. Superior vena cava-pulmonary artery anastomosis is not liable to bacterial endarteritis.

4. Superior vena cava–pulmonary artery anastomosis is not followed by an increase of blood pressure in the main pulmonary artery. Blalock's operation may be followed by pulmonary hypertension (McGaff *et al.,* 1962).

5. Superior vena cava–pulmonary artery anastomosis is a simpler operation.

Glenn (1958) successfully accomplished this anastomosis in a boy of 7 years of age with transposition, single ventricle, and pulmonary stenosis. Clinical and laboratory studies after the operation indicated significant improvement in the exercise tolerance and in the arterial oxygen saturation. Sanger *et al.* (1959) operated on a boy 11 years of age with transposition and pulmonary stenosis. The patient survived the operation and the cyanosis disappeared. Reevaluation of the patient 3 years later (Robicsek *et al.,* 1962) showed that improvement was maintained and that the anastomosis was patent with good blood flow to the lungs with no demonstrable ill effects on the heart and circulation. Bakulev and Kolesnikov (1959) reported their results on 41 patients (type not specified). Fourteen patients died during the operation or in the early postoperative period. Long-term results up to 2 years after the operation in 16 cases, showed good results in 14 and slight improvement in 2. Bickford and Edwards (1960) operated on 2 patients with tricuspid atresia with considerable improvement in cyanosis. Of the 11 patients operated on by Mitri *et al.* (1962), 1 had transposition of the great arteries with pulmonary stenosis, while 2 had transposition with tricuspid atresia. Six patients improved, 6 had a fair result (1 with pulmonary stenosis and transposition), 1 did not improve, while the remaining patient, with transposition and tricuspid atresia, died of thrombosis at the site of the anastomosis. Young *et al.* (1963) operated on 25 patients with different types of cyanotic congenital heart disease with a mortality rate of 20%. Their only patient with transposition died at operation. They pointed out that the degree of clinical improvement afforded by this operation had been encouraging. Reed *et al.* (1963) anastomosed the superior vena cava to the pulmonary artery in 7 patients with complete transposition of the great arteries. Pulmonary stenosis was an associated defect in 5. Three cases with pulmonary stenosis survived with considerable improvement, while the remaining 4 died at or immediately after the operation. Of the 15 patients who underwent anastomosis between the superior vena cava and the right pulmonary artery by Keirle *et al.* (1963), 3 had transposition with pulmonary stenosis. These 3 patients survived the operation and at follow-up evaluations all had maintained their initial improvement in color. Helmsworth *et al.* (1964) operated on 4 babies with transposition and pulmonary stenosis. All survived with appreciable improvement. A cavopulmonary artery anastomosis was successfully performed on one of the patients with transposition of the great arteries by Hallman and Cooley (1964). Eight patients with transposition and pulmonary stenosis underwent an anastomosis between the superior vena cava and the distal right pulmonary artery by Glenn *et al.* (1965). Of these 8, pulmonary stenosis produced by banding of the pulmonary artery 8 months to 3 years before the shunting procedure was present in 3. A Blalock–Hanlon procedure was performed at the same operation on 3. There were 2 operative deaths. Laboratory studies indicated a postoperative rise in the systemic arterial saturation and a fall in hematocrit level. In 1966, Glenn *et al.* collected, through personal communications and from the literature, 537 cases in which the shunt was employed. Transposition of the great arteries was present in 68 cases; 58 with pulmonary stenosis and 10 without it. Of the 58 with pulmonary stenosis, the stenosis was surgically produced by a pulmonary artery band 18 months or more before establishment of the shunt in 5. Four of the banded patients survived shunting for more than 1 year while the fifth died at operation. Virtually no communication existed between the left and right sides of the heart. A systemic artery–pulmonary artery shunt was done 2 years before the shunt in 3 patients, all of whom survived the second operation for more than 1 year. In 2 patients the shunt did not function and was immediately replaced or supplemented by a systemic artery–pulmonary shunt; neither patient survived. In 3 others an atrial septal defect was performed, 1 year after, 3 weeks after, and at the same time as the shunt; in one instance this was in conjunction with a pulmonary valvulotomy. All 3 patients survived longer than a year. The mortality rate in the group with pulmonary stenosis was 16% (9 operative and no late deaths). Of the 48 surviving patients,

39 were alive more than 1 year; 42 were reported as having obtained an "excellent" or "good" result. Of the 10 patients without pulmonary stenosis, 9 were under 2 years of age. In 4 patients, ranging in age from 10 days to $3\frac{1}{2}$ years, an atrial septal defect was made, in two cases at the same time as the shunt and in two others more than a month before. One of the four died 10 weeks after creation of the shunt, with thrombosis of the anastomosis, while the 3 others were classed more than a year later as having "excellent" or "good" results. One patient survived who had a banding of the left pulmonary artery simultaneously with creation of the shunt. There were 6 operative deaths (60%). Sachs *et al.* (1968), performed a cavopulmonary anastomosis on a 3-year-old patient with transposition and pulmonary stenosis. The patient died 36 hours after surgery of thrombosed shunt. Robicsek *et al.* (1969) experimentally produced cavopulmonary anastomosis in dogs. In addition, the right pulmonary veins were detached from the left atrium and implanted into the central stump of the superior vena cava. The authors suggested that the procedure drains the circulation of the right lung into the systemic atrium and could be used as a palliative procedure for patients with transposition and pulmonary stenosis. Achtel *et al.* (1969) anastomosed the superior vena cava to the right pulmonary artery in 16 children with cyanotic heart disease of which 5 had transposition with pulmonary stenosis. Of these 5 patients with transposition, 1 died later with infarction of the right lower lobe of the lung. The authors pointed out that a syndrome of pulmonary infarction both isolated and in association with intractable heart failure develops following cavopulmonary anastomosis. Patency of the azygos vein probably decreases the blood flow through the anastomosis abetting stasis and thrombosis. In their view, since resection of the anastomosis is difficult, this shunt should not be employed when the possibility of surgical correction exists. On the other hand, Martin *et al.* (1970) pointed out that the shunt does not preclude performance of total corrective operation. Six patients with transposition, pulmonary stenosis, and "incorrectable" ventricular chambers were treated by superior vena cavopulmonary artery shunt by Pontius (1970). There was no surgical mortality but one unexplained late death occurred. Trusler *et al.* (1971) pointed out that since a cavopulmonary anastomosis is essentially irreversible, this method is most useful in cases in which a corrective procedure is difficult or impossible. Of the reported 58 children with a cavopulmonary shunt, 22 had transposition with ventricular septal defect and pulmonary stenosis. The majority of their patients were over 2 years of age. There were no postoperative deaths in the group with transposition. Color and exercise tolerance improved greatly after operation in 21; in 1 patient improve-

ment was lessened when the innominate vein became thrombosed adjacent to the site of ligation of a left superior vena cava. No child in this group showed evidence of clinically significant elevation of superior vena caval pressure, but 2 children developed a right pleural effusion following operation.

Palacios-Macedo et al. (1961), and Young et al. (1963) pointed out that the only but certainly major drawback of this operation is the fact that if thrombosis of the anastomosis occurs early in the postoperative course due to technical error, the patient is very likely to succumb to the cerebral complications of superior vena cava obstruction. Moreover, Mitri et al. (1962) found that the development of varying degrees of superior vena caval obstruction syndrome following this operation was the rule rather than the exception. Edwards and Bargeron (1963) described a technique for delayed ligation of the azygos vein 1 week after the operation. They pointed out that this allows temporary decompression of the vena cava through the azygos vein and prevents excessive elevation of the superior vena caval pressure with cerebral edema. Moreover, delayed ligation permits maximum flow through the shunt after the dangers of cerebral edema have passed. Canent et al. (1964) studied the cardiopulmonary dynamics of the circulation through the right lung in 6 patients with cyanotic congenital heart disease who had undergone surgery with anastomosis of the superior vena cava to the right pulmonary artery. They found that episodes of increased pulmonary vascular resistance may be of etiological significance in the clinical picture of superior vena caval obstruction syndrome which can occur postoperatively. Similarly increased pulmonary vascular resistance associated with sustained increased intrathoracic pressure may play an important role in the postoperative complication of right chylothorax. Glenn et al. (1970) evaluated the lung perfusion in patients who had undergone cavopulmonary anastomosis for a variety of congenital malformations of the right side of the heart. Transposition of the great vessels was diagnosed in 8 cases. Lung scans using 131 iodinated macroaggregates of albumin and 133 xenon gas were obtained. Scans were performed 1 to 10 years postoperatively. Except in those cases with elevated pulmonary vascular resistance, greater than about 80% of the injected isotope was detected in the right lung. The authors pointed out that on long-term follow-up, patients with a cavopulmonary anastomosis continue to receive significant and stable benefit.

In the present series 8 patients underwent a cavopulmonary anastomosis; 2 in Group II, and 6 in Group IV. The ages ranged between 3 and 10 years when the shunt was performed. Of the 2 with an intact ventricular septum, 1 developed chylothorax and died in the immediate postoperative course. The second patient, who survived the operation, had an atrial septal defect surgically created 3 years before the cavopulmonary shunt. There were no surgical deaths or complications among the 6 in Group IV. In one of these 6, a Baffe procedure was performed several years before the cavopulmonary shunt. Cyanosis and effort tolerance improved in all survivors and none showed signs of superior vena caval obstruction.

PULMONARY VALVOTOMY OR INFUNDIBULECTOMY

Eight patients in this series underwent pulmonary valvotomy or infundibulectomy; 1 in Group I, 1 in Group II, and 6 in Group IV. Six patients were above 2 years of age, and 2 were under 1. Three survived and 5 died in the immediate postoperative course. All the survivors were in Group IV. Improvement in the cyanosis and effort tolerance was slight among the survivors and 1 developed slight postoperative pulmonary incompetence.

Transventricular pulmonary valvotomy was first performed by Brock (1948) and Sellors (1948). Brilliant results were obtained after pulmonary valvotomy or infundibulectomy in isolated pulmonary stenosis. The value of this operation as a palliative therapy for complete transposition of the great arteries with pulmonary stenosis is doubtful. It is generally agreed that a shunt procedure with or without a surgical atrial septal defect or atrial septostomy is the palliative operation of choice for these patients. The literature contains few reports on the results of pulmonary valvotomy in transposition of the great arteries. Rothlin and Senning (1965) resected peripheral pulmonary artery stenosis and created an atrial septal defect on a 6½-month-old infant. Improvement was maintained during the 20-month follow-up period. One of the patients of Somerville *et al.* (1969) underwent pulmonary valvotomy but the result of the operation was not discussed by the authors.

Methods of Diminishing the Pulmonary Blood Flow

PULMONARY ARTERY BANDING

Muller and Dammann (1952), and Dammann and Muller (1953) pointed out that the creation of pulmonary stenosis in the group of congenital heart disease characterized by pulmonary hypertension and increased pulmonary blood flow, e.g., ventricular septal defect and single ventricle, although not curative, should prevent heart failure and result in a more efficient circulation. It should also prevent the changes which take place in the pulmonary arteries in the presence of a long standing pulmonary hypertension. Another use of the operation has been suggested by experimental work of Blank *et al.* (1958). These investigators found that restoration of an elevated pulmonary arterial pressure to its normal level in dogs may result in regression of medial hypertrophy and intimal proliferation of the pulmonary vascular bed. Moreover, Dammann *et al.* (1961) produced evidence that banding of the pulmonary artery in the presence of significant pulmonary vascular disease and significant pulmonary hypertension may improve the pulmonary vascular bed.

The results of pulmonary artery banding in the group of patients with uncomplicated ventricular septal defect, who are in intractable heart failure, have been most gratifying (Fowler *et al.*, 1958; Morrow and Braunwald, 1961; Albert *et al.*, 1961; William *et al.*, 1962; Craig and Sirak, 1963). On the other hand, the mortality rate in the group with complicated defects (single ventricle, transposition of the great arteries or truncus arteriosus) has been high. Of the 23 patients who were operated upon for pulmonary artery constriction reported by William *et al.* (1962), 2 had transposition of the great arteries. One of these survived the operation and showed diminished cyanosis and increased activity and was followed up for 20 months afterward. In the other patient, all attempts to band the pulmonary artery resulted in a fall of the aortic pressure and oxygen saturation. The banding was abandoned and the patient died 3 days postoperatively. Haller (1962) combined pulmonary artery banding with creation of an atrial septal defect in 3 patients, who showed improvement. Craig and Sirak (1963) reported their results on 38 patients who had undergone surgery for pulmonary artery banding. Of the 20 with complicated defects, who were operated upon because of intractable heart failure, multiple episodes of pneumonia, and general growth failure, 6 had complete transposition of the great arteries. Of these 6, 5 died after operation but the sixth survived and was alive but deeply cyanosed 28 months after the operation, which was combined with creation of an atrial septal defect. They reported that mortality rate of the group with combined defects (excluding single ventricle) was 72%. Of the 10 patients who underwent banding of the pulmonary artery by Coles *et al.*, (1963), 2 had complete transposition of the great arteries. In one of these two an operative procedure to increase the mixing of arterial and venous blood was carried out as well as pulmonary artery banding. In the second patient a large ventricular septal defect was present, and only banding of the pulmonary artery was performed. Both patients survived and improved. Glotzer *et al.* (1963) banded the pulmonary artery of a 5-month-old infant with transposition in heart failure. Marked improvement in the general condition was maintained for nearly 2 years after which, because of marked cyanosis, creation of atrial septal defect was undertaken. Helmsworth *et al.* (1964) banded the pulmonary artery and excised the atrial septum of 10 patients with transposition. Seven patients died after operation. Of the 3 survivors, 2 were still alive 9 years and 8½ years after operation while the third was lost to the follow-up. The authors believed that although the general result was good in one of the two longest survivors, prevention of pulmonary hypertension was accomplished in both. Of the 16 infants under the age of 2 years with complete or "corrected" transposition operated upon by Sterns *et al.* (1964b), the pulmonary artery was banded in 5. Four survived while the fifth died in the first postoperative day. Autopsy showed a patent ductus arteriosus coexisting with complete transposition of the great arteries. One of the 4 survivors died of undetermined cause at home 2 months after surgery. The 3 survivors, of whom one had a single ventricle, appeared to have benefited by the operation. Gerbode *et al.* (1964) banded the pulmonary artery of 2 infants with transposition. One died as a result of operation and one died later at surgical creation of an atrial septal defect. Starr *et al.* (1964) banded the pulmonary artery of 6 patients with transposition, massive pulmonary overcirculation, and slight cyanosis. The only survivor in this group required creation of an atrial septal defect a few months later because of increasing cyanosis. Of the 5 who died, 3 had banding of the pulmonary artery alone. Of these 3, 1 had a large ventricular septal defect, another had a large patent ductus arteriosus, and the third had a ventricular septal defect, patent foramen ovale, and coarctation of the aorta. The remaining 2 patients had banding of the pulmonary artery as the initial procedure but tolerated this so poorly that they were returned to the operating room for creation of an atrial septal defect. Both died of cardiac arrest at surgery and autopsy revealed a large ventricular septal defect in one and a ventricular septal defect and a large ductus in the other. Reed (1965) banded the pulmonary artery of 1 patient with transposition and coupled this procedure with creation of an atrial septal defect in an additional 8 patients. One died as a result of central nervous system damage and another of bilateral "pneumonia." Initial postoperative improvement has been maintained or has increased in all 7 survivors. Among the 71 patients with transposition reported by Brom *et al.* (1965), the pulmonary artery was banded in 10. An atrial septal defect was also created in 3 of these 10. All patients survived the operative procedure. Rothlin and Senning (1965) banded the pulmonary artery and created an atrial septal defect in 4 patients with transposition with 4 survivors. Of the 7 who underwent banding of the pulmonary artery by

Trusler and Mustard (1968), 2 with associated single ventricle survived. Idriss *et al.* (1968) banded the pulmonary artery of 14 children with transposition; 2 surgical deaths occurred. Of these 14 children, 5 were banded following creation of an atrial septal defect, and 3 following balloon atrial septostomy. Waldhausen *et al.* (1969) reported their results of banding of the pulmonary artery of 10 patients with transposition and ventricular septal defect (dextroposition in 9 and levoposition in 1). The ages of the patients ranged from 5 weeks to 19 months. In one of these patients, tricuspid atresia was also present. Seven had had initial balloon atrial septostomy. There was 1 operative and 2 late deaths. All survivors showed signs of postoperative improvement. Of the 146 patients who underwent banding of the pulmonary artery at the Hospital For Sick Children, London, 15 had transposition of the great arteries with a ventricular septal defect (Stark *et al.*, 1969). Of these 15 patients, 13 were infants. Hospital deaths occurred in 10, and a late death in 1. Pulmonary artery banding as the only procedure was performed on 7 patients with 1 survivor. An initial atrial septal defect was created at the same time in 4 with 2 survivors. The pulmonary artery was banded a few days or weeks after creation of an atrial septal defect in 2 cases with 1 survivor. In 1 case, a successful Blalock-Hanlon was performed 1 month after banding. Additional information on the results of banding of the pulmonary artery at the Hospital For Sick Children, London, apparently in another group of patients with transposition was reported by Stark *et al.* (1970). There were 15 infants and 18 children who underwent this operation. Atrial septostomy by the Blalock–Hanlon or Rashkind procedure was performed prior to banding in 22 patients, at the same operation in 5, and after banding of the pulmonary artery in 3. In 3 patients atrial septostomy was not performed. In the infant group there were 2 hospital and 3 late deaths. In the older group there were 2 hospital and 1 late deaths. The authors found that in infants it was always possible to lower the pulmonary arterial pressure below 45 mm Hg. On the other hand, the pulmonary arterial pressure in over 1-year-old children could not always be lowered because of a high incidence of pulmonary vascular disease. The authors pointed out that the indications for banding of the pulmonary artery in transposition with a ventricular septal defect are (1) a pulmonary artery/systemic artery systolic pressure ratio greater than 0.8 in infants or children, and (2) intractable congestive heart failure. In children, who already have some elevation of the pulmonary vascular resistance, the operation is performed to prevent further development of pulmonary vascular disease. Hunt *et al.* (1971) presented the results of banding of the pulmonary artery in 111 children with cardiac malformations associated with excessive pulmonary blood flow. There were 16 patients with transposition of the great arteries; with ventricular septal defect in 14, and intact ventricular septum in 2. At the time of the banding operation, a Blalock–Hanlon procedure was also done in 8 patients, each with a ventricular septal defect. Six of these 8 patients survived. In the other 6 patients with a ventricular septal defect, a Blalock–Hanlon procedure was not done at the same time of banding and only one patient survived. The 2 patients with an intact ventricular septum also died after banding of the pulmonary artery. The 7 patients with a ventricular septal defect who survived banding appeared to have benefited clinically with presumed reduction in excessive pulmonary blood flow and decreased pulmonary vascular resistance. Oldham *et al.* (1972) performed pulmonary artery banding in 7 patients with transposition and ventricular septal defect. All patients had congestive heart failure inadequately responsive to vigorous medical management. Five survived the operation with improvement. Repeat cardiac catheterization in some patients demonstrated a reduction in pulmonary artery pressure. The pulmonary vascular resistance was unchanged or minimally reduced. Left ventricular volume, mass, and systolic output were significantly reduced from preoperative values but remained higher than normal. One patient required surgical creation of an atrial septal defect in the follow-up period. A corrective procedure consisting of closure of the ventricular septal defect, removal of the pulmonary artery band, and correction of the remaining defects were performed in 3 with 2 survivors. The authors pointed out that the indications for banding of the pulmonary artery are (1) excessive pulmonary blood flow with pulmonary hypertension and congestive heart failure, and (2) prevention of progressive changes in the pulmonary vessels causing irreversible progressive pulmonary hypertension. They emphasized that pulmonary artery banding remains an effective technique in staged treatment of patients with complex congenital cardiac defects.

Trusler and Mustard (1972) used a premarked band of 4 mm wide Teflon impregnated with Silastic to band the pulmonary artery of patients with a ventricular septal defect with or without transposition. For transposition patients, band circumference of 26–30 mm allowed a sufficient but not excessive pulmonary blood flow. The optimum circumference of pulmonary artery band estimated by body weight varied from 26 mm in a 2 kg infant to 29 mm in a 5 kg infant. The circumference of the pulmonary artery band in millimeters is 24 plus the infants weight in kilograms. The authors used this technique on 18 infants with transposition and a large ventricular septal defect. A Blalock–Hanlon procedure or the modification of Edwards and Bargeron (1964) was done at the same time. There were 4 deaths; 1 related directly to the band, 2 caused by the atrial septal procedure, and 1 secondary to gastric perforation.

In the present series 19 patients underwent banding of the pulmonary artery; 1 in Group I and 18 in Group III. At the same time of the banding, an atrial septal defect was surgically created in 8 and the right pulmonary veins repositioned in 2. There were 2 operative and 1 late death in this group. A Blalock–Hanlon procedure was not done at the same time of the banding operation in 9 patients. Only 4 of these 9 patients survived; the remaining 5 died in the immediate postoperative course. The 11 survivors in this series appear to have benefited from banding of the pulmonary artery. Subsequently, 2 of these 11 patients underwent a Blalock–Taussig anastomosis, and 1 the Mustard procedure. Repeat cardiac catheterization before the Mustard procedure in the last patient demonstrated spontaneous closure of the ventricular septal defect.

At the time of this writing it seems that almost all patients with transposition and a large ventricular septal defect and pulmonary hypertension should undergo banding of the pulmonary artery or total surgical correction during the first year of life. Creation of an atrial septal defect by the Rashkind or Blalock–Hanlon procedures should be performed before or at the same time of banding since the surgical risk is higher when atrial septostomy is not performed. The surgical mortality of pulmonary artery banding during the first year of life should not be more than 25%. A patent ductus arteriosus or coarctation of the aorta, if present, should be dealt with at the same time of banding. The value of banding of the pulmonary artery in children over the age of 1 year is not yet established. More information is still needed to attest to the validity of the conclusion of Stark *et al.* (1970), that in older children with transposition, pulmonary vascular disease can be arrested at the stage that it had reached at the time of banding of the pulmonary artery. Spontaneous closure of isolated ventricular septal defects after pulmonary artery banding has been reported in 3 separate case reports (Stark *et al.*, 1970; Nghiem *et al.*, 1969; Edgett *et al.*, 1968). It appears that the patient in this series is the first reported transposition case in which spontaneous closure of a ventricular septal defect occurred after banding of the pulmonary artery.

Methods of Augmenting the Shunt

CREATION OF AN ATRIAL SEPTAL DEFECT

The work of Hanlon and Blalock (1948), regarding the age survival in relation to the associated defects, has been discussed in Chapter 18. In a

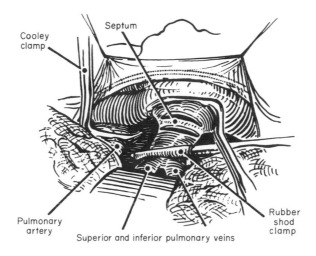

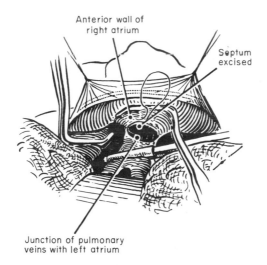

Fig. 20.1. Diagrammatic illustration of the Blalock-Hanlon operation. The approach is through the fifth right interspace with the infant lying on the left side. The pericardium is incised beneath the phrenic nerve, and the pulmonary veins and pulmonary artery are isolated and taped. A curved clamp includes both pulmonary veins and a generous portion of the right and left atrial walls. The pulmonary artery is occluded and suitably placed incisions are made in the left and right atria. The cut edges of the atrium are closed with a running suture. The clamp is removed and the tapes removed from the pulmonary veins and the artery. From W. T. Mustard (1965), from *Advan. Surg.*, Claude E. Welch, ed.; by permission Year Book Medical Publishers.

later paper, Blalock and Hanlon (1950) discussed the various defects that may provide means of mixing between the systemic and the pulmonary circulations in cases of transposition, and concluded that the combination of an atrial septal defect and a ventricular septal defect gives the best prognosis for those having transposition of the great arteries. Three different types of surgical operations were suggested: (1) construction of extracardiac shunts, either venous or arterial, (2) creation of an atrial septal defect, and (3) creation of an atrial septal defect plus an extracardiac arterial shunt. The one which is discussed here is the creation of an atrial septal defect, an operation well known as the Blalock–Hanlon operation (Fig. 20.1). This surgical procedure has proved to be life saving in the seriously ill infants with transposition of the great arteries. Subsequent modifications of the original technique have been reported by Ochsner *et al.* (1961), Moss *et al.* (1961), Sautter (1963), Schuster *et al.* (1963), Trusler *et al.* (1964), Hallman and Cooley (1964), Lindesmith *et al.* (1965), Fonkalsrud (1966), Fonkalsrud and Tocornai (1967, 1968), and Raston and Konez (1971). Factors which increase the flow through the atrial septal defect in experimental transposition were discussed by Leeds *et al.* (1955).

Blalock and Hanlon (1950) treated 12 patients with complete transposition of the great arteries by the creation of an atrial septal defect. Only 3 survived and appeared to have benefited by the operation. The remaining 9 patients died, most of them less than 24 hours after the operation. They reported that a disquieting aspect of the surgical therapy of transposition was that a number of survivors were only moderately improved, the arterial saturation generally remaining below 75%. In some instances, the red cell count increased after operation. Ash *et al.* (1959) reported the results of operation on 17 of their patients with complete transposition of the great arteries. Of the 10 patients in whom a defect of the atrial septum was created, 4 survived with improvement. Collins *et al.* (1959) reported their results on 17 patients with transposition who were operated upon between 1 week and 7 months of age. An atrial septal defect was created in 13, with 9 survivors. Ochsner *et al.* (1961, 1962) reported the results of the creation of an atrial septal defect in 45 patients with transposition. The majority were under 1 year of age and the overall mortality rate was 33%. Of the 129 patients who underwent surgical procedures for transposition of the great vessels by Hallman and Cooley (1964), 100 had creation of an atrial septal defect with an overall mortality rate of 29%. The mortality rate of the 70 in the first year of life was 33% (Hallman and Cooley, 1963; Cooley and Hallman, 1964). Improvement was seen among survivors. Starr *et al.* (1964) reported their experience with 21 patients undergoing emergency palliative surgery for transposition of the great arteries with pulmonary overcirculation. Creation of an atrial septal defect as the only operative procedure was performed in 14 patients; 4 deaths ensued. Satisfactory clinical results were observed in the survivors. They pointed out that those patients suffering predominantly from severe cyanosis may expect a good result from a Blalock–Hanlon operation. Those patients suffering from pulmonary overcirculation and only minimal cyanosis are poor candidates for palliative surgery and must be considered for total correction if survival is to be obtained. Trusler *et al.* (1964) utilized an open technique with inflow caval occlusion with moderate hypothermia to create an atrial septal defect in 28 infants and children with transposition of the great arteries. The overall mortality was 50%. Of the 12 infants for whom operation was necessary during the first 2 weeks of life, only 2 survived. On the other hand, 4 of the 16 children operated on between the ages of 2 weeks and 3 years died. Despite the initial improvement afforded by the surgical procedure, 3 sudden late deaths occurred. The authors pointed out that this technique is not adequate for infants during the first 2 weeks of life but it may be preferable in older age groups. Lindesmith *et al.* (1965) created an atrial septal defect during inflow occlusion of the cavae and baffled the inferior vena cava through the defect in 9 patients with transposition of less than 2 months of age. There were 2 early and 2 late deaths. All survivors did extremely well. A further report on the results of surgical creation of an atrial septal defect by inflow occlusion was made by Lindesmith and associates (1966). Of the 23 neonates who underwent this operation in which the inferior vena cava was also baffled through the created defect, 16 survived.

The results of creation of an atrial septal defect as a palliative surgical procedure in transposition has been reported by other workers. Thus, Reed (1965) operated upon 4 patients with 3 survivors, Rothlin and Senning (1965) on 9 with 5 survivors, and Brom *et al.* (1965) on 22 with 11 survivors. Of the 19 patients who underwent the Blalock–Hanlon operation by Morgan *et al.* (1965), 10 died in the immediate postoperative course. The authors pointed out that the surgical mortality was low when the operation was done without prior cardiac catheterization or angiocardiography. Thus, of the 12 patients who were not investigated by cardiac catheterization or angiocardiography prior to operation, 4 died. On the other hand, of the 7 patients who were investigated before surgery, 6 died. Based on this experience the authors believed that cardiac catheterization and angiocardiography should be omitted in typical cases. The results of the Blalock–Hanlon procedure on 90 infants and children at the Johns Hopkins Hospital between the years 1948 and 1964 were reported by Cornell and associates (1966). Fifty-four patients died at operation or in the immediate postoperative course. Thirty-three deaths were directly attributable to hemorrhagic pulmonary edema secondary to occlusion of the right pulmonary veins at the time of surgery and lung congestion, which results from overflow of blood to the lungs in patients without pulmonary stenosis. Clinical improvement of the 36 survivors was definite although often not dramatic. Sixteen patients survived more than 10 years after operation and 7 of these had lived at least 13 years. Venables (1966) reported the results of creation of an atrial septal defect in 30 infants with transposition. Creation of atrial septal defects under inflow occlusion was abandoned in favor of the Blalock–Hanlon technique after three attempts because of two episodes of coronary air embolism and one of accidental cardiac perforation. There were 11 deaths which appeared to be related to the procedure. In 4 infants there was no change in the clinical status suggesting that no effective defect had been created. These infants died at intervals ranging between 5 weeks and 16 months after surgery. The survivors improved and their condition remained stable. Kirchhoff (1967) performed the Blalock–Hanlon operation on 24 children with transposition. Twelve died in the immediate postoperative course and 2 after 4 weeks. Plauth *et al.* (1968) reported the results of surgical creation of an atrial septal defect by the Blalock–Hanlon operation in 45 infants with transposition. All patients were severely cyanotic, dyspnoic, with inadequate mixing at the atrial and no mixing, or only poor exchange, at the ventricular level. Twenty-seven of 32 patients (84%) operated upon at increased environmental pressure and 8 out of 13 (62%) operated upon under normobaric conditions survived. Atrial septal defects in all infants operated upon under hyperbaric conditions were created under direct vision by means of inflow occlusion. The techniques used in the normobaric group consisted of various modifications of the Blalock–Hanlon operation. Among those who left the hospital postoperatively, there were 5 late deaths. The authors attributed the improved results obtained under hyperbaric condition to (1) early referral to the hospital, (2) a team with a special interest in neonatal cardiology handles these patients, (3) the metabolic needs of the babies before, during, and after operation are analyzed and met with appreciably more skill than in the past, and (4) a significant contribution to the survival of these infants is the increased availability of oxygen provided in the hyperbaric environment. Of the 8 infants who underwent surgical creation of an atrial septal defect (inflow occlusion in 7, and Blalock–Hanlon in 1) by O'Donovan *et al.* (1968), 7 survived. Banding of the pulmonary artery was performed at the same time in 1 case, and after 12 months in another. Aberdeen and Carr (1968) pointed out that in their experience the survival rate over the age of 3 months was about 95%, but for the group under the age of 6 weeks survival was about 33%. The high mortality in the younger group was related mainly to pulmonary complications. Of the 43 infants below the age of 3 months who underwent this operation, 19 survived while of the 22 above the age of 3 months 21 survived. Trusler and Mustard (1968) abandoned the inflow occlusion method for surgical creation of an atrial septal defect in view of the high mortality rate in comparison with the Blalock–Hanlon procedure. Of their 28 patients who underwent the Blalock–Hanlon operation, 12 were 14 days of age or less with 3 survivors. Sixteen were over 14 days of age with 12 survivors. Deverall et al. (1969) studied the results of 178 consecutive atrial septectomies by the Blalock–Hanlon technique. There were 80 hospital deaths. The hospital mortality rate was 57% in the earlier years of the study and 35% in the last 5 years of the study. In children more than 6 weeks of age, the mortality rate fell from 46 to 18%. The mortality rate in children aged 6 weeks or less fell from 69 to 61%. Of the 80 hospital deaths there were 26 operative deaths, and 54 postoperative deaths. The most common cause of operative death was hemorrhage due to technical error and the most common cause of postoperative death was respiratory failure. Twenty-four children died after leaving the hospital and the most common causes of death in this group were subsequent heart surgery and congestive heart failure. Zamora et al. (1970) reported the results of the Blalock–Hanlon operation on 28 infants with transposition. Eighteen infants had an intact ventricular septum and 16 required the operation within the first 2 months of life. Of the 10 patients with a ventricular septal defect, a pulmonary artery band was performed at the same time as the Blalock–Hanlon in 8, and 8 months before it in 1. There were 3 operative and 1 late deaths. With the exception of one child with an intact ventricular septum and pulmonary stenosis, all others improved. Litwin et al. (1971) reported the results of 105 consecutive surgical atrial septectomies. Of these 105, the operation was carried out as an isolated procedure in 77. Surgical septectomy was performed when the systemic arterial oxygen saturation was less than 60% on the basis of poor mixing or when the mean pressure gradient between the two atria was markedly elevated. The operation was done under hyperbaric conditions and the inflow occlusion technique was used. Of the 77 patients, there were 58 individuals with an intact ventricular septum or very small ventricular septal defect, 8 with a sizeable ventricular septal defect, 8 with ventricular septal defect and moderate pulmonary stenosis, and 3 with other conditions. Among the 61 survivors (79%) followed for an average of 31 months, there was an increase in the mean systemic arterial oxygen saturation from a preoperative value of 58 to 79% postoperatively. The most impressive improvement occurred in those with an intact ventricular septum. The authors pointed out that a late fall in arterial oxygen saturation was often indicative of diminishing pulmonary blood flow on the basis of increasing pulmonary stenosis or pulmonary vascular obstructive disease.

Azzolina *et al.* (1972) pointed out that in Blalock–Hanlon operation, clamping of the right pulmonary artery or its branches as well as the right pulmonary vein is involved, and the right lung is excluded from the circulation. To eliminate the drawback of clamping the right pulmonary veins and artery, a looped vascular suture is placed across the interatrial groove for traction. An exclusion clamp is placed in such a way as to encompass the anterior wall of the right pulmonary veins, that portion of the left atrial wall between the entrance of the right pulmonary veins and the interatrial groove, and a sufficient portion of the posterolateral wall of the right atrium adjacent to the septum. Two longitudinal parallel incisions are made adjacent to and on each side of the interatrial line. Pulling on the traction suture while barely loosening the exclusion clamp permits a larger portion of the interatrial septum to be excised. The authors used this technique in 50 patients with transposition, of whom 16 were under 12 months of age. The overall operative mortality within 30 days of operation was 10%. All deaths occurred in the group of 16 patients under 12 months of age.

In the present series, 113 patients underwent surgical creation of an atrial septal defect. The original technique of Blalock–Hanlon was used in 101 patients, and the inflow occlusion technique in 12. An isolated atrial septal defect was created in 101 patients. In the remaining 12 patients, atrial septectomy was undertaken in combination with another surgical procedure. The surgical results were studied with reference to five age groups as follows: 0–1 month, 1–3 months, 3–6 months, 6–12 months, and more than 1 year. The surgical results of atrial septectomy in the isolated or combined surgical groups are summarized in Tables 20.3, 20.4 and 20.5. The overall surgical mortality was 56%. Of the 12 who underwent surgical creation of an atrial septal defect by the inflow occlusion technique, 11 died at or immediately after surgery. The surgical mortality in this group was 92% (Table 20.6). Of the 101 patients who underwent the Blalock–Hanlon procedure, 53 died as a result of the operation and the surgical mortality was 52%. The surgical mortality in the isolated atrial septal defect group was 57% and the combined surgical group was 50%. The highest surgical mortality (72%) occurred during

TABLE 20.3

113 Surgical Atrial Septal Defect; Blalock–Hanlon and Inflow Occlusion [a]

Group	Isolated atrial septal defect 0-1 m		1-3 m		3-6 m		6 m-1 y		Above 1 y		Combined surgical procedures 0-1 m		1-3 m		3-6 m		6 m-1 y		Above 1 y		Survived	Died	% Death	Late deaths	Follow up
	D	A	D	A	D	A	D	A	D	A	D	A	D	A	D	A	D	A	D	A					
Group I (68 Patients)	36	12	4	6	1	2	2	0	0	3	1	0	1	0	0	0	0	0	0	0	23	45	66	9	14
Group II (7 Patients)	1	2	2	1	0	0	0	0	0	1	0	0	0	0	0	0	0	0	0	0	4	3	43	1	3
Group III (32 Patients)	6	3	3	4	0	2	1	2	2	1	1	1	0	1	0	2	1	1	0	1	18	14	44	5	13
Group IV (6 Patients)	0	0	0	2	0	1	0	0	0	1	2	0	0	0	0	0	0	0	0	0	4	2	33	2	2
Total (113 Patients)	43	17	9	13	1	5	3	2	2	6	4	1	1	1	0	2	1	1	0	1	49	64	56	17	32

[a] A, alive; D, deceased; m, month; y, year.

TABLE 20.4
Surgical Atrial Septal Defect; The Blalock–Hanlon Operation [a,b]

Group	Isolated atrial septal defect										Combined surgical procedures										Late deaths	Follow up
	0-1 m		1-3 m		3-6 m		6-1 y		Above 1 y		0-1 m		1-3 m		3-6 m		6-1 y		Above 1 y			
	D	A	D	A	D	A	D	A	D	A	D	A	D	A	D	A	D	A	D	A		
I (60 Patients)	32	11	3	6	0	2	2	0	0	3	1	0	0	0	0	0	0	0	0	0	8	14
II (6 Patients)	0	2	2	1	0	0	0	0	0	1	0	0	0	0	0	0	0	0	0	0	1	3
III (29 Patients)	4	3	3	4	0	2	1	2	2	1	0	1	0	1	0	2	1	1	0	1	5	13
IV (6 Patients)	0	0	0	2	0	1	0	0	0	1	2	0	0	0	0	0	0	0	0	0	2	2
Total (101)	36	16	8	13	0	5	3	2	2	6	3	1	0	1	0	2	1	1	0	1	16	32

[a] 101 patients.
[b] Abbreviations same as in Table 20.3.

TABLE 20.5
SURGICAL ATRIAL SEPTAL DEFECT BY THE INFLOW OCCLUSION TECHNIQUE [a,b]

Group	Isolated atrial septal defect										Combined surgical procedures										Late deaths	Follow up
	0–1 m		1–3 m		3–6 m		6–1 y		Above 1 y		0–1 m		1–3 m		3–6 m		6–1 y		Above 1 y			
	D	A	D	A	D	A	D	A	D	A	D	A	D	A	D	A	D	A	D	A		
I (8 Patients)	5	1	1	0	0	0	0	0	0	0	0	0	1	0	0	0	0	0	0	0	1	0
II (1 Patient)	1	0	0	0	0	0	0	0	0	0	0	0	0	0	0	0	0	0	0	0	0	0
III (3 Patients)	2	0	0	0	0	0	0	0	0	0	1	0	0	0	0	0	0	0	0	0	0	0
IV (None)	0	0	0	0	0	0	0	0	0	0	0	0	0	0	0	0	0	0	0	0	0	0
Total (12)	8	1	1	0	0	0	0	0	0	0	1	0	1	0	0	0	0	0	0	0	1	0

[a] 12 patientss.
[b] Abbreviations same as in Table 20.3.

TABLE 20.6

RESULTS OF SURGICAL CREATION OF AN ATRIAL SEPTAL DEFECT

	Total	Survived	Died	% Death
0–1 Month	66	18	48	72
1–3 Months	24	14	10	42
3–6 Months	7	7	0	0
6 Months–1 year	7	3	4	56
Above 1 year	9	7	2	22
Total	113	49	64	56
Inflow occlusion	12	1	11	92
Blalock–Hanlon procedure	101	48	53	52
Isolated atrial septal defect	101	43	58	57
Combined surgical procedures	12	6	6	50

the first month of life, and the lowest (22%) above the age of 1 year (Table 20.6). The surgical mortality in the 4 groups was 66% in Group I, 43% in Group II, 44% in Group III, and 33% in Group IV (Table 20.3). Of the 49 survivors in the whole group, there were 17 late deaths and 32 were followed up for a period from 5 to 6 years. The cause of death in the follow up period was heart surgery in 13, heart failure in 2, pneumonia in 1, and sudden death in 1. Of the 32 who were still alive, 15 underwent successful Mustard's procedure, 3 have had a Blalock-Taussig or cavopulmonary anastomosis, and 13 are alive and well without further surgery.

At the time of this writing the Blalock–Hanlon procedure should be used if creation of an atrial septal defect is indicated in children older than 6 months of age. In view of the increasing thickness of the atrial septum above this age, adequate septostomy by the Rashkind procedure may not be possible. The surgical mortality of this operation above the age of 6 months should be 10–15%.

ANASTOMOSIS OF THE RIGHT PULMONARY VEINS TO THE RIGHT ATRIUM, AND THE SUPERIOR OR INFERIOR VENA CAVA TO THE LEFT ATRIUM

In 1948, Hanlon and Blalock experimentally anastomosed the right pulmonary veins to the right atrium in dogs. Lillehei and Varco (1953) thought that if an operation could be developed to completely transpose the pulmonary and the systemic veins, it would have these advantages: (1) the coronary vessels would be provided with oxygenated blood, and (2) a virtually curative operation could be provided in patients without septal defects. By doing so, complete transposition is transformed into a

form of corrected transposition. They described four types of partial correction of the veins.

1. Anastomosis of the right superior and inferior pulmonary veins to the right atrium.
2. Anastomosis of the right pulmonary veins to the right atrium and anastomosis of the inferior vena cava to the left atrium.
3. Anastomosis of the cardiac end of the left innominate vein to the left atrium with ligation of the superior vena cava.
4. Anastomosis of the superior vena cava to the left atrium with a polythene tube maintaining a temporary blood flow between the superior vena cava and the right atrium.

The authors diverted the right pulmonary venous return into the right atrium in 4 patients with 2 successes. Four other patients, in whom the right pulmonary veins were anastomosed to the right atrium and the inferior vena cava to the left atrium, died immediately after operation. The authors concluded that it is potentially hazardous to perform pulmonary venous–right atrial anastomosis alone, unless large internal shunts are known to exist. In the absence of the latter, the rapidly lethal effects that result from unbalancing the two basically independent circulations which exist in complete transposition, constitute sufficient reason for only recommending procedures designed to achieve hemodynamic equilibrium.

Murphy *et al.* (1955) reported their results of surgical palliation in complete transposition of the great arteries. Transplantation of the right pulmonary veins to the right atrium was performed in 10 patients, while in 13 others, in addition to this procedure, the inferior vena cava or the superior vena cava was transplanted to the left atrium. Of these 23 patients 4, in whom only the pulmonary veins were transplanted into the right atrium, survived with improvement.

Baffes (1956) found that if the right pulmonary veins were transplanted into the right atrium and the superior vena cava into the left atrium, the anatomical relations of the superior vena cava are such that it is readily compressed by the right main bronchus, the right pulmonary artery, and the transposed right pulmonary veins, as it passes between these structures to the left atrium. He thought it would be better to utilize the inferior vena cava in spite of its extremely short length in humans, as it is in such a position that no other structures will compress it after it has been transferred into the left atrium. In addition, the amount of blood returning to the heart through the inferior vena cava is approximately the same as that delivered through the pulmonary veins, thus the systemic

and pulmonary circulations tend to remain balanced after transposition of these major vessels. He successfully used a homologous aortic graft to transplant the inferior vena cava to the left atrium, and at the same time transplanted the right pulmonary veins to the right atrium in 1 patient. His further experience with this operation has been reported by Potts *et al.* (1956) ; and Miller and Baffes (1957). The results of this operation on 35 patients were reported by Baffes (1957), and on 38 patients by Baffes *et al.* (1957). Thirteen patients died in the immediate postoperative period and 23 survived. Four of the survivors died after leaving the hospital; 2 of infectious processes and two of "pulmonary arteriosclerosis." The symptoms of the remaining 19 patients were satisfactorily alleviated. The authors pointed out that as these grafts do not grow, as large a graft as possible should be introduced. In addition, the azygos vein is left intact, so that, should any relative obstruction of the inferior vena cava occur with the growth of the patient, there would be sufficient available collateral circulation to prevent the formation of hepatic congestion or ascites. Among the 117 patients with a homologous aortic graft reported by Paul *et al.* (1960), pre- and postoperative physiological studies were performed on 8. They found that the maximum increase in the systemic arterial oxygen saturation was from 39 (preoperatively) to 84% (postoperatively). Calculations indicated that the pulmonary venous blood entering the aorta may increase as much as threefold after operation. The authors pointed out that severe pulmonary artery hypertension if associated with significantly increased pulmonary blood flow, was not a deterrent to dramatic clinical and physiological improvement. Three patients with the pulmonary vascular resistance of more than 10 units survived with definite but less improvement. The authors emphasized that left ventricular outflow tract obstruction is not a contraindication to this operation, provided that the pulmonary blood flow is normal or increased. Baffes *et al.* (1960) and Baffes (1962) reported the results of surgery on 148 cases of transposition. Of these 148 patients, 117 were treated by utilizing a homologous aortic graft to transfer the inferior vena cava to the left atrium (Paul *et al.*, 1960). In the second group of 31 patients a Teflon graft was used instead of homologous one. A temporary occluding ligature about the pulmonary artery as soon as thoracotomy was accomplished, protects the right lung from engorgement during surgical manipulation. The mortality rate in the second group was 35.5% and in the first group was 29%. Among the 83 survivors, the result was good in 58, fair in 18, poor in 2, and 5 were lost to the follow-up. Hastreiter *et al.* (1966) reported the clinical and hemodynamic findings in 17 patients

with transposition treated by the Baffes operation. Seventy-one percent of these patients had surgery before 1 year of age, and the hemodynamic studies were performed $2\frac{1}{2}$ to $8\frac{1}{2}$ years later. The authors pointed out that when adequate surgical relief of cyanosis is accomplished, the future hemodynamic course of these patients appears to be determined by the type and size of the associated anatomical lesions. Patients with absent or small ventricular septal defect did not develop pulmonary hypertension. Left ventricular outflow tract obstruction developed over the years in some patients with a large ventricular septal defect. The authors emphasized that complete transposition, even when associated with a large ventricular septal defect, does not necessarily result in pulmonary vascular obstruction in patients whose hypoxia has been palliated in early life. In addition, the hemodynamic behavior of their patients with transposition and ventricular septal defect did not appear to differ significantly from that of patients with a ventricular septal defect without transposition of the great arteries. Until 1968, a total of 202 children with transposition underwent the Baffes procedure at the Children's Memorial Hospital in Chicago (Paul *et al.*, 1968). These authors pointed out, however, that because of the extensive nature of the surgery and the availability of other less complex procedures, the Baffes operation was much less frequently employed.

Of the patients operated on by the Baffes procedure other than those reported from Chicago by Baffes and his group, Ferguson (1958) operated on 2; 1 patient died 7 hours after the operation while the other was well and alive 4 months postoperatively. Ash *et al.* (1959) operated on 4 patients with transposition. Transplantation of the superior vena cava to the left atrium and the right superior pulmonary vein to the right atrium was effected in 1 patient with survival for 5 months after the operation. In 2 other cases, the right pulmonary veins were transplanted to the right atrium; 1 died 14 hours after operation and the other died suddenly several months later after contracting a mild infection. A Baffes operation was performed on a fourth patient with survival for 36 hours after operation. Hallman and Cooley (1964) used the Baffes technique successfully in 2 cases while Brom *et al.* (1965) had 10 survivors among 15 cases.

In the present series 12 patients underwent the Baffes procedure with 5 survivals and 7 deaths. There were 3 patients in Group I, 7 in Group III, and 2 in Group IV. Of the 6 patients below the age of 1 year, 4 died and 2 survived. Of the 6 patients above the age of 1 year, 3 died and 3 survived. All 5 survivors showed considerable improvement in cyanosis and effort tolerance. No late deaths occurred in this group and they were followed for periods between 2 and 6 years. During the follow up period, 2 underwent Mustard's operation, 1 cavopulmonary anastomosis, and 2 were alive and well.

Anastomosis of the superior vena cava to the left atrium was performed in this series on 1 patient at the age of 4½ months. This patient died after completion of the operation.

REPOSITIONING OF THE RIGHT PULMONARY VEINS

In 1964, Edwards *et al.* transposed the atrial septum to redirect the right pulmonary veins into the right atrium for palliative treatment of transposition of the great arteries. The operation is performed through a right anterolateral incision. The pulmonary artery is isolated and temporarily occluded and the right pulmonary veins are encircled with umbilical tape. An exclusion clamp is placed across the interatrial septum including the right common pulmonary vein. Two parallel incisions are made inside the jaws of the clamps. One of these parallel incisions enters the right atrium, while the other enters the common right pulmonary vein. All of the atrial septum inside the clamp, except a small ridge about 2 mm wide, is removed. The small rim of atrial septum which remains is sutured to the wall of the left atrium. After the sutures are tied the atrial septum has been transposed to the left of the entrance of the right pulmonary vein. Finally, the free margins of the incised pulmonary vein and right atrium are approximated, and the exclusion clamp and vascular snares removed. The authors believed that when an atrial septal defect is created by the Blalock–Hanlon method a right-to-left shunt becomes predominant until pulmonary blood flow becomes so high that pulmonary arterial pressure approximates systemic arterial pressure. This additional overloading of the pulmonary circuit probably increases cardiac work and definitely increases pulmonary congestion. The authors added that this operation produces an effective left-to-right shunt into the right atrium and at the same time decompresses the pulmonary vascular bed that has proved so lethal in these children. The authors successfully used this technique on 3 infants with transposition. The systemic arterial oxygen saturations improved to well over 70% in all 3 children, and they maintained this improvement in the follow-up. In 1965, Edwards and Bargeron further reported on 5 additional cases. Of the whole group of 8 patients, there was an early death and 2 late deaths. Morgan *et al.* (1965) attempted the Edwards procedure in 2 infants, both of whom were moribund at the time of surgery and died in the immediate postoperative period. Trusler and Kidd (1967) suggested that the absence of lung flooding during the postoperative phase is responsible for the relative success of the procedure. Trusler and Mustard (1968) pointed out that the Edwards operation tends to reduce pulmonary blood flow to a level dependent upon the amount of blood returning to the pulmonary circulation through the bronchial collaterals or communication in the atrial or ventricular septa. Dramatic reduction of the pulmonary plethora occurs after this operation. These authors operated on 7 infants, 5 less than 2 weeks of age, with 1 death. Two of the 6 survivors became increasingly cyanotic due to a marked diminution in pulmonary blood flow. Over a year later both developed cerebral thrombosis, but their condition was subsequently improved by the creation of an atrial septal defect. Two others continued well without any further surgery. The remaining 2 children maintained an increased pulmonary blood flow and higher systemic oxygen saturation as the result of enlargement of the patent foramen ovale by blind instrumentation at the time of the Edwards procedure. The authors used the Edwards procedure in combination with banding of the pulmonary artery on 4 children, all of whom survived. Cardiac catheterization in 1 of these 4 children both before and after the procedure showed a rise in arterial oxygen saturation despite a fall in pulmonary blood flow. Ankeney and O'Grady (1968) used the Edwards operation on 16 patients with transposition; 7 with an intact ventricular septum and 9 with a ventricular septal defect. Of the 5 deaths in this group, 4 had an intact ventricular septum and 1 had a ventricular septal defect. A further report on the Edwards procedure was made by Ehrenstein et al. (1969). These authors operated on 20 patients with transposition; 6 with an intact ventricular septum and 14 with a ventricular septal defect. Five patients died at the operation or in the early postoperative course; 3 with an intact septum and 2 with a ventricular septal defect. The surgical result indicated to the authors that congestive heart failure is relieved and hypoxia is reduced in children with large ventricular septal defects and increased pulmonary blood flow. The authors pointed out that in such patients, a concomitant pulmonary artery banding has not been necessary. On the other hand, satisfactory palliation was not achieved with repositioning the pulmonary veins in patients with an intact septum. An additional report on the Edwards operation was made by Trusler (1971). This operation was performed on eleven infants with intact ventricular septum, 9 of whom were less than 2 weeks old. Nine survived, and in 6 of these the transposition had been successfully corrected. The procedure was combined with banding of the pulmonary artery in

14 infants; 12 survived. The author pointed out that this procedure, shunting all of the right pulmonary venous blood into the right atrium, produces a more obligatory mixing than the Blalock–Hanlon or other procedures, and at the same time tends to reduce pulmonary blood flow. By this reduction the Edwards operation may enhance the effect of banding.

In this series 11 patients underwent the Edwards procedure; 9 in Group I, and 2 in Group III. Pulmonary artery banding was also carried out on the 2 patients in Group III. The surgical results on 9 of the 11 patients in this series, and on 2 others with a ventricular septal defect have been discussed by Trusler and Mustard (1968). The remaining 2 patients in this series who have not been reported by Trusler and Mustard, were both neonates with an intact ventricular septum. Both died in the early postoperative course. In summary, of the 9 patients with an intact septum in this series, 6 survived and 3 died. The 2 with a large ventricular septal defect survived combined banding of the pulmonary artery and the Edwards procedure.

As pointed out by Trusler and Mustard (1968), it seems that the best indication for the Edwards procedure would be in combination with banding of the pulmonary artery of patients with a large ventricular septal defect. Since this operation alone does not lower the pulmonary arterial pressure in patients with a large ventricular septal defect, banding of the pulmonary artery of these children during the first 6 months of life is mandatory to reduce pulmonary vascular obstruction.

CREATION OF VENOUS OR ARTERIAL OR VENOARTERIAL
EXTRACARDIAC SHUNT

In 1950, Blalock and Hanlon published their pioneer work on the creation of extracardiac shunts in patients with complete transposition of the great vessels. Five different types of operation were described, their object being to divert some blood to the side of the heart opposite to its point of origin.

1. Anastomosis between the distal end of the right superior pulmonary vein (proximal end ligated) and the side of the superior vena cava.
2. Division of the left innominate vein and anastomosis of its proximal end to the side of the left main pulmonary artery.
3. Division of the pulmonary artery to the right upper lobe and anastomosis of its proximal end to the side of the inferior vena cava.
4. Division of the pulmonary artery to the right upper lobe, anastomo-

sis of its proximal end to the side of the superior vena cava, and anastomosis of its distal end to the proximal end of the right subclavian artery.

5. Division of the right main pulmonary artery, anastomosis of its
proximal end to the side of the superior vena cava, and anastomosis of its
distal end to the proximal end of the right subclavian artery.

Blalock and Hanlon operated on 9 patients using these techniques. One
patient died during operation, while the remaining 8 survived completion
of the operation only to die within a few minutes, or at most, several days
after. In most cases, pulmonary edema was the terminal feature. The fa-
talities in this group suggested to the authors that the procedures employed for treatment of transposition were basically unsound. They pointed out that on theoretical grounds one might doubt the advisability of
creating shunts which would upset the balance of the two sides of the circulation. It was proposed to anastomose the proximal end of the right
subclavian artery and the distal end of the pulmonary artery to the right
upper lobe, after the creation of an atrial septal defect. A large part of
the additional blood sent to the right lung through the subclavian artery
returns to the right atrium through the atrial septal defect. By doing this,
the danger associated with a unidirectional shunt is avoided, since the
atrial septal defect equalizes the pressures on the two sides of the circulation. This double procedure was used in 12 patients all of whom survived
the operative procedure, but 4 died shortly afterward. Most of the survivors seem to have improved.

Moss *et al.* (1961) advocated a palliative operation to permit more
extensive mixing of the pulmonary and systemic circulations in patients
with transposition and increased pulmonary blood flow. The operation
consists of creating an atrial septal defect and of end to end anastomosis
between the proximal portions of the azygos vein and the apical segmental branch of the right pulmonary artery. They used this technique on 6
babies with transposition; 3 died immediately after operation, and 3 survived with improvement.

Stimulation of the Bronchial Collateral Circulation

Vidone and Liebow (1957) found that ligation of all pulmonary arteries and veins to one lobe stimulates the development of an extensive arterial supply from the aorta, and a venous collateral circulation drains the
lungs by means of augmented precapillary connections with the pulmonary veins into the right side of the heart. They suggested that in the treatment of transposition of the great arteries this operation, therefore, would

have the effect of introducing an autogenous oxygenator into the right-sided systemic circuit. The lungs would receive desaturated blood from the transposed aorta by way of expanded bronchial arteries and after oxygenating it, return it to the right heart via expanded bronchial veins. Toole *et al.* (1960) used this technique once but the patient died 11 months after operation.

Anatomic Correction of Transposition

Blalock and Hanlon (1950) pointed out that the most direct approach to the treatment of complete transposition of the great arteries would be to disconnect the aorta and the pulmonary artery from the heart and reattach them to their proper ventricles. They pointed out, however, that the coronary arterial circulations would still arise near the origin of the aorta which would receive poorly oxygenated blood from the right ventricle.

Using a perfusion pump and a biological oxygenator (monkey lung), Mustard *et al.* (1954) operated on 7 patients with transposition of the great vessels by transplanting the aorta and the left coronary artery to the left ventricle and the pulmonary artery with the right coronary artery to the right ventricle. No patient survived the operation.

Bjork and Bouckaert (1954) described an experimental technique of switch-over anastomosis utilizing grafts without interruption of the circulation. No extracorporeal circulation or hypothermia was required. An anastomosis was established between the aorta, as close to the coronary artery as possible, and the left pulmonary artery using an aortic graft. Another graft was anastomosed between the main pulmonary artery and the aorta distal to the left subclavian artery. Subsequently the aorta and the pulmonary artery were divided between the grafts. The authors pointed out that a switch-over anastomosis cannot be used in cases with a normal pressure in the pulmonary artery, since this would only result in circulatory arrest due to the low pressure in the left ventricle taking over the systemic circulation, or a pulmonary edema within a few hours due to the high pressure in the right ventricle taking over the pulmonary circulation.

Cross *et al.* (1954) thought that external shunting procedures with plastic shunts, affords a simple approach to surgery on the vessels at the base of the heart. They experimentally cross-anastomosed the proximal aorta to the distal pulmonary artery and the proximal pulmonary artery to the distal aorta in dogs. Attempts to use the shunts were made in 2 of their patients with transposition of the great arteries. In both, the heart failed before the shunts could be tested.

Kay and Cross (1955) suggested a sequence of anastomosis between the aorta and the pulmonary artery which would result in complete re-transposition of the aorta and the pulmonary artery but not of the coronary arteries. The right pulmonary artery is first anastomosed to the ascending aorta. The aortic arch is cut beyond the right pulmonary artery and anastomosed to the main pulmonary artery. Finally, the left pulmonary artery is anastomosed to the proximal aorta and the right pulmonary artery with a graft. Using this technique, the authors operated on 2 infants with complete transposition of the great arteries. Both died immediately after operation.

Senning (1959) transposed the aorta with its coronary arteries to the left ventricle and the pulmonary artery to the right ventricle. The pulmonary artery with its valve is dissected from the left ventricle. The resulting hole which is limited on the right by the aorta and the interventricular septum, and on the left by the anterior mitral valve cusp where it meets the atrial wall in the annulus fibrosus, is sutured, thus fusing the anterior mitral cusp to the aortic root. A right ventriculotomy is made over the outflow tract. Part of the right aortic border is dissected from the right ventricular wall. A prothesis is sutured to the right of the aorta. Thus the aorta communicates directly with the left ventricle through the ventricular septal defect and then the pulmonary root is sutured into the right ventricle. Senning used this method in 3 patients with transposition of the great arteries, 2 with a ventricular septal defect and 1 with an intact ventricular septum. All 3 patients died immediately after completion of the operation.

Idriss et al. (1961) transposed the aorta with the coronary arteries to the left ventricle and the pulmonary artery to the right ventricle. The aorta is dissected to the level of the ligamentum arteriosum or the ductus arteriosus. The coronary arteries and the pulmonary arteries are dissected free. The aorta is cross-clamped with a Pott's coarctation clamp producing ischemic cardiac arrest. The aorta is then transected, first, about 5 mm distal to the coronary ostia and, second, proximal to the coronary ostia. An isolated aortic segment about 8 mm in length is thus produced containing the ostia of both coronary arteries. The pulmonary artery is transected 1 mm distal to the valve commissures. The aortic segment containing the coronary ostia is anastomosed to the left ventricular stump and a second anastomosis is established between the aortic segment and the distal aorta. Finally, the pulmonary artery is anastomosed to the right ventricle. The authors pointed out that the basic features that make it possible to transfer both coronary arteries with the aorta, are the intact aortic segment and the turning maneuver. The intact segment acts in real-

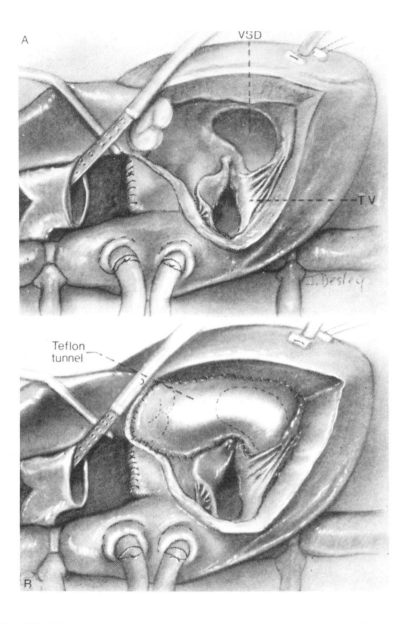

Fig. 20.2. Diagrammatic illustration of the Rastelli operation. (A) Pulmonary artery is divided and cardiac end oversewn. Interior of right ventricle demonstrates relationship of ventricular septal defect (VSD), tricuspid valve (TV), and aortic valve. (B) Left ventricle is connected to aorta by tunnel between ventricular septal defect and aortic orifice, made with Teflon patch. (C) Aortic homograft is sutured

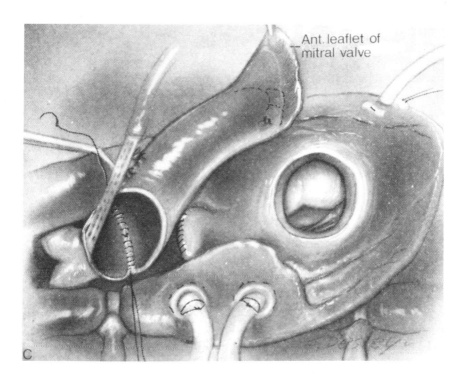

between distal end of pulmonary artery and "window" in anterior wall of right ventricle. (D) Complete repair shows anterior leaflet of homograft mitral valve used as gusset to close apical portion of ventriculotomy. From Rastelli *et al.* (1969b), by permission of the American Heart Association, Inc.

ity as a graft lengthening the coronary arteries, thus obviating the difficulty associated with the individual transfer of these vessels. They operated on 2 patients with complete transposition with an intact ventricular septum. The right and left ventricular pressures of the first patient were 108/8 and 37/8 mm Hg, respectively, and of the second patient 52/0 and 62/5 mm Hg, respectively. Both died immediately after operation, the first of left ventricular failure and the second of bleeding.

In 1969, Rastelli pointed out that the pre-bypass attempts for anatomic correction of transposition were doomed to failure for various reasons: (1) lengthy multisuture procedures which were required while the circulation was unsupported, (2) the coronary arteries were not, or only partially, transferred, (3) associated defects were not repaired, and (4) the patients operated on were very young. He emphasized that the anatomical approach is theoretically sound and the need for alternate procedure

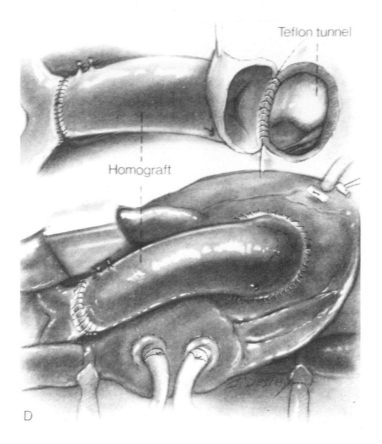

D

to the Mustard repair is stressed by the problems encountered when this latter technique is used to repair transposition associated with a ventricular septal defect. When subvalvular pulmonary stenosis is present in addition to the ventricular septal defect, the mortality rate after surgical correction becomes prohibitive (Rastelli *et al.,* 1969b) for the following reasons: (1) incomplete relief of the subvalvular stenosis, (2) the location of the obstruction in the left ventricular outflow tract makes a satisfactory surgical exposure impossible, (3) even if exposure were satisfactory, the nature of the obstruction would often defy surgical repair in cases associated with a hypoplastic left ventricular outflow tract, a small pulmonary valve ring, and obstructive anomalies of the mitral valve, and (4) resection of subvalvular obstruction can cause complete atrioventricular block. He devised a technique that would bypass these obstacles altogether. No attempt at relieving the subvalvular obstruction is made and the pulmonary artery is divided above the valve and the cardiac end is oversewn (Fig. 20.2) . Redirection of left ventricular outflow is achieved by repairing the ventricular septal defect in such a way as to make the left ventricle empty into the aorta. For this purpose, a tunnel is constructed by suturing a teflon patch between the ventricular septal defect and the aortic orifice. The area of the ventricular septal defect must be equal to or larger than that of the aortic orifice in order to avoid obstruction to left ventricular outflow. If the ventricular septal defect is not large enough, the defect can be enlarged by excision of part of its anterosuperior aspect in the region of the septal band. The connection of the right ventricle to the pulmonary artery is made by way of a homograft that includes the ascending aorta, the aortic valve, and the anterior leaflet of the mitral valve. The homograft is anastomosed to the distal end of the pulmonary artery and proximally to a large "window" opened in the anterior wall of the right ventricle around the ventriculotomy. The anterior leaflet of the mitral valve is used as a gusset to complete the closure of the apical aspect of the ventricular opening. The author pointed out that the area of the right ventricular wall that is excised should be devoid of main coronary arteries, and the intracardiac tunnel connecting the left ventricle to the aorta must not impinge on the right ventricular "window." Rastelli et al. (1969) used this technique successfully on 3 patients with a ventricular septal defect and subvalvular pulmonary stenosis. The ages of these patients were 14½, 15, and 2 years and 4 months, respectively. Postoperative cardiac catheterization in 1 patient demonstrated a residual pressure gradient of 24 mm Hg between the pulmonary artery and the right ventricle. The authors pointed out the fact that transfer of coronary arteries is not required contributes to the success of this operation. Realignment of the right ventricle with the pulmonary circulation and the left ventricle with the systemic circulation affords a more physiological repair than that achieved with intra-atrial transposition of the venous return, since it obviates the need for the right ventricle and the tricuspid valve to function in the high pressure systemic circuit. They added that repair of transposition with a ventricular septal defect without left ventricular outflow tract obstruction, could also be carried out with the same technique. McGoon et al. (1970) further reported on the results of this operation on 11 patients at the Mayo Clinic. Nine had a ventricular septal defect and subvalvular pulmonary stenosis. Two hospital deaths occurred among this group, and both patients were less than 4 years of age. In 2 patients the ventricular septal defect was small or absent. In one of these 2 patients, the stenosis was caused by a pulmonary artery band. To permit a desired repair a ventricular septal defect was enlarged or created. Both patients died after surgery; one of occlusion of the left anterior descending coronary artery during suturing of the homograft, and one of technical problems. Imamura *et al.* (1971) used this technique successfully on a 12-year-old patient with a ventricular septal defect and pulmonary valvular stenosis. The patient was doing well 15 months after the operation. Clarkson *et al.* (1972) used the Rastelli procedure on 1 patient with pulmonary valvular stenosis, and 1 with pulmonary valve atresia at 3 and 6 years of age, respectively. Both patients died postoperatively. The authors pointed out that the first of these operations was performed 3 years before this procedure was described by Rastelli *et al.* (1969a). McGoon (1972) pointed out that 40 Rastelli operations for transposition of the great arteries and pulmonary stenosis have been performed at the Mayo Clinic.

Deverall *et al.* (1971) suggested the following plan for total repair of transposition and pulmonary stenosis. A direct attack is performed on the pulmonary stenosis with hemodynamic. correction of transposition when (1) the ventricular septum is intact or the septal defect is small, (2) left ventricular outflow obstruction is at pulmonary valve level even though the ventricular septal defect is larger, and (3) probably if corrective surgery is indicated in a child less than 5 years of age. Anatomic correction is preferred in older children in whom a large ventricular septal defect coexists with subvalvar obstruction or when the rotation of the heart is such to make right atrial access impracticable.

In the present series a graft operation was performed on 9 patients, and a switch-over anastomosis on 10. These operations were pre-bypass attempts at total correction of transposition. All patients died on the operating table or in the immediate postoperative course.

Intraventricular Correction of Transposition

Intraventricular repair of complete transposition of the great arteries was first described by Senning (1966), who reported the case of a 4-year-old child with complete transposition, pulmonary stenosis, and three atria. A right ventriculotomy exposed a huge ventricular septal defect, through which the left ventricular outflow tract obstruction was resected. The pulmonary and systemic circulations were crossed by means of a screw-blade-shaped Dacron patch, which also closed the ventricular septum. The child did well and was in excellent condition after surgery. McGoon (1972a) used the same technique on a 2-year-old boy with transposition, pulmonary stenosis, large ventricular septal defect, and dextrocardia with solitus atria, and an 11-year-old boy with transposition, ventricular septal defect, and a patent ductus arteriosus. A very large ventricular septal defect extending from the tricuspid annulus to the anterior heart wall existed in both. Both patients underwent replacement of the basal portion of the ventricular septum with a prosthetic patch in such a way that the reconstructed septum had a spiral configuration. The outflow of the left ventricle thus ended in the aorta and that of the right ventricle in the pulmonary artery. The first patient made an uneventful recovery and was followed up for 2½ years. Postoperative cardiac catheterization showed correction of the defects save for hemodynamically significant subpulmonary stenosis. The second patient died 48 hours after surgery. At autopsy, the left ventricular outflow tract was adequate (1 cm in diameter), but the right ventricular outflow tract had narrowed to a diameter of 7 mm. Death was believed due to a combination of subpulmonary stenosis and pulmonary vascular obstructive disease. The author pointed out that a prerequisite to this repair is the presence of an extra large ventricular septal defect that represents complete absence of the basal portion of the ventricular septum, both posteriorly and anteriorly. Absence of the anterior septum offers the opportunity to correct the hemodynamic abnormality resulting from transposition by the surgical placement of a spiraling prosthetic conal septum so that a given ventricle will empty into its appropriate great artery. A boomerang-shaped patch is preferable to avoid encroachment on the outflow tracts of either ventricles. In patients who have only a posteriorly located ventricular septal defect or even no ventricular septal defect, a large ventricular septal defect could be created. In the author's view, if late follow-up of patients who have undergone the Mustard procedure show a significant incidence of tricuspid insufficiency or right ventricular failure, there may be reason to explore the application of this technique.

Hemodynamic Correction of Transposition

Albert (1954) pointed out that transposing the aorta and the pulmonary artery into their normal positions is not a satisfactory procedure because the coronary arteries would continue to receive venous blood. If, however, the systemic and pulmonary venous returns were transposed, the lesions in effect would be corrected. He devised an operation in which an incision in the interatrial septum is made to produce flaps, and by shifting and resuture of these flaps to a new position, transposition of the venous returns can effectively be done. A C shaped incision is made in the interatrial septum around the lateral, inferior, and superior margins, leaving an intact base medially and the coronary sinus undamaged inferiorly. Another incision is made in this flap of septum starting at the center of the periphery and extending toward the center of the base. The two flaps of the interatrial septum thus created are sutured around the orifices of the vena cava in such a way as to divert the blood from them to the left ventricle, and the blood from the pulmonary veins to the right ventricle.

Based on the principle of Albert (1954), several workers proposed similar operations for interatrial transposition of the venous returns. Merendino *et al.* (1957) used a prosthesis made of Ivalon to divert the pulmonary venous blood to the right atrium, and the systemic venous blood and the coronary sinus blood to the left atrium. The whole of the interatrial septum was excised and replaced by a prosthesis. They operated on 2 patients using this technique. The first patient died on the operating table and the second a few hours after completion of the operation.

Kay and Cross (1957) used a U-shaped right atrial flap to divert the caval and the coronary sinus blood to the left ventricle and the pulmonary venous blood to the right ventricle. An incision is made in the right atrial wall along the projected course of the superior vena cava. This incision is extended to include a U-flap of the atrial wall just proximal to the inferior vena cava. The superior vena cava is then reconstructed down to the U-flap. Two large openings are then made in the atrial septum. The left atrial wall is then grasped on the valvular side of the ostia of the pulmonary veins and sutured about the cephalad opening into the atrial septum. The U-flap to which the cavae communicate is then sutured about the caudal opening in the atrial septum. The right auricular appendage is then opened and used to reconstruct the lateral wall of the right atrium. The authors used this technique on 2 infants with transposition. Both died after operation; the first of collapse of the left lung and the second of complete heart block.

Creech *et al.* (1958) with the aid of a heart–lung machine, used a kidney-shaped patch of polyvinyl sponge to retranspose the circulation within the atria. Again the whole atrial septum had to be excised. One patient was operated on by this method only to succumb 12 hours after operation. With the use of cardiopulmonary bypass, Collins *et al.* (1959) inserted a prosthetic atrial septum in 2 infants with transposition of the great arteries in order to divert the caval blood to the left ventricle and the pulmonary venous blood to the right ventricle. Both infants died.

Senning (1959) thought that the use of a prosthesis or grafts, may lead to obstruction of the blood later when the child is growing. He described the following operation, which is performed under extracorporeal circulation. A long incision is made in the right atrium in front of and parallel to the venae cavae. The right pulmonary veins are incised as close as possible to the left atrium. By a U-shaped incision, the atrial septum is made into as big a posterior flap as possible. Separation of the pulmonary veins from the left atrium is achieved by suturing the atrial septal flap to the posterior wall of the left atrium in front of the pulmonary veins. The anterior edge of the posterior part of the original right atrial wall is sutured to the lower rim of the created atrial septal defect. The venous return from the venae cavae as well as the coronary sinus blood is thus directed to the mitral valve. Finally, the anterior part of the right atrial wall is sutured to the lateral incisional edge of the right pulmonary veins. The "anterior atrium" consists of the posterior part of the original left atrium with the entrance of the pulmonary veins, limited posteriorly against the left atrium by the atrial septal flap and communicating widely behind the venae cavae with the anterior remainder of the original atrium. Senning operated on 4 patients with complete transposition by this method. Three died in the immediate postoperative course while the fourth, age 9½ years, survived the operation. Cardiac investigation later showed arterial oxygen saturation of 97% and no evidence of blood shunts (Jonsson et al., 1959; Senning et al., 1962). Kirklin et al. (1961) used the Senning operation on 9 infants in intractable congestive heart failure and 2 young children with transposition. Three infants and 1 of the older children survived. One infant died later at home of apparently unrelated causes. Of these 11 patients, a ventricular septal defect was present in 9. Aronstam et al. (1963) reported a 16-month-old baby with complete transposition with an intact ventricular septum who was completely cured by the Senning technique. Helmsworth et al. (1964) operated on a 10-week-old baby with an intact ventricular septum who was still surviving 9 months after the surgical procedure. Ongley (1964) stated that Kirklin had had 9 successes on 27 children using the Senning type of complete repair. On the other hand, Hallman and Cooley (1964) did not have any success on their 4 patients. Rothlin and Senning (1965) reported the results of this operation on 4 older children with transposition. The 3 survivors had an intact ventricular septum with normal pulmonary arterial pressure. The fourth patient with a ventricular septal defect and pulmonary stenosis did not survive the operation. Fontan et al. (1965) used the Senning operation successfully on a 4-year-old child with transposition and an intact ventricular septum. The authors pointed out the combination of an interatrial septal defect and low left ventricular pressure represents the best and almost the only indication for Senning operation. Of the 6 patients with transposition totally corrected by Nauta et al.

(1965), utilizing the Senning operation, 3 died immediately after surgery, 2 patients died after 1 and 3 months, respectively, and 1 patient was in good condition 1 year after operation. A further report on the results of this operation on 9 children with transposition was made by Senning (1966). Of the 6 patients with an intact ventricular septum, 4 showed normal arterial oxygen saturation, 1 had signs of a right-to-left shunt, and 1 died of pulmonary complications. The remaining 3 patients had a ventricular septal defect and left ventricular outflow tract obstruction. They all died in the immediate postoperative course. The cause of death in this group was considered due to difficulties with repair of the accessory anomalies, rather than to atrial reconstruction. Complete repair of the Senning type was performed on one of the patients of Venables (1966). A pericardial patch was used to divert venous inflow. The operation was followed by death from intractable intrathoracic hemorrhage unrelated to the repair itself. Rastelli *et al.* (1969b) used the Senning operation on 5 patients with transposition and pulmonary stenosis with no survivors.

In this series the Senning technique was used on 3 infants and a 4½-year-old child. Two were in Group I, and 2 in Group III. All 4 died on the operating table.

Glotzer *et al.* (1960) proposed a one-stage intracardiac procedure for total transposition of the venous returns. The interatrial septum is excised completely and a crimped knitted Dacron patch is sutured about the orifices of the pulmonary veins posteriorly. The other end of the patch is cut to appropriate size and is sutured to the tricuspid annulus, thus creating an artificial atrial septum in a new plane. They experimented with this method in 10 dogs and applied it clinically on a 14-day-old infant. Death, however, occurred from overtransfusion associated with an error in management of perfusion.

Shumacker (1961) pointed out that the use of the atrial septum itself to transpose the venous returns as described by Albert (1954) is unlikely to prove suitable for human beings in view of the small size of the septum and the frequency with which the amount of available septal tissue is further decreased because of the presence of an atrial septal defect. He thought that the creation of the interatrial tunnel exclusively by means of a prosthesis as suggested by Merendino *et al.* (1957) and Creech *et al.* (1958) appears unwise since it would not grow with the increasing size of the patient and heart. On the other hand, if the graft used constitutes only a portion of the repair, viable autogenous tissue will make up the rest. He suggested an operation which deviates the vena caval and coronary sinus blood flow into the left ventricle by the creating of a tunnel constructed by means of a double-pedicled right atrial flap and reconstruction of the anterior right atrial wall, so as to permit pulmonary venous blood to flow through the tricuspid valve into the right ventricle. The right atrial wall is reconstructed by means of a graft rather than by direct suture. Alternatively, a plastic extension of an appropriate size and shape could be added to the right side of the atrial flap. In this way a narrow atrial flap could be used which may permit reconstruction of the anterior wall of the right atrium by direct suture closure. The first method was used in a 10½-month-old infant and the second method in a 1-month-old infant. Both died immediately after operation, the first because of difficulty in securing hemostasis, and the second because of the small caliber of the venous drainage tubes and the consequent poor perfusion rate. In 1969, Shumacker and Girod reported a patient who was successfully operated upon by the double right atrial wall flap method at the age of 1 year. The patient was doing well 7 years after surgery. Cardiac catheterization showed no significant residual defects and the systemic arterial oxygen saturation was 94%.

Rey-Balter *et al.* (1961) described an experimental technique on the same lines as that of Albert (1954). The interatrial septum is incised in a Z-shaped fashion to form two flaps; one superior with a base directed posteriorly and one inferior with a base located anteriorly. The left atrial appendage is invaginated and, together with the atrial flaps, are utilized in such a way so that a tunnel is formed which connects the venae cavae with the mitral valve and the pulmonary veins with the tricuspid valve.

Bernard *et al.* (1962) devised a one-stage intracardiac procedure utilizing a plastic graft for interatrial transposition of the venous returns. The right atrium is opened with a T-shaped incision, the top of the T running about 1 inch from and parallel to the atrioventricular groove from the base of the appendage to a point ½ inch above the entrance of the inferior vena cava. The shaft of the T extends from the midpoint of this incision in a slightly caudal direction to end at the interatrial groove below the entrance of the pulmonary veins. The atrial septum is excised as widely as possible. The pulmonary venous blood is diverted to the right ventricle by means of a suitably sized graft. The prosthesis is so designed that the pulmonary venous return drains through it to the anatomic right ventricle, while the systemic venous blood flows around it to enter the anatomic left ventricle. The right atrium is reconstructed by direct suture. The authors used this technique in a girl 16 years of age with an intact ventricular septum and an atrial septal defect. Postoperative investigation showed functional correction with a small bidirectional shunt at atrial level. In addition, there was a small gradient between the right atrium and the part of the left atrium connected to the left ventricle at the site where the prosthesis partially obstructed the atrial defect. The patient was doing well 1 year after operation. The authors pointed out that obstruction can be avoided by completely excising the atrial septum and, if necessary, enlarging the atrium by inserting a plastic roof. A similar operation was performed on a girl 12 years of age by Burakovskii and Konstantinov (1965).

Wilson *et al.* (1962) excised the atrial septum of an infant with transposition of the great arteries and used a baffle of compressed Ivalon sponge to shunt the cavae with the coronary sinus to the left atrium and the pulmonary veins to the right atrium. After completion of operation the systemic arterial saturation increased to 100%. The following day, however, the patient developed edema and expired. The authors thought that with the heart shrinking considerably in size after operation, there would not be adequate room for all of the pulmonary and systemic venous return to pass through the area previously occupied by the atrial septum. Pulmonary as well as vena caval return will eventually become compromised more than can be tolerated and pulmonary edema will ensue.

Baffes (1962) thought that the methods in which both circulations have been made to cross the atrial septal defect interfered with adequate passive drainage of the pulmonary veins. To obviate this disadvantage he suggested the use of an Ivalon patch to shunt the entire pulmonary venous return across the atrial septal defect. Transposition of the systemic venous return is achieved in the same operation by distal right pulmonary artery–superior vena cava anastomosis, and by direct suture of the inferior vena cava to the under surface of the left atrium.

Intonti (1964) devised an experimental method in which he created two new atrial cavities. The systemic atrium conveyed all the systemic venous blood to the left ventricle, and a pulmonary atrium which conveyed all the oxygenated blood to the right ventricle. The author used this technique on 14 dogs, but the method was not applied clinically.

In 1964, Mustard outlined a method of total correction of transposition of the great arteries as a two-stage procedure. In the first stage an atrial septal defect is created in infancy. The second stage is carried out when the child is 2 or 3 years old. A longitudinal incision is made in the right atrium near the septum and the entire septum is carefully excised. A baffle of pericardium is sewn in place to redirect the pulmonary veins to the tricuspid valve and the venae cavae to the mitral valve (Fig. 20.3). This graft is sutured with a running stitch in such a fashion that the left atrium, which is to become the functional right atrium, was not encroached upon beyond the orifices of the pulmonary veins. After comple-

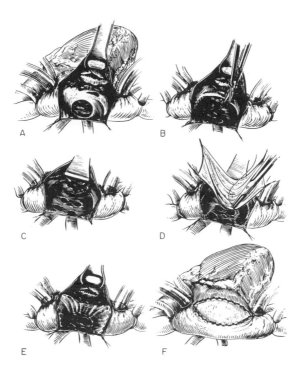

Fig. 20.3. Diagrammatic illustration of the Mustard procedure. (A) The venae cavae are cannulated and a curved atriotomy incision is performed. (B,C) After the atrial septal defect is exposed the remaining portion of the septum is completely excised, with care to suture and endothelialize the entire cephalad surface of the intraatrial septum. The coronary sinus is opened into the left atrium. (D) The baffle is sutured, in place, commencing at the superior margin of the inferior pulmonary vein on the left by a double-armed suture. (E) The suturing of the baffle must be quite close to the orifices of the left pulmonary veins to allow adequate flow from the venae cavae to reach the mitral valve. (F) The new left atrium is enlarged by either a prosthesis or by pericardial graft. From W. T. Mustard (1969), by permission of "Pediatric Surgery," Volume 1, Year Book Medical Publishers.

tion of the suturing of the pericardial graft, which placed both cavae and coronary sinus into the left atrium and all pulmonary veins into the right atrium, the atriotomy is closed. Mustard used this technique on a 2-year-old girl, who had an atrial septal defect created at the age of 3 weeks. A small ventricular septal defect was closed by direct sutures prior to insertion of the pericardial baffle. Postoperatively the systemic arterial oxygen saturation increased to 95%. Subsequent cardiac catheterization and angiocardiography demonstrated physiological correction of the condition. Mustard and associates (1964) used this technique on 7 addition-al patients with 5 survivors and 2 deaths. One of the 5 survivors was suc-cessfully operated on in one stage. Four patients made a rapid convalesc-ence to healthy activity and on recatheterization normal hemodynamics were demonstrated. Prolonged convalescence was noted in 2 cases; in one the newly created left atrium was not as large as it should have been, while in the other pulmonary infection delayed convalescence. One death was due to advanced pulmonary vascular disease and the other to techni-cal error.

In the author's view the Mustard operation was the breakthrough in total surgical correction of transposition of the great arteries. The earliest application of this operation was performed by the Great Ormond Street group with spectacular results. In 1965, Aberdeen *et al.* operated on 9 children with transposition with 7 survivals. Death was caused in 2 pa-tients by the shock-lung in one, and technical problems in the other. The cases were selected to include mainly older children with transposition and those with a near-normal pulmonary vascular resistance. The ventri-cular septum was intact in 5, and a ventricular septal defect was present in 4. Supraventricular arrhythmia occurred at some time in the first weeks after operation in 5 cases and 3 children went home still in atrial flutter. Immense clinical improvement was seen in all survivors. Reed *et al.* (1966) used the Mustard operation successfully on 3 children with transposition and an intact ventricular septum. The pulmonary artery was also debanded in 1. Postoperatively, the patients became asymptomatic but a wandering pacemaker developed in one patient 11 months after the operation. Hightower *et al.* (1966) have had 9 survivors among 13 oper-ated on by the Mustard operation. Their material included 5 with an in-tact ventricular septum with 4 survivors, 5 with a ventricular septal defect with 3 survivors, and 3 with left ventricular outflow tract obstruction with 2 survivors. Of their 5 patients with ventricular septal defect, pulmonary hypertension at systemic levels was present in 4. Cooley *et al.* (1966) op-erated on 17 children with transposition. Of the 9 without pulmonary stenosis or ventricular septal defect, 7 survived the surgical procedure. On the other hand, of the 8 with a ventricular septal defect or pulmonary stenosis, only 2 survived. The cause of hospital death in this group was hemorrhage and cardiac arrest in 3, pulmonary edema in 2, technical problems in 2, and sudden cardiac arrest in 1. There was 1 late death secondary to heart failure and pulmonary arteriosclerosis in this group. One-half of the patients who died following total repair exhibited diffuse medial hypertrophy of the small muscular arteries and focal intimal scle-rosis. The authors pointed out that the surgical mortality following correction of transposition is most closely corrected with a high pressure in the left ventricle, and that they do not recommend total correction in patients with a systolic pressure of 70 mm Hg or more in the left ventricle. Clark and Barratt-Boyes (1967) reported 2 patients who were successfully treated by the Mustard operation. In the immediate postoperative course, each developed severe pulmonary edema which was found to be caused by mediastinal blood clot invaginating the wall of the right atrium against the intra-atrial baffle. The authors pointed out that pulmonary edema caused by incorrectly placed baffle obstructing the pulmonary venous return could be detected by measuring the pressure in the pulmonary veins and new "left" atrium after completion of the procedure. To prevent postoperative tamponade at the time of intracardiac correction, particular care must be paid to hemostasis and the area lateral to the right atrium must be adequately drained. The occurrence of pulmonary edema despite these precautions would be an indication for reexploration. Shankar *et al.* (1967) reported 5 patients who underwent the Mustard operation; 1 with a ventricular septal defect, and 4 with an intact ventricular septum. Debanding of the pulmonary artery was also performed on 2. Four patients survived the procedure, while 1 with a ventricular septal defect died. Atrial arrhythmias occurred in the postoperative course of 2. Hemodynamic and angiocardiographic studies in 3 survivors showed a small atrial shunt in 2. The normal size of the surgically created new atria suggested that the pericardial baffle grew as the body increased in size. Results of corrective surgery by the Mustard operation at the Hospital For Sick Children, London, were reported by Aberdeen and Carr (1968). Of the 49 children who underwent this operation, 35 had an intact ventricular septum, 13 had a ventricular septal defect, and 1 had ventricular septal defect and pulmonary stenosis. There were 8 deaths in the whole group; 5 with an intact septum, 2 with a ventricular septal defect, and 1 with ventricular septal defect and pulmonary stenosis. Two late deaths occurred. Among other complications of the procedure, narrowing of the superior vena cava occurred in 3, narrowing of the inferior vena cava in 1, and pulmonary edema and insufficiency in 4. One-half of the cases had abnormal rhythms in the first postoperative day or two. Persistent arrhythmias occurred in 12 survivors; nodal rhythm in 6, atrial flutter in 2, and third-degree atrioventricular block in 4. The two late deaths were attributed to atrial flutter in 1, and nodal rhythm in 1. The authors pointed out that damage to the sinoatrial node may occur during placement of the superior vena caval cannula. The node may be compressed by the partial occlusion clamp or even damaged by a suture sealing the atrium around the cannula. The node or the sinus node artery may be damaged during the suturing of the pericardial patch around the superior vena caval cannula. Damage to the atrioventricular node may be caused during the placement of the atrial septal pedicle flap or pericardial graft in this region. Placement of the patch posterior to the coronary sinus distorts this structure and increases the incidence of postoperative arrhythmias. For this reason the authors fix the suture line with superficially placed sutures in front of the coronary sinus. Until 1968 Mustard had operated on 26 children with an intact ventricular septum with 19 survivors, 7 with a large ventricular septal defect with 1 survivor, and 4 with a ventricular septal defect and pulmonary stenosis with 1 survivor. Rastelli *et al.* (1969b) summarized the experience of the Mayo Clinic with complete correction of transposition and pulmonary stenosis in 23 patients. A ventricular septal defect was present in all but one. The Mustard operation was used in 18 patients; 7 with pulmonary valve stenosis, and 11 with subvalvular pulmonary stenosis. Thirteen patients survived; 7 with valvular and 6 with subvalvular stenosis. The authors pointed out that the primary reason for this high mortality rate is incomplete relief of the subvalvular stenosis. Dobell *et al.* (1969) operated on 10 infants with transposition by Mustard's procedure with 6 survivals. Nine of these 10 patients had had balloon atrial septostomy in early life. An intact ventricular septum was present in 9, and a ventricular septal defect in 1. The cause of the 4 deaths was septicemia in 1, and hyperkalemia in 3. The authors pointed out that the procedure is technically feasible in the young child and early hemodynamic correction may hold more hope of salvage than repeated palliative procedures. The experience of The Johns Hopkins Hospital with Mustard's procedure was reported by Haller *et al.* (1969a). Nine children between the ages of 2 and 6 underwent this surgical procedure. All had an intact ventricular septum with moderate pulmonary stenosis in 2. One patient died of progressive pulmonary insufficiency 12 days after surgery but the others survived. Mechanical ventillation, with tracheostomy in 7, was used for 3 to 10 days after surgery in all. Postoperative nodal rhythm developed in all and 6 patients were paced for 2 to 10 days after surgery. To help prevent the complications of pulmonary venous congestion due to unrecognized obstruction from redundancy of the pericardial baffle, and postoperative atrioventricular dissociation, Haller and associates (1969b) described two modifications for the Mustard operation. By extending the incision of the coronary sinus into the left atrium, the possibility of direct injury to the atrioventricular conduction bundle is diminished. The second modification consists of tailoring the pericardial baffle after it has been sewn in position rather than attempting to prefashion it. Mazzei and Mulder (1971), however, reported the case of a 3½-year-old boy who developed superior vena caval syndrome secondary to a Mustard repair. The central portion of the pericardial baffle underwent constrictive changes presumably due to bacterial infection of the baffle. The authors pointed out that the need for tailoring the pericardial baffle may have predisposed this area to infecion. Reed (1969) suggested that a "bow tie" configuration for the pericardial tissue baffle is better suited to the geometry of the anatomic features of intra-atrial repair of transposition than a rectangular segment. To avoid the complication of pulmonary venous congestion, which may follow the Mustard operation, Replogle and Lin (1972) described the following technique. Following insertion of the pericardial baffle, the right atrium is incised posteriorly across the interatrial groove to the origin of the right pulmonary veins. A Dacron patch is inserted to enlarge the outflow tract of the pulmonary veins to the tricuspid valve. In 2 patients with a previous Baffes procedure operated on for total correction, Yao and Mustard (1969) found the venous orifices too close to each other to allow adequate and safe baffling of the pulmonary veins. It was elected to redirect the right pulmonary veins as well as the venae cavae into the physiological right atrium. Dillard et al. (1969) pointed out that palliative procedures generally work well when properly applied but many infants are not suitable candidates for any of these operations. In their view there are many patients who urgently need complete correction at early ages when most surgical teams have found perfusion techniques to carry a prohibiive mortality. They emphasized that complete correction could be accomplished during the first 6 months of life. They operated on 7 infants ranging in age from 3 days to 11 months with 4 survivors with an intact ventricular septum. Their method included deep hypothermia, deep ether anesthesia, infusion of low molecular weight dextran, and the creation of respiratory alkalosis by relative hyperventilation during cooling. A transverse atriotomy extending through the posterior portion of the atrial septum and longitudinal closure enlarges the critically small septum and permits correction. On the other hand, Lindesmith et al. (1969) expressed the view that total correction in the small infant is considered by most surgeons to be unsatisfactory and for this reason surgical correction must, in most cases, be considered a two-stage procedure. They used the Mustard operation on 16 children who had had palliative atrial septectomy in infancy with 15 survivors. The only death in the series was a patient with a preoperative left ventricular pressure of 115 mm Hg and a right ventricular pressure of 90 mm Hg. Varying degrees of postoperative conduction disturbances occurred in all patients, but none required electrical pacemaking in this interval. Daicoff and associates (1969) operated on 6 patients with left ventricular outflow tract obstruction; 4 with a ventricular septal defect and 2 with an intact ventricular septum. The approach to the pulmonary valve and subvalvular region was through a longitudinal incision in the pulmonary artery. This allowed ready access to the pulmonary valve and provided for adequate exposure of the subvalvular region. There were 5 survivors; the only death in this series, a patient with a large ventricular septal defect, was caused by a cerebrovascular accident. Postoperative cardiac catheterization in 3 patients demonstrated a significant reduction in the severity of pulmonary stenosis. Nineteen patients with complete transposition were operated upon by the Mustard technique by Indeglia *et al.* (1970). Of these 19 patients, an intact ventricular septum was present in 13, a ventricular septal defect in 5, and an intact ventricular septum and subvalvular pulmonary stenosis in 1. Previous palliative procedures had been performed on 18; surgical septectomy in 16, and balloon atrial septostomy in 2. In addition, 4 patients with a ventricular septal defect, and 1 with an intact ventricular septum had a pulmonary artery band at the time of the Blalock–Hanlon procedure. Of the 13 patients with an intact ventricular septum, 9 survived the operation. One late death occurred. Of the 5 patients with a ventricular septal defect, 3 died in the immediate postoperative period and the 2 surviving patients died after discharge from the hospital. The one patient with an intact ventricular septum and pulmonary stenosis died in the immediate postoperative course. The most common postoperative complication was pulmonary problems. The severity of these problems were related to left ventricular or pulmonary artery pressures before surgery. Constriction of the superior systemic venous inlet was observed in 7 of the 10 autopsies performed. Clinical superior vena caval obstruction occurred in 2 patients. In one of these 2 patients the obstruction was so severe that a second operation was necessary within 3 hours. The superior ridge of the resected atrial septum was found to significantly obstruct the upper systemic venous inlet. This obstruction was adequately relieved by extending an incision from the superior vena cava into the transverse sinus, including part of the posterior wall of the anatomic right and left atria and by interposing a segment of a prosthetic patch within that area. Transient and intermittent paroxysmal supraventricular tachycardia, and sinus bradycardia were observed in 3 patients. Of the 3 late deaths, 2 with intermittent tachycardia in the immediate postoperative course died suddenly. The third death occurred 10 months after surgery in a patient with lung problems, caused by stenosis of the trachea at the site of a prolonged endotracheal intubation and tracheostomy. Pontius (1970) operated on 4 children with a ventricular septal defect. A preliminary atrial septectomy had been performed on all and a pulmonary artery band on 1. The ventricular septal defect was closed by suture through a ventriculotomy. Two patients survived the procedure. Pulmonary vascular disease was found in the 2 patients who failed to survive. Monties *et al.* (1970) reported the results of the Mustard repair on 4 children. Three had an intact ventricular septum and 1 a ventricular septal defect and pulmonary valve stenosis. One patient with an intact septum died postoperatively, the others survived with a satisfactory result. Waldhausen *et al.* (1970) reported the results of the Mustard operation on 12 patients with an intact ventricular septum. Ten of these patients had been palliated in infancy by balloon atrial septostomy, while 2 patients had atrial septectomy by the Blalock–Hanlon technique. The proper size of the baffle was ascertained by removing the caval tapes leaving the physiological left atrium open and by observing the ballooning out of the baffle. Any leaks discovered were repaired. In the last patients the new physiological left atrium was enlarged by the use of a large diamond-shaped pericardial graft placed in such a manner as to increase the distance between the superior and inferior vena caval orifice, thus enlarging the area between superior and inferior portions of the baffle. This maneuver eliminated the possibility of obstruction to the blood flow within the new physiological left atrium. All 12 patients survived the operation. All developed episodes of nodal rhythm in the early postoperative period, and 1 required transient cardiac pacing. Postoperative pulmonary complications were frequent and 3 patients had respiratory failure and required tracheostomy and mechanical ventilation. There was one late death caused by improper placement of the baffle and pulmonary venous obstruction. All survivors improved. The low arterial oxygen tension observed in most survivors was attributed by the authors to thebesian venous drainage into the arterial side of the heart, intrapulmonary shunting, or interatrial shunting. In 1971, Waldhausen and associates further reported on their experience with the Mustard operation on 32 patients, An atrial septal defect was created in infancy in all but 1 case. Eighteen patients had an intact ventricular septum and correction was performed between the ages 8 months and $9\frac{1}{2}$ years. The only death in this group occurred 9 months after surgery. Eight of the 9 patients with a ventricular septal defect had required banding of the pulmonary artery in infancy. Correction was performed between $2\frac{1}{4}$ and 6 years of age. Three of these patients died during the postoperative period, and 1 patient died 9 months after operation. Two patients had transposition and intact ventricular septum and pulmonary stenosis. Correction was done at $2\frac{1}{3}$ and $3\frac{3}{4}$ years. Both patients did well. Three patients had transposition with a ventricular septal defect and

age for performing Mustard's operation in uncomplicated cases is probably in infancy and perhaps at about 6 months of age. There were 2 other
reports from Great Ormond Street and in each a complication of the
Mustard procedure was discussed. In the first report, Stark *et al.* (1971,
1972) studied 113 survivors from a total of 143 patients who underwent
the Mustard operation. Four patients showed clinical signs of superior
vena caval obstruction 1 to 33 months after operation. Three patients developed pulmonary venous obstruction 6 weeks to 6 months after the operation. Only 1 patient was reoperated to relieve the pulmonary venous
obstruction but he did not survive. Because of these complications, a
Dacron patch had been used instead of pericardium in their last 20 consecutive cases. The second report was by Tynan and Aberdeen (1971)
and Tynan *et al.* (1972). These authors found 17 patients with tricuspid
incompetence among 173 patients corrected by the Mustard operation.
In 14 there was little hemodynamic or clinical disturbance, but 3 with severe incompetence died. Preoperative angiograms showed that 6 of 14
patients had had tricuspid regurgitation before surgery. After surgery tricuspid incompetence was related to arrhythmias but not to the closure of
ventricular septal defects. They suggested that the determinants of tricuspid incompetence after the Mustard operation are preexisting inadequacy
of the tricuspid valve and the presence of postoperative arrhythmias. The
authors thought that their data threw doubt on the long-term adequacy of
the tricuspid valve as the systemic atrioventricular valve in transposition,
particularly, in the presence of an arrhythmia. Wagner *et al.* (1971)
from Buffalo Children's Hospital, used the Mustard procedure in 40
children with transposition between the ages of 2 months and 7½ years.
Eight patients were under 1 year of age. Twenty-three younger patients
were operated on under surface-induced hypothermia and circulatory arrest. Open heart surgery was done at a temperature of 20°C during complete circulatory arrest of up to 60 minutes (Subramanian *et al.*, 1971).
Eighteen children had uncomplicated transposition and 4 of them died in
the postoperative period. In 22 children a ventricular septal defect with
or without pulmonary stenosis was associated. Seven of them died. The
overall mortality was 27% and not related to the age. The authors electively offered the Mustard procedure under deep hypothermia to any
child with transposition around the first birthday or earlier if arterial oxygen saturation was below 65% in spite of balloon atrial septostomy or if
pulmonary artery hypertension was found by routine cardiac catheterization at the age of 6 months. Similarly, Dillard *et al.* (1971) used deep hypothermia and total circulatory arrest during the Mustard procedure for 9
patients with transposition. The average age of these 9 patients was 5.3

months. Eight had an intact ventricular septum and 1 had a ventricular septal defect. All except one had had previous balloon atrial septostomy. Three died of a hypoplastic right ventricle in 1, severe pulmonary vascular disease in 1, and postoperative problems in 1. Follow-up periods ranged from 7 to 36 months with an average of 24 months. All patients showed marked improvement of growth and development with normal cardiac function. The authors concluded that infants with transposition and an intact ventricular septum are ideal candidates for total repair under hypothermia. Barrett-Boyes *et al.* (1971), from Auklund, New Zealand, used deep hypothermia by surface cooling and limited cardiopulmonary bypass during the Mustard procedure on 13 infants with transposition. Under halothane anesthesia these infants were cooled to a temperature of 26°C on a circulating water blanket and the temperature was lowered further to 22°C by a short period of total body perfusion. After a period of circulatory arrest, which averaged 48 minutes at 22°C during which the intercardiac repair was carried out, rewarming to 32°C was achieved by 20 minutes of total body perfusion and final rewarming to 36°C by surface means. All 13 infants with transposition operated on in this manner had had initial palliation by balloon atrial septostomy. Of the 3 with a ventricular septal defect, there were 2 hospital deaths. Of the 10 infants with intact ventricular septum, 9 survived the operation. None in this group received assisted ventilation postoperatively. The authors pointed out that the major advantages of this technique lies in the provision of a complete bloodless, relaxed, and quiet heart during a period of circulatory arrest of sufficient duration to allow accurate and rapid repair of complex defects. On the other hand, Pierce *et al.* (1971) employed cardiopulmonary bypass in 12 infants with transposition. Each infant had balloon atrial septostomy at the initial catherization. Their weight at total repair ranged from 5.1 to 10 kg. Of these 12 patients, 8 had an intact ventricular septum. These 8 patients underwent a Mustard type of repair and all survived the operation. Four patients had a ventricular septal defect which was associated with pulmonary stenosis in 2 and aortic arch atresia and a patent ductus in 1. The patient with aortic atresia had had pulmonary artery banding, ligation of patent ductus arteriosus, and aortic arch reconstruction at the age of 10 months. These 4 patients with a ventricular septal defect underwent a Mustard procedure, plus closure of ventricular septal defect, removal of pulmonary artery band, and repair of pulmonary stenosis as indicated. Three patients survived the operation. The only death was in a patient with associated pulmonary stenosis. The authors pointed out that a comparison of the results of representative series of open heart operations that have been performed in infants for transposition and other serious conditions do not indicate a clear advantage to cardiopulmonary bypass or to deep hypothermia. They did not believe that there was an advantage to employing hypothermia for routine open heart operations in infants, because its use is associated with marked metabolic aberration which includes poorly understood hepatic and endocrine dysfunction. Moreover, these metabolic abnormalities, combined with the additional time required, added danger of air embolism, and the risk of heart block may outweigh the advantages of the operative field with less blood returning and with less cardiac movement obtained by using deep hypothermia. A further report from Aukland, New Zealand, on the results of the Mustard operation on 56 patients was made by Clarkson *et al.* (1972). The hospital mortality in 45 "simple" cases, where the only associated lesion requiring correction in 5 patients was a patent ductus arteriosus, was 15.5%. In 11 "complex" cases, where there were more complex lesions requiring attention at the time of the repair, the hospital mortality was 54.5%. All patients discharged from the hospital were clinically well at the time of review which extended to 5 years postoperatively. In simple cases, hospital mortality was 20.8% in 24 children over 2 years of age and 9.5% in 21 patients less than 2 years of age. They attributed in part this reduced mortality in younger patients to increasing experience with the profound hypothermia technique. After initial palliation by balloon septostomy the authors carry out the Mustard operation on patients with intact ventricular septum electively between 3 and 6 months of age or earlier than this when mixing is inadequate. They pointed out that with this management there is no place for repeat balloon septostomy or septectomy. In addition, both the late mortality during the waiting period and the not insignificant morbidity associated with cerebrovascular accidents are reduced to a minimum. The authors added that in cases with a large ventricular septal defect their results following palliation by septectomy and pulmonary artery banding have been disappointing. Moreover pulmonary artery banding did not provide absolute protection against the development of obstructive pulmonary vascular disease. For cases with a large ventricular septal defect, the authors advocate balloon septostomy followed by early one-stage intracardiac repair. Bonchek and Starr (1972) pointed out that the Mustard procedure was their initial surgical intervention in all patients with transposition in whom balloon atrial septostomy fails regardless of the age of the patient. Of the 12 patients operated upon successfully, 3 were under 6 months old, 5 from 13 to 21 months, and 4 between 2¼ and 10 years. An intact ventricular septum was present in 7, large ventricular septal defect in 1, small ventricular septal defect in 1, and intact septum and pulmonary stenosis in 3. Two hundred patients (average age 39 months) underwent correction of transposition of the great arteries at the Hospital For Sick Children, London, between 1965 and 1971 (Breckenridge et al., 1972). Previous atrial septectomy or septostomy had been performed in 81%. Intact ventricular septum was present in 138 cases, ventricular septal defect in 44 cases and ventricular septal defect and left ventricular outflow tract obstruction in 14 cases. The mortality rate for the 200 children was 26.5% (18% in hospital, 8.5% late), and in the three groups it was 18, 43, and 50% respectively. In the last 59 patients the authors used right thoracotomy and Dacron instead of pericardium for the interatrial patch, and these figures were 13, 14, and 50%. Lack of improvement in the last group was attributed to difficulty in relieving left ventricular outflow tract obstruction. Unfavorable long-term prognosis even after balloon atrial septostomy induced the authors to correct 40 infants under 1 year of age. In 31 infants with intact ventricular septum, the mortality rate was 6% and in 9 patients with ventricular septal defect it was 56%. Eleven children with uncomplicated transposition of the great arteries repaired by the Mustard procedure were studied by atrial pacing, cardiac catheterization, and cineangiography by Rodriguez-Fernandez et al. (1972). In 6 of the 11 patients, pericardium was used to fashion the interatrial baffle. In 5, the baffle was constructed of knitted Dacron fabric. According to these authors, this material prevents the possibility of postoperative pericardial shrinkage producing obstruction and avoids the problem of using pericardium in patients with post Blalock–Hanlon pericardial adhesions. One patient had partial thrombotic occlusion of the inferior vena cava and complete obstruction of the superior vena cava at the vena cava–atrial junction. This patient was repaired by a Dacron baffle. In 10 patients in whom the new right atrium was entered at cardiac catheterization sequential pressures in the superior vena cava, physiological right atrium and inferior vena cava showed no evidence of obstruction to systemic venous return. In addition, all 10 had normal bilateral pulmonary capillary wedge pressure. In 3 patients, pulmonary stenosis with a gradient that ranged from 20 to 38 mm Hg across the outflow tract of the left ventricle was demonstrated. In 7 children dye-dilution curves indicated small right-to-left shunts. In all 7, superior vena cava cineangiograms showed leaks in the baffle at the superior atrial junction. Nine patients had persistent postoperative ectopic cardiac rhythms. Atrial pacing in 5 suggested sinus node damage in 4 and A-V junctional conduction tissue damage in 1. Berman et al. (1972) reported the results of cardiac catheterization in 9 patients who had the Mustard operation for transposition and intact ventricular septum 3–24 months previously. Eight were asymptomatic, while 1 infant had evidence of pulmonary venous obstruction. The pulmonary capillary wedge, pulmonary arterial, and pulmonary venous pressures were normal in 8, while 1 (aged 6 months) had a diastolic gradient between the pulmonary venous atrium and the right ventricle. Bidirectional atrial shunting was evident in 3, and a left-to-right atrial shunt was documented in 5 others. In all instances, the atrial defect could be traversed by the catheter. Because of the apparent high incidence of residual atrial communications, the authors advocate postoperative studies on all patients who have undergone the Mustard operation regardless of the symptoms.

The causes of dysrhythmia after the Mustard operation were discussed in three recent publications. The first two have already been reviewed in Chapter 13. El-Said *et al.* (1972) studied dysrhythmias after Mustard operation in 60 patients who survived the surgery. Only 3 patients consistently had sinus rhythm after the operation. Three types of dysrhythmias were described: active dysrhythmia, passive dysrhythmia, and A-V conduction defect. Five patients died of arrhythmia in the follow-up period. Of these 5 patients, 2 died in the early recovery period, 1 died suddenly 4 months after surgery, 1 died 4 years after operation with persistent A-V junctional rhythm and repeated attacks of atrial flutter, and 1 died 5 years postoperatively with progressive dysrhythmia. In the hearts recently operated upon, fresh hemorrhages and acute inflammation surrounded the sutures embedded in the atrial myocardium. This reaction to the sutures and the pericardial patch extended focally into the sinus nodal tissue. The S-A node in the 3 patients who died 4 months or more after surgery was not readily identified. Its usual site was occupied by fat and connective tissue. The S-A nodal artery was either completely occluded or altered by marked intimal sclerosis and medial hypertrophy. The authors thought that the insertion of the pericardial graft affects the S-A node in several ways: direct trauma, foreign body reaction to the sutures, and damage to the artery of the S-A node. Excision of the atrial septum with its internodal tracts and fixation of the patch to the area where the A-V node lies may be contributory factors. To protect the S-A node and its arterial supply, the authors recommend (1) cannulation through the right atrial appendage rather than through the superior vena cava, (2) the incision in the right atrial wall made anterior to the sulcus terminalis to avoid injuring the S-A nodal artery, and (3) the superior part of the pericardial patch fixed away from the superior vena cava. Isaacson *et al.* (1972) studied apparent interruption of the atrial conduction pathways after the Senning operation, the Mustard procedure or the creation of an atrial septal defect in the hearts of 49 patients with transposition of the great arteries, and the findings were correlated with postoperative dysrhythmias. The authors emphasized that the sinus node itself was not directly injured by surgical procedures in any of the 49 hearts. They indicated that surgical trauma to the regions of the atrial conduction pathways is associated with postoperative dysrhythmias. Disturbance of all three pathways was almost always associated with postoperative dysrhythmias, the most common dysrhythmias being nodal rhythm. When two of the three pathways appeared to have been interrupted, and one of the two was the middle pathway, nodal rhythm always existed. Injury to the posterior pathway alone was not associated with postoperative dysrhythmia. Waldo *et al.* (1972) correlated the incidence of early postoperative arrhythmias with the intraoperative electrophysiological studies in 24 patients with transposition of the great arteries undergoing the Mustard procedure. During surgery, the heart was paced from the sinus node to continuously evaluate A-V conduction. The course of the His bundle was electrophysiologically delineated. The anterior internodal tract was excluded from the atrial septectomy, and the suture line of the baffle and its integrity were evaluated electrophysiologically. In the immediate postoperative period, 23 patients had sinus rhythm which was maintained, except for periods of benign A-V junctional rhythm in 11 patients. Surgical trauma to the A-V nodal region in 1 patient was associated with A-V junctional tachycardia. Three patients developed transient tachyarrhythmias. The authors pointed out that intraoperative monitoring to immediately detect A-V conduction abnormalities, electrophysiological delineation of the His bundle, and preservation of the anterior internodal tract were associated with a low incidence of serious early postoperative arrhythmias.

McGoon (1972b) suggested the following principles for management of patients with transposition. All should undergo early balloon septostomy. Those with an intact ventricular septum who thereafter demonstrate adequate mixing should be considered for the Mustard operation during the second or, at the latest, third year of life. If the infant remains more cyanotic with an arterial oxygen saturation of less than 60% the Mustard operation is indicated even during the first months of life. In cases with a ventricular septal defect and severe pulmonary hypertension very early operation is indicated at 6 to 8 months of age because of the probability of rapidly progressive pulmonary vascular obstructive disease. The poor results with early pulmonary arterial banding and later repair and "debanding" warrant such a trial with early closure of the ventricular septal defect and intra-atrial transposition of the venous return. For infants and young children with a ventricular septal defect and pulmonary stenosis and who are severely incapacitated excellent palliation is afforded by a systemic-to-pulmonary artery shunt. Corrective operation by the Rastelli method usually can be deferred until 5 years of age.

From 1963 to December 1971 Mustard (1972) had operated on 106 patients with transposition; 77 with an intact ventricular septum with 18 deaths, 3 with an intact ventricular septum and pulmonary stenosis with no deaths, 16 with a ventricular septal defect with 10 early and 2 late deaths, and 10 with a ventricular septal defect and pulmonary stenosis with 3 early deaths.

The oldest reported patient who underwent Mustard's operation successfully was a 36-year-old woman with an intact ventricular septum, partial anomalous pulmonary venous drainage into the right atrium, and subvalvular pulmonary stenosis (Gerbode et al., 1967).

Lindesmith and associates (1972) pointed out that when transposition of the great vessels is associated with ventricular septal defect and pulmonary hypertension or pulmonary stenosis attempts at correction have resulted in high mortality rates. They reported 8 patients with transposition and pulmonary hypertension or pulmonary stenosis in whom the anatomical or physiological defects were not completely corrected and in whom the Mustard procedure was used as a palliative operation. Of their 8 patients, an intact ventricular septum and pulmonary hypertension were present in 1, ventricular septal defect in 1, ventricular septal defect and pulmonary hypertension in 3, ventricular septal defect and pulmonary stenosis in 2, and ventricular septal defect and pulmonary stenosis and hypertension in 1. Six patients survived with considerable improvement in their condition. The authors concluded that the Mustard operation as a palliative procedure seems indicated in patients whose size or clinical status renders them unacceptable candidates for total correction.

In the present series 34 patients underwent surgical repair by the Mustard procedure (Tables 20.7–20.10) ; 20 in Group I, 4 in Group II, 6 in Group III, and 4 in Group IV. Two patients in Group I had a previous Baffes operation. Debanding of the pulmonary artery was also performed on 1 patient in Group III. Hospital deaths occurred in 12 patients, 4 in Group I (20%), 1 in Group II (25%), 3 in Group III (50%), and 4 in Group IV (100%). The overall hospital mortality was 35%. Nine deaths occurred within 24 hours after completion of the operation and the causes of death included postoperative bleeding, lung problems, and kidney failure. Two patients died on the second postoperative day and the cause of death was lung problems in 1, and brain hemorrhage in 1. One patient died in the third postoperative day of the shock-lung. Of the

3 patients who died in Group III, a large ventricular septal defect was found in 2, and a small defect (2.5 mm) was found in 1. The pulmonary vascular changes were classified as grade 3 in all. One patient in Group IV with a pulmonary subvalvular diaphragm was found at autopsy to have grade 4 pulmonary vascular disease. Disturbances of cardiac rhythm in the postoperative course occurred in 15 patients; atrial flutter in 7, nodal rhythm in 6, nodal tachycardia in 1, and nodal rhythm followed by complete atrioventricular dissociation in 1. The course of these arrhythmias was benign and of a short duration in 11. Of the remaining 4, 1 patient required an implanted pacemaker for a slow nodal rhythm which later changed to complete atrioventricular dissociation. One patient developed intermittent attacks of atrial flutter for 1½ years after surgery until he finally died of congestive heart failure. One patient is still in atrial flutter 3½ years after operation, although the heart rate is satisfactorily controlled on digitalis. In the fourth patient a 2:1 atrial flutter had to be cardioverted in the fourth postoperative month. Late deaths occurred in 3 patients. One patient with an intact ventricular septum developed heart failure and recurrent 2:1 flutter. He died 1½ years after the operation but an autopsy examination was not performed. The second patient, with an intact ventricular septum remained cyanotic and developed an attack of supraventricular tachycardia and cardiac arrest 4 months after surgery. At cardiac catheterization a bidirectional shunt at atrial level and almost complete mixing of the two blood streams were found. The patient underwent a second operation, 7 months after the first one, but he died of technical problems a few hours later. At autopsy the original baffle had completely detached from the suture line and had become adherent to the left atrial wall completely occluding the two pulmonary veins of the left lung. The third patient, with a ventricular septal defect, died 8 months postoperatively after a tracheostomy tube had been taken out. This patient was reported by Shaher et al. (1966). At autopsy the trachea was narrowed 2.5 cm below the tracheostomy site; the area of narrowing is 1 cm long and the lumen was 0.3 in diameter. A patent ventricular septal defect 7 × 8 mm was found posterior and inferior to the crista. The two stitches used for closure had pulled out and were covered by endothelium. The pericardial graft was completely covered by endothelium. There were two defects in the graft. Each defect was divided into two halves by a suture which had pulled out of the atrial wall. One defect was situated below the entrance of the superior vena cava and the other above the entrance of the inferior vena cava. The pulmonary veins entered by a common channel into the right-sided atrium. The diameter of this channel, which was slightly narrowed, measured 10 × 10 mm. All

TABLE 20.7

Mustard Operation [a,b]

Patient	Age at ASD	Age at Mustard	RV p	LV or PA p	Pul. vasc. disease	Comment
1	6 Months	1 y, 4 m	80/0–7	33/0–9		Survived
2	1 Month	1 y, 4 m	87/50	45/0–6	Normal	Died after 8 hours
3	1 Week	1 y, 7 m	85/4	46/2		Survived
4	1 Month	1 y, 8 m	99/6	31/2		Survived
5	2 Months	1 y, 11 m	122/7	65/4	No autopsy	Died after 1½ years, atrial flutter
6	7 Weeks	2 y	100/0		1	Died after 36 hours, pulmonary problems
7	4 Weeks	2 y	80/0	25/0		Survived
8	3 Weeks	2 y	90/10	32/10		Died of shock lung 3rd postoperative day
9	7 Weeks	2 y, 2 m	76/3	44/2		Survived
10	13 Months	2 y, 4 m	80/5	35/6	2	Died after 22 hours, high potassium level
11	1 Year	3 y	90/10	30/10		Survived
12	3 Months	3 y, 10 m	81/6	25/6		Died after 8 months at subsequent correction
13	6 Months	4 y, 7 m	90/6	25/6		Survived
14	3 Years	5 y, 2 m	98/6	33/5		Survived
15	Baffe 5 years	6 y	85/0	35/0		Survived
16	4 Weeks	6 y, 6 m	100/5	30/10		Survived
17	Blalock 4 years	9 y, 5 m	90/0–6	62/0–5	Biopsy 3	Survived, Blalock was not functioning
18	6 Weeks	11 y	90/50	22/0		Survived
19	—	12 y, 7 m	72/6	23/0		Survived
20	Baffe 6 years	13 y, 5 m	80/0	30/0		Survived

[a] Group I, 20 patients.

[b] ASD, atrial septal defect; LV, left ventricle; P, pressure; PA, pulmonary artery; Pul. vasc, pulmonary vascular; RV, right ventricle. All other abbreviations same as in Table 20.3.

TABLE 20.8

MUSTARD OPERATION [a,b]

Patient	Age at ASD	Age at Mustard	RV p	LV or PA p	Pul. vasc. disease	Comment
21	16 Days	1 y, 2 m	100/6	40/5	Normal	Died 1st postoperative day
22	10 Days	2 y	83/10	64/11	—	Survived
23	1 Year	3 y	90/3	56/3	—	Survived
24	BAS 6 months	3 y, 5 m	90/10	60/5	—	Survived

[a] Group II, 4 patients.

[b] BAS, balloon atrial septostomy. All other abbreviations as in Tables 20.3 and 20.7.

TABLE 20.9
MUSTARD OPERATION [a,b]

Patient	Age at ASD	Age at Mustard	RV p	LV or PA p	Pul. vasc. disease	Comment
25	3 Months	1 y, 3 m	95/0–11	102/0–12	3	Died 15 hours later, pulmonary problems
26	4 Months	1 y, 17 m	71/4	71/4	3	Died 8 months after surgery at removal of endotrachial tube
27	3 Weeks	2 y	78/6	40/0–5		Survived
28	2 Months	2 y, 1 m	80/0	87/0	3	Died 6 hours later, ventricular septal defect 7.5 mm
29	—	4 y, 4 m	80/0	PA80/40	3	Died 24 hours later
30	2 Months PA band same time	7 y	77/6	135/0		Survived, PA debanded, ventricular defect spontaneously closed

[a] Group III, 6 patients.
[b] Abbreviations same as in Tables 20.3 and 20.7.

TABLE 20.10

MUSTARD OPERATION [a,b]

Patient	Age at ASD	Age at Mustard	RV p	LV p	Pul. vasc. disease	Comment
31	—	3 y, 9 m	92/2	100/0	—	Died in operating room, no autopsy
32	—	3 y, 10 m	95/9	95/9	2	Died after 20 hours, subdural and mediastinal hemorrhage
33[c]	2 y, 11 m	4 y, 6 m	127/23	114/20	4	Died 36 hours later, cortical hemorrhage
34	—	6 y, 2 m	90/0	94/0	—	Died after 16 hours, no autopsy

[a] Group IV, 4 patients.
[b] Abbreviations same as in Tables 20.3 and 20.7.
[c] Autopsy demonstrated pulmonary subvalvar diaphragm.

TABLE 20.11

Hemodynamics before and after Mustards Operation [a,b]

Group	Patient	Age	Hb	Pressures (mm Hg)							Percentage O₂ saturation								Comments
				RA mean	RV	Ao	PV mean	LA mean	LV	PA	SVC	RA	RV	Ao	PV	LA	LV	PA	
I	1	1 y, 4 m	14.8	5	80/0	80/50	—	7	33/0	—	55	65	73	75	94	94	88	—	—
		1 y, 5 m	9.4	—	—	109/42	—	5	32/0	—	74	—	—	96	—	72	69	—	—
	2	2 y, 2 m	14.8	3	76/3	90/52	8	—	44/2	—	50	62	68	67	99	91	92	—	—
		2 y, 4 m	11.7	4	100/0	100/71	17	4	60/3	—	78	97	94	94	—	84	86	—	L–R S
	3	3 y, 5 m	17.0	4	81/6	81/58	13	4	25/6	—	69	79	77	75	100	95	82	—	—
		4 y, 2 m	—	4	86/4	86/67	—	4	28/3	—	58	83	83	83	97	83	84	—	Bidirectional S
	4	3 y	—	5	90/10	90/55	—	5	30/10	—	59	74	77	70	97	91	93	—	—
		7 y	12.9	—	120/5	120/75	—	7	32/5	—	74	—	94	91	—	70	71	—	—
	5	6 y, 6 m	13.7	7	100/5	80/40	—	7	30/10	—	60	81	69	70	94	92	90	—	—
		10 y	—	—	100/10	100/60	—	2	20/4	20/16	74	—	93	93	—	74	75	76	—
	6	9 y, 2 m	21.6	2	90/6	90/60	—	2	62/5	—	41	48	59	44	99	94	90	—	Blalock S
		9 y, 11 m	11.9	4	82/0	89/67	—	3	76/0	77/48	72	98	98	98	—	83	83	82	L–R S
II	7	2 y	16.7	6	83/10	83/51	12	6	64/11	—	45	50	62	58	—	84	88	—	—
		2 y, 1 m	11.2	2	82/3	88/61	10	3	49/0	—	60	96	93	94	96	68	68	—	L–R S
	8	2½ y	18.6	5	90/10	100/10	—	5	60/5	—	57	80	79	82	98	91	88	—	—
		6 y	13.1	4	102/6	123/6	—	2	55/4	12/3	64	92	93	92	—	67	69	68	LV infundibulum 12/3
III	9	13 d	21.2	5	60/0	65/44	—	—	—	—	—	42	46	44	—	—	88	—	Small VSD
		2 y	12.0	—	—	78/60	—	6	40/0	—	—	—	—	96	—	—	70	—	—
	10	6 y, 6 m	22.4	7	77/6	75/45	—	7	135/0	—	38	61	41	48	92	89	87	—	PA band, VSD closed spontaneously
		7 y	10.5	—	90/0	90/60	—	10	60/10	—	37	50	72	70	—	—	57	—	Bidirectional S

a After the Mustard operation right atrium and left atrium signify the cardiac chambers supplying the right and left ventricles respectively.

b Ao, aorta; d, days; Hb, hemoglobin; L, left; LA, left atrium; LV left ventricle; m, months; PA, pulmonary artery; PS, pulmonary stenosis; PV, pulmonary vein; R, right; RA, right atrium; RV, right ventricle; S, shunt; SVC, superior vena cava; VSD, ventricular septal defect; y, years.

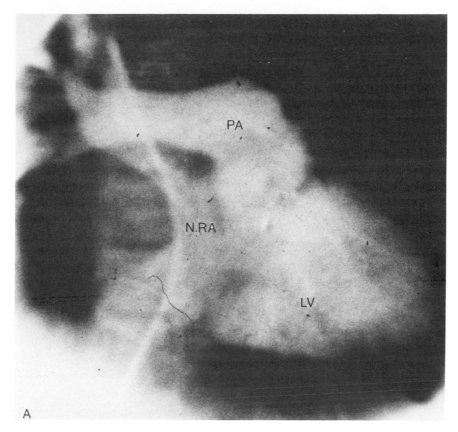

Fig. 20.4. Angiocardiography after the Mustard procedure. (A) Contrast medium injected into the superior vena cava opacifying new right atrium (N.RA), left ventricle (LV), and pulmonary artery (PA). (B) Contrast medium injected into the superior vena cava showing constriction (arrow) of the upper venous inlet. (C) Contrast medium injected into inferior vena cava (IVC) opacifying new right atrium (N.RA), left ventricle (LV), and pulmonary artery (PA). (D) New left atrium (N.LA) opacifying after opacification of the lungs. (E) Right ventricular angiogram demonstrating origin of the aorta (Ao) from the right ventricle (RV) and slight tricuspid incompetence (arrow).

survivors showed tremendous improvement in growth, development, and effort tolerance. Cyanosis disappeared immediately after surgery but clubbing of the fingers took about 6 months to 1 year before it finally did so. Cardiac catheterization was carried out on 10 of the survivors (Table 20.11); 6 in Group I, 2 in Group II, and 2 in Group III. The result on 4 of these patients has been published by Kidd and Mustard (1966). The systemic arterial oxygen saturation was normal in 8. In 2 with systemic

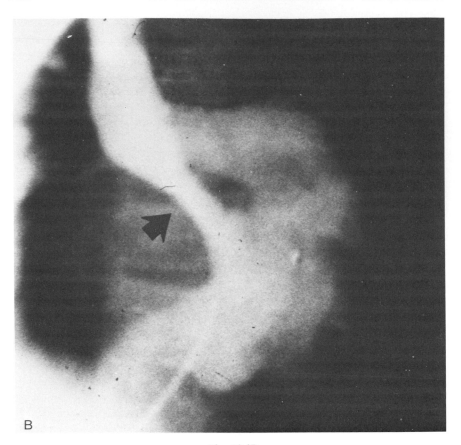

Fig. 20.4B

arterial desaturation, (Cases 3 and 10) a bidirectional shunt was discovered at atrial level. This bidirectional blood shunt was caused by detachment of the baffle in Case 3 and a defect in it in Case 10. Other than these two cases with a bidirectional atrial shunt, a small left-to-right shunt at the atrial level was found in 3 (Cases 2, 6 and 7). In 2 patients there was a 3 mm Hg gradient between the superior vena cava and the new right atrium. The new left atrium was entered through a small defect in the baffle in 3, and retrogradely through the tricuspid valve in 1. A gradient of pressure difference between pulmonary vein and the new left atrium (average 9.5 mm Hg) was found in 3 patients. A left ventricular outflow tract gradient of 43 mm Hg was found in 1 patient in Group II (Case 8). Venous angiography showed slight narrowing of the superior vena cava in 2 patients but the new atria had an adequate size (Fig. 20.4). Slight tricuspid incompetence was demonstrated by right ventricular angiography in 1 with chronic atrial flutter.

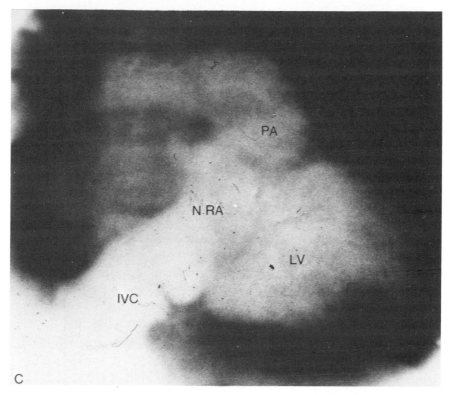

Fig. 20.4C

At the time of this writing it would seem that the operation of choice for hemodynamic correction of transposition of the great arteries is the Mustard operation. It would appear that given adequate postoperative intensive care, the operation could be performed on very young children or infants with good results. It seems that the main risk at surgery is not from suturing of the baffle, but from correction of the associated defects, and the presence of pulmonary vascular disease. The two problems of postoperative disturbances of the cardiac rhythm and narrowing of the systemic or pulmonary venous ostia have been minimized by various modifications of the original operation. Serious complications secondary to contraction of the baffle have not been observed in this series or in most reported cases. Postoperative angiocardiography has demonstrated good sized atria in most patients. So far the trend had been toward performing this operation on younger children with uncomplicated transposition. It seems that more surgeons feel that the operation should be performed if balloon atrial septostomy fails regardless of the age of the patient.

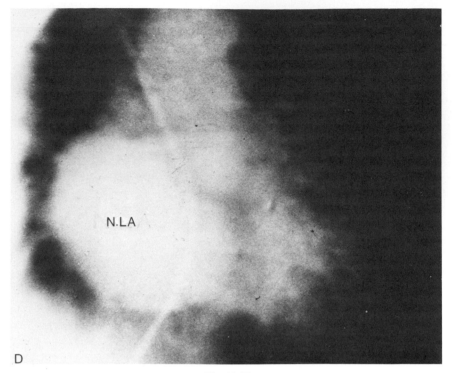

Fig. 20.4D

Selection of Patients for Surgery

FIRST STAGE

Balloon atrial septostomy should be performed on all patients when first seen during the first 6 months of life.

SECOND STAGE

There are two schools of thought concerning the second stage. Advocates of the first school recommend elective total surgical correction of transposition of any child around the first birthday or earlier if the arterial oxygen saturation is 65% or less in spite of a balloon atrial septostomy or if pulmonary hypertension is found by routine cardiac catheterization at the age of 6 to 8 months. Advocates of the second school recommend the following.

1. Patients with an intact ventricular septum with or without left ventricular outflow tract obstruction should undergo repeat cardiac catheri-

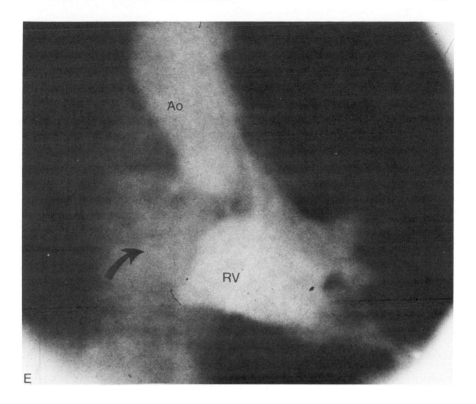

Fig. 20.4E

zation followed by the Mustard procedure between the ages of 2 and 3 years.

2. Patients with a ventricular septal defect should undergo repeat cardiac catheterization between 6 to 8 months and banding of the pulmonary artery performed if pulmonary hypertension is found. Patients without pulmonary hypertension have a small ventricular septal defect and should be treated as those with an intact ventricular septum and totally corrected between 2 and 3 years of age. Patients with a pulmonary artery band should be corrected at about the age of 4 or 5 years.

3. When indicated patients with a ventricular septal defect and pulmonary stenosis should undergo a Waterston anastomosis during the first year of life or a Blalock–Taussig anastomosis after this age. Most authors do not recommend a cavopulmonary anastomosis for this condition. Total surgical correction could be postponed until the patient is old enough to undergo safe definitive correction. For patients with pulmonary valvular stenosis, a Mustard procedure is performed between the ages of 4 and 5 years of age. For patients with a subvalvular tunnel, with or without valvular stenosis, a Rastelli operation is performed at about the age of 5 years.

References

Aberdeen, E. (1971a). Mustard's operation in transposition of the great arteries. *In* "The History and Progress in Treatment of Congenital Heart Defects." (B. S. L. Kidd and J. D. Keith, eds.) , p. 162. Charles C. Thomas, Springfield, Illinois.

Aberdeen, E. (1971b). Correction of uncomplicated cases of transposition of the great arteries. *Brit. Heart J. Suppl.* 33, 66–68.

Aberdeen, E., and Carr, I. (1968). Transposition of the great arteries. "Modern Trends in Cardiac Surgery." Vol. 2, p. 182. Butterworth, London.

Aberdeen, E., Waterston, D. J., Carr, I., Graham, G., Bonham-Carter, R. E., and Subramanian, S. (1965). Successful "correction" of transposed great arteries by Mustard's operation. *Lancet* i, 1233.

Achtel, R. A., Kaplan, S., Benzing, G., III, and Helmsworth, J. A. (1969) . Superior vena cava to right pulmonary artery anastomosis. Long term results. *Ann. Thorac. Surg.* 8, 511.

Albert, H. M. (1954). Surgical correction of transposition of the great vessels. *Surg. Forum* 5, 74.

Albert, H. M., Fowler, R. L., Craighead, C. C., Glass, B. A., and Atik, M. (1961). Pulmonary artery banding. A treatment for infants with intractable cardiac failure due to interventricular septal defects. *Circulation* 23, 16.

Ankeney, J. L., and O'Grady, T. J. (1968). The treatment of transposition of the great vessels. *Ann. Thorac. Surg.* 5, 262–276.

Aronstam, E. M., Hewlett, T. H., Orbison, J. A., Franklin, R. B., and Dixon, L. M. (1963). Surgical correction of transposition of the great vessels. A successful complete correction. *Ann. Surg.* 158, 282–284.

Ash, R., Johnson, J., Koop, E., Friedman, S., and Rashkind, W. (1959). Cardiovascular surgery in a children's hospital. II. Cyanotic lesions. A review of 193 operations. *J. Pediat.* **54**, 348.

Astley, R., and Parsons, S. (1952). Complete transposition of the great vessels. *Brit. Heart J.* **14**, 13.

Azzolina, G., Eufrate, S. A., and Pensa, P. M. (1972). Closed interatrial septostomy: modified technique and results. *Ann. Thorac. Surg.* **13**, 338.

Baffes, T. G. (1956). A new method for surgical correction of transposition of the aorta and pulmonary artery. *Surg. Gynecol. Obstet.* **102**, 227.

Baffes, T. G. (1957). Experiences in the surgical correction of transposition of the aorta and the pulmonary artery. *Amer. Surg.* **23**, 1065.

Baffes, T. G. (1962). Closed treatment of transposition of the great arteries. *In* "Congenital Heart Disease" (D. P. Morse, ed.), p. 197. Blackwell, Oxford.

Baffes, T. G., Ricker, W. L., DeBoer, A., and Potts, W. J. (1957). Surgical correction of transposition of the aorta and the pulmonary artery. *J. Thorac. Surg.* **34**, 469.

Baffes, T. G., Lev, M., Paul, M. H., Miller, R. A., Riker, W. J., DeBoer, A., and Potts, W. J. (1960). Surgical correction of transposition of the great vessels—a five year survey. *J. Thorac. Cardiovasc. Surg.* **40**, 298.

Baker, C., Brock, R. C., Campbell, M., and Suzman, S. (1949). Morbus Coeruleus. A study of 50 cases after the Blalock-Taussig operation. *Brit. Heart J.* **11**, 170.

Bakos, A. P. (1950). The question of the function of the right ventricular myocardium: an experimental study. *Circulation* **1**, 724.

Bakulev, A. N., and Kolesnikov, S. A. (1959). Anastomosis of superior vena cava and pulmonary artery in the surgical treatment of certain congenital defects of the heart. *J. Thorac. Surg.* **37**, 693.

Barnard, C. N., Schrire, V., and Beck, W. (1962). Complete transposition of the great vessels. Successful complete correction. *J. Thorac. Cardiovasc. Surg.* **43**, 768.

Barrett-Boyes, B. G., Simpson, M., and Neutze, J. M. (1971). Intracardiac surgery in neonates and infants using deep hypothermia with surface cooling and limited cardiopulmonary bypass. *Circulation* **43** (Suppl. 1), 25.

Berman, M. A., Talner, N. S., and Stansel, H. C., Jr., (1972). Residual atrial-level shunts following Mustard's procedure for transposition of the great arteries. *Circulation* **45** and **46**, Suppl. 11, 97.

Bernhard, W. F., Jones, J. E., Friedberg, D. Z., and Litwin, S. B. (1971). Ascending aorta-right pulmonary artery shunt in infants and older patients with certain types of cyanotic congenital heart disease. *Circulation* **43**, 580–584.

Bickford, B. J., and Edwards, F. R. (1960). Cavo-pulmonary anastomosis. *Thorax* **15**, 165.

Bjork, V. O., and Bouckaert, L. (1954). Complete transposition of the aorta and the pulmonary artery. An experimental study of the surgical possibilities. *J. Thorac. Surg.* **28**, 632.

Blalock, A. (1947). The technique of creation of an artificial ductus arteriosus in the treatment of pulmonic stenosis. *J. Thorac. Surg.* **16**, 244.

Blalock, A., and Hanlon, C. R. (1950). The surgical treatment of complete transposition of the aorta and the pulmonary artery. *Surg. Gynecol. Obstet.* **90**, 1.

Blalock, A., and Taussig, H. B. (1945). The surgical treatment of malformations of the heart in which there is pulmonary stenosis or pulmonary atresia. *J. Amer. Med. Ass.* **128**, 189.

Blank, R., Muller, W. H., Jr., and Damman, J. F., Jr. (1958). Changes in pulmonary vascular lesions after restoring normal pulmonary artery pressure. *Surg. Forum* **9**, 356.

Bonchek, L. I., and Starr, A. (1972). Total correction of transposition of the great vessels as initial surgical management. *Ann. Meet. Soc. Thorac. Surgeons. San Francisco, California.*

Braunwald, E., Morrow, A. G., and Friedman, W. F. (1966). Ligation of the main pulmonary artery and systemic-pulmonary arterial anastomosis. A new palliative operation for complete transposition of the great arteries. *Circulation* **34**, 55.

Breckenridge, I. M., Oelert, H., Stark, J., Graham, G. R., Bonham-Carter, R. E., and Waterston, D. J. (1972). Mustard's operation for transposition of the great arteries. *Lancet* **i**, 1140.

Brock, R. C. (1948). Pulmonary valvulotomy for the relief of congenital pulmonary stenosis. Report of three cases. *Brit. Med. J.* **1**, 1121.

Brom, A. G., Schaar, H. V. D., and Nauta, J.: (1965). The surgery of transposition of the great vessels. *Arch. Dis. Child.* **40**, 128.

Burakovskii, V. I., and Konstantinov, B. A. (1965). Radical surgical correction in complete transposition of aorta and pulmonary artery. A clinical and experimental study. *Eksp. Khir. Anesteziol.* **4**, 18–24.

Canent, R. V., Jr., Spach, M. S., and Young, W. G., Jr. (1964). Cardiopulmonary dynamics in patients with anastomosis of the superior vena cava to the right pulmonary artery. *Circulation* **30**, 47.

Carlon, C. A., Mondini, P. G., and DeMarchi, R. (1951). Surgical treatment of some cardiovascular disease (A new vascular anastomosis). *J. Int. Coll. Surg.* **16**, 1.

Clarke, C. P., and Barratt-Boyes, B. G. (1967). The cause and treatment of pulmonary edema after the Mustard operation for correction of complete transposition of the great vessels. *J. Thorac. Cardiovasc. Surg.* **54**, 9–15.

Clarkson, P. M., Barratt-Boyes, B. G., Neutze, J. M., and Lowe, J. B. (1972). Results of a ten year period of palliation followed by corrective surgery for complete transposition of the great arteries. *Circulation* **45**, 1251.

Cleland, W. P., Goodwin, J. F., Steiner, R. E., and Zoob, M. (1957). Transposition of the aorta and pulmonary artery with pulmonary stenosis. *Amer. Heart J.* **54**, 10.

Coles, J. C., Gergely, N. F., and Buttigliero, J. (1963). Banding of the pulmonary artery. *Clin. Pediat.* **2**, 316.

Collins, H. A., Harberg, F. J., Soltero, L. R., McNamara, H. A., and Cooley, D. A. (1959). Cardiac surgery in the newborn. *Surgery* **45**, 506.

Cooley, D. A., and Hallman, G. L. (1964). Cardiovascular surgery during first year of life: Experience with 450 consecutive operations. *Amer. J. Surg.* **107**, 474.

Cooley, D. A., and Hallman, G. L. (1966). Intrapericardial aortic-right pulmonary arterial anastomosis. *Surg. Gynecol. Obstet.* **122**, 1084–1089.

Cooley, D. A., Hallman, G. L., Bloodwell, R. D., and Leachman, R. D. (1966). Two stage surgical treatment of complete transposition of the great vessels. *Arch. Surg.* **93**, 704–714.

Cornell, W. P., Maxwell, R. E., Haller, J. A., and Sabiston, D. C. (1966). Results of the Blalock-Hanlon operation in 90 patients with transposition of the great vessels. *J. Thorac. Cardiovasc. Surg.* **52**, 525–532.

Craig, T. V., and Sirak, H. D. (1963). Pulmonary artery banding. An analysis of 38 cases. *J. Thorac. Cardiovasc. Surg.* **45**, 599.

Creech, O., Jr., Mahaffey, D. E., Sayegh, S. F., and Sailors, E. L. (1958). Complete transposition of the great vessels. A technique for intracardiac correction. *Surgery* **43**, 349.

Cross, F. S., Kay, E. B., and Jones, R. D. (1954). A simple shunting technique for surgery of the aortic and pulmonary valves and proximal great vessels. An experimental study. *J. Thorac. Surg.* **28**, 229.

Daicoff, G. R., Schiebler, G. L., Elliott, L. P., Van Mierop, L. H. S., Bartley, T. D., Gessner, I. H., and Wheat, M. W. (1969). Surgical repair of complete transposition of the great arteries with pulmonary stenosis. *Ann. Thorac. Surg.* **7**, 529–538.

Dammann, J. F., Jr., and Muller, W. H., Jr. (1953). The role of the pulmonary vascular bed in congenital cardiac disease. *Pediatrics* **12**, 307.

Damman, J. F., Jr., McEachen, J. A., Thompson, W. M., Jr., Smith, R., and Muller, W. H., Jr. (1961). The regression of pulmonary vascular disease after the creation of pulmonary stenosis. *J. Thorac. Cardiovasc. Surg.* **42**, 722.

Danielson, G. K., Mair, D. D., Ongley, P. A., Wallace, R. B., and McGoon, D. C. (1971). Repair of transposition of the great arteries by transposition of venous return. Surgical considerations and results of operation. *J. Thorac. Cardiovasc. Surg.* **61**, 96–103.

Deverall, P. B., Tynan, M. J., Carr, I., Panagopoulos, P., Aberdeen, E., Bonham-Carter, R. E., and Waterston, D. J.: (1969). Palliative surgery in children with complete transposition of the great arteries. *J. Thorac. Cardiovasc. Surg.* **58**, 721–729.

Deverall, P. B., Bargeron, L. M., Jr., Barcia, A., and Kirklin, J. W. (1971). Transposition of the great arteries with pulmonary stenosis: surgical considerations. *In* "The Natural History and Progress in Treatment of Congenital Heart Defects." (B. S. L. Kidd and J. D. Keith, eds.) , p. 175. Charles C. Thomas, Springfield, Illinois.

Dillard, D. H., Mohri, H., Merendino, K. A., Morgan, B. C., Baum, D., and Crawford, E. W. (1969). Total surgical correction of transposition of the great arteries in children less than six months of age. *Surg. Gynecol. Obstet.* **129**, 1258–1266.

Dillard, D. H., Mohri, H., and Merendino, K. A. (1971). Correction of heart disease in infancy utilizing deep hypothermia and total circulatory arrest. *J. Thorac. Cardiovasc. Surg.* **61**, 64–69.

Dobell, A. R. C., Gibbons, J. E., and Busse, E. F. G. (1969). Hemodynamic correction of transposition of the great vessels in infants. *J. Thorac. Cardiovasc. Surg.* **57**, 108–114.

Donald, D. E., and Essex, H. E. (1954). Pressure studies after inactivation of the major portion of the canine right ventricle. *Amer. J. Physiol.* **176**, 155.

Edgett, J. W., Jr., Nelson, W. P., Hall, R. J., Jahnke, E. J., and Aaby, G. V. (1968). Spontaneous closure of a ventricular septal defect after banding of the pulmonary artery. *Amer. J. Cardiol.* **22**, 729.

Edwards, W. S., and Bargeron, L. M., Jr. (1963). The importance of the azygos in superior vena cava–pulmonary artery anastomosis. *J. Thorac. Cardiovasc. Surg.* **46**, 811.

Edwards, W. S., and Bargeron, L. M., Jr. (1965). More effective palliation of transposition of the great vessels. *J. Thorac. Cardiovasc. Surg.* **49**, 790.

Edwards, W. S., Bargeron, L. M., Jr., and Lyons, C. (1964). Reposition of right pulmonary veins in transposition of great vessels. *J. Amer. Med. Ass.* **188**, 522.

Edwards, W. S., Mohtashemi, M., and Holdefer, W. F., Jr. (1966). Ascending aorta to right pulmonary artery shunt for infants with tetralogy of Fallot. *Surgery* **59**, 316–321.

Johnson, J., Kirby, C. K., Greifenstein, F. E., and Castillo, A. (1949). The experimental and clinical use of vein grafts to replace defects of the large arteries. *Surgery* **27**, 945.

Jonsson, B. C., Ovenfors, C. O., and Senning, A. (1959). Surgically corrected case of transposition of the great vessels. *Acta Chir. Scand. Suppl.* **245**, 297.

Kagan, A. (1952). Dynamic responses of the right ventricle following extensive damage by cauterization. *Circulation* **5**, 816.

Kaplan, S., Helmsworth, J. A., Ahearn, E. N., Benzig, G., Daoud, G., and Schwartz, D. C. (1968). Results of palliative procedures for tetralogy of Fallot. *Ann. Thorac. Surg.* **5**, 489–497.

Kay, E. B., and Cross, F. S. (1955). Surgical treatment of transposition of the great vessels. *Surgery* **38**, 712.

Kay, E. B., and Cross, F. S. (1957). Transposition of the great vessels corrected by means of atrial transposition. *Surgery* **41**, 938.

Keirle, A. M., Helmsworth, J. A., Kaplan, S., and Ogden, A. E. (1963). Experience with anastomosis of superior vena cava to pulmonary artery (Glenn procedure). *Circulation* **27**, 753–757.

Kidd, L., and Mustard, W. T. (1966). Hemodynamic effects on a totally corrective procedure in transposition of the great vessels. *Circulation* **33**, 28–33.

Kirchhoff, P. G. (1967). Zur Palliativoperation nach Blalock-Hanlon. *Thoraxchir. Vask. Chir.* **15**, 644–646.

Kirklin, J. W., Devloo, R. A., and Weidman, W. H. (1961). Open intracardiac repair for transposition of the great vessels: 11 cases. *Surgery* **50**, 58.

Leeds, S. E., Culiner, M. M., and Strauss, S. H. (1955). Experimental transposition of the great vessels. Some factors which increase the flow through the atrial septal defect. *J. Thorac. Surg.* **30**, 642–648.

Lillehei, C. W., and Varco, R. L. (1953). Certain physiologic, pathologic and surgical features of complete transposition of the great vessels. *Surgery* **34**, 376.

Lindesmith, G. G., Meyer, B. W, Jones, J. C., and Gallaher, M. (1965). Palliative procedure for treatment of transposition of the great vessels. *Circulation* **31** (Suppl. 1), 21–24.

Lindesmith, G. G., Gallaher, M. F., Durnin, R. E., Meyer, B. W., and Jones, J. C. (1966). Collective review: cardiac surgery in the first month of life. *Ann. Thorac. Surg.* **2**, 250.

Lindesmith, G. G., Meyer, B. W., Stanton, R. E., Gallaher, M. E., Stiles, Q. R., and Jones, J. (1969). Surgical treatment of transposition of the great vessels. *Ann. Thorac. Surg.* **8**, 12–19.

Lindesmith, G. G., Stiles, Q. R., Tucker, B. L., Gallaher, M. E., Stanton, R. E., and Meyer, B. W. (1972). The Mustard operation as a palliative procedure. *J. Thorac. Cardiovasc. Surg.* **63**, 75–80.

Lindskog, G. E., Liebow, A. A., and Glenn, W. W. L. (1962). "Thoracic and Cardiovascular Surgery with Related Pathology," p. 586. Appleton Century Crofts, New York.

Litwin, S. B., Plauth, W. H., Jr., Jones, J. E., and Bernhard, W. F. (1971). Appraisal of surgical atrial septectomy for transposition of the great arteries. *Circulation* **43** (Suppl. 1), 7.

McGaff, C. J., Ross, R. S., and Braunwald, E. (1962). The development of elevated pulmonary vascular resistance in man following increased pulmonary blood flow from systemic–pulmonary anastomosis. *Amer. J. Med.* **33**, 201.

McGoon, D. C. (1972a). Intraventricular repair of transposition of the great arteries. *J. Thorac. Cardiovasc. Surg.* **64**, 430.

McGoon, D. C. (1972b). Surgery for transposition of the great arteries. *Circulation* **45**, 1147.

McGoon, D. C., Rastelli, G. C., and Wallace, R. B. (1970). Discontinuity between right ventricle and pulmonary artery: Surgical treatment. *Ann. Surg.* **172**, 680–689.

Martin, S. P., Anabtawi, I. N., Selmonsky, C. A., Folger, G. M., Ellison, L. T., and Ellison, R. G. (1970). Long-term follow up after superior vena cava–right pulmonary artery anastomosis. *Ann. Thorac. Surg.* **9**, 339.

Mazzei, E. A., and Mulder, D. G. (1971). Superior vena cava syndrome following complete correction (Mustard repair) of transposition of the great vessels. *Ann. Thorac. Surg.* **11**, 243–245.

Merendino, K. A., Jesseph, J. E., Herron, P. W., Thomas, G. I., and Vetto, R. E. (1957). Interatrial venous transposition: A one-stage intracardiac operation for the conversion of complete transposition of the aorta and pulmonary artery to corrected transposition. Theory and clinical experience. *Surgery* **42**, 898.

Miller, R. A., and Baffes, T. G. (1957). Early postoperative results following partial correction of transposition of the great vessels. Abstracts of the 30th Scientific Sessions. *Circulation* **16**, 916.

Mitri, M., Murphy, D. R., Dobell, A. R. C., and Karn, G. M. (1962). Cavo-pulmonary anastomosis in the management of certain irreparable congenital heart lesions. *Surgery* **52**, 513.

Monties, J. R., Baille, Y., Goudard, A., *et al.* (1970). La correction chirurgicale de la transposition complete des gros vaisseaux (a propos de 4 cas operes). *Arch. Mal. Coeur. Vaiss.* **63**, 1406–1413.

Morgan, A. D., Krovetz, L. J., Schiebler, G. L., Shanklin, D. R., Wheat, M. W., Jr., and Bartley, T. D. (1965). Diagnosis and palliative surgery in complete transposition of the great vessels. *Ann. Thorac. Surg.* **1**, 711–722.

Morrow, A. G., and Braunwald, N. S. (1961). The surgical treatment of ventricular septal defect in infancy. The technique and results of pulmonary artery constriction. *Circulation* **24**, 34.

Moss, A. J., Maloney, J. V., Jr., and Adams, F. H. (1961). Transposition of the great vessels: surgical palliation during infancy. *Ann. Surg.* **153**, 183.

Muller, W. H., Jr., and Dammann, J. F., Jr. (1952). Treatment of certain malformations of the heart by the creation of pulmonary stenosis to reduce pulmonary hypertension and excessive pulmonary blood flow. *Surg. Gynecol. Obstet.* **95**, 213.

Murphy, T. O., Gott, V., Lillehei, W., and Varco, R. L. (1955). The results of surgical palliation in 32 patients with transposition of the great vessels. *Surg. Gynecol. Obstet.* **101**, 541.

Mustard, W. T. (1964). Successful two-stage correction of transposition of the great vessels. *Surgery* **55**, 469.

Mustard, W. T. (1968). Recent experiences with surgical management of transposition of the great arteries. *J. Cardiovasc. Surg.* **9**, 532–536.

Mustard, W. T. (1971). Total correction in transposition of the great arteries. *In* "The Natural History and Progress in Treatment of Congenital Heart Defects." (B. S. L. Kidd and J. D. Keith, eds.), p. 159. Charles C. Thomas, Springfield, Illinois.

Mustard, W. T. (1972). Personal communications.

Mustard, W. T., Chute, A. L., Keith, J. D., Sirek, A., Rowe, R. D., and Vlad, P. (1954). A surgical approach to transposition of the great vessels with extracorporeal circuit. *Surgery* **36**, 39.

Mustard,, W. T., Keith, J. D., Trusler, G. A., Fowler, R., and Kidd, L. (1964). The surgical management of transposition of the great vessels. *J. Thorac. Cardiovasc. Surg.* **48**, 953–958.

Nauta, J., Bruins, C., Dekker, A., Van der Schaar, H., and Brom, A. G. (1965). Surgical treatment of transposition of the large vessels. *Pac. Med. Surg.* **73**, 69–74.

Nghiem, Q. X., Harris, L. C., and Tyson, K. R. T. (1969). Spontaneous closure of a ventricular septal defect after pulmonary artery banding. *J. Pediat.* **75**: 694, 1969.

Noonan, A., Nadas, A. S., Rudolph, A. M., and Harris, G. B. C. (1960). Transposition of the great arteries. A correlation of clinical, physiologic and autopsy data. *N. Engl. J. Med.* **263**, 592.'

Nuland, S. B., Glenn, W. W. L., and Guilfoil, P. H. (1958). Circulatory bypass of the right heart. III. Some observations on long-term survivors. *Surgery* **43**, 184.

Ochsner, J. L., Cooley, D. A., Harris, L. C., and McNamara, D. G. (1961). Treatment of complete transposition of the great vessels with the Blalock-Hanlon operation. *Circulation* **24**, 51.

Ochsner, J. L., Cooley, D. A., McNamara, D. G., and Kline, A. (1962). Surgical treatment of cardiovascular anomalies in 300 infants younger than one year of age. *J. Thorac. Cardiovasc. Surg.* **43**, 182.

O'Donovan, T. G., Barnard, C. N., and Gotsman, M. S. (1968). The surgical relief of transposition of the great vessels in infancy. *Thorax* **23**, 256–260.

Oldham, H. N., Jr., Kakos, G. S., Jarmakani, M. M., and Sabiston, D. C., Jr. (1972). Pulmonary artery banding in infants with complex congenital heart defects. *Ann. Thorac. Surg.* **13**, 342.

Ongley, P. A. (1964). Cyanotic congenital heart disease. Selection of patients for operation and treatment of complications. *Pediat. Clin. N. Amer.* **11**, 269.

Palacios-Macedo, X., Perez-Alvarez, J. J., Ortiz-Marquez, J., and Hernadez-Peniche, J. (1961). Some experimental observations on the superior vena cava–pulmonary artery anastomosis. *J. Thorac. Cardiovasc. Surg.* **41**, 186.

Patino, J. F., Glenn, W. W. L., Guilfoil, P. H., Hume, M., and Fenn, J. E. (1956). Circulatory bypass of the right heart. II. Further observations on vena caval–pulmonary artery shunts. *Surg. Form* **6**, 189.

Paul, M. H., Miller, R. A., and Baffes, T. G. (1960). Physiologic studies in patients with partial surgical correction of transposition of the great vessels. Abstracts of the 33rd Scientific Sessions. *Circulation* **22**, 795.

Paul, M. H., Miller, R. A., and Potts, W. J. (1961). Long term results of aortic–pulmonary anastomosis for tetralogy of Fallot. An analysis of the first 100 cases eleven to thirteen years after operation. *Circulation* **32**, 525.

Paul, M. H., Muster, A. J., Cole, R. B., and Baffes, T. G. (1968). Palliative management for transposition of the great arteries. *Ann. Thorac. Surg.* **6**, 321–329.

Pierce, W. S., Raphaely, R. C., Downes, J. J., and Waldhausen, J. A. (1971). Cardio-pulmonary bypass in infants: indications, methods, and results in 32 patients. *Surgery* **70**, 839.

Plauth, W. H., Jr., Nadas, A. S., Bernhard, W. F., and Gross, R. E. (1968). Transposition of the great arteries. Clinical and physiological observations on 74 patients treated by palliative surgery. *Circulation* **37**, 316–330.

Pontius, R. G. (1970). Surgery for transposition of the great arteries without intact ventricular septum. *Arch. Surg.* **101**, 327–331.

Potts, W. J., and Gibson, S. (1948). Aortic pulmonary anastomosis in congenital pulmonary stenosis. Report of forty-five cases. *J. Amer. Med. Ass.* **137**, 343.

Potts, W. J., and Smith, S. (1949). New surgical procedures in certain cases of congenital pulmonary stenosis. *Arch. Surg.* **59**, 491.

Potts, W. J., Smith, S., and Gibson, S. (1946). Anastomosis of the aorta to a pulmonary artery. Certain types in congenital heart disease. *J. Amer. Med. Ass.* **132**, 627.

Potts, W. J., McQuiston, W. O., and Baffes, T. G. (1956). Causes of death in one thousand operations for congenital heart disease. *Arch. Surg.* **73**, 508.

Rastelli, G. C. (1969). A new approach to 'anatomic' repair of transposition of the great arteries. *Mayo Clin. Proc.* **44**, 1–12.

Rastelli, G. C., McGoon, D. C., and Wallace, R. B. (1969a). Anatomic correction of transposition of the great vessels with ventricular septal defect and pulmonary stenosis. *J. Thorac. Cardiovasc. Surg.* **58**, 545.

Rastelli, G. C., Wallace, R. B., and Ongley, P. A. (1969b). Complete repair of transposition of the great arteries with pulmonary stenosis. A review and report of a case corrected by using a new surgical technique. *Circulation* **39**, 83–95.

Raston, H., and Konez, J. (1971). A new method of closed atrio-septectomy for palliative treatment of complete transposition of the great vessels. *J. Thorac. Cardiovasc. Surg.* **61**, 705–709.

Redo, S. F. (1964). Shunting procedures for cyanotic congenital cardiac defects. *Amer. J. Surg.* **107**, 469.

Reed, W. A. (1965). Selection of palliative operation for transposition of the great vessels. *Circulation* **31**, 25–30, 1965.

Reed, W. A. (1969). Total correction of transposition of the great vessels. A modified technique. *J. Thorac. Cardiovasc. Surg.* **58**, 84–86.

Reed, W. A., Kittle, C. F., and Heilbrunn, A. (1963). Superior vena cava–pulmonary artery anastomosis. *Arch. Surg.* **86**, 87.

Reed, W. A., Lauer, R. M., and Diehl, A. M. (1966). Staged correction of total transposition of the great vessels. *Circulation* **33**, 13–18.

Replogle, R. L., and Lin, C. Y. (1972). Surgical correction of transposition of the great vessels: A technical suggestion. *J. Thorac. Cardiovasc. Surg.* **63**, 196–198.

Rey-Balter, E., Blanco, G., and Bailey, C. P. (1961). Transposition of the great vessels. New experimental technique for its complete correction. *J. Thorac. Cardiovasc. Surg.* **41**, 509.

Robicsek, F., Temesvari, A., and Kadar, R. L. (1956). A new method for the treatment of congenital heart disease associated with impaired pulmonary circulation. *Acta Med. Scand.* **154**, 151.

Robicsek, F., Magistro, R., Foti, E., Robicsek, L., and Sanger, P. W. (1958). Vena cava–pulmonary artery anastomosis for vascularization of the lung. *J. Thorac. Surg.* **35**, 440.

Robicsek, F., Sanger, P. W., and Taylor, F. H. (1962). Three year follow up of a patient with transposition of the great vessels, atrial septal defect, and pulmonary stenosis treated by vena cava–pulmonary artery anastomosis. *J. Thorac. Cardiovasc. Surg.* **44**, 817.

Robicsek, F., Sanger, P. W., Taylor, F. H., and Najib, A. (1963). Complete bypass of the right heart. *Amer. Heart J.* **66**, 792.

Robicsek, F., Daugherty, H. K., Tam, W., Sanger, P. W., and Bagby, E. (1969). A new procedure for the palliation of transposition of the great vessels. An experimental study. *Ann. Thorac. Surg.* **7**, 21–26.

Rodbard, S., and Wagner, D. (1949). By-passing the right ventricle. *Proc. Soc. Exp. Biol. Med.* **71**, 69.

Rodriguez-Fernandez, H. L., Kelly, D. T., Collado, A., Haller, A., Jr., Krovetz, L. J., and Rowe, R. D. (1972). Hemodynamic data and angiographic findings after Mustard repair for complete transposition of the great arteries. *Circulation* **46**, 799.

Rose, J. C., Broida, H. P., Hufnagel, C. A., Gillespie, J. F., Rabil, P. J., and Freis, E. D. (1955a). A method for the study of the circulation using a mechanical left ventricle. *J. Appl. Physiol.* **7**, 580.

Rose, J. C., Cosimano, S. V., Jr., Hufnagel, C. A., and Massulo, E. A. (1955b). The effects of exclusion of the right ventricle from the circulation in dogs. *J. Clin. Invest.* **34**, 1625.

Rothlin, M., and Senning, A. (1965). Zur chirurgischen Behandlung der Transposition der grossen arterien. *Deut. Med. Woehenschr.* **90**, 417–421, 433.

Sachs, B. F., Pontinus, R. G., and Zuberbuhler, J. R. (1968). The clinical use of the superior vena cava–pulmonary artery shunt: A report of 20 cases. *J. Pediat. Surg.* **3**, 364.

Sanger, P. W., Robicsek, F., and Taylor, F. H. (1959). Vena cava–pulmonary artery anastomosis. III. Successful operation in case of complete transposition of the great vessels with interatrial septal defect and pulmonary stenosis. *J. Thorac. Surg.* **38**, 166.

Sautter, R. D. (1963). Enlargement of atrial septal defect: Simplified technic. *J. Thorac. Cardiovasc. Surg.* **46**, 386.

Schuster, S. R., Kiernan, E., Rosencranz, J., and Bozer, A. (1963). New technique for creation of atrial septal defect with clinical application. *J. Thorac. Cardiovasc. Surg.* **46**, 510.

Sellors, T. H. (1948). Surgery of pulmonary stenosis. A case in which the pulmonary valve was successfully divided. *Lancet* **i**, 988.

Senning, A. (1959). Surgical correction of transposition of the great vessels. *Surgery* **45**, 966.

Senning, A. (1966). Surgical correction of transposition of the great vessels. *Surgery* **59**, 334–336.

Senning, A., Ikkos, D., and Rudhe, U. (1962). Surgical treatment of transposition of the great vessels: open correction. *In* "Congenital Heart Disease" p. 200. (D. P. Morse, ed.). Blackwell Oxford.

Shaher, R. M., Keith, J. D, and Mustard, W. T. (1966). Necropsy findings eight months after total correction of complete transposition of the great vessels by the interatrial baffle technique. *Can. Med. Ass. J.* **94**, 1127.

Shankar, K. R., Lauer, R. M., Diehl, A. M., and Reed, W. A. (1967). Transposition of the great vessels. Hemodynamic changes after physiologic total correction. *Amer. J. Surg.* **114**, 760–764.

Shumacker, H. B., Jr. (1951). Suggestions concerning the use of the subclavian which arises from the aorta in the treatment of the tetralogy of Fallot. *Yale J. Biol. Med.* **23**, 486.

Shumacker, H. B., Jr. (1961). New operation for transposition of the great vessels. *Surgery* **50**, 773.

Shumacker, H. B., Jr., and Girod, D. A. (1969). Transposition of the great vessels. Long term follow up of corrected case. *J. Thorac. Cardiovasc. Surg.* **57**, 747–752.

Shumacker, H. B., Jr., and Mandelbaum, I. (1962). Ascending aortic–pulmonary artery shunts in cyanotic heart disease. *Surgery* **52**, 675.

Sirak, H. D., and Britt, C. I. (1962). Technic for taking down Pott's anastomosis. *Circulation* **25**, 111.

Somerville, J., Yacoub, M., Ross, D. N., and Ross, K. (1969). Aorta to right pulmonary artery anastomosis (Waterston's operation) for cyanotic heart disease. *Circulation* **39**, 593–602.

Stark, J., Aberdeen, E., Waterston, D. J., Bonham-Carter, R. E., and Tynan, M. (1969). Pulmonary artery constriction (banding): a report of 146 cases. *Surgery* **65**, 808.

Stark, J., Tynan, M., Tatooles, C. J., Aberdeen, E., and Waterston, D. J. (1970). Banding of the pulmonary artery for transposition of the great arteries and ventricular septal defect. *Circulation* **41** (Suppl. 2), 116.

Stark, J., Tynan, M. J., Ashcroft, K. W., Aberdeen, E., and Waterston, D. J. (1971). Obstruction of pulmonary veins and superior vena cava after Mustard operation for transposition of the great arteries. *Circulation* **44**, (Suppl. 2), 91.

Stark, J., Tynan, M. J., Ashcroft, K. W., Aberdeen, E., and Waterston, D. J. (1972). Obstruction of pulmonary veins and superior vena cava after the Mustard operation for transposition of the great arteries. *Circulation* **45** (Suppl. 1), 116.

Starr, A., Campbell, T. J., Wood, J., McCord, C., Herr, R., and Menashe, V. (1964). Transposition of the great vessels. Recent experiences with the Blalock-Hanlon procedure. *Amer. J. Surg.* **108**, 198.

Starr, I., Jeffers, W. A., and Meade, R. H., Jr. (1943). The absence of conspicous increments of venous pressure after severe damage to the right ventricle of the dog, with a discussion of the relation between clinical congestive failure and heart disease. *Amer. Heart J.* **26**, 291.

Sterns, L. P., Baker, R. M., and Edwards, J. E. (1964). Complete transposition of the great vessels. Unusual longevity in a case with subpulmonary stenosis. *Circulation* **29**, 610.

Sterns, L. P., Bitash, A. F., and Lillehei, C. W. (1964b). Cardiovascular surgery in infancy. *Amer. J. Cardiol.* **13**, 153.

Subramanian, S., Wagner, H., Lambert, E., and Vlad, P. (1971). Early correction of congenital heart defects under surface induced deep hypothermia. *Circulation* **44**, (Suppl. 2), 230.

Toole, A. L., Glenn, W. W. L., Fisher, W. H., Whittemore, R., Ordway, N. K., and Vidone, R. A. (1960). Operative approach to transposition of the great vessels. *Surgery* **48**, 43.

Trusler, G. A. (1971). Palliative operations for transposition of the great vessels. *In* "The Natural History and Progress in Treatment of Congenital Heart Defects." (B. S. L. Kidd and J. D. Keith, eds.), P. 153. Charles C. Thomas, Springfield, Illinois.

Trusler, G., and Kidd, L. (1967). Surgical palliation in complete transposition of the great vessels. *Circulation* **36** (Suppl. 4), 252.

Trusler, G. A., and Mustard, W. T. (1968). Selection of palliative procedures in transposition of the great vessels. *Ann. Thorac. Surg.* **5**, 528.

Trusler, G. A., and Mustard, W. T. (1972). A method of banding the pulmonary artery for large isolated ventricular septal defect with and without transposition of the great arteries. *Ann. Thorac. Surg.* **13**, 351.

Trusler, G. A., Mustard, W. T., and Fowler, R. S. (1964). The role of surgery in the treatment of transposition of the great vessels. *Can. Med. Ass. J.* **91**, 1096.

Trusler, G. A., MacGregor, D., and Mustard, W. T. (1971). Cavo-pulmonary anastomosis for cyanotic congenital heart disease. *J. Thorac. Cardiovasc. Surg.* **62**, 803.

Tynan, M., and Aberdeen, E. (1971). Tricuspid incompetence following the Mustard operation for transposition of the great arteries. *Circulation* **44** (Suppl. 2), 92.

Tynan, M., Aberdeen, E., and Stark, J. (1972). Tricuspid incompetence after the Mustard operation for transposition of the great arteries. *Circulation* 45, (Suppl. 1), 111.

Venables, A. W. (1966). Complete transposition of the great vessels in infancy with reference to palliative surgery. *Brit. Heart J.* 28, 335.

Vidone, R. A., and Liebow, A. A. (1957). Anatomical and functional studies of the lung deprived of pulmonary arteries and veins with an application in the therapy of transposition of the great vessels. *Amer. J. Pathol.* 33, 539.

Wagner, H., Vlad, P., Lambert, E., and Subramanian, S. (1971). Surgical correction of transposition of the great arteries. *Circulation* 44 (Suppl. 2), 237.

Waldhausen, J. A., Boruchow, I., Miller, W., and Rashkind, W. J. (1969). Transposition of the great arteries with ventricular septal defect. Palliation by atrial septostomy and pulmonary artery banding. *Circulation* 39 and 40 (Suppl. 1), 215.

Waldhausen, J. A., Pierce, W. S., Rashkind, W. J., Miller, W. W., and Friedman, S. (1970). Total correction of transposition of the great arteries following balloon atrioseptostomy. *Circulation* 41 (Suppl. 2), 123–129.

Waldhausen, J. A., Pierce, W. S., Park, C. D., Rashkind, W. J., and Friedman, S. (1971). Physiologic correction of transposition of the great arteries. *Circulation* 43, 738.

Waldo, A. L., Krongrad, E., Bowman, F. O., Jr., Kaiser, G. A., Husson, G. S., and Malm, J. R. (1972). Electrophysiological considerations during total repair of transposition of the great vessels. *Circulation* 45 and 46, Suppl. 11, 34.

Waterston, D. H. (1962). Treatment of Fallot's tetralogy in children under one year of age. *Rozhl Chir.* 41, 181–185.

William, V. L., Cooper, T., Mudd, J. G., and Hanlon, C. R. (1962). Treatment of ventricular septal defect by constriction of pulmonary artery. *Arch. Surg.* 85, 745.

Wilson, H. E., Nafrawi, A. G., Cardozo, R. H., and Aguillon, A. (1962). Rational approach to surgery for complete transposition of the great vessel: analysis of the basic hemodynamics and critical appraisal of previously proposed corrective procedures, with a suggested approach based on laboratory and clinical studies. *Ann. Surg.* 155, 258.

Yao, J. K. Y., and Mustard, W. T. (1969). Operative technique for transposition of the great vessels with previous Baffes procedure. *Surgery* 65, 873–875.

Young, W. G., Jr., Sealy, W. C., Houck, W. S., Jr., Whalen, R. E., Spach, M. S., and Canent, R. V., Jr. (1963). Superior vena cava–right pulmonary artery anastomosis in cyanotic heart disease. *Ann. Surg.* 157, 894.

Zamora, R., Moller, J. H., Lucas, R. V., Jr., and Castaneda, A. R. (1970). Complete transposition of the great vessels: Surgical results of emergency Blalock-Hanlon operation in infants. *Surgery* 67, 706–710.

AUTHOR INDEX

Numbers in *italics* refer to the pages on which the complete references are listed.

SUBJECT INDEX